Clinical Empathy

Mohammadreza Hojat

Clinical Empathy

The Heart of Patient Care

Springer

Mohammadreza Hojat
Sidney Kimmel Medical College
Thomas Jefferson University
Philadelphia, PA, USA

ISBN 978-3-031-87412-3 ISBN 978-3-031-87413-0 (eBook)
https://doi.org/10.1007/978-3-031-87413-0

This Springer imprint is published by the registered company Springer Nature Switzerland AG
The registered company address is: Gewerbestrasse 11, 6330 Cham, Switzerland

In dedication to those who devote their professional lives to understanding human suffering, eliminating pain, eradicating disease and infirmity, curing human illnesses, and improving the physical, mental, and social well-being of their fellow human beings.

Foreword

I am delighted to write this foreword to the third edition of *Clinical Empathy: The Heart of Patient Care* by Mohammadreza Hojat. Professor Hojat is an eminent academic and psychologist who has been at the forefront of research and teaching in clinical empathy for over 20 years, and his experience, wisdom, and insights into the topic shine out from every page.

Professor Hojat published his first paper on empathy in healthcare in 2001. Since then, he has pursued an impressive career in research and teaching on clinical empathy producing an extensive body of research. His work on the measurement, development, erosion, enhancement, and correlates of empathy in healthcare education and patient care has received broad media coverage, including in the *New York Times*, *Wall Street Journal*, *Philadelphia Inquirer*, and on American television.

Empathy in healthcare has gained much attention in recent years, with a growing body of research showing that it has beneficial effects on both patients and physicians. Despite this, it remains a controversial topic, with a great variation in how it is defined. There is often confusion between empathy and sympathy, and Chapter 1 of the book tackles this head on and helpfully gives a historical account of the various definitions of empathy, and how it differs from sympathy. The remaining four chapters that make up the first section of the book then give a broad overview of human empathy, in relation to its evolution and survival value, what is now known about the genetics of empathy, and the psychodynamics of empathy in the development of prosocial and altruistic behaviors. In short, section one is a thorough treatise on what is known about the importance of empathy in human development and society. This gives the reader solid foundational knowledge on the topic of empathy, before moving on to more clinical considerations.

Chapters 6–15 then make up the second section of the book which focuses on clinical empathy, covering areas such as empathy and health; the importance of both verbal and nonverbal aspects of empathy; the measurement of empathy by the Jefferson Scale of Empathy and its validity; the interpersonal dynamics of empathy; the relationship between clinician empathy and choice of speciality; gender differences in empathy; effects on clinical outcomes; barriers to clinical empathy; the neuroscience of empathy; and future aspects of healthcare including digital and AI approaches and the challenges posed to clinical empathy.

Professor Hojat's writing is academically robust yet highly readable and engaging, and it is obvious that he believes passionately in the power of empathy in healthcare, and indeed in broader society. But the researcher must always rise above personal viewpoints, and put forward their case on the basis of rigorous research and evidence. Professor Hojat does that in abundance throughout the pages of this book. The book is a tour de force of the topic of clinical empathy that should be read (and re-read) by doctors and healthcare professionals at all stages of their career.

Stewart W. Mercer, Ph.D.
Professor of Primary Care and Multimorbidity,
Usher Institute, University of Edinburgh, UK
Creator of the Consultation and Relational Empathy (CARE)

Preface

All human beings are in truth akin,
all in creation share one origin.
When fate allots a member pangs and pain,
no ease for other members then remains.
If, unperturbed, another's grief canst scan,
thou are not worthy of the name of human.

—Saadi (classic Persian poet, 1210–1290 AD)

Although the primary purpose of this book is to describe the antecedents, development, measurement, correlates, group differences, enhancement, erosion, and consequences of clinical empathy in the context of health professions education and patient care, some of the material presented may seem to go beyond that purpose. For the sake of a more comprehensive analysis, one cannot isolate such a complex and dynamic entity as clinical empathy from a string of determining factors (e.g., its evolutionary, genetic, developmental, and psychodynamic aspects) and multiple consequences (e.g., physical, mental, and social well-being; educational and clinical outcomes). Thus, to achieve a broader understanding of clinical empathy in health professions education and patient care, I discuss the issue in a broader perspective of a dynamic system, the function of which rests on the following five premises:

- Human beings are social creatures.
- The human need for affiliation, intimacy, and social support has survival value.
- Interpersonal relationships can fulfill the human need for affiliation, intimacy, and social support.
- The interpersonal relationship between clinician and patient is a special case of a "mini" social support system that can fulfill the need for affiliation, intimacy, and support.
- An empathic clinician–patient relationship can improve the physical, mental, and social well-being of the patient as well as the clinician.

Human beings are designed by evolution to form meaningful interpersonal relationships through verbal and nonverbal communication. Human beings possess a system of needs for social affiliation—for bonding and attachment, for forming a social network, for feeling felt, for understanding, and for being understood. The grand principle is the same whether the individual is an infant, a child, an adolescent, or an adult, or whether the individual is male or female, healthy or ill: *Being connected is beneficial to the human's physical, mental, and social well-being; it has survival value.*

The aforementioned principle is indeed the theme underlying all chapters of this book. In some chapters, it may seem that I take my eyes off the intended target of health professions education and patient care, but I always return to the underlying theme to link the discussion to the patient–clinician relationship. When appropriate, I use the terms "clinician" and "client," rather than "doctor," "physician," or "patient," to make the discussion more general and thus applicable to all healthcare disciplines and professions, not to medicine and physicians alone.

Clinical empathy is viewed in this book from a multidisciplinary perspective that includes evolution; neurology; clinical, social, developmental, and educational psychology; sociology; medicine; and all other health professions that involve patient care. Some theoretical aspects of antecedents, development, and outcomes of empathy are discussed, and relevant experimental studies and empirical findings are presented in support of the theoretical discussion.

The book is written for a broad audience that includes physicians, residents, medical students, and students and practitioners of all other health professions, including the disciplines of nursing, dentistry, pharmacy, psychology, and clinical social work, and other health professions students and practitioners who are involved in patient care. In particular, faculty involved in the education and training of health professionals can use the book as a reference in their courses in the art (and science) of patient care.

Because the book is intended to serve as a reference source on the topic of clinical empathy, on many occasions, I have cited multiple references for critical issues for those who need to learn more beyond what I have presented in this book. Although a critical review of the literature was not among the intended purposes of the book, occasionally when appropriate, I reported additional information such as measuring instruments used, and described the study design and sample used in the cited research to help readers judge the merit of the findings.

It is my hope that it can help to improve our understanding of clinical empathy in the context of health professions education and patient care. A problem that is well understood is a problem that is half solved. Thus, the more the health professions students, teachers, and practitioners understand the importance of clinical empathy, the better the patients are served.

***

The first edition of this book, *Empathy in Patient Care: Antecedents, Development, Measurement, and Outcomes*, was published in 2007. It contributed to a surge of interest in clinical empathy research in medicine and other health profession disciplines, evident by the increasing number of publications on clinical empathy, using the *Jefferson Scale of Empathy,* in health professions education and patient care research.

The second edition of the book, *Empathy in Health Professions Education and Patient Care,* published in 2016, was an expanded and updated version of the original edition. In addition to the broad attention to the previous two editions of the book by educators, researchers, students, and practitioners in health professions disciplines, the following factors prompted me to embark on another journey to prepare this third expanded edition of the book.

First and foremost, clinical empathy, I believe, is a core element of professionalism in healthcare, and as the heart of the art of patient care, received exponential attention in recent years by leaders, administrators, and educators in academic health centers; practitioners of patient care; students and researchers in health professions education; and the public media. Further, the rapid rate of using computer diagnostic and therapeutic technology, telemedicine, digital patient care, and artificial intelligence led to a new wave of research on the impact of these changes on clinical empathy and the patient–clinician interpersonal relationship.

Second, another major advancement in clinical empathy research has been the increasing volume of published research in health professions students and practitioners in the USA and abroad in which the *Jefferson Scale of Empathy* (JSE) was used. Indeed, this wave of national and international research evokes great pleasure for me and my research team as we witness the impact of our work in the advancement of empirical research on clinical empathy in health professions education and patient care. I have included findings of some of this accumulating volume of research by national and international researchers in the annotated bibliography in this edition of the book (see Appendix A).

This third edition of the book is divided into two parts. The first part consists of Chaps. 1 through 5, in which empathy is discussed from a broader perspective in the general context of human relationships. This part lays the foundation for the second part, without which the discussion of clinical empathy would look like a structure without solid, supportive pillars.

In the second part, consisting of Chaps. 6 through 15, the focus shifts more specifically to clinical empathy in the context of health professions education and patient care. The two parts are closely interrelated, evident by frequently referring readers to different chapters in the book to avoid redundancies. Each chapter begins with an abstract, presenting the major highlights of the text, and ends with a recapitulatory paragraph that provides a precis of the chapter.

Chapter 1 presents a historical background about the concept of empathy and discusses the ambiguity associated with the definitions and conceptualization of clinical empathy. The long-standing confusion between empathy and sympathy is discussed and specific features of each construct are listed to distinguish the two. In addition, distinctions are made between cognition and emotion and between understanding and feeling, as specific features of empathy and sympathy, respectively. Finally, the implications of such distinctions are outlined to clarify their different consequences in the context of patient care.

Chapter 2 is based on the assumption that human beings are evolved to connect together for survival. The importance of making and breaking human connections in health and illness is discussed. The beneficial effects of a social support system on health and the detrimental effects of isolation, loneliness, and disconnection are presented to underscore the nature, mechanisms, and consequences of interpersonal relationships. The chapter concludes with the notion that the positive relationship between clinician and patient/client is formed by the drive for human connectedness and serves as a special kind of social support system with all its beneficial healing power.

In Chapter 3, empathy is viewed from an evolutionary perspective, and the psycho-socio-physiological function of empathic engagement is described. In addition, the chapter discusses the genetic studies of empathy. The chapter ends with the notion that the foundation of the capacity for empathy developed during the evolution of the human species, and empirical data support heritability of empathy from one generation to another.

Chapter 4 discusses the psychodynamics of empathy by emphasizing the importance of prenatal, perinatal, and postnatal factors in the development of prosocial and altruistic behaviors. In particular, the early rearing environment is discussed, especially the effects of the mother's availability and loving responsiveness in the development of internal working models that provide a framework for later interpersonal relationships. Experimental studies are presented to show that early relationships with a primary caregiver influence the regulation of emotions, an important factor in interpersonal relationships in general, and in empathic capacity in particular.

Chapter 5 briefly describes several instruments that researchers have used most often to measure empathy in children and adults. The contents of the items in these instruments indicate that these instruments are useful for measuring empathy in the general population; thus, their content relevance (or face and content validities) is limited in the context of health professions education and patient care. The chapter concludes with the notion that a psychometrically sound instrument, developed specifically to measure clinical empathy in the context of health professions education and patient care, was urgently needed to measure clinical empathy among students and practitioners of the healthcare professions.

In Chapter 6, the starting chapter of the second part of the book, empathy in patient care is discussed in relation to the World Health Organization's definition of health and the triangular bio-psycho-social paradigm of health and illness. In that context, clinical empathy is defined, and four key features in the definition are emphasized: cognition, understanding, communication, and intention to help. The chapter concludes with the point that the patient's recognition of the clinician's empathy through verbal and nonverbal communication plays an important role in the outcome of empathic engagement.

Chapter 7 describes in detail the developmental phases and psychometric properties of the Jefferson Scale of Empathy (JSE), which was developed specifically to measure empathy among students and practitioners in medicine and other health professions. A large volume of empirical evidence is presented from our research team and from other national and international researchers in support of the validity and reliability of the three versions of the JSE. Supporting data from a nationwide landmark project on clinical empathy in the US osteopathic medical students reported in this chapter (and described in detail in Chap. 14) add to our confidence about internal and external validity, utility, reproducibility, and generalizability of the JSE in health professions students and clinicians. The chapter ends with the thought that the accumulating empirical evidence from the USA and abroad in support of the JSE's psychometrics should instill more confidence in those who are searching for a psychometrically sound instrument for measuring clinical empathy.

Chapter 8 discusses the interpersonal dynamics involved in an empathic relationship between clinician and patient, and proposes that both can benefit from empathic engagement. The chapter presents several experimental studies that describe how role expectations, the tendency to bind with others for survival, uncritical acceptance of and compliance with authority figures, and the effects of the clinical environment can influence clinicians' and patients' behavior in clinical encounters. In addition, the chapter argues that clinician–patient encounters are unique due to such psychological mechanisms as identification, transference, and countertransference, plus placebo effects, cultural factors, personal space, and boundaries. The chapter ends with the notion that for achieving a better empathic engagement, the clinician should learn to listen with the "third ear" and to see with the "mind's eye."

Chapter 9 describes the link between clinical empathy; psychological and social variables; clinical performance; career interest; and choice of specialty. The chapter reports a number of desirable personality attributes conducive to relationship building that are positively correlated with clinical empathy, and a number of undesirable personal qualities detrimental to interpersonal relationships that are negatively correlated with clinical empathy. Data reported in this chapter suggest that high clinical empathy scores are associated with greater clinical competence and more interest in people-oriented specialties as opposed to technology- or procedure-oriented specialties.

Chapter 10 discusses gender differences in clinical empathy in favor of women observed in a large number of studies of students and practitioners in the health professions. While the contribution of social learning in gender differences cannot be ignored, I propose that other factors can provide plausible explanations for gender differences in social skills and capacity for empathy. The ancestral history in mate selection, parental investment, division of labor, and hormonal and physiological factors have endowed women with a greater propensity for social skills and empathic engagement. It is argued that women may be endowed at an early age with a greater sensitivity to social stimuli and a better understanding of emotional signals that can result in a greater capacity for empathic engagement. This argument is reflected in studies reporting gender differences in the practice styles of male and female health professionals.

Chapter 11 reports the theoretical link between clinical empathy and positive patient outcomes. It provides evidence concerning the quality of clinician–patient relationships that can lead to more trusting relationships between clinician and patient. Such quality in turn could lead to more accurate diagnoses, and to patients having greater satisfaction with their healthcare providers, better compliance with clinicians' advice, firmer commitment to treatment plans, and a reduced tendency to file malpractice litigations. This chapter describes the mechanism linking clinical empathy to optimal clinical outcomes and pathways connecting physician empathy to patient outcomes. Based on the reported empirical studies, and particularly findings that showed significant associations between physician's level of clinical empathy and tangible clinical outcomes in diabetic patients, it is concluded that empathy should be considered an important component of the overall clinicians' competence that must be assessed and enhanced in health professions education and practice of patient care.

Chapter 12 describes obstacles to the enhancement of empathy in health professions education and practice, including the cynicism that students develop during their professional education, the changes evolving in the market-driven healthcare system, and the current overreliance on computerized patient care. The chapter also presents some empirical evidence suggesting that clinical empathy is amenable to change by targeted educational programs and describes a variety of approaches used in psychological and health education research to enhance empathy. In particular, some approaches used for enhancing empathy in the context of patient care are briefly described, including interpersonal skill training; perspective taking; role playing; exposure to role models; imagining, exposure of students to activities resembling patients' experiences while hospitalized or during encounters with healthcare providers; the study of literature and the arts; development of narrative skills and reflective writing; and the Balint approach to training physicians. The chapter presents an overall view that clinical empathy can be taught through targeted educational programs, but the challenge is to sustain the improvement for a longer time.

Chapter 13 describes a new wave of research in social cognitive neuroscience exploring the neurological underpinnings of clinical empathy. Research findings from neuroimaging studies and on the mirror neuron system hold promise for helping to understand the neurological underpinnings of clinical empathy. Relying on the conceptualization of empathy (Chaps. 1 and 6), and findings from neuroimaging research, showing neurological impairment linked to deficiencies in empathy, it can be assumed that particular cortical regions of the brain may be implicated in empathic responses. The importance of making a clear distinction between empathy (predominantly a cognitive attribute) and sympathy (predominantly an affective reaction) in exploring the neurological underpinnings of empathy is discussed. However, challenges exist in developing a research paradigm to evoke empathic responses on one occasion and sympathetic reactions on another to examine similarities and differences in brain activities in the two situations. It is argued that exploring neurological underpinnings of empathy as opposed to sympathy is important for finding ways to maximize clinical empathy and regulate sympathy in patient care.

Chapter 14 briefly describes the *Project in Osteopathic Medical Education and Empathy* (POMEE), which is a unique landmark study in which nationwide representative samples of osteopathic medical students in the USA participated. It investigated clinical empathy, its associations with emotional empathy; attitudes toward osteopathic medicine; selected demographic variables; career interest and personal quality measures, such as attitudes toward interprofessional collaboration; orientation toward lifelong learning; and burnout experiences. Changes in clinical empathy in different years of medical school education were also examined, and findings were compared with those from allopathic medical students. National norms for clinical empathy and other personal quality measures used in the project were developed for the first time in national samples of medical students.

In Chapter 15, the final chapter, clinical empathy in the context of health professions education and patient care is viewed from the broad perspective of the systems theory. I suggested that a systemic paradigm of empathy in patient care includes the following subsets that interactively operate in the system: clinician related, non-clinician related, social learning, and educational subsets. The elements within each subset and the interactions of the elements within and between subsets during clinical encounters that lead to functional (positive) or dysfunctional (negative) patient outcomes are discussed. Finally, an outline of an agenda for future research on several topics involving clinical empathy in patient care is presented, including additional research on correlates of clinical empathy, the use of indicators of clinical empathy in admissions decisions of applicants to health professions schools, post-graduate medical education programs, and the assessment of practicing clinicians. Also, further research was suggested to examine the impact of telemedicine and computerized healthcare on forming empathic engagement in patient care, and the impact of artificial intelligence technologies on the development and assessment of clinical competence of physicians-in-training and in-practice. The chapter concludes that the implementation of remedies for enhancement of empathy is a mandate, and that any attempt to enhance empathic understanding among people is a step toward building a better civilization.

It is my hope that the instruments we developed—different versions of the JSE—and research conducted in clinical empathy by our team and by other national and international researchers can continue to generate greater motivation and inspire more researchers to undertake more inquest on the topic. Such endeavors will improve our understanding of the concerns, pain, and suffering of our fellow human beings in general, and enhance health professionals' empathic engagement in patient care, in particular. As the entire text of this book communicates, empathic understanding can not only enhance the quality of patient–clinician relationships and improve outcomes of patient care, but also serve as a means for achieving global peace and harmony in all humans, everywhere, regardless of any so-called divisive factors.

Mohammadreza Hojat
Philadelphia, PA
October, 2025

A Personal Odyssey

Life is full of surprises!

—(A popular cliché)

A mother and her young daughter sat in the examination room, waiting for the doctor to show up. They looked anxiously at the closed door, expecting a stranger in a white coat to open it at any moment. Time seems to stand still when a patient is waiting for a doctor to come. It is interesting that patients always view a doctor as the most trusted of all strangers unless an adverse event occurs, usually during the first encounter.

At the recommendation of the pediatrician, the mother brought her teenaged daughter to this pediatric cardiologist to be examined for heart palpitations. The pediatrician had indicated that, at that age, occasional palpitations were not necessarily a serious cause for concern: They could be a result of too much caffeine for a coffee-lover like that young girl, a sign of test-taking anxiety at school, or a sign of a transitory emotional state. However, to eliminate the possibility of a serious heart condition, the pediatrician referred the girl to an expert in cardiology.

Here they were waiting for the expert to deliver the final verdict—either a clean bill of health or a long-term treatment that eventually could involve surgical procedures. The fear of the unknown that always haunts human beings was escalating with the passage of time. Finally, the doctor entered the room shadowed by a young woman also wearing a white coat. He pointed to her and said, "This is my resident." No greetings were exchanged, and the doctor seemed indifferent and in a rush. The encounter was cold. Without looking at the mother or the girl, he opened the medical chart the pediatrician had sent him and announced that additional tests were needed. The test he suggested was a heart monitor the girl would wear 24 hours a day, seven days a week, for at least a month. After each abnormal heartbeat, the device would transmit the recorded signals to a monitoring center via a telephone line connected to the monitor.

When the anxious mother asked the doctor how her daughter could be hooked up to a heart monitor for a month without missing her classes, the cardiologist said the monitor was light and could be attached to a belt around her waist and connected to a watch-like device on her wrist. The only additional information he offered was that the monitor could be rented for a month and that the expense might not be covered by insurance. He seemed to be more concerned about how the monitor would be paid for than about the mother's and daughter's need for comforting comments.

> The doctor informed the mother that the next appointment would be in a month or so, after the heart monitor test was completed. The anxious mother expected, to no avail, more information about her young daughter's condition, some sign from the doctor that would make her daughter, who was looking hopelessly into the doctor's emotionless eyes, feel a little hopeful at least. As the doctor and his resident were leaving the examination room (where no examination had been performed), the mother, with a despairing look, asked the doctor: "Is my daughter's heart condition really serious enough to need constant monitoring for a month? Couldn't her condition be transitory?" The doctor looked at his resident and mumbled, "We've got another doctor in here," and the two left the room, leaving mother and daughter feeling desperate and confused. The mother did not trust the expert, never rented the monitor, and the heart palpitation stopped abruptly when the daughter stopped drinking coffee. However, memories of cold encounters can last forever.

It is interesting that an adverse event occurring when a person is in a heightened state of emotional arousal tends to leave a deeper scar in the sufferer's mind than it would otherwise. Or it may be that a lack of empathic understanding has a more lasting effect by generating undesirable emotional arousal. Is it true that negative experiences often have a more lasting trace than positive ones? Is it any wonder that many patients hate to go to a doctor's office? (By the way, that mother happened to be my wife, and the young patient was my daughter).

Also interesting to note is that the gift of presence of a lovingly responsive and empathic human being can become a panacea to another's pain and suffering. Here is a personal observation:

> The baby startled first at the touch of the immunization needle in her tiny thigh, then came bursts of cries. The mother anxiously rushed to her baby's side, held her tight in her arms, gently put the baby on her chest, while patting her back started to talk in a calm motherly voice: "Oh my little girl … don't cry baby, it's over …" The little girl gazed at her mother's eyes, stopped crying, cuddling in the security of her mother's arms as if her pain had gone away to the sky …

I accompanied my wife and my daughter that day to the pediatrician's office, observed this event, and wondered: What is in the mother's tender loving care that soothes her baby's pain? Could it be a miraculous outcome of an empathic understanding?

The aforementioned events, plus my long-standing curiosity about and fascination with the two opposing poles of human connectedness versus lack of connectedness—namely interpersonal relationship versus loneliness—compelled me to embark on a journey that would lead to a better understanding of why empathy is so important in patient care.

***

Since my college years, I have been curious about why people behave as they do in making or breaking human connections. What are the foundations on which human beings build, or fail to build, the capacity to form meaningful interpersonal relationships? Has human evolution included development of the ability to form interpersonal connections? What roles do genetic predisposition, rearing environment, quality of attachment with significant others, personal qualities, educational experiences, and social learning play in achieving personal and professional success, in clinician–patient encounters, or in student–teacher relationships, or even in achieving likeability or attaining the qualities of professional, educational, or political leadership?

While earning my master's degree at the University of Tehran, I attempted to satisfy my curiosity about the personal attributes leading to popularity and success by examining the qualities of popular students using a sociometric methodology. I found that the human attribute of likeability, or popularity, was rooted in the early rearing environment and was also linked to positive personality traits, such as sociability and self-esteem. Furthermore, academic and likability can be the end results of these social skills. This research culminated in my master's thesis, *An Empirical Study of Popularity*.

While earning my doctoral degree at the University of Pennsylvania several years later, I continued to pursue my research interests, which eventually resulted in my doctoral dissertation, *Loneliness as a Function of Selected Personality, Psychosocial and Demographic Variables*. During this period, I studied factors contributing to loneliness, an indication of an inability to form meaningful interpersonal relationships. The findings showed that perceptions of the early relationship with a primary caregiver, early experiences in the family environment, early relationships with peers, a set of personality factors, and later living environment could predict experiences of loneliness (i.e., impaired capacity to make meaningful connection with others) in adulthood.

From the results of both studies, I learned that a common set of psychosocial attributes can contribute to the development of a capacity (or incapacity) to make (or break) human connections. These psychosocial attributes that are conducive to making human connections are similar to the elements of "emotional intelligence" that lead to the development of capacity for empathic understanding, such as social competency and the ability to understand the views, feelings, and emotions of others.

***

As a psychologist by academic training, I entered a new territory of medical education research more than four decades ago. At the beginning, I was not sure whether my interests, knowledge, skills, and academic background in psychology could serve the purpose of medical education research. However, I soon discovered that the field of medical education research was a rich and challenging territory at the crossroads of several disciplines, including psychology, education, and sociology as well as medicine. As a result of learning more about the field, I became convinced that both the art of medicine and the alleviation of human suffering would flourish by incorporating ideas from the behavioral and social sciences into the education of physicians.

I started my career in medical education research at a great academic medical center, Sidney Kimmel Medical College at Thomas Jefferson University, where I was charged with administrative and research responsibilities for the Jefferson Longitudinal Study of Medical Education. This study retrieves data about Jefferson's medical students and graduates from the most comprehensive, extensive, and uninterrupted longitudinal database of medical education maintained in a single medical school (Gonnella, Callahan, Veloski, DeSantis, & Hojat, 2022). The Jefferson Longitudinal Study was initiated under the supervision of Joseph S. Gonnella,

M.D., a decade before I joined the faculty. Joe was then the Director of the Office of Medical Education, who initiated the study because he had a vision concerning the need to empirically assess the outcomes of medical education at a time when most medical faculty and leaders in academia did not believe in the value of such an extensive (and expensive) study and thus were unwilling to devote resources to such investment.

My involvement with the Jefferson Longitudinal Study not only opened up a new window of opportunity for me but also proved to be an extremely interesting beginning to my professional life. I enjoyed the freedom bestowed on me to add new dimensions (e.g., personality and psychosocial measures) to the Jefferson Longitudinal Study database to address psychosocial aspects of academic success in medical school. Given my academic background in psychology, to me, that green light which allowed me to include personality and psychosocial measures in the longitudinal study was analogous to offering a cool glass of water to a thirsty man in the heat of a desert! The job provided me with a golden opportunity to incorporate my ideas about psychosocial attributes into research on the contribution of those attributes to the academic attainment and professional development of physicians-in-training, to the professional success of physicians in-practice, and to clinical outcomes, the ultimate goal of health professions education. So far, this highly productive research enterprise has resulted in more than 200 publications in peer-reviewed journals (Gonnella, Callahan, Veloski, DeSantis, & Hojat, 2022).

Meanwhile, my long-term interest in why people behave as they do in making or breaking human connections shifted to a more specific interest in empathy in health professions education and patient care. Then the question became the following: Why are some health professionals more capable than others of forming empathic relationships with their patients? More important, how can clinical empathy be conceptualized and quantified in the context of health professions education and patient care by a psychometrically sound instrument? How does the capacity for empathy develop? What are the antecedents and consequences of clinical empathy?

All the elements of the above-mentioned interrelated chain of events brought me to the uncharted terrain of empathy in health professions education and patient care. Interestingly, empathy has proved to be an extremely rich area of research, requiring a multidisciplinary approach that links views, concepts, theories, and data from diverse disciplines, such as evolutionary psychiatry; ethology; developmental, clinical, and social psychology; psychoanalysis; sociology; neuroscience; cognitive sciences; philosophy; art; and literature. What prompted me to embark on a search for the answers to my questions about clinical empathy was fascination with the richness of this uncharted territory combined with my long-time interest in the mysteries of interpersonal relationships, my academic background in the behavioral and social sciences, and my professional experience in medical education research.

If a fortune-teller had told me at the beginning of my college years that I would end up with a career as a researcher in medical education, I would have laughed uproariously in disbelief! And that wise fortune-teller probably would have responded by saying, "Well, young man! Life is full of surprises." It is indeed!

Acknowledgments

I am indebted to many for their influence on my thoughts, for inspiring me to pursue this line of research, and for their encouraging and supporting my research ideas and activities. Because of space constraints, I cannot name them all.

There is a popular saying in the Persian language: "Forever remain my masters those from whom I have learned." Following this piece of advice, I must begin with my mother—that angel from whom I heard before taking my first breath, who taught me to say my first word, who is engraved vividly in my mind as the foremost symbol of love, care, and empathic understanding.

Then there are others: among them, those who are the most valuable of all human resources, the teachers. There are many of them, but I would like to mention two of my undergraduate psychology teachers, Professor Reza Shapurian, Ph.D. (who joined the eternity after publication of the original edition of this book), and Professor Amir Hooshang Mehryar, Ph.D. (now enjoying the golden years of retirement and still an active scholar). Both of them not only opened up a window for me to the study of human behavior but also instilled self-confidence in me by asking me, when I was a novice undergraduate student, to write a critical review of their book for publication.

There are others who trained me on the job and supported me in my professional development, particularly in medical education research. Foremost among them is Joseph S. Gonnella, M.D., who is one of the best and brightest role models of an exemplary clinician-academician, teacher, leader, scholar, and researcher in medical education, whom I consider my mentor in medical education research. His great advice to me that "perfectionism is an obstacle to progress" has made my research career productive. Joe has continued to be a source of inspiration to me, unceasingly providing me with his intellectual input and instrumental support to pursue my research on clinical empathy in medical education and patient care. I must confess that it was indeed his idea to empirically study patient outcomes of physician empathy (and to use diabetes as the disease of choice, since it has well-defined criteria for patient improvement) that led to the publication of our two key studies on linking physician empathy to clinical outcomes, which enjoyed broad media coverage (these studies are cited in Chapter 11). Joe is now enjoying his golden age of retirement.

The Jefferson physician empathy project was supported in part for a few years at its inception by a grant from the Pfizer Medical Humanities Initiative, Pfizer Inc., New York. At the beginning, I could not imagine that a modest financial support could lead to such an important project. Also, I would like to acknowledge funding provided by Dr. Yoshihisa Asano, founder and chairman emeritus of Noguchi Medical Research Institute in Tokyo, Japan, to partially support our continuous research on clinical empathy in health professions education and patient care.

Several colleagues reviewed different chapters of this book and made valuable suggestions for improvement. Joe Gonnella was kind enough to review all the chapters and his valuable feedback has been incorporated in the text. Herbert Adler, M.D., Ph.D., Clinical Professor of Psychiatry and Human Behavior, Sidney Kimmel Medical College, reviewed Chaps. 8 and 13; Abdolmohammad Rostami, M.D., Ph.D., Chairman and Distinguished Professor, Department of Neurology, Sidney Kimmel Medical College at Thomas Jefferson University, reviewed Chapter 13; Charlie Pohl, M.D., Professor of Pediatrics, Senior Vice Provost of Student Affairs, and Director of the Asano-Gonnella Center for Research in Medical Education and Health Care, Sidney Kimmel Medical College at Thomas Jefferson University, and Vittorio Maio, Pharm. D., Professor of Population Health, and Managing Director of the Asano-Gonnella Center for Research in Medical Education and Health Care, Thomas Jefferson University, reviewed Chapter 14; Alice Eagly, Ph.D., Distinguished Professor of Psychology, Northwestern University, and Judith A. Hall, Ph.D., Distinguished Professor, Northeastern University, reviewed Chapter 10; and Nuno Sousa, M.D., Ph.D. Professor of Neuroscience at University of Minho, Portugal, reviewed Chapter 13. All of these colleagues made valuable comments to improve the chapters they reviewed, but I take full responsibility for any possible shortcomings in those chapters. Jennifer DeSantis, M.Ed., my research assistant, contributed to statistical analyses of POMEE data (Chapter 14) and reviewing that chapter. I am also grateful to Pamela Walter, M.F.A., Writer and Editor at Thomas Jefferson University, for her valuable help in editorial polishing of the text. Shira Carroll, Empathy Project Coordinator, helped me in preparing the tables, some of the graphical presentations, formatting the text, and checking the consistency of the text format. Jocelyne Waller helped in preparing the list of doctoral dissertations in which the JSE was used (reported in Appendix A), and in checking entries of Appendix A to conform with the APA publication guidelines. Anne Therese Namocatcat prepared the book cover design and some of the color figures. Timothy Flanagan helped in making all graphical works ready for production team.

Finally, I would like to thank my wife, Mimi, who made all needed accommodations (including canceling family trips and vacations!) to enable me to uninterruptedly continue completing this book, and my children, Arian, Anahita, and Roxana, who frequently asked me about the status of the book, and have always been my inspiring source of hope, joy, and energy.

Competing Interests The author has no competing interests to declare that are relevant to the content of this book.

About the Author

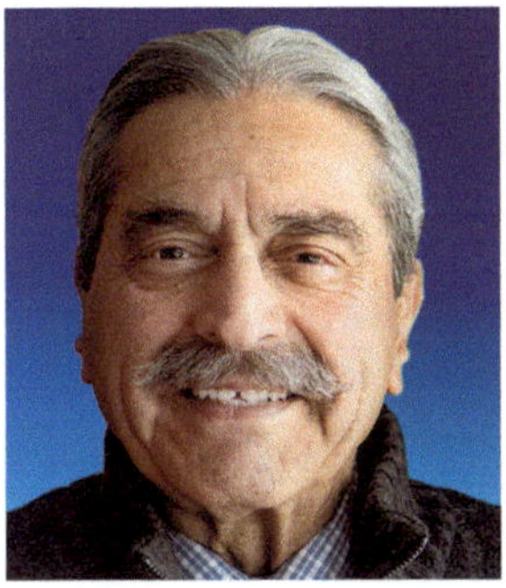

Mohammadreza Hojat, Ph.D., Research Professor, Department of Psychiatry and Human Behavior, and Director of the Jefferson Longitudinal Study of Medical Education, Asano-Gonnella Center for Research in Medical Education & Health Care, Sidney Kimmel Medical College at Thomas Jefferson University in Philadelphia, PA, USA. He received his bachelor's degree in educational psychology from Pahlavi University (currently University of Shiraz), his master's degree in psychology from the University of Tehran in Iran, and his doctoral degree in psychological services from the University of Pennsylvania. Dr. Hojat is a licensed psychologist in the Commonwealth of Pennsylvania, and has published more than 290 articles in peer-reviewed journals and 13 book chapters on educational, psychological, and social issues. Dr. Hojat has led the development of 10 psychometrically sound instruments (including the Jefferson Scale of Empathy) for the assessment of health professions education and patient outcomes, and professional development of health professionals-in-training and in-practice. Dr. Hojat's research on measurement, development, erosion, enhancement, group differences, and correlates of empathy in health professions education and patient care has received broad media coverage, featured in the *New York Times, Wall Street Journal, Philadelphia Inquirer*, the *National Public Radio*, and television program segments. Dr. Hojat received the Lifetime Achievement Award for his research in clinical empathy at the Global Empathy in Healthcare Network Symposium 2025, University of Leicester, United Kingdom. Dr. Hojat has served as a co-editor of the following books: "*Loneliness: Theory, Research, and Applications*" (Sage Publications, 1987), "*Assessment Measures in Medical School, Residency, and Practice: The Connections*" (Springer, 1993), and "*Fifty Years of Findings from the Jefferson Longitudinal Study of Medical Education*" (Springer, 2022), and a monograph on "*Personality Assessments and Outcomes in Medical Education and Practice of Medicine*" (2014, AMEE Guide No. 79). The original edition of his clinical empathy book "*Empathy in Patient Care: Antecedents, Development, Measurement, and Outcomes*" was published in 2007 which was expanded in 2016 under a new title "*Empathy in Health Professions Education and Patient Care.*" This is the third updated and expanded edition of his seminal book.

Experts' and Reviewers' Remarks About the Book

Excerpts from Foreword to the First Edition

Empathy is a critical component of being truly human and an essential characteristic of a good physician. Yet critics assert that modern physicians lack empathy. If that is true, the selection process may be at fault ... Sadly, current medical school education squeezes empathy out of the students who learn the body and forget the spirit/mind ... We humans are social beings who need to live with others and who depend on interpersonal relationship for support. That need for human relationship, Hojat finds essential to the patient-physician dyad, as much as to the work of the ministry. Basing his conclusions on data obtained by the research instruments he utilized and perfected, Dr. Hojat does not just talk about empathy, he measures it. A Ph.D. psychologist of estimable attainment, Dr. Hojat has been drawn to viewing empathy as integral to the practice of medicine. The whole aim of his longitudinal study is to select medical students who will be empathic practitioners and to keep them empathic throughout life. Dr. Hojat's strong views on human connection are echoed by the phrase "a friend a day keeps the doctor away!" Hojat finds the roots of empathy nourished by the mother-child relationship, even as he elucidates the nature-nurture conflict. Emotional support in childhood must be enormously fruitful, and nurturing of infants crucial in establishing a model. Dr. Hojat wisely provides an agenda for future research, ranging from selecting prospective medical students for their empathy to evaluating neurobiological components of empathy and compassion. But it may be a long time before the personal qualities of prospective medical students will trump their scientific know-how or their desirably high scores in the MCAT. Gentleness does not loom as captivating as high science grades to most deans of admissions. Hojat's utopia wisely provides goals which medical practitioners and teachers can ponder and try to reach for their daily activities. We are in his debt.

Howard Spiro, M.D.
Emeritus Professor of Medicine
Yale University School of Medicine, New Haven, CT
1924-2012

Excerpts from Foreword to the Second Edition

It was in a 1964 decision (Jacobellis vs. state of Ohio) in which he was trying to define obscenity that Supreme Court justice Potter Stewart famously said, "I shall not today attempt to define the kinds of {obscene} material I understood to be embraced. *But I know [it] when I see it.*" Much the same can be said for defining and researching empathy, especially in the context of health professions education and patient care ... For a concept with so many different definitions, empathy's history is surprisingly brief, the word having entered the lexicon in the late nineteenth and early twentieth centuries. This is not to say that caring, concern, and compassion for patients, all mentioned in various definitions of empathy, didn't exist prior to 1900. On the contrary, one can trace the philosophy and practice of these skills to ancient Greek physicians ... A few researchers have attempted, and even fewer have succeeded in operationalizing empathy in a comprehensive theoretical framework and measuring it in valid and reliable ways. The good news is that this is exactly what Dr. Hojat has done in the expanded and updated edition of *Empathy in Health Professions Education and Patient Care*. Building on his closely reasoned view of empathy and the exact literature ... this expanded edition provides the reader with updates to the field including exciting developments in the neuroscience of empathy, physiological correlates and heritability, psychodynamics, communication, gender, and the relationship of empathy to personal characteristics such as career choice, knowledge acquisition, and clinical competence. Included in the expanded edition are also updated chapters on the development and use of the Jefferson Scale of Empathy (JSE) as well as results from a worldwide network of scholars who have used it in their research. In short, this book is a treasure trove of information and practical wisdom about studying empathy that is unparalleled in depth, breath, and scholarship ... Dr. Hojat's recent research on the role of empathy in diabetes stands out as a telling example of the scientific maturation of research on empathy and the movement from descriptive studies to predictive models. The same can be said of his work in medical education and his finding that there is a decided decrease in empathy in the third year of medical school, a finding that is both significant and actionable. As a communication researcher, educator, and sometimes patient, I am especially grateful to Dr. Hojat for his long-standing interest and focus on this topic and for the path he has blazed in bringing clarity and precision to the science and practice of empathy.

Richard M. Frankel, Ph.D., M.D. (Hon)
Professor of Medicine and Geriatrics
Indiana University School of Medicine
Indianapolis, IN

Remarks by Experts on the Third Edition

Professor Hojat has been a leader in empathy research and practice for over two decades. In this excellent book, he combines personal insights with the science and evidence supporting the therapeutic value of human connection, the methods and benefits of measuring empathy, and how empathic connections benefit patients and practitioners. It is a must read for medical and other healthcare students, teachers, and curriculum developers.

Jeremy Howick, Ph.D.
Professor of Empathic Healthcare, and Director of the Stoneygate and Center for Excellence in Empathic Healthcare,
Leicester Medical School, University of Leicester, UK.

There is no doubt that Dr. Hojat is *the* world's expert on empathy and its application to clinical settings. Any practicing health professional, and those teaching in the health professions, should have this book on hand as a ready, thorough source of information on all aspects of empathy. This updated third edition is heavily researched and is an essential read for anyone who seeks to understand the importance of establishing an empathic bond of trust with their patients. I can think of no other source concerning empathy that is as clearly written and comprehensive as this third edition.

Bruce W. Newton, Ph.D.
Retired Professor and Chair of Anatomy
Campbell University Jerry M. Wallace School of Osteopathic Medicine
Lillington, NC

In this third edition of his book on empathy, Hojat does an outstanding job of outlining the causes and consequences of low and high clinical empathy (summarized in his Figure 15.1). Thus, laying a comprehensive foundation to predict how this empathy might be fostered in healthcare professionals and their students. And he considers deeply the ways in which provider empathy enhances the well-being of both patients and the providers themselves. As Hojat points out, major challenges of future research in this important field include (1) sustaining and prolonging methods to promote higher clinical empathy in healthcare professional education throughout these providers' careers and (2) discovering how these and new efforts might be employed globally to produce more compassionate cultures and societies and, thus, improve public health. Similarly, (3) how can we determine whether using clinical empathy as a selection criterion for admission to healthcare provider training programs improves patient care and, most optimistically, (4) might it become possible "that empathic understanding can not only enhance the quality of patent-clinician relationships and improve outcomes of patient care, but also serve as a means for achieving global peace and harmony in all humans, everywhere, regardless of any so-called divisive factors" (p. xv).

Lon J. Van Winkle, Ph.D.
Professor of Medical Humanities
Rocky Vista University, Englewood, CO
Emeritus Professor of Biochemistry
Midwestern University, Downers Grove, IL

Remarks by Experts on Previous Editions

This book is unique in combining an encyclopedic overview of empathy with a fine-grained, precise way of measuring it. Clinicians, researchers, students, and educators will find in this book both a resource for work already done and a blueprint for what still needs to be done. The latest edition [of the book] grounds the clinical art of empathic caring in the newly recognized contributions of brain imagery and social cognitive neuroscience. Furthermore, it updates the accumulating empirical evidence for the clinical effects of empathy that has been facilitated by the widespread use of the Jefferson Scale of Empathy, a generative contribution to clinical research by this book's author. In addition, the book is so coherently structured that each chapter contributes to an overall understanding of empathy, while also covering its subject so well that it could stand alone.

Herbert Adler, M.D., Ph.D.
Clinical Professor of Psychiatry and Human Behavior
Sidney Kimmel Medical College at Thomas Jefferson University
Philadelphia, PA

Dr. Hojat has provided a definitive resource for the evolving area of empathy research and education. For those engaged in medical student or resident education and especially for those dedicated to efforts to improve the patient experience, this book is a treasure trove of primary work in the field of empathy.

Leonard H. Calabrese, D.O.
Professor of Medicine
Cleveland Clinic Lerner College of Medicine
Case Reserve University
Cleveland, OH

This book is a scholarly achievement in the field. All will benefit from its comprehensiveness.

Joseph S. Gonnella, M.D.
Emeritus Dean and Distinguished Professor of Medicine
Sidney Kimmel Medical College at Thomas Jefferson University
Philadelphia, PA

This book is an outstanding contribution to the scholarly and clinical understanding of empathy. Most importantly, it combines conceptual rigor with an empirical foundation. Dr. Hojat has devoted himself to developing ways of measuring empathy, and in this book he combines his own findings with an encyclopedic knowledge of other relevant empirical work. This book will be important for any serious student of empathy, including medical educators who are seeking to truly transform professional training.

Jodi Halpern, M.D., Ph.D.
Author, "From Detached Concern to Empathy: Humanizing Medical Practice"
Chancellor's Chair and Professor of Bioethics
University of California, Berkeley, CA

It is my firm belief that empathy as defined and assessed by Dr. Hojat in his seminal book has far reaching implications for other areas of human interaction, including business, management, government, economics, and international relations.

Amir H. Mehryar, Ph.D.
Emeritus Professor of Behavioral Sciences and Population Studies
Institute for Research and Training in Management and Planning
Tehran, Iran

Professor Hojat offers all of us in healthcare education an uplifting *magnum opus* that is sure to greatly enhance how we conceptualize, measure, and teach the central professional virtue of empathy. Hojat's book provides students and professionals across health care with the most scientifically rigorous, conceptually vivid, and comprehensive statement ever produced, providing once and for all what we all know intuitively – empathy is healing both for those who receive it and those who give it. This book is filled with great science, great philosophizing, and great 'how to' approaches to education. Every student and practitioner in healthcare today should read this and keep it by the bedside in a permanent place of honor.

Stephen G. Post, Ph.D.
Professor of Preventive Medicine
Founding Director of the Center for Medical Humanities, Compassionate Care, and Bioethics
School of Medicine, Stony Brook University
Stony Brook, NY

This book should be essential reading for all those engaged in medical education. The author writes clearly and covers the broad area of empathy, with theoretical depth and practical suggestions based on his own research and that of others. He is a foremost leader in this field and his book sets a standard for all to follow.

Marvin Zuckerman, Ph.D.
Emeritus Professor of Psychology
University of Delaware
1928–2018

Excerpts From Book Reviews

This is an extraordinarily well developed, researched, and validated summary on the value and use of the concept of empathy in the health professions. It serves as an excellent review for admissions committees of all health disciplines, career counselors in the undergraduate areas and for those considering residency training, and as a tool for those in health profession leadership roles in counseling graduate clinicians who have experienced difficulties in their interpersonal relations and patient-clinician relations.

Vincent F. Carr
Doody's Book Reviews, August, 2016

Hojat presents an excellent compilation of research and theory regarding the doctor-patient relationship in general and the importance of connectedness and empathy in that relationship specifically. As in all good research, defining constructs is the primary step. Hojat makes a clear distinction between empathy and sympathy—the former cognitive, the latter emotional. Hojat's review of the psychometric testing of the JSE is detailed but easy to follow. Hojat tells the reader early on that he believes personality attributes determine behavior. This belief is the foundation for the development of the JSE, an instrument that measures attitudes, not behaviors … Chapter 7 on the development of the JSE can stand alone as a text for teaching scale and instrument development … He discusses several characteristics of modern medical education and practice that can interfere with empathy and how empathy can be enhanced in both training and practice … Hojat grounds his argument for the importance of empathy in the doctor-patient relationship in theory and empiricism. This important text has a place in every medical school. It also will be widely used in health services research because of the rigorous research process it models.

Mary Ann Cook
PsycCRITIQUES, 2007, *52* (20).

Hojat, who is a preeminent researcher in the field, has written a comprehensive survey of empathy in medical practice, including its history, development, scope, methodologies, and results of empirical studies … Hojat begins by carefully distinguishing empathy from related concepts or qualities, like sympathy and compassion, and by clarifying the cognitive, as opposed to affective, nature of empathy … Hojat begins by sketching the evolutionary and neurological substrates of empathy, including the recent discovery of a system of mirror neurons of emotions. In this system it appears that certain neurons activated when a person experiences an emotion are similarly activated when he or she sees another person experiencing the same emotion, thus suggesting an empathic response. Hojat then summarizes research literature on empathy in the clinical setting. The Jefferson Scale of Empathy (JSE), developed by Hojat, is among the most useful and well-validated self-report survey instruments … Hojat presents the results of numerous studies using the JSE and other instruments to assess medical student and physician empathy … There is also a considerable body of evidence showing that physicians' empathic engagement with patients is associated with better health outcomes. The chapter on empathy enhancement (i.e., "teaching" empathy) is especially relevant to medical education. Many studies suggest that medical students suffer a gradual decline in empathy over the years of professional training. Hojat reviews various educational techniques that have been employed to enhance clinical empathy, including, for example, communication skills training, systematic shadowing of role-model physicians, reflective writing, and targeted study of literature and the arts … Dr. Hojat has performed an important service by providing us with this lucid, well-organized, and comprehensive study of clinical empathy. Moreover, his own research program serves as an elegant model for future investigators.

Jack Coulehan, M.D., MPH
Journal of Continuing Education in the Health Professions, 2010, *30*(30), 205.

This book seeks to restore empathy to medical practice, to demonstrate how important it is for doctors to listen to their patients, to experience and understand what their patients are feeling. The book's chapters have been wisely divided into two sections: I. Empathy in human relationships and II. Empathy in patient care. The author, who originally developed the Jefferson Scale of Empathy, has provided a detailed description of the scale in his book. JSE is a psychometrically sound instrument that is specifically developed to measure empathy in the context of patient care and is being used internationally… Empathy is a powerful communication skill that is often misunderstood and underused. Initially, empathy was referred to as "bedside manner"; now, however, authors and educators consider empathetic communication a teachable, learnable, skill that has tangible benefits for both clinician and patient … What is the difference between empathy and sympathy? Whereas empathy is used by skilled clinicians to enhance communication and delivery of care, sympathy can be burdensome and emotionally exhausting and can lead to burnout … Many medical schools have now developed curricula with a strong focus on physician-patient communication and empathy … Reading of the book for those who would like to know what empathy is, what its role in patient care is, and how to measure it in clinical setting is highly recommended.

Reza F. Ghosehtani, M.D.
European Journal of Dermatology, 2007, *17*(4), 355.

Mohammadreza Hojat, a prominent researcher in medical education, makes the case that empathy is not a mere abstraction but a psychological attribute that has concrete clinical benefits. He argues that empathic engagement with patients is an essential response to a deep human need for social connection—a need that is often deepened among the ill and can be harnessed for therapeutic ends … Empathy is placed in the contexts of biological, psychological, and developmental research, and its importance in the clinical encounter is forcefully laid out. Later chapters, which have more applied focus, present a psychometric measure of empathy that is tailored to research and patient care. Here Hojat shows how empathy enhances clinician-patient encounters and thus can lead to positive clinical outcomes. The concluding chapters examine how individual differences in empathy are related to gender, specialty choice, and clinical competence and what methods can be used to foster the use of empathy among professionals. Acknowledging the limitations of existing work on the subject of empathy, Hojat proposes several directions for future research and policy. If the capacity for empathy is a better predictor of clinical performance than academic results, for example, should it be factored into the admissions process for medical schools and residencies? Among the strengths of this book are its thorough and up-to-date reviews of varied specialist literatures and its author's consistently humanist voice. Although his tone is more empirical than poetic, the author never loses sight of the practice of empathy as an easily learned toolkit of interpersonal skills ... Hojat energetically advocates for more research.

Nick Haslam, Ph.D.
The New England Journal of Medicine, 2007, *356* (17), 1792.

This book is an excellent overview about antecedents, development and measurement of empathy, and in particular about the importance of empathy in patient care. In the whole book theoretical aspects are discussed, and relevant studies and empirical findings are presented in support of the theoretical discussion. Many references cited for critical issues for further review are alphabetically listed at the end of the book. Empathy can contribute to the physical, mental, and social well-being of both patient and clinician … All medical schools should incorporate new classes and methods in the curricula to improve empathy skills among students and residents, for future better physician-patient relationship and better patient outcome ... As the author wrote, although studies that confirm a correlation between physician-patient empathic engagement and patient outcomes in medical care are convincing, more empirical evidence is needed to verify a direct link between measures of empathy in the context of patient care and objective indicators of patient outcomes.

Mirjana Huic
Croatian Medical Journal, 2007, *48*, 271-275.

This carefully written discussion of empathy in patient care will be useful to those interested in any kind of practitioner-client relationship. One underlying principle is "Being connected is beneficial to the human body and mind." The author's more specific focus is on the development of empathy among medical students and its impact on patient outcomes. Hojat, a psychologist, headed the Jefferson Longitudinal Study of Medical Education and focuses here on the Jefferson Scale of Empathy (JSE). Cognition, understanding, and communication are three key measures in the JSE … He also writes about personal attributes that can either contribute to or interfere with empathy in therapeutic relationships. Using systems theory and triangular biopsychosocial approach of health psychology, Hojat suggests that empathic engagement leads to physical, mental, and social well-being … Summing up: Recommended. Upper-level undergraduates and above.

M. K. Snooks
Choice, 2007, *44* (9), 1565.

Empathy is at the heart of all human cooperative endeavors … Empathy is woven into fabric of the humanities and all the social sciences … Dr. Hojat, a psychologist, comes to the problem of empathy as an investigator in medical education with a long-range mission of improving our system of medical care and thereby improving the health and well-being of all of us. Hojat's research program evolved under the umbrella of the Jefferson Longitudinal Study of Medical Education. These efforts are fueled by a serious demoralization evident within health professions (diminished prestige, loss of autonomy, and deep personal dissatisfaction are among the outcomes of paradigmatic shift in health care system) ... Despite the impressive breadth of scholarship (about 1100 references), Hojat's work is bounded by a particular perspective and a particular context, namely medical education. Hojat is committed to the scientific measurement of physician empathy and to enhancing empathy through 'dedicated educational programs and through demonstration of its beneficial effects on patient outcomes.' Although written for a broad audience, Hojat's book itself looks like and read like a graduate-level textbook. The text is segmented into small sections titled in bold captions, each chapter concluding with a brief synopsis. The book's instructional intent is also evident in its extensive literature review and, most clearly, in its detailed explication of the steps taken to establish the validity and reliability of the Jefferson Scale of Empathy, Hojat's signal accomplishment … Hojat has established with uncommon rigor the psychometric soundness of his measuring instruments. One would be hard-pressed to find instruments that have been as rigorously documented, even among peer-reviewed research journal papers. Hojat's concern with precision comes, of course, with a price. The context is medical education, and the language of the test items relates to doctor-patient relationships, limiting its usefulness. When measures of empathy developed by other investigators were discussed, Hojat faulted many of them for their psychometric limitations … Hojat's work will probably be seriously examined and debated by medical education and policy makers. Psychodynamically-oriented professionals who may be put off by Hojat's insistent objectivity and narrow conceptualization of empathy will be challenged by this work and by societal pressures to make a clearer and more convincing case for their point of view.

Charles Saltzman

Psychodynamic Practice, 2008, *14* (3), 342-345.

Accessible from: *https//doi.org/10.1080/14753630802196430*

Contents

Part I
Empathy in Human Relationships

Chapter 1
Descriptions and Conceptualization

To be one in heart is enchanting, more than to be one in tongue.

—Rumi (Persian mystical poet and philosopher, 1207–1273 AD)

Abstract

- Empathy, a translation of the German word *Einfühlung*, has been described as an elusive and slippery concept with a long history marked by ambiguity and controversy.
- There has been an ongoing debate about the construct of empathy, described sometimes as a cognitive attribute featuring *understanding of experiences* of others (cognitive empathy); at other times, as an emotional state of the mind featuring *sharing of feelings* (emotional empathy); and at still other times as a concept involving both cognition and emotion.
- Distinctions are made in this chapter between cognition and emotion and also between their corresponding underlying mechanisms of understanding and feeling.
- The unsettled issue of the differences between empathy and sympathy in the context of patient care is addressed by viewing empathy in patient care as a predominantly cognitive attribute featuring understanding of others' concerns (cognitive empathy, or clinical empathy) that has a positive and linear relationship with patient outcomes and by viewing sympathy (synonymous to emotional empathy) as a primarily emotional concept featured by sharing emotions and feelings that has a curvilinear relationship (an inverted U shape) with patient outcomes.

M. Hojat, *Clinical Empathy*, https://doi.org/10.1007/978-3-031-87413-0_1

- Distinctions between cognition and emotion, understanding and feeling, and empathy and sympathy are utterly important because of their implications not only for relevant conceptualization and valid measurement of empathy in patient care but for their different consequences in patient outcomes as well.

Introduction

The concept of empathy has received a lot of attention in the past few decades in public media, academia, national and international politics, arts, ethics, health professions education, and patient care (Coplan, 2014). Despite the popularity of the concept, there is no consensus on the definition of empathy among researchers (Matravers, 2014). The notion of "empathy" has a long history marked by ambiguity, discrepancy, disputation, and controversy among philosophers and behavioral, social, and medical scholars (Aring, 1958; Basch, 1983; Preston & deWaal, 2002; Wispe, 1978, 1986). Because of conceptual ambiguity, empathy has been described as an "elusive" concept (Basch, 1983)—one that is difficult to define and hard to measure (Kestenbaum, Farber, & Sroufe, 1989). Eisenberg and Strayer (1987a, p. 3) described empathy as a "slippery concept … that has provoked considerable speculation, excitement, and confusion." Also, because of the ambiguity associated with the concept of empathy, Pigman (1995) suggested that empathy has come to mean so much that it means nothing! More than seven decades ago, Theodore Reik (1948, p. 357), the prominent psychoanalyst, made a similar comment: "The word empathy sometimes means one thing, sometimes another, until now it does not mean anything at all."

Because of the conceptual ambiguity, Wispe (1986) suggested that the outcomes of empathy research might not be valid because empathy means different things to different investigators, who may believe they are studying the same thing but actually are referring to different things! As a result, Lane (1986) suggested that empathy might not even exist in reality after all. Later, Levy (1997) proposed that the term should be eliminated and replaced by a less ambiguous one.

Despite the conceptual ambiguity, it is interesting to note that empathy is among the most frequently mentioned humanistic dimensions of patient care (Linn, DiMatteo, Cope, & Robbins, 1987). Many successful clinicians know intuitively what empathy is without being able to define it. In that respect, empathy may be analogous to love, which many of us have experienced without being able to define it! Thus, while we all have a positive image of the concept of empathy and a preconceived idea about its positive outcomes in interpersonal relationships in general and in patient care in particular, we wonder how to define it operationally. Needless to say, no concept can be subject to scientific scrutiny without an operational definition.

The Origin and History of the Term *Empathy*

The concept of empathy (not the English term) was first discussed in 1873 by Robert Vischer, a German art historian and philosopher who used the word *Einfühlung* to address an observer's feelings elicited by works of art (Hunsdahl, 1967; Jackson, 1992). According to Pigman (1995), the word was used to describe the projection of human feelings onto the natural world and inanimate objects. However, the German term was originally used not to describe an interpersonal attribute but to portray the individual's feelings when appreciating a work of art, specifically when those feelings blurred the distinction between the observer's self and the art object (Wispe, 1986).

In 1897, the German psychologist–philosopher Theodore Lipps brought the word *Einfühlung* from aesthetics to psychology. In describing personal experiences associated with the concept of *Einfühlung*, Lipps indicated that "when I observe a circus performer on a hanging wire, I feel I am inside him" (cited in Carr, Iacoboni, Dubeau, Mazziotta, & Lenzi, 2003, p. 5502). In 1903, Wilhelm Wundt, the father of experimental psychology, who established the first laboratory of experimental psychology in 1879 at the University of Leipzig in Germany, used *Einfühlung* for the first time in the context of human relationships (Hunsdahl, 1967). In 1905, Sigmund Freud (1960) used *Einfühlung* to describe the psychodynamics of putting oneself in another person's position (Pigman, 1995).

The English term "empathy" is a neologism coined by psychologist Edward Bradner Titchener (1909) as an English equivalent or the translation of the meaning of *Einfühlung*. The term empathy derives from the Greek word *empatheia*, which means appreciation of another person's feelings (Astin, 1967; Wispe, 1986). Although Titchener (1915) used the term empathy to convey "understanding" of other human beings, Southard (1918) was the first to describe the significance of empathy in the relationship between a clinician and a patient for facilitating diagnostic outcomes. Thereafter, American social and behavioral scientists have often used the concept of empathy in relation to the psychotherapeutic or counseling relationship and in the discussion of prosocial behavior and altruism (Batson & Coke, 1981; Carkhuff, 1969; Davis, 1994; Eisenberg & Strayer, 1987b; Feshbach, 1989; Feudtner, Christakis, & Christakis, 1994; Hoffman, 1981; Ickes, 1997; Stotland, Mathews, Sherman, Hansson, & Richardson, 1978). Empathy also has been discussed frequently in the psychoanalytic literature (Jackson, 1992) and in social psychology, counseling, and clinical psychiatry and psychology (Berger, 1987; Davis, 1994; Eisenberg & Strayer, 1987b; Ickes, 1997).

Definitions, Descriptions, and Features

A review of the literature indicates that more disagreement than agreement exists among researchers about the definition of empathy. Presenting a long list of definitions and descriptions of empathy would take us far beyond the intended scope of the book, and space constraints do not allow such an extensive review. I have deliberately chosen a few definitions and descriptions that seem to be most relevant to health professions education and can also provide a framework for the conceptualization and definition of empathy in the context of patient care that will be presented in Chap. 6.

Carl Rogers (1959, p. 210), the founder of client-centered therapy, suggested the following often-cited definition of empathy as an ability "to perceive the internal frame of reference of another with accuracy *as if* one were the other person but without ever losing the '*as if*' condition" (emphasis added). In addition, Rogers (1975) described the experience of empathy as entering into the private perceptual world of another person and becoming thoroughly at home in it. Similarly, in one of the first psychoanalytic studies of empathy, Theodore Schroeder (1925, p. 159) suggested that "empathic insight implies seeing *as if* from within the person who is being observed" (emphasis added).

George Herbert Mead (1934, p. 27) suggested the following definition of empathy more than nine decades ago: "The capacity to take the role of another person and adopt alternative perspectives." More than six decades ago, Charles Aring (1958) described empathy as the *act* or *capacity* of appreciating another person's feelings *without* joining those feelings. Robert Hogan (1969, p. 308) defined empathy as "the intellectual or imaginative apprehension of another's condition or state of mind *without* actually experiencing that person's feelings" (emphasis added). Clark (1980, p. 187) defined empathy as "the unique capacity of the human being to feel the experience, needs, aspirations, frustrations, sorrows, joys, anxieties, hurt, or hunger of others *as if* they were his or her own" (emphasis added). These definitions by Hogan and Clark are in line with Rogers's (1959) "as if" condition in describing empathy and with Aring's (1958) "without joining" feature of empathy described earlier. I will assert later in this chapter that the "as if" condition is a key feature that distinguishes empathy from sympathy.

Wispe (1986, p. 318) described empathy as "the attempt by one self-aware self to comprehend nonjudgmentally the positive and negative experiences of another self." Baron-Cohen and Wheelwright (2004) described empathy as the "glue" of the social world that draws people to help one another and stops them from hurting others. Levasseur and Vance (1993, p. 83) described empathy as follows: "Empathy is not a psychological or emotional experience, nor a psychic leap into the mind of another person, but an openness to, and respect for, the personhood of another." Similarly, Shamasundar (1999) described empathy as related to open-mindedness and tolerance for ambiguity and complexity.

Mead (1934) described empathy as an element of social intelligence. This description resembles the notion of emotional intelligence introduced originally by Salovey and Mayer (1990) and later by Goleman (1995) who proposed that empathy, as an ability to recognize emotions in others, is one domain of emotional intelligence. The proposition that empathy has a significant overlap with measures of emotional intelligence and social skills has been supported (Schutte et al., 2001).

Greif and Hogan (1973) described empathic development as a parallel function of moral maturity. Schafer (1959, p. 343) defined empathy as "the inner experience of sharing and comprehending the momentary psychological state of another person." Stefano Bolognini (1997, p. 279) described empathy as "a state of complementary conscious-preconscious contact based on separateness and sharing." William Ickes (1997, p. 183) defined empathy as "a state of our mind upon which we reflect." Bellet and Maloney (1991, p. 183) defined empathy as "the capacity to understand what the other person is experiencing from within the other person's frame of reference, i.e., the capacity to place oneself in another's shoes." Hamilton (1984, p. 217) defined empathy as a "vehicle for understanding one another in a meaningful way."

Levasseur and Vance (1993, p. 82) described empathy as "a mode of caring," adding that "Empathy is not for those who are flourishing or happy. ... Empathy is for those who need help or are suffering or struggling in some way." Similarly, Shamasundar (1999) suggested that the intensity of empathic resonance is deeper for negative states, such as sadness, anger, hostility, and illness. These descriptions portray the importance of empathy in situations where others are suffering or are sad. Thus, the importance of empathic relationships in clinical encounters is apparent.

Empathy has been described as the neural matching mechanism constituted of a mirror neuron system in the brain that enables us to place ourselves in the "mental shoes" of others (Gallese, 2001, 2003). Briefly, mirror neurons are brain cells (not visual cells) that are activated when we observe another person who is performing a goal-directed action as if we are performing that act (Carr et al., 2003; Gallese, 2001; Iacoboni et al., 1999). Brain imaging studies have shown that watching on a television screen a needle prick a specific hand muscle influences the same hand muscle in the observer (Singer & Frith, 2005). These brain studies suggest the possibility that, in the future, empathy may be defined in neurological terms and be measured by physiological indicators (see Chap. 13 for a more detailed discussion).

Empathy Viewed from the Cognitive and Emotional Perspectives

In general, empathy has been described as a cognitive or an emotional (affective) attribute or a combination of both. Cognition requires mental activities involved in acquiring and processing information for better understanding, and emotion is sharing of the affect manifested in subjectively experienced feelings (Colman, 2001). Two types of empathy, cognitive empathy and emotional empathy, fit these descriptions of cognition and emotions, respectively. I believe that emotional empathy is conceptually synonymous to sympathy and vicarious empathy, which will be addressed later.

Cognitive Perspective

Rosalind Dymond (1949) viewed empathy as a cognitive ability to assume the role of another person. Heins Kohut (1971, p. 300) described empathy as "a mode of *cognition* that is specifically attuned to the perception of a complex psychological configuration" (emphasis added). Basch (1983) also described empathy as a complex cognitive process involving cognitive functions, such as judgment and reality testing. MacKay, Hughes, and Carver (1990, p. 155) described empathy as "the ability to understand someone's situation without making it one's own."

Cognitive activities, such as perspective taking and role taking, are among the features some authors have presented in their definition of empathy. For example, Dymond (1949, p. 127) defined empathy as "the imaginative transposing of oneself into the thinking, feeling, and acting of another, and so structuring the world as he [she] does." Blackman, Smith, Brokman, and Stern (1958) defined empathy as an ability to step into another person's shoes and to step back as easily into one's own shoes again when needed. Similarly, Decety and Jackson (2004) described empathy as subjective experience of similarity between feelings experienced by self and others without losing sight of whose feelings belong to whom. Those who advocate the cognitive view of empathy place more emphasis on understanding and social insight than on emotional involvement (Rogers, 1975).

Emotional Perspective

Some authors have defined empathy as an emotional response generating identical feelings and sharing emotions between people. For example, Batson and Coke (1981, p. 169) defined empathy as "an emotional response elicited by and congruent with the perceived welfare of someone else." Rushton (1981, p. 260) defined empathy as "experiencing the emotional state of another." Eisenberg (1989) described it as "an emotional response that stems from the apprehension of another's emotional state or condition and is congruent with the other's emotional state or condition" (p. 108). Halpern (2001, p. xv) described empathy as "a form of emotional reasoning with risks of error that such reasoning involves." Katz (1963, p. 26) defined it as "the inner experience of feeling oneself to be similar to, or nearly identical with the other person." Kalisch (1973, p. 1548) defined it as "the ability to enter into the life of another person, to accurately perceive his [her] current feelings and their meaning"; and Hoffman (1981, p. 41) defined it as "a vicarious affective response to someone else's situation rather than one's own." However, Underwood and Moore (1982) suggested that an emotional perspective is not a sufficient condition to define empathy. In my view, clinical empathy is aligned more with cognitive rather than emotional conceptualization of empathy.

A number of researchers, however, believe that empathy involves both cognition and emotion (Baron-Cohen & Wheelwright, 2004; Davis, 1994). For example,

Bennett (2001, p. 7) defined empathy as "a mode of relating in which one person comes to know the mental content of another, both *affectively* and *cognitively*, at a particular moment in time and as a product of the relationship that exists between them." Mark Davis (1994, p. 12) defined empathy as "a set of constructs having to do with the responses of one individual to the experiences of another. These constructs specifically include the process taking place within the observer and the affective and non-affective outcomes which results from those processes." Hodges and Wegner (1997, p. 313) suggested that "empathy can have either an emotional component … or a cognitive component, or both."

Cognition and Emotion

Silvan Tomkins (1962, 1963) viewed cognition and emotion as two separate systems working side by side to process incoming data. The processing of cognitive information often involves specific mental activities, such as reasoning and appraisal (Tausch, 1988). In contrast, emotional mental processing often entails an affective response experienced spontaneously without involvement of the higher mental processes that are activated in reasoning (Basch, 1996). Therefore, *reasoning* and *appraisal* are the features of cognitive responses, and *spontaneity* and *arousal* are the hallmarks of emotional responses (Tucker et al., 2005) (see Table 1.1). Solomon's (1976) description of the wisdom of "reason" against the treachery of the "passions" is somewhat analogous to the nature of a cognitive response as opposed to an emotional one.

Basic emotions and their expressions, as Charles Darwin (1965) was first to note, are universally similar regardless of cultural factors, personal background, or educational experiences. On the contrary, the processing of cognitive information is not culture-free and is heavily dependent on personal background, learning, and educational experiences. Thus, the contribution of learning is more significant in a cognitive response (e.g., empathy) than it is in an emotional reaction (e.g., sympathy) (see Table 1.1). Manifestation of cognitive behaviors is more *effortful*, and its behavioral roots are more *advanced* (Schulte-Ruther, Markowitsch, Fink, & Piefke, 2007). The same is true of empathy. Expression of emotion is *effortless*, and its behavioral roots are more *primitive*. The same is true of sympathy (see Table 1.1). An emotional response is colored more by subjective judgments, leading to a less accurate interpretation than would result from a cognitive response.

At the neuroanatomical level, different brain mechanisms appear to be involved in the processing of cognitive and emotional input (Nathanson, 1996). Cognitive mental processing is primarily an *advanced intellectual process* that often involves social perception, analysis of information, and generation of appropriate responses based on one's understanding of another person and the situation. Emotional responses consist primarily of more *primitive* mental processes, wherein the person responds, through a process of contagion, with emotions similar to the emotions of

Table 1.1 Features of cognitive (clinical) empathy and emotional empathy (sympathy)

Feature	Cognitive (Clinical) Empathy	Emotional Empathy (Sympathy)
Contribution of learning	More significant	Less significant
Contribution of cognition	More significant	Less significant
Contribution of affects	Less significant	More significant
Contribution of innate or genetic factors	Less innate	More innate
Objectivity vs. subjectivity	More objective	More subjective
Likelihood of accuracy	More accurate	Less accurate
Behavioral roots	Advanced	Primitive
Required efforts	More effortful	More effortless
Relation to clinician's performance	Linear	Inverted U shape
Reaction time	Nonspontaneous	Spontaneous
Patient's emotions	Appreciated without joining	Perceived by joining
Feeling felt	The kind and quality of the patient's feelings	The degree and quantity of the patient's feelings
Brain processing area	Predominantly neocortex	Predominantly limbic system
Psychological regulatory process	Appraisal	Arousal
Neurological regulatory process	Parasympathetic (inhibitory)	Sympathetic (excitatory)
Psycho-physiological state	Energy conserving	Energy consuming
Behavioral motivation	Altruistic	Egoistic
State of mind	Intellectual	Emotional
Typical expression to patient	I understand your suffering	I feel your pain
Key mental processing	Cognitive/intellectual/understanding	Affective/emotional/feeling

Reproduced from Hojat, Maio, Pohl, & Gonnella, 2023, ©Authors, Open Access

others who are present (Mehrabian, Young, & Sato, 1988). Thus, emotion often is contagious in interpersonal exchanges, but cognition is not (Doherty, 1997).

Despite these differences between cognition and emotion, some authors do not make such distinctions and assign equal weight to both cognition and emotion in the construct of empathy (Bennett, 2001). Freud (1958a, 1958b), for example, emphasized the intellectual or cognitive component while recognizing emotion as another important aspect of empathy in forming empathic relationships between clinician and patient.

It is indeed virtually impossible to treat emotion and cognition as two completely independent entities because one cannot fully exist without the other. For practical reasons, however, the distinction between the two is important, particularly in clinical empathy in the context of patient care, to avoid confusion between the concepts of understanding and feeling (and thus between empathy and sympathy). I will discuss this further in the following sections.

Understanding and Feeling

The distinction between cognition and emotion provides a context for distinguishing between the two other corresponding interrelated concepts of understanding and feeling, which are often used interchangeably. In the context of patient care, however, it is useful to define understanding as the awareness of meaning (Sims, 1988) and to define feeling as the perception of emotions. All meaningful social relationships are based on both mutual understanding of one another and feeling of emotions.

Understanding is often based on *tangibility* and *objectivity*, whereas feeling is more a product of *subjectivity* and thus can be subject to *prejudice. Accuracy in judgment* is more likely to emerge from effortful mental activities associated with understanding than from spontaneous and effortless emotional arousal. Understanding is more likely to be based on learning and requires active efforts, whereas feeling is more likely to be *innate* and *effortless* (Wispe, 1986). A higher mental processing is involved when attempting to understand another person's concerns, whereas a primitive mental processing is involved in feeling another person's emotions (see Table 1.1). Clinical empathy is associated more with cognitive response and understanding, whereas sympathy is associated more with emotions and affects. To be empathic, according to Bellet and Maloney (1991, p. 1831) "the physician does not have to experience the intense feelings or emotions that grip the patient … but only to understand these feelings and relate to them while maintaining a sense of self." According to Shamasundar (1999), the less empathic connection between individuals, the more difficult it is to reach a mutual understanding of each other regardless of the use of a larger and more precise vocabulary.

Empathy and Sympathy

Both empathy and sympathy are important components of interpersonal relationships. Sympathy derives from the Greek *sym* (being with) and *pathos* (suffering, pain) (Black, 2004). The two distinct concepts of empathy and sympathy are often mistakenly tossed into the same terminological basket in empathy research—a mistake that has created conceptual confusion and debates for years but has never been settled (Black, 2004; Chismar, 1988; Gruen & Mendelsohn, 1986; Wispe, 1986; Zhou, Valiente, & Eisenberg, 2003). The two constructs of empathy and sympathy in the context of patient care reflect different human qualities that have different measurable influences on clinicians' professional behavior, utilization of resources, and clinical outcomes (Nightingale, Yarnold, & Greenberg, 1991; Yarnold, Greenberg, & Nightingale, 1991).

We showed in an empirical study that it is possible to differentiate and quantify empathic and sympathetic responses to patient care (Hojat, Spandorfer, Louis, & Gonnella, 2011). In that study, we asked medical students to respond to clinical scenarios by using one scale pertaining to empathic engagement (for measuring a student's inclination toward *understanding* the patient's pain and suffering); and using another scale pertaining to sympathetic response (to measure the student's tendency to *feel* a patient's pain and suffering). Findings indicated that inclination toward empathic engagement was significantly correlated with a validated measure of cognitive empathy (Jefferson Scale of Empathy, Hojat et al., 2002, see Chap. 7), and sympathetic responses were significantly associated with measure of emotional empathy measured by subscales of the Interpersonal Reactivity Index (Davis, 1983, 1994, see Chap. 7).

According to Decety and Jackson (2004, p. 85) "an essential aspect of empathy is to recognize the other person as like self while maintaining a clear separation between self and other." The key feature of empathy is the preponderance of *cognitive* information processing that distinguishes it from the predominantly *emotional* mental processing involved in sympathy (Brock & Salinsky, 1993; Streit-Forest, 1982; Wolf, 1980). Trout (2010, p. 21) made the following distinction "Empathy has as a goal to accurately understand another's inner states …by taking his perspective. Sympathy, on the other hand, is focused not on accurate understanding but on feeling." Although one cannot claim that empathy and sympathy are fully independent from cognition and emotion, one can argue that the degree of cognitive and emotional involvement is different in the two concepts of empathy and sympathy. Figure 1.1 is a graphic presentation showing the relative contribution of degree of cognition and emotion in empathy and sympathy on the X (emotion) and Y (cognition) axes, and the overlap between them (compassion). As it is shown in the figure, empathy is in the area of higher degree of cognition than emotion. Conversely, sympathy is in the area of higher degree of emotion than cognition. Compassion, I propose, resides in the area of the overlap between empathy and sympathy, where both of these attributes are expressed in a moderate amount. Consistent with this conceptualization, Marsh (2012) describes compassion as the ability to recognize fearful perspectives in others (p. 197).

Empathy is a *cognitive* attribute, whereas sympathy is an *emotional* state of mind (Gruen & Mendelsohn, 1986). Empathy refers to one person's attempt to comprehend

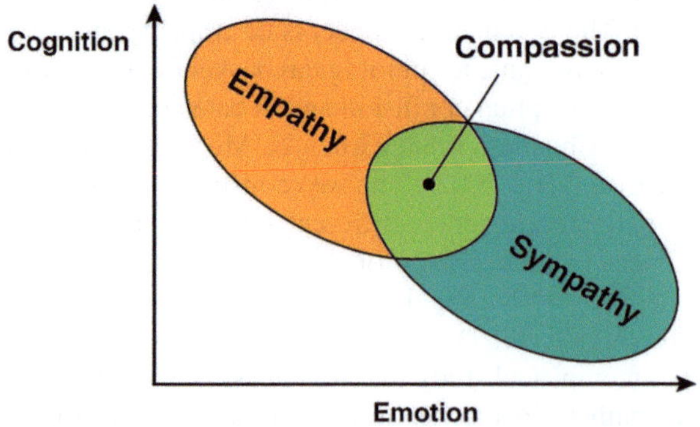

Fig. 1.1 Empathy and sympathy as related to cognition and emotion

nonjudgmentally another person's experiences (Wispe, 1986). Self-awareness is augmented in empathy, but it is reduced in sympathy. Whereas the aim of empathy is to *understand* another person's pain, suffering, and concerns better, the aim of sympathy is to *feel* another person's pain, suffering, and emotions better (see Table 1.1). The empathic relationship implies a *convergence* of understanding between two people, and the sympathetic relationship implies a *parallelism* in the feelings between the two (Buchheimer, 1963). According to Kohut (1984), empathy is a "value-neutral" mode of observation. Similarly, Olinick (1984) believed that empathy is an affect-free phenomenon, whereas sympathy involves an affect-laden perception.

The underlying behavioral motivation in empathy is likely to be altruistic, but it is more likely to be egoistic in sympathy (Table 1.1). The ultimate goal of altruistically motivated helping behavior is to reduce another person's distress without any expectation of reward, whereas the goal in egoistically motivated helping behavior may involve reducing one's own level of stress, to avoid adverse feelings, or to receive rewards (Coke, Batson, & McDavis, 1978). A genuine attempt to understand the experiences of another person—or *empathic understanding*—increases the likelihood of altruistic helping behavior. However, feeling the emotions of others, or sympathetic sharing of emotions, leads to physiological arousal, thus increasing the likelihood of egoistic behavior to reduce emotional arousal and avoid aversive experiences.

In clinical encounters, empathy involves an effort to *understand* the patient's experiences without joining them, whereas sympathy involves an effortless feeling of *sharing* or joining the patient's pain and suffering (Aring, 1958). Titchener (1915), who first coined the term empathy, distinguished empathy from sympathy by describing empathy as a tendency to perceive another person's experiences and by describing sympathy as "feeling together" with another person. McKellar (1957, pp. 220–221) suggested that "One can, however, empathize without necessarily experiencing sympathy for the other person; empathy involves understanding rather than 'siding with.'" Wilmer (1968) described empathy as entering into the sufferer's mind and understanding that person's pain from within as if the pain were ours but remains the sufferer's. In contrast, sympathy, according to Wilmer, is sharing feelings together with the patient as if the pain was ours and remains so.

Hinshelwood (1989) wrote that empathy in contrast to sympathy involves a sophisticated mental operation in which two interacting people are clearly separated, but one conceives of the other person's mental landscape without losing sight of reality and his or her own identity. Similarly, Black (2004) described empathy as a sophisticated and conscious act and sympathy as an involuntary propensity that makes affective attunement possible.

Understanding the *kind* and *quality* of the patient's experiences is the territory of empathy, whereas feeling the *degree* and *quantity* of the patient's pain and suffering falls within the terrain of sympathy. A patient will feel *felt* if the clinician understands the kind and quality, not the degree and quantity, of the patient's experiences (Greenson, 1960). Whereas empathy is an internal cognitive process that should be communicated, sympathy seems to be more transparent. Benjamin Disraeli described the transparency of feelings in the following statement: "Never apologize for showing feelings. When you do so, you apologize for the truth" (retrieved March 2015 from http://www.quotationspage.com/quote/2563.html).

Empathy has been described as the art of understanding (Agosta, 1984; Starcevic & Piontek, 1997). This notion of empathic understanding is reflected in different features attributed to empathy, such as perspective taking, role-playing, standing in another person's shoes, tolerance, openness, uncritical judgment, and unconditional acceptance. The difference between empathy and sympathy is more than a semantic one because each involves different mental activities during information processing (Gruen & Mendelsohn, 1986). The predominantly cognitive nature of empathy and the primarily emotional nature of sympathy imply additional differences between the two terms that go beyond semantics. A cognitive response (in empathy) is more likely to be nonspontaneous because it is influenced by the regulatory process of *appraisal*. An affective reaction (in sympathy) is more likely to be spontaneous because it is influenced by the psychological regulatory process of *arousal* (Siegel, 1999). Sympathy (synonymous to emotional empathy) as opposed to cognitive empathy (a feature of clinical empathy, see Chap. 6) can predispose clinicians to professional exhaustion and burnout while cognitive empathy can lead to a feeling of personal accomplishment (Williams, 1989).

Also, empathy as a cognitive response is characterized by an *inhibitory* energy-conserving state in the *parasympathetic* branch of the neurological regulatory process. However, sympathy as an emotional reaction is characterized by an *excitatory* energy-consuming state related to the *sympathetic* neurological regulatory process (Siegel, 1999) (Table 1.1). Despite the differences between empathy and sympathy, they cannot be completely independent from one another. For example, in one of our studies (Hojat, Mangione, Kane, & Gonnella, 2005), we found a moderate correlation ($r = 0.48$, $p < 0.01$) between cognitive empathy (measured by the Jefferson Scale of Empathy) and emotional empathy (which is synonymous to sympathy) measured by scores on the Empathic Concern scale of the Interpersonal Reactivity Index (Davis, 1983, 1994, see Chap. 7). A correlation of this magnitude indicates that the overlap between the two concepts is approximately 23 % (coefficient of determination: $r^2 = 0.48^2 = 23\%$). More empirical research is needed to examine the degree of overlap between measures of empathy and sympathy. Similar patterns of relationships between empathy and sympathy were observed in an earlier study (Hojat et al., 2001).

Empathy and Sympathy in the Context of Patient Care

The distinction between sympathy (also known as emotional empathy, or vicarious empathy) and empathy (also known as cognitive empathy, or clinical empathy in the context of patient care) has important implications for the clinician–patient relationship because joining the patient's emotions, a key feature of sympathy, can impede clinical decision making, and ultimately patient outcomes. A clinician should sense the patient's feelings only to a limited extent to improve objectivity in his or her understanding of the patient without impeding professional judgment (Starcevic & Piontek, 1997). When experiencing empathy, individuals are able to disentangle themselves from others, whereas individuals experiencing sympathy have difficulty maintaining a sense of whose feelings belong to whom (Decety & Jackson, 2006).

Ehrlich and Jaffe (2002) indicated that empathy must be distinguished from sympathy and sentimentalism because neither of the latter two concepts is desirable in the context of patient care. Starcevic and Piontek (1997) argued that because a clinician, as a separate human being, can never fully share the patient's feelings, perfect sympathy can never be achieved. Furthermore, as Truax and Carkhuff (1967) suggested, it would be undesirable for the clinician to feel the patient's emotions too strongly. Black (2004) pointed out that sympathy is a concept that psychoanalysts avoid, in contrast to empathy, which they use with pride. Wilmer (1968) compared the outcomes of pity, defined by as awareness of pain and suffering of another person, coupled with feeling sorry for the person (Chochinov, 2007; Jeffrey, 2016; Newton 2023), sympathy, and empathy in the patient care context and concluded that "pity rarely helps, sympathy commonly helps, empathy always helps." (Wilmer, 1968, p. 264). Conceptual clarity and consequential outcomes of these terms have practical implications for health professions education and patient care.

Because of the emotional nature of sympathy, its overabundance can be overwhelming and therefore can impede the clinician's performance and patient outcomes. This notion about the restraints in sympathetic clinician–patient relationships and clinical outcomes implies that the relationship between sympathy and a clinician's performance is likely to be *curvilinear*—an inverted U function similar to that between anxiety and performance on achievement tests. Although a certain amount of anxiety can improve performance, too much anxiety can hinder it by disrupting cognitive functioning. Thus, to a certain degree, sympathy can be beneficial in clinician–patient encounters—beyond that, however, it can interfere with clinical objectivity and professional effectiveness. The relationship between empathy and a clinician's performance, however, is considered to be *linear*. That is, the more empathic the relationship, the better the clinical outcomes. Therefore, the general conclusion is that sympathy must be restrained or regulated in clinical situations, whereas empathy needs no restraining boundary.

The differences in features between empathy and sympathy are summarized in Table 1.1. I already described some of these differences in this chapter when discussing the concepts of cognition and emotions, and of understanding and feelings that correspond to empathy and sympathy, respectively.

Maximizing Empathy, Regulating Sympathy

In the context of patient care, when expressed in abundance, empathy would be an "enabling" factor, whereas sympathy, in excess, would be a "disabling" factor. Thus, it seems desirable to maximize empathy and regulate (or optimize) sympathy in patient care for optimal patient outcomes. As I indicated previously, the two concepts of empathy and sympathy have mistakenly been used interchangeably, as if one can replace the other without any serious consequences. However, in the context of patient care, the two terms must be used in their proper context because of their different consequences in patient outcomes. It is my hope that the differences described in Table 1.1 can help to settle the longstanding debate about empathy and sympathy in the context of health professions education and patient care. I will return again to the issues of empathy's definition and the differences between empathy and sympathy in the context of patient care in Chap. 6.

Recapitulation

Empathy is a vague concept that has been described sometimes as a cognitive attribute, sometimes as an emotional state of mind, and sometimes as a combination of both. The ambiguity associated with the definition of empathy may obstruct our view to clearly see what we intend to study and may hinder our ability of how to measure it in the context of patient care. Also, we should realize that fundamental differences exist between cognition and emotion, between understanding and feeling, and between clinical empathy and emotional empathy (synonymous to sympathy). Moreover, these have important implications not only for the conceptualization and measurement of clinical empathy, but also for the assessment of patient outcomes, development of proper research design, remedies to enhance clinical empathy (see Chap. 12), and accurate interpretation and appropriate implementation of research outcomes. Research findings on empathy will continue to be subject to serious challenges if differentiations remain unsettled between concepts of cognition and emotion, between mechanisms of understanding and feeling, and between empathy and sympathy.

Chapter 2
Human Connection in Health and Illness

Hear the reed's complaining wail!
Hear it tell its mourning tale!
Torn from spot it loved so well,
Its grief, its sighs our tears compel.

—Rumi (Persian mystical poet and philosopher, 1207–1273 A.D.)

It is not good for the man to be alone.

—(Genesis 2:18)

Abstract

- Humans are evolved to connect together for survival. Among the factors that fulfill the human need for affiliation and connectedness are social institutions, such as marriage, family, and the social support network, including clinician–patient empathic relationships.
- Human connection serves to promote health and prevent illness. Conversely, an absence of satisfactory human connection, experienced as loneliness, is detrimental to physical, mental, and social well-being.
- The mechanisms involved in linking the quality of human connection to health or illness are not well understood. However, empathic engagement that involves a multisystem of psychoneuroimmunology can provide some explanations for the beneficial effects of human connections.
- The clinician–patient relationship is formed in part by the drive for connectedness, which increases with illness. The empathic connection between clinician and patient can serve as a special kind of social support system with all of its beneficial effects.

M. Hojat, *Clinical Empathy*, https://doi.org/10.1007/978-3-031-87413-0_2

Introduction

Human beings are evolved to be social. We are, according to Larson (1993), "pre-wired" to be connected by evolutionary design for the sake of survival. Our survival depends on our ability to understand others and to communicate our understanding. Social relationships provide opportunities for empathic engagement, which in turn reinforces human connections, a cycle that has always been in motion in the evolution of humankind. In the often-cited list of basic needs proposed by psychologist Henry Murray (1938), the need for "affiliation" and the needs for "understanding" and "succorance" (to be gratified by being understood; seeking empathy, affection, and support) are included among the human being's basic psychosocial needs. Without fulfillment of those needs, Murray said, self-actualization cannot be fully achieved. In this chapter, I describe the importance of human ties in health and illness and discuss the consequences of making and breaking human connections on one's physical, mental, and social well-being. Also, I will attest that the human factors involved in clinician–patient empathic engagement make it the epitome of human connection.

The Need for Connectedness

The need for affiliation is a powerful motivator that guides human interactions in health and illness (Lieberman, 2007). Human connection is the bedrock of empathic growth. The urge for connectedness arises from the human need for affiliation. That basic need prompts us to fall in love, marry, establish a family, raise children, associate with other people, enjoy the company of others, and develop interpersonal relationships. The need for affiliation has survival advantages and is deeply rooted in the evolutionary history of humankind.

Human connection leads not only to psychological pleasure but also to biophysiological changes and activities in the endocrine system (Uchino, Cacioppo, & Kiecolt-Glaser, 1996). For example, female students living together in university dormitories noticed that their menstrual cycles had become synchronized, and this hormonal synchronization occurred not only among roommates but among networks of close friends as well (McClintock, 1971).

People interacting with one another often show behavioral synchronization, usually unconsciously, that is reflected in such nonverbal clues as facial mimicry, imitation, and the motor mirroring reaction (see Chaps. 3 and 13). These signals are not necessarily learned; they seem to be the outcomes of a pre-wired built-in behavioral repertoire that facilitates interpersonal exchanges (see Chap. 8).

The Making of Connections

It is now widely recognized that making connections has a powerful effect on the maintenance of health and that breaking connections can lead to the development of illness (Cohen, 1988). This recognition is not new, however. Early research by the French sociologist Emile Durkheim on factors contributing to suicide found that erosion of the capacity for social integration and human connection was the triggering factor for social miseries, including people's attempt to end their lives (Durkheim, 1951).

In their widely cited epidemiological research, Berkman and Syme (1979) showed that the absence of human connections was significantly linked to an increase in disease and mortality. So much evidence has been accumulating that it is now beyond doubt that being connected and feeling acknowledged are beneficial to physical, mental, and social well-being—the three pillars of health defined by the constitution of the World Health Organization (WHO, 1948) (see Chap. 6). Social connections in epidemiological research are typically defined in terms of marital status, family, friends, peer relationships, and membership in social or religious groups (Cacioppo et al., 2002). In this context, marriage, family, peer relations, and belonging to social or religious groups, as well as clinician–patient empathic engagement, have a common denominator: They connect people together and serve as social support systems.

Marriage and the Family

Traditionally, the family is built on the covenant of marriage for the purpose of bringing couples together, to make a commitment to share their concerns, feelings, and experiences in health and illness and in happiness and sadness "till death do us part." Thus, marriage and the family are important social support systems that can fulfill the human needs for affiliation, intimacy, and connectedness.

The social support system originates in the family, which is regarded as a secure base for the development of the capacity for human connection from cradle to grave. The relationships inside the family between parents and children, spouses, and among other family members become a prototypical working model, or a representational model of human connections outside the family, extending to friends, peers, colleagues, and others (see Chap. 4).

Consistent with the notion that fulfillment of the need for affiliation promotes health, research has shown that the mortality rate of death for medical causes is significantly lower for married couples than it is for single, separated, divorced, and widowed individuals (Goodwin, Hunt, Key, & Samet, 1987; Ortmeyer, 1974; Wiklund, Oden, & Sanne, 1988). In addition, married people are the healthiest group, with the lowest rates of chronic disease and disabilities, followed by single, widowed, divorced, and separated people in that order (Verbrugge, 1979).

The proportion of elderly people living in an assisted living or nursing home facility was highest among those who were single or divorced and lowest among married elderly people (Verbrugge, 1979). Research also indicates that married patients with cancer live longer than their single counterparts (Goodwin et al., 1987).

Numerous studies indicate that spouses, children, other family members, and a network of friends play important roles in prevention of disease and maintenance of health. Among patients who underwent coronary angiography and had at least one blocked coronary artery, those who were not married or lacked a companion to talk to regularly were significantly more likely to die within 5 years after the procedure (Williams et al., 1992).

It has been suggested that a stable marriage and close family relationships can free a person from becoming entrapped in serious psychopathology (Valliant, 1977). Consistent with this finding, empirical data from a longitudinal study conducted in Sweden found that single people and those living alone had an elevated risk of dementia compared with married people living with their spouses (Fratiglioni, Wang, Ericsson, Maytan, & Winblad, 2000). In summarizing his family studies, Lewis (1998) pointed out that marriage and family have beneficial effects because couples often express their affects openly to one another, and family members frequently communicate empathically, in particular.

It is interesting to note that although making a connection through marriage is beneficial for both men and women, men benefit more from marriage than women do. In addition, although breaking the marital connection is harmful for both men and women, men seem to suffer more than women from separation, divorce, and spousal death (Glynn, Christenfeld, & Gerin, 1999). Gender differences in sociability, interpersonal skills, social behavior, and empathic capacity (see Chap. 10) can provide plausible explanation for the differential effects of making and breaking human connections in men and women.

It should also be noted that because breakdown of human connections resulting from disruption of marriage, separation, and divorce is detrimental to physical, mental, and social well-being (Bloom, Asher, & White, 1978; Verbrugge, 1979), fragmentation of this important social institution raises a red flag for public health in society at large. Such a trend toward the breakdown of the family places additional responsibility on healthcare providers to fill the gap and serve as part of a social support system. Having a supportive clinician who listens empathically to the patient's personal illness narrative with a "third ear" and sees patient's concerns with the "mind's eye" helps the patient sort out those experiences and is, in itself, therapeutic (see Chap. 8 for more description on the third ear and the mind's eye).

Social Support

Social support is defined as a multidimensional construct of social relationships that enhances well-being (Rodriguez & Cohen, 1998). It has also been described as the interpersonal resource people use to share understanding and emotions and to develop a sense of belonging (Wellman, 1998). A social support system provides psychological and material resources that benefit an individual's ability to cope with stress (Blumenthal et al., 1987; Cohen, 2004). A social support network of peers and friends is important for the well-being of both children and adults (Cohen, 2004; Hartup & Stevens, 1999). A substantial volume of accumulated evidence indicates the extent to which supportive social relationships are related to individuals' physical, mental, and social well-being (Berkman, 1995). The positive effect of social support on increasing longevity is as strong as the negative effects of obesity, cigarette smoking, and hypertension on life expectancy (Sapolsky, 2004). It has been reported that Vietnam veterans who benefitted from social support were significantly less likely to develop posttraumatic stress disorders (PTSD) than those with low level of support systems (Boscarino, 1995). Because of the benefits of a social support system in promoting health and well-being, Berkman (1995) suggested that social support networks, such as family, friends, and community, should be incorporated into treatment interventions. A review of 81 studies showed that social support was significantly associated with health beneficial effects on cardiovascular, endocrine, and immune systems (Uchino et al., 1996). According to Morgan (2002), a functional social support system requires empathy for more optimal health benefits.

Beneficial Outcomes of Making Connections

The association between social connection and health outcomes is fairly well established in epidemiological research (Glynn et al., 1999). Dean Ornish (1998) described the healing power in coronary artery disease of intimacy and social relationships, beyond drugs and surgery, as follows: "Our heart *is* a pump that needs to be addressed on a physical level, but our hearts are more than just pumps. A true physician is more than just a plumber, technician, or mechanic. We also have an emotional heart, a psychological heart, and a spiritual heart. Our language reflects that understanding." (p. 11).

Cohen (1988) reported that when research participants were exposed to the common cold virus, the perceived social connections served as a protective factor against the virus. Sociability and social activity were found to predict longer survival among women with breast cancer (Hislop, Waxler, Coldman, Elwood, & Kan, 1987), and it is widely recognized that one factor that contributes to improving the health of patients with cancer is social connection (Holland, 2001). The aforementioned studies support the notion that meaningful social relationships, manifested in empathic engagement, can enhance human immunocompetence to a miraculous degree.

Although the well-known Framingham Heart Study concentrated primarily on physiological and lifestyle factors in heart disease (Levy, 1999), this and several other large-scale epidemiological studies provide strong support for the proposition that human connection is beneficial to health, and a lack of it is an independent risk factor leading to illness. For example, in a study of the mortality rate caused by heart disease among Italian American residents in two adjacent towns in eastern Pennsylvania, the researchers found that the death rate among the residents of Roseto was higher than it was among the residents of Bangor (Egolf et al., 1992; Wolf, 1992). The researchers attributed this difference in mortality rates to changes in the social support system and to lower family and community cohesiveness among Italian Americans in Roseto as a result of becoming a more “Americanized” community.

Remarkable recoveries from life-threatening diseases have been linked to the power of social connections, such as an enduring marriage, family relationships, and friendships (Hirshberg & Barasch, 1995). In a study of Japanese people who emigrated to the USA, Marmot and Syme (1976) found that those immigrants who maintained their traditional family ties had a low prevalence of heart disease similar to their counterparts living in Japan, but those who became acculturated by adopting the Western lifestyle were 3–5 times more likely to suffer from heart problems.

Another epidemiological study, conducted in Alameda County near San Francisco, found that perception of a lack of social network (family, friends, religious and other group affiliations) significantly increased the mortality rate during the 9-year follow-up period (Berkman, 1995; Berkman, Leo-Summers, & Horwitz, 1992; Berkman, Glass, Brissette, & Seeman, 2000; Berkman & Syme, 1979). Using residents of the same county, researchers found that during their 5-year study, the mortality rate for breast cancer was twice as high among the women who lacked a strong social connection (Raynolds, Boyd, & Blacklow, 1994).

Investigators in the Tecumseh Community Health Study conducted in Michigan found that during a period of 10–12 years, the morbidity rates for stroke, other cardiac problems, cancer, arthritis, and lung disease increased 2–3 times during the study period as a result of participants’ weakening of social support systems (House, Robbins, & Metzner, 1982). Blazer (1982) found that people who expressed dissatisfaction with their social support system were more than three times as likely as their satisfied counterparts to die sooner of disease.

These and other epidemiological studies indicate that the risk of a physical illness doubles, at least, when a person’s social connections become weak or fragmented (Kaplan, Salonem, & Cohen, 1988; Orth-Gomer & Johnson, 1987; Schoenbach, Kaplan, Fredman, & Kleinbaum, 1986; Seeman, Berkman, & Kohout, 1993). On the basis of the findings just described, it appears that vigilance, inquiries, and advice about patients’ social connections not only can help clinicians find remedies that will improve their patients’ health status but also can confirm the importance of empathic connection between clinician and patient as a prototype of a support system that in itself is therapeutic.

Pennebaker (1990) suggested that a social support system has a potent benefit because it serves as an outlet for people to talk about their concerns and feelings. Similarly, the healing power of “opening up” during consultations with a health care provider is facilitated by the provider’s active listening and empathic interpersonal connection with the patient (see Chap. 8). Pennebaker, Kiecolt-Glaser, and Glaser (1988) reported that self-disclosure during a clinician–patient encounter can have beneficial effects on the patient’s immune system. The clinician’s empathic understanding can strengthen the clinician–patient connection that leads the patient to self-disclose at deeper levels, which in turn results in a more positive health outcome. In support of this notion, Greenberg, Watson, Elliot, and Bohart (2001) suggested that an empathic relationship can help strengthen the self and free a person from isolation and loneliness.

The precise mechanisms that promote health as an outcome of human connection are not well understood. However, research suggests that some neurobiological (e.g., endocrine and immune functions) and psychological mechanisms (e.g., stress-buffering effects, emotional support) are involved (Uchino et al., 1996). Berkman (1995) also confirmed that the immune and neuroendocrine systems are involved in the linkage of social connection and health outcomes. In a review article, Cohen (1988) concluded that health-promoting effects of social ties reflected in social integration (e.g., marriage, network of family and friends, group activities, and religious affiliation) are the combined outcomes of psychosocial factors (e.g., regulation of emotions, cognitive processes, lifestyle, and health behaviors) as well as biophysiological functions (e.g., neuroendocrine, immune, and cardiovascular systems).

Social connections are protective because of the satisfaction that results from human relationships—an important health-promoting factor. For example, Berkman (2000) emphasized that satisfaction with one's spouse, children, relatives, and friends is more important than the frequency of contact with them. In other words, the perceived *quality* of one's social connections is more important than the *quantity* of such connections in maintaining health. Similarly, Seeman and Syme (1987) showed that the size of one's social network is less important than the quality of the interpersonal relationships within that network in lowering the risk of coronary artery disease. Evidence has been accumulating that social support serves as a protective "buffer" against fear and anxiety associated with stress (Cohen, 1988; LaRocco, House, & French, 1980), which in turn could prolong the lives of patients with breast cancer (Spiegel, Bloom, Kraemer, & Gottheil, 1989).

The health-promoting aspects of human connection could be a consequence of certain patterns of psycho-physiological response involving the relaxing effect of affiliation, decreased sympathoadrenal activity, and hormonal and metabolic activities associated with human contact (Uvnas-Moberg, 1997). It appears that perceptions of interpersonal connection affect the nervous, endocrine, and immune systems (collectively called psychoneuroimmunology) and that the combined effects of the interactions of these systems contribute to either health (when connections are satisfactory) or illness (when connections, such as negative or stressful relationships are dissatisfactory).

According to the aforementioned studies, the risk of illness should be lower among people who have strong social connections in several domains, including the perception of support from their health care providers. This is important for health care providers to know, because Berkman (2000) suggested that one type of satisfactory social relationship can fill the gap for another. Thus, empathic engagement in clinician–patient encounters can serve as a substitute for, or an additional source of human connection, with all its beneficial outcomes.

Detrimental Outcomes of Breaking Connections

Making and breaking human connections obviously will have opposite consequences for health. An inadequate social network is associated with a high degree of loneliness experiences (Seeman & Syme, 1987). Lonely people obviously are deprived of the protective effects of human connections. According to House, Landis, and Umberson (1988), social isolation is a significant risk factor for morbidity and mortality comparable to obesity, sedentary lifestyle, and even smoking. A detailed discussion of loneliness and its corrosive effects on human well-being is beyond the intended scope of this book. However, because loneliness reduces the likelihood of empathic engagement, I will briefly discuss its detrimental outcomes as well as its link to empathy.

Loneliness, defined as the perception that one lacks meaningful connections with others, is a complex phenomenon that is an outcome of many factors, including the early rearing environment, insecure attachment relationships in childhood, a dysfunctional social network, a nonfacilitative living environment, social forces, and the lack of interpersonal skills (Hojat & Crandall, 1989). These same factors also contribute to a deficient capacity for empathy (see Chap. 4).

Loneliness not only impedes psychosocial well-being but also has a negative effect on physical health through the pathway of the immune system (Kennedy, Kiecolt-Glaser, & Glaser, 1988). It has been shown that human disconnectedness, experienced as loneliness, leads to a compromised immune system and thus increases a person's vulnerability to infection and disease. For example, medical students who were lonely had poor immune function, as measured by decreases in the proportions of T-helper lymphocytes and in the number and function of natural killer cells (Kiecolt-Glaser et al., 1984).

Disconnected people lack social skills and are similar to people with deficient empathic capacity. For example, in one of our recent studies with medical students (Hojat, Mangione, Kane, & Gonnella, 2005), we found that scores on the Jefferson Scale of Empathy (see Chap. 7) were negatively correlated with scores on the UCLA Loneliness Scale (Russell et al., 1980) but were positively correlated with sociability scores on the Extraversion subscale of the Zuckerman–Kuhlman Personality Questionnaire (Zuckerman, 2002).

Research shows that lonely people are likely to score low on measures of positive aspects of personality that are conducive to relationship building (e.g., self-esteem, extraversion) (Hojat, 1982a, 1982b, 1983; Shapurian & Hojat, 1985). Conversely, lonely people are likely to score high on negative aspects of personality that are detrimental to interpersonal relationships (e.g., depression, anxiety, neuroticism, tough-mindedness) (Hojat, 1982a, 1982b, 1983; Hojat, Shapurian & Mehryar, 1986; Hojat & Shapurian, 1986; Shapurian & Hojat, 1985). Disconnected people are less likely to trust others, as is indicated by a significant correlation between scores on the UCLA Loneliness Scale and scores on a scale measuring misanthropy or faith-in-people (Hojat, 1982a). The findings that lonely people lack the skills required to achieve interpersonal connections and tend not to trust others suggest that loneliness is not conducive to forming empathic relationships. In a 2015 study (Hojat, Michalec et al., 2015), we found that medical students who were recognized by their classmates as positive influencers, compared to others, scored significantly lower on the UCLA Loneliness Scale, but scored higher on the JSE. In a study by Papadakis et al. (2005), it was found that impaired peer relationships during medical school could predict later disciplinary action by medical boards against physicians. Thus, capacity to connect can have a lasting effect on physicians' professional behavior.

In his book with the telling title, *The Broken Hearts: The Medical Consequences of Loneliness*, James Lynch (1977, p. 181) proposed that "the lack of human companionship, the sudden loss of love, and chronic human loneliness are significant contributors to serious disease (including cardiovascular disease) and premature death." For example, being surrounded by family or friends reduced the likelihood of premature death by half among elderly patients compared to the rate of death among those who were lonely (Penninx et al., 1997).

Another study found that living alone was an independent risk factor in recurrent major cardiac events (Case, Moss, Case, McDermott, & Eberly, 1992). However, it is reported that feeling alone is more detrimental to health than living alone (Berkman, 2000; Hojat, 1992). A growing body of evidence in epidemiologic and psychosomatic medicine suggests that disconnectedness is a significant stressor that can be a causative element in the onset or exacerbation of a large and diverse number of medical illnesses, including asthma, cancer, congestive heart failure, diabetes mellitus, infectious hepatitis, leukemia, peptic ulcer, hypertension, hyperthyroidism, and rheumatoid arthritis and in the onset of medical catastrophes, such as sudden death after bereavement (for a review, see Hojat & Vogel, 1989). The perceived distress emerging from dissatisfaction with the social network adversely affects the psychoneuroimmune system, which leads to the progression of illness and deterioration of health (Keller, Shiflett, Schleifer, & Bartlett, 1994).

A number of studies have documented that patients who are lonely, single, or lack a confidant have a higher mortality rate after a myocardial infarction (Berkman, Leo-Summers, & Horwitz, 1992; Case et al., 1992). Low levels of social resources were identified as important risk factors, independent of important medical prognostic factors, in patients medically treated for coronary artery disease (Williams et al., 1992). The harmful outcomes associated with the lack of interpersonal connections result in a reduced ability to adapt to environmental changes, which can inflict damage on the cardiovascular, metabolic, and immune systems (McEwen, 1998).

Results of a study indicated that myocardial stunning was an outcome of emotional stress resulting from the death of a family member or close friend in 47 % of the patients with stress-related cardiomyopathy (Wittstein et al., 2005). The authors suggest that exaggerated sympathetic stimulation (or "broken heart" syndrome) as a result of overwhelming emotional stress after loss of a loved one might be central to the myocardial stunning.

Windholz, Marmar, and Horowitz (1985) reported that bereaved spouses were at greater risk for deteriorating health and had a higher mortality rate. In a longitudinal study of volunteers of mammography, Fox, Hyner, and Lyle (1994) found that experiencing the death of a spouse or another close family member within the previous 2 years significantly increased the risk of breast cancer in women. To summarize, misery will knock on the door when human connection is broken in women by death of a loved one, divorce, separation, or loneliness. Empathic engagement can overhaul the misery of human disconnectedness.

Human Connections in Therapy

Human connection can generate an interpersonal dynamic that has a healing effect. For example, group therapy is a method of therapy conducted with a group of patients who often have similar problems. Support groups composed of patients or former patients who get together to discuss illness-related experiences represent another therapeutic approach. The unique elements of these types of therapies are interpersonal connection, mutual understanding, and sharing of experiences and concerns, all of which are elements of empathic engagement as well. Shamasundar (1999) postulated that participants in such groups experience relief from anxiety and distress through the process of diluting emotional states during empathic engagement that occurs while sharing experiences with others. In multiple studies, Spiegel (1990, 1994), Spiegel and Bloom (1983), and Spiegel, Bloom, and Yalom (1981) demonstrated that by providing members with social support, group therapy and support groups lead to longevity for patients with cancer. In a series of articles, Spiegel (1993, 1994, 2004) and Spiegel et al. (1989) demonstrated that the perception of belongingness associated with group membership could significantly increase the longevity of patients with metastatic breast cancer.

In one clinical study, patients with metastatic breast cancer were encouraged to express their feelings about their illness in a group (Spiegel et al., 1989). On the average, those patients lived approximately 18 months longer than did members of a control group. The researchers concluded that group support and expression of feelings can mobilize patients' vital resources more effectively. A similar phenomenon occurs during empathic clinician–patient engagement.

In a meta-analytic study, Bohart, Elliot, Greenberg, and Watson (2002) confirmed that group therapy led to slightly better patient outcomes than did individual therapy. A study with addicted physicians found that a peer-led self-help program similar to Alcoholics Anonymous (AA) was successful in treating the physicians' addiction (Galanter, Talbott, Gallegos, & Rubenstone, 1990). The authors identified three factors that contributed to the program's positive outcomes—shared beliefs, group cohesiveness, and mutual understanding—all of which are elements of empathic engagement. Development of an empathic understanding among participants in group therapy or support groups as a result of sharing common goals and experiences could be a contributing factor to changes that occur in group behavior (Shamasundar, 1999). Feelings of being understood generate connectedness that diminishes patients' feelings of loneliness and perceptions of alienation that lead to the therapeutic alliance (Book, 1991).

The phenomenon known as mass psychogenic illness often occurs at a group level among members of a network consisting of family members, friends, coworkers, and classmates who share similar experiences and concerns (Colligan & Murphy, 1982). The empathic relationship has been identified as a factor that contributes to the contagion of group psychogenic illness (Colligan & Murphy, 1982). Also, contagious yawning triggered by seeing or imagining another person's yawning has been linked to the ability to empathize with others (Platek, Critton, Myers, & Gallup, 2003; Platek, Mohamed, & Gallup, 2005). For example, after-dinner yawning that triggers others at the dinner table to yawn may be akin to mass psychogenic behavior that is analogous to interpersonal mimicry or synchronized posture elicited by empathic engagement (Boruch, 1982). The notions that yawning can increase oxygenation of the brain when needed, or can help to draw attention have not been confirmed empirically. According to Newberg and Waldman (2010), yawning evokes neural activities in the brain that are involved in social awareness and empathy. Platek et al. (2005) proposed that contagious yawning is an expression of cognitive processes involved in awareness of self and others and may be driven by the mirror neuron system (see Chap. 13). Contagious yawning could be explained as a means of nonverbal communication and part of neural network involved with social interaction and empathy.

The Gift of Being Present

The human drive for connectedness increases during times of illness-related distress because illness often makes patients feel disconnected (Platt & Keller, 1994). Therefore, the availability of social support for patients is crucially important. As Morgan (2002) indicated, social support is somewhat synonymous with treatment in the context of health care. Being present when a person is in need of help is, in itself, a social support factor and is a therapeutic remedy described as the "gift of presence" (Nicholas, 2002). The clinician's presence is especially supportive when an empathic relationship is formed between clinician and patient.

The presence of a supportive ally, such as an empathic health care provider, serves as a buffer against the cardiovascular stress response (Christenfeld & Gerin, 2000). In particular, the presence of a woman who provides social support has been found to be more significant than the social support provided by a man (Christenfeld & Gerin, 2000). In an experiment on the influence of social support provided by men and women, study participants were assigned to deliver a short speech on euthanasia (Glynn et al., 1999). The researchers found that when the support was provided by women, who were in the audience and nodding in agreement, the magnitude of the systolic blood pressure was reduced in both male and female speakers. However, a cardiovascular effect of that magnitude was not observed in the speakers when men in the audience nodded in agreement. From the results of this experiment, the researchers concluded that the gift of the presence of supportive individuals, especially supportive women, would probably lead to fewer heart conditions (Glynn et al., 1999). (See Chap. 10 for a discussion of gender differences in medical practice.) These findings also suggest the important role that nurses (most of whom have traditionally been women) often play in providing care and support to the patients (e.g., the concept of caring versus curing described in Chap. 8).

The Empathic Clinician–Patient Relationship as the Epitome of Human Connection

The term "social support" applies to a broad range of conceptualizations of social network structures and their health-promoting functions (Blumenthal et al., 1987; Cohen & Matthews, 1987). In that regard, the clinician–patient relationship can be conceptualized as a special kind of social support system. Cohen (2004) suggested that social support can provide three types of resources: (a) instrumental, involving the provision of material aids; (b) emotional, involving the expression of empathy, caring, and reassurance; and (c) informational, involving the provision of relevant information to help the individual understand the problem better and cope with difficulties. An empathic clinician–patient relationship provides all of the aforementioned resources, and research shows that empathic understanding of pain and suffering enhances cooperative relationships (Goubert et al., 2005).

The patient's perception of the clinician's support is a complex phenomenon that is a function of the nature of the patient's help-seeking behavior, desire for affiliation, and the clinician's feedback loop through empathic communication. When a trusting relationship is established and is further reinforced by empathic engagement, constraints in the relationship will diminish and a heart-to-heart human communication will prevail (see Chap. 11). This kind of human connection, characterized by full trust, can be formed between lovers as well as between clinicians and their patients.

The relevance and importance of the notion of social support in clinician–patient relationships becomes more evident, considering that patients exhibit an increased desire for affiliation that is naturally expected when people are in distress (Taylor, Klein, Gruenewald, Gurung, & Fernandes-Taylor, 2003). In his research, Stanley Schachter (1959) demonstrated that stress increases our desire to affiliate. In the experiment, participants in a high-stress condition (they were told they would receive painful shocks) were twice as likely as other participants to wait in the company of others than to wait alone to participate in the experiment. Moreover, it has been shown that the presence of others can reduce the experience of pain and suffering (Romano, Jensen, Turner, Good, & Hops, 2000).

One plausible explanation is that human connectedness has a fear-reducing effect that contributes to positive health outcomes (House et al., 1988). Accordingly, it has been suggested that a positive encounter between a clinician and a patient, in itself, has a potential healing power (Novack, 1987; Spiro, 1986). Because of this powerful impact, Balint (1957) described clinicians as the most frequently used therapeutic agents in the history of medicine.

The positive influence of clinician–patient encounters on patient outcomes has been called "Factor X," an unknown factor in healing human suffering (White, 1991). The patient's social support system in general and the nature and quality of the clinician–patient relationship in particular are among the components of the human factor in health and illness. In the process of interpersonal connection, empathy has a mediating role in improving the strength of the connections by increasing a sense of common identity and reducing prejudice (Stephan & Finlay, 1999). Thus, empathy paves the road to the interpersonal connection between clinicians and patients, which is a special kind of social support system, with all of its beneficial healing powers.

Recapitulation

The human tendency to seek connections has an evolutionary root and a survival advantage. Abundant evidence indicates that satisfying the need for affiliation and human connectedness through marriage, family, peers, friends, community, and other social support networks leads to physical, mental, and social well-being. Conversely, breaking social connections leads to loneliness and its detrimental health outcomes. The opportunity for empathic engagement is one underlying reason for the health-promoting outcomes of human connections. Because the drive for human connection increases during times of distress and illness, the presence of an empathic clinician is a gift for the patient that epitomizes the human connection.

Chapter 3
An Evolutionary Perspective, Sociophysiology, and Heritability

Empathy can lead to the evolution of fairness.
—(Karen Page & Martin Novak, 2002, p. 1101)

Abstract

- For a better grasp of empathy, we need to understand its evolutionary roots and its sociophysiological functions.
- During the course of evolution, human beings have been endowed with an innate capacity to express and understand emotions from nonverbal cues, which contributed to survival and is conceptualized as primitive empathy.
- Evidence showing infant's reactive crying, facial mimicry, physiological synchronicity in interpersonal interactions, and universal expression of emotions indicate that aspects of interpersonal behaviors cannot be attributed only to social learning.
- Twin studies suggest that heritability is also a significant component of empathy more likely in emotional empathy than cognitive empathy.

Introduction

In Chap. 2, I described human beings as social creatures that evolved to be connected with other human beings because social groupings provided increased defense against predators (Plutchik, 1987). Empathic engagement, particularly at the time of distress, was viewed in that chapter as a special kind of social support system. In this chapter, I discuss empathy as having an evolutionary root with a sociophysiological function and a heritability component. Long before they developed

M. Hojat, *Clinical Empathy*, https://doi.org/10.1007/978-3-031-87413-0_3

the capacity for verbal communication and invented language, our ancestors could relay their feelings, intentions, and expectations by nonverbal means, such as facial expressions, imitation, motor mimicry, and bodily postures. Nonverbal empathic communication has a longer history in the course of human evolution than does verbal communication. Thus, if the brain has areas for verbal communication and language (e.g., Broca's and Wernicke's areas), it must have areas for nonverbal communication and understanding of emotions. Because empathy implies understanding of feelings, emotions, and inner experiences, any means of communicating these concepts would be relevant to studies on the capacity for empathy.

Empathic exchanges, according to Buck and Ginsburg (1997a, p. 481), involve "a genetically based, spontaneous communication process that is fundamental to all interpersonal interactions and that includes innate sending and receiving mechanisms (visual, auditory, or chemical displays, and pre-attunements to such displays); empathy involves communicative genes." If one assumes that empathy is based on an *innate* mechanism and involves "communicative genes," then it must have an evolutionary root, a neuroanatomical structure, and a sociophysiological function.

An Evolutionary Perspective

Evolution lays out the historical path along which humankind has traveled to reach the present point. To understand human behavior, we must understand its evolution. According to the notion of evolution espoused by Charles Darwin (1965, 1981) human beings have evolved during a long evolutionary history of struggle for existence that resulted in the survival of the fittest. During that long history, emotions and their expressions and social cognition evolved for their adaptive advantages in dealing with the fundamental task of survival (Ekman, 1992).

Allport (1924) suggested that the expression of emotion originated from experiences *common* to all human beings. Similarly, Ekman (1992) proposed that our cognitive appraisal of situations that evoke emotions (e.g., those that threaten our survival) is primarily determined by our ancestral past. Carl Gustav Jung (1964) proposed the notion of "collective unconscious" as a transpersonal residue of experiences inherited from one generation to the next. These views imply the existence of a common evolutionary root in the expression of emotion and in cognitive appraisal that are vehicles of empathic communication.

In her thought-provoking article on the biological perspective of empathy, Leslie Brothers (1989) proposed that the capacity for empathy improves fitness for survival. The capacities our ancestors developed to read emotions from nonverbal clues (e.g., facial expression, bodily movement, tone of voice) provided a means of distinguishing foes from friends and danger from safety. The ability to understand social signals conveyed by facial expressions and bodily movements provides a competitive advantage over adversaries and protects against being deceived by them (Brothers, 1989).

Obviously, people who were armed with the capacity to understand other people's states of mind could escape danger more easily than others who lacked that skill; thus, they were more fit for survival. People who failed to develop the capacity for empathy because of genetic predisposition, inappropriate psychosocial experiences, a nonfacilitative rearing environment, or arrested neurological development were less likely to survive. Natural selection, therefore, favored empathy (Humphrey, 1983; Ridley & Dawkins, 1981). Parallel to sensitivity in detecting social signals, human beings developed the skills of deception and manipulation to conceal their emotions and intentions from predators. Studying these evolutionary adapted skills can enhance our understanding of empathy in interpersonal exchanges.

Evolutionary adaptation is linked not only to the physiological activities but also to such social behaviors as mate selection (Buss, 2003), reproductive strategies (Buss, 1995; Buss & Schmitt, 1993), parental investment (Trivers, 1972) (see Chap. 10), and prosocial behavior, altruism, and empathy (Buck & Ginsburg, 1997a; Ridley & Dawkins, 1981). During the history of human evolution, capacities have gradually evolved to achieve the ultimate purpose of life—survival or the preservation of genes. Dawkins (1999) proposed that the engine of the survival machine is driven by the "selfish gene," which determines whether to protect, fight, or flee to increase the probability of survival. All of these actions require understanding of others' intentions. However, Buck and Ginsburg (1997b, p. 19) argued that "some genes are selfish, and function to support the survival of the individual organism, but other genes are social functioning to support the survival of species."

Buck and Ginsburg's notion was supported by Hamilton (1964) who, in discussing the evolutionary concept of exclusive fitness, proposed that human beings are not programmed exclusively and egoistically to protect their own individual genes but are programmed inclusively and altruistically to protect the survival of others who share similar characteristics. The capacity for empathy evolved to serve that purpose.

In support of this notion, de Quervain et al. (2004) used positron emission tomography (PET) to study the neural basis of *the social brain* with regard to intrinsic rewards for prosocial behaviors (e.g., cooperation and observing social norms) and punishment for violating them. The researchers found that people derive intrinsic satisfaction from punishing norm violators, which suggests that such altruistic punishment for the sake of the group's survival has been a decisive force in the evolution of human social behavior. A reward-related region of the brain, the dorsal striatum, has been implicated in the processing of rewards that accrue for socially desirable behavior (de Quervain et al., 2004), including inclination for empathic engagement.

The idea of a "non-selfish" gene that protects the survival of the group suggests that the unit of observation for the purpose of survival may be the group of individuals with common characteristics, rather than the individual. Perhaps this is a reason why empathic engagement becomes stronger with similar rather than dissimilar individuals. The chance of group survival increases with prosocial and altruistically motivated behaviors. The evolutionary basis of empathy, according to Hoffman

(1978), can be linked to altruistic behavior in helping others to survive, sometimes even at a cost to the self.

Altruistic behaviors have puzzled evolutionary scholars who believe that the purpose of the struggle for existence is preservation of the individual's genes. However, the notion of a "non-selfish" gene can explain the underlying motivation for altruism. For example, sacrificing one's own life for the good of the country (patriotic behavior) was dramatically illustrated by Japan's kamikaze pilots during World War II. Political suicidal missions can also be explained by the concept of a "non-selfish" gene aiming at group rather than individual survival. Empathy may have a role in such self-sacrificing behaviors, rooted in the understanding of pain and suffering of others who share some common features.

The issue of whether unconscious (or conscious) efforts to survive are selfishly and egoistically directed toward the preservation of individual genes or are selflessly and altruistically directed toward maintaining the group's genes has been hotly debated by evolutionary scholars. Although the details of such a debate are beyond the intended scope of this book, we should always remember that we are the product of millions of years of evolutionary adaptation for the purpose of either individual or group survival. Empathy is a by-product of this evolutionary adaptation.

Nonverbal Means of Empathic Communication

Through the process of evolution, the human brain has evolved to send and receive messages through nonverbal cues, such as facial expressions, motor mimicry, bodily gestures, change of facial skin color, sweating, and trembling, as well as through vocal sounds, such as voice pitch, crying, and laughter; thus, happiness, friendliness, and well-intended behaviors could be distinguished from sadness, disagreement, and hostile intent (Adolphs, Tranel, Damasio, & Damasio, 1994; Siegel, 1999). As a result of this evolutionary process, according to Darwin (1965), basic affects such as happiness, sadness, anger, fear, and disgust, and the nonverbal means of expressing them can be understood and communicated easily regardless of language or cultural barriers.

The ability to send and receive communicative signals in interpersonal encounters is a means of survival. In interpersonal behavior, described by Westerman (2005, p. 22) as "a person's contributions to doing something with other people," expression of emotions plays a major role. The ability to understand other people's emotions from external signals, such as facial expressions and bodily gestures, also is a core ingredient in inferring others' inner feelings and intentions, thus facilitating forming an empathic relationship (Ekman & Friesen, 1974; Zahn-Waxler, Robinson, & Emde, 1992). Empathy can be conveyed through lexical as well as kinetic means of communication (Mayerson, 1976). It has been suggested that behavioral or nonverbal cues, because of difficulty to conceal them, may be even more effective in conveying emotional messages than lexical or verbal communication which can be easily faked (Bayes, 1972). Nonverbal means of communication, according to Mehrabian (1972), include observable actions such as facial expressions; emotional expressions; hand and arm gestures; postures; bodily positions; various movements of the body, head, hand, and legs; eye contact and gaze aversion; as well as subtle aspects of speech, such as speech errors, slip of the tongue, pauses, long silence, speech rate, and deliberate choice of words. Better understanding of these nonverbal cues in interpersonal or clinical encounters can enhance empathic engagement.

Facial Expression, Mimicry, Imitation, and Bodily Posture

The human face presents fascinating and meaningful clues about a person's physical and mental status. The facial muscles, controlled by the central nervous system, have the unique ability to produce a wide variety of expressions (Dawson, 1994; Siegel, 1999). Because facial expressions and bodily postures are the external manifestation of the internal world, they facilitate empathic communication, especially in clinician–patient encounters. For example, the degree of rapport between clinician and patient, according to Goldstein and Michaels (1985, p. 107), is correlated with the occurrence of "shared posture." Observing facial expression unconsciously triggers similar expression (and muscle tone measured by electromyography) in the observer (Dimberg, Thunberg, & Elmehed, 2000) (See "mirror neuron system" in Chap. 13 describing a similar phenomenon).

Experimental evidence suggests that the human brain is designed to be attentive to emotional signals emitted via facial expressions. For example, studying the "still-face" procedure, Tronick, Als, Adamson, Wise, and Brazelton (1978) found that young children become distressed and withdrawn when their mothers assume an emotionless face, rather than revealing their emotions (see Chap. 4). Evidence also indicates that infants can imitate human facial gestures, such as sticking out the tongue, protruding the lips, and opening the mouth (Meltzoff & Moore, 1977, 1983). Also, emotional expressions can be mimicked (Field, Woodson, Greenberg, & Cohen, 1982; Kugiumutzakis, 1998). Thus, mimicry is a nonverbal means of communicating experiences, which occurs when one observes another person's expression and responds with a similar motor representation (Hess, Blairy, & Phillippot, 1999). For example, we all tend to assume the postural strains of athletes or dancers during moments when we are absorbed in observing their actions (Davis, 1985). Furthermore, most of us have either experienced or observed that while spoon-feeding their infants, parents often open their own mouth *as if* they are spoon-feeding themselves! These examples suggest that mimicry is a nondeliberate imitation that serves the function of communication.

Mimicry and the ability to imitate facial gestures and to understand facial expressions have been conceptualized as a type of primitive empathy, rooted in the history of human evolution (Bavelas, Black, Lemery, & Mullett, 1986). Mimicry and imitation behaviors can be explained by the principle of ideomotor action postulated by William James (1890) and the perception-action coupling proposed by Preston and deWaal (2002) (see Chap. 13), suggesting that observing another person's behavior increases a tendency in the observer to behave similarly.

Because mimicry and its associated somatosensory outcomes can help us to understand another person's experiences (Wicker et al., 2003), their relevance to empathy is evident (Chartrand & Bargh, 1999). According to Davis (1985), appraising the concept of mimicry is important when analyzing the components of empathy. Mimicry and facial expression generate changes in the autonomic nervous system associated with feelings that correspond to the facial expression (Decety & Jackson, 2004). Basch (1983) proposed that unconscious, automatic imitation of another person's facial expressions (facial mimicry) and bodily gestures (motor mimicry) generates an automatic and synchronized response in the observer that leads to better understanding of experiences identical to those experienced by the observed individual.

Carr, Iacoboni, Dubeau, Mazziotta, and Lenzi (2003) proposed that individuals with a high degree of empathy compared with others exhibit more unconscious mimicry of other people's facial expressions and bodily postures. Chartrand and Bargh (1999) described this phenomenon as the "chameleon effect"—the mere perception of another person's behavior can automatically increase the likelihood of imitating the perceived behavior. Lakin, Jefferis, Cheng, and Chartland (2003) reported that the chameleon effect is a kind of social glue that represents the evolutionary significance of nonconscious mimicry and serves to foster interpersonal relationships. Chartrand and Bargh suggested that the chameleon effect is the mechanism behind motor mimicry that satisfies the human need for connection and affiliation. Furthermore, they reported that individuals with high empathy scores on the Interpersonal Reactivity Index (Davis, 1983) (see Chap. 5) exhibited the chameleon effect to a greater degree than others with low empathy scores. Chartrand and Bargh (1999) reported that a number of researchers have conceptualized mimicry in terms of empathy.

Imitation of another person's behavior is a different type of mimicry that generates a tendency to repeat an observed action (Meltzoff & Prinz, 2002). Imitation of an action implies striving to achieve the goal of that action (Baldwin & Baird, 2001). This indicates that in observing a behavior, either positive or negative, the underlying intention is also inferred, which is perhaps more important in prompting imitative behavior. This explains why role models in health professions education and practice are important motivators of professional behavior. In his theory of violence, Berkowitz (1984) postulated that violence shown in public media contributes to imitating aggressive and criminal behaviors, which can be explained by the principle of ideomotor action (James, 1890) and the perception-action model (Preston & deWaal, 2002) (see Chap. 13).

One indicator of recognizing emotions early in life is the observation that newly born infants will cry in response to the sound of another infant's cry (Sagi & Hoffman, 1976; Simner, 1971). This reactive crying does not occur in response to either a loud sound or a vocal sound that lacks the affective components of the other infant's cry, or even to the recorded crying of the newborn infant itself. According to Hoffman (1978), the human infant's reactive crying is based on a built-in mechanism that is an early precursor of empathic understanding.

Sociophysiology

The link between human physiology and social interaction has attracted the attention of scholars for a long time. For example, more than six decades ago, Boyd and DiMascio (1957) studied the concept of the "sociophysiology" of social behavior and found a relationship between emotions expressed in clinical interviews and autonomic physiologic responses, such as heart rate, skin resistance, and facial temperature. The notion of "interpersonal physiology" in clinician–patient interactions was first introduced in a study by DiMascio, Boyd, and Greenblatt (1957), who found that patients' and therapists' heart rates and skin temperatures were synchronized during clinical interviews. Goldstein and Michaels (1985, p. 68) reported that synchronization typically occurs between individuals who have "good rapport" with one another. Accuracy in perception of negative emotions was found to be a function of physiological synchrony between the perceiver and the target person (Levenson & Ruef, 1992). It is suggested that empathy can emerge as a result of the autonomic nervous system, which tends to simulate another person's physiological state (Ax, 1964). In other words, an empathic engagement reflected in good interpersonal rapport facilitates physiological synchronization during clinical interviews.

In another early experiment, investigators noticed that the physiological responses of healthy young soldiers were different when interacting with an officer (who was a psychiatrist) compared with a person who was an enlisted man (Reiser, Reeves, & Armington, 1955). The researchers concluded that the sociophysiology of the relationship in clinician–patient encounters could be a function of the client's view regarding the care provider's prestige or status (Reiser et al., 1955). In their study, Chartrand and Bargh (1999) found that greater time in contact with elderly people was associated with poorer memory and more forgetfulness, indicating that even mental status of others can be adapted by frequent observations.

In a review article, Adler (2002) proposed that the experience of an empathic relationship in clinical encounters reduces the secretion of stress hormones and concluded that "the immediate effect of a caring relationship flows from the physiologic consequences of feeling cared about, because the neurobiology of such a relationship promotes an endocrine response pattern that favors homeostasis and is the antithesis of the fight–flight response" (p. 878).

A physiological feedback loop is set in motion during clinical interviews that is a reflection of mutual understanding. Observing emotion in another person has been reported to result in a similar display of emotion in the observer (Lanzetta & Englis, 1989). Similarly, emotional distress in one person can automatically trigger similar distress in another person when the two are interacting (Eisenberg, 1989). A study of physiological changes, such as heart rate, during interpersonal interactions revealed that a clinician's interpersonal style (e.g., praising or criticizing) can influence the patient's physiological reaction (Malno, Boag, & Smith, 1957). For example, these investigators observed that patients' heart rates rose significantly when the clinician had had a "bad" day. The results of a study indicate that physiological synchronicity (e.g., in heart rate and muscle activity) between people can lead to more accurate perceptions of their feelings (Decety & Jackson, 2006).

Maurer and Tindall (1983) observed that patients' perceptions of the therapist's empathic understanding increased when therapist's arm and leg positions were congruent (mirror image) of the patients. Mimicry, imitation, and body posture synchronization serve as an adaptive function to facilitate interpersonal interaction (Chartrand & Bargh, 1999). Schaflen (1964) observed that the more people in group share similar viewpoints, the more they tend to mimic one another's postures. It is also reported that patients perceive more empathic engagement when the clinicians mimicked their body posture; the effect is reciprocal if the clinician and client are acquainted with each other (La France, 1979). It has also been observed that students' ratings of their teacher's involvement in class activities improved when there was more postural synchronicity between students and their teacher (La France, 1982).

Kaplan and Bloom (1960, p. 133) proposed the idea that the empathic process involves not only placing oneself in another person's "psychological" shoes but also placing oneself in that person's "physiological" shoes. However, Szalita (1976, p. 145) suggested that in empathic engagement with patients, "it is good to be able to put yourself into someone else's shoes, but you have to remember that you don't wear them." In a study of couples examined by using functional magnetic resonance imaging (fMRI), Singer et al. (2004) found that couples who scored higher on the Empathy Scale (Hogan, 1969) (see Chap. 5) and the Empathic Concern Scale of the Interpersonal Reactivity Index (Davis, 1983) (see Chap. 5) showed more intense brain activity when they observed their partner experiencing pain.

These findings suggest that empathic resonance involves shared physiological-neurological activities between people who are interacting. The notion of shared physiology between interacting people is intriguing (Ax, 1964; Kaplan & Bloom, 1960; Levenson & Ruef, 1992), and it opens up a window for studying the "physiological dance" that takes place in empathic engagement. More research is needed to investigate the underlying mechanisms involved in the psycho-socio-physiology of social behavior and the relevance of shared physiologic responses to empathic understanding and sympathetic feelings (see Chap. 13).

Heritability

Mumford (1967) regarded empathy as a genetically determined quality that can be enhanced or inhibited by positive or negative life experiences, respectively (cited in Szalita, 1976). A standard approach to research on heritability is the "twin study." In this research design, genetically identical or monozygotic (MZ) twins (who share 100% common genes) are compared with fraternal or dizygotic (DZ) twins (who share approximately 50% of their genes). Heritability can be determined with regard to a particular trait when MZ twins are more highly correlated than DZ twins on the trait, assuming a similar rearing environment. In a sample of 278 MZ and 378 DZ twins, strong genetic influences were found in 78% of the twins younger than 11 years of age and in 66% of those aged 11 years or older concerning the heritability of social cognitive skills relevant to empathy (Scourfield, Martin, Lewis, & McGuffin, 1999).

In a study involving 114 MZ and 116 DZ twins, the researchers found a significant heritability component of 72% on a derived index of empathic concern (Matthews et al., 1981). In yet another study involving 94 MZ and 90 DZ twins, the investigators found modest evidence of heritability in empathy (Zahn-Waxler et al., 1992). In another study of 573 adult twin pairs of both sexes, empathy, as measured by the Emotional Empathy Scale (Mehrabian & Epstein, 1972) (see Chap. 5), had a relatively broad heritability estimate of 68% (Rushton et al., 1986). In a study of 174 pairs of MZ twins and 148 pairs of DZ twins, it was found that 42% of prosocial behavior was due to the twins' genes, 23% to twins' shared environment, and the remaining to the twins' non-shared environment (Rushton, 2004).

In a recently reported ongoing longitudinal study, initiated in 1998 (Stern, Bailey, Castello, ... Allen, 2024), a sample of 184 seventh and eighth grade students in the USA were followed up from age of 13 into parenting age for almost 25 years. Assessments of mother–child empathic care, attachment quality, and frequent evaluations of supportive behavior observed in empathic responses to peer and own children (in female participants who had children [$n = 70$]) predict capacity to provide similar empathic care to peer, friends, and offspring. Thus, supporting the notion of transmission of empathy across three generations; and possibility of heritability of empathic capacity (Stern, Castello, Kansky,... Allen, 2021).

Knafo, Zahn-Waxler, Van Hule, Robinson, and Rhee (2008) studied the genetic and environmental influences on empathy among 409 young twins and noticed increased contribution of genes, but decreased effects of environment with age. The results of another study (Davis, Luce, & Kraus, 1994) using the Interpersonal Reactivity Index (Davis, 1983) (see Chap. 5) showed evidence of significant heritability for the subscales of Empathic Concern and Personal Distress (indicators of emotional empathy of the Interpersonal Reactivity Index, (Davis, 1983) but not for the Perspective Taking subscale (an indicator of cognitive empathy of the Interpersonal Reactivity Index). Studying genetic variations in empathy, Kazmierczak, Rybicka & Syty (2024) reported that the effects of genes were stronger for prediction of emotional empathy (e.g., empathic concern and personal distress) than cognitive empathy (e.g., perspective taking). These findings generally suggest that indicators of the so-called emotional empathy, which is more akin to sympathy, seem to have a higher heritability component than the cognitive empathy. This prediction of more heritability component in emotional empathy (synonymous to sympathy, see Chaps. 1 and 6) than cognitive empathy was also confirmed in a review and meta-analytic study by Abramson, Uzefovsky, Toccaceli et al. (2020).

Recapitulation

In this chapter, I presented an evolutionary perspective on precursors of empathy through nonverbal behavior such as facial mimicry, imitation, and body posture. Data from twin studies were also presented to suggest that the capacity for empathy could be heritable to some extent (more in emotional than cognitive empathy). Research findings on the sociophysiology of interpersonal behavior, linking empathy to unconscious mimicry, imitation, and postural synchronicity, were discussed to show that an empathic relationship in general, and empathic engagement in patient care in particular, resemble a synchronized dance between the involved parties which is orchestrated by sociophysiological factors to harmonize the dynamic exchanges and optimize interpersonal communication.

Chapter 4
Psychodynamics and Development

Love, and lack of it, changes the young brain forever.

—(Thomas Lewis, Fari Amini, & Richard Lannon, 2000, p. 89)

The key to the heaven is under mother's footsteps.

—(A popular Persian saying)

The hand that rocks the cradle rules the world.

—(A popular cliché)

Abstract

- Empathy is nurtured in a facilitative early rearing environment, particularly in relation to the quality of a child's relationship with the mother or primary caregiver.
- Evidence suggests that nature has endowed the mother with the innate ability to be the most important participant in the development of a child's capacity for empathy; i.e., the newborn's preference for its mother's voice; maternal investment in child-rearing, lactation and breast-feeding; and attachment relationships.
- Experimental findings obtained by using the "still-face" and "visual cliff" paradigms indicate that infants can understand and react to their primary caregiver's emotional state.
- The foundation for a child's mental representation (internal working models) of the world is the early relationship with the mother that becomes an influential force in the regulation of emotions and empathic behavior throughout life.
- Associations are discussed between empathy and facial imitation and mimicry in childhood, as well as theory of mind.
- Some developmental roots are described to better understand the factors that foster or arrest the capacity for empathy in childhood.

M. Hojat, *Clinical Empathy*, https://doi.org/10.1007/978-3-031-87413-0_4

Introduction

The search for the roots of the capacity for empathy is of paramount importance in understanding the course or the arrest of its development. In this chapter, I describe some of the factors that contribute to the nourishment of empathy. The central notion emphasized throughout the chapter is that empathy is nurtured in the early rearing environment in relation to the quality of the early attachment relationship with a primary caregiver (Henderson, 1974; Schaflen, 1964).

The Nature–Nurture Debate

The issue of whether nature or nurturing contributes more to prosocial behavior has been debated for a long time. Proponents of nature place great emphasis on the notion that genetic makeup has an undeniable role in the development of human behavior. The developments in the Human Genome Project have provided more fuel in support of their argument (Collins, 1999).

However, proponents of nurture use Watsonian and Skinnerian approaches to classical conditioning and operant learning as evidence that human behavior can be molded according to the principles of behavior modification, and they believe that environmental and experiential factors have a more prominent role than genes do in the development of prosocial or antisocial behavior. The often-cited statement made by John Brutus Watson (1924, p. 82), the founder of the school of behaviorism in psychology, supports the nurture notion:

> Give me a dozen healthy infants, well formed, and my own special world to bring them up, and I will guarantee to take any one at random and train him to become any type of specialist I might select—doctor, lawyer, artist, merchant-chief, and yes, even beggar and thief, regardless of his talents, penchants, tendencies, abilities, vocations, and race of his ancestors.

Although some experts still believe that nurturing matters more than nature does in determining human behavior (Hoover, 2000), most scholars nowadays are of the opinion that it is the interaction of nature and nurturing that contributes to the development of social behavior. Human beings are born with a potential for "engageability," which is triggered to a certain degree by, and will develop to a certain extent depending on, environmental and experiential factors (Neubauer & Neubauer, 1990).

Although many genetics-oriented scientists were excited about the discoveries of the Human Genome Project (Collins, 1999), determining the basis of human behavior proved to be a more complicated matter than simply mapping the human genome. For example, findings in a study of 44,788 sets of twins indicated that environmental and lifestyle factors as well as inherited genes make significant contributions to the development of different types of cancers (Lichtenstein et al., 2000). Abundant research evidence has accumulated in support of the proposition that the family environment and parental care play an important role in the development of adults' prosocial behavior, including the propensity for empathic relationships.

The Family Environment

The family is the oldest and the most important social institution in the history of human civilization. It is "the seedbed of commitment, love, character, and social as well as personal responsibility" (Ashcroft & Straus, 1993, p. 1). The United Nations Convention on the Rights of the Child, adopted unanimously by the General Assembly, recognized that for full and harmonious development, children must grow up in a facilitative family environment in an atmosphere of happiness and love provided by their parents (Grant, 1991; Hojat, 1993, 1997). The calming experience of feeling felt and the echoes of love spring to life in the family first, then expand to embrace a broader social network, even the entire human race (Eibel-Eibesfeldt, 1979).

The family environment early in life not only shapes the quality of later interpersonal relationships (Fonagy, 2001) but also sows the seed for the growth of the capacity for empathic engagement. The way we are brought up in the early periods of our lives influences "all our later relationships, all our later days" (Neubauer & Neubauer, 1990, p. 81). The child whose emotional needs are unmet or denied in the family will not develop a sense of trust, a problem that will have a lasting negative influence on later social relationships (Rempel, Holmes, & Zanna, 1985). The capacity for empathy also can be negatively influenced by unmet emotional needs in the family (Eisenberg & Strayer, 1987; Perry et al., 2001) because, as Guzzetta (1976) proposed, empathy springs from interpersonal relationships within the family. Development of empathy, according to Barnett (1987), occurs in a family environment in which parental warmth and responsiveness satisfy the child's emotional needs and provide opportunities for the child to observe and experience warm interpersonal responses in a variety of situations.

The family's importance in the development of the capacity for empathy has led to health care researchers' apt description of the clinician's family of origin as the bedrock for the development of interpersonal skills in patient care (Farber, Novack, & O'Brien, 1997; Mengel, 1987).

The Parents

Empathy has a rich and complex developmental history (Shapiro, 1974). It arises from early sensory and tactile communication between mother and child (Schwaber, 1981). In a review of the literature on parental behavior that contributes to the development of empathy in children, Mehrabian, Young, and Sato (1988) concluded that the parents of children with a strong capacity for empathy were more verbally explicit about their feelings, offered more emotional support, and were more tolerant. Early interactions with parents, according to Roe (1957), determine the child's future vocational choice in people-oriented versus other occupations.

Human beings differ from all other animals in the length of their dependency on a caregiver for survival and protection. This period of dependency is crucial for neurological development (e.g., the process of myelination) (Davison & Peters, 1970) and social growth. The critical period of susceptibility opens a window of opportunity during which activation of specific brain functions is essential for ongoing development of different areas of the brain related to social behavior (Siegel, 1999). That window will close after a certain period of time.

The importance of the critical period of neurological development was first noticed by Hubel and Wiesel who found that suturing one eye closed in kittens during the first few weeks after birth caused a sharp decline in the number of cells in the visual cortex (Hubel, 1967; Hubel & Wiesel, 1963). The investigators found that up to 5 years after the eye was opened, only a minimal amount of the visual cortex had recovered (Hubel & Wiesel, 1970). Hubel (1967) noticed that when kittens were not exposed to horizontal lines during a certain critical period of development, their visual cortex was unable to process horizontal input later in life.

Abundant evidence supports the existence of a sensitive period of neurological development. For example, baby chimpanzees reared in darkness during that sensitive period will be blind for the rest of their lives (Chow, Riesen, & Newell, 1957). MacLean (1967) found that if certain neural circuits were not formed during a crucially receptive period in the brain's development, the circuits were unlikely to ever be fully developed. The assumption is that the repeated activation of specific neuronal pathways as a result of early experiences reinforces the strength of connections between groups of neurons. The neurons that create interconnections through early experiences, according to Hebbian neuron cell assembly theory (Hebb, 1946; Keysers & Perrett, 2004), fire together later in life, so to speak, because "neurons that fire together wire together" (see Chap. 13).

In addition to physical stimulation, emotionally rich interactions in early life contribute to neurological development. One early experiment on the importance of early life experiences to human survival was conducted in the thirteenth century by Emperor Frederick II who wanted to know what language children would speak if no one talked to them. Thus, "he bade foster mothers and nurses to suckle the children, to bathe and wash them, but in no way to prattle with them. ... But he labored in vain, because the children died" (Ross & McLaughlin, 1949, pp. 366–367).

Supportive parenting fosters capacity for empathy (Soenens, Duriez, Vansteenkiste, & Goossens, 2007) because in addition to passing along genetic predisposition, supportive parents serve as the model of empathic understanding for their children (Chase-Lansdale, Wakschlag, & Brooks-Gunn, 1995; Krevans & Gibbs, 1996). Parental warmth has been hypothesized to promote children's capacity for empathy and prosocial behavior (Hoffman, 1982; Janssens & Gerris, 1992). Children of empathic parents reacted vicariously to others' negative emotions (Robinson, Zahn-Waxler, & Emde, 1994; Trommsdorff, 1995). Cross-sectional and longitudinal research, using structural equation modeling, has confirmed that parents' expression of positive emotions is the mechanism that mediates a causal relationship between parental warmth and children's empathic capacity (Zhou et al., 2002). On the contrary, Zahn-Waxler and Radke-Yarrow (1990) suggested that family risk factors such as parental depression, marital discord, and parental maltreatment, particularly in the first two years of life, could contribute to the arrest of empathy development in children and can be manifested in the adults' deficit in interpersonal relationships.

The Hand that Sows the Seeds

Parents usually provide the love and affection their children need for healthy development. Research has shown that a supportive relationship with both parents is predictive of high empathy scores as well as social sensitivity in children (Adams, Jones, Schvaneveldt, & Jenson, 1982). However, although both parents must share childcare responsibilities for their children to achieve ideal social development, some findings suggest that the mother's role may be more crucial than that of any other caregiver, including the father.

For example, in a study of Harvard University graduates who were followed up for 35 years, Russek and Schwartz (1997) found that 91 % of the graduates who retrospectively perceived the lack of a warm and friendly relationship with their mother had serious health problems in midlife (e.g., coronary artery disease, high blood pressure, alcoholism) compared with 45 % of the graduates who retrospectively perceived their relationship with their mother as having been warm and friendly. The corresponding figures for their perceived relationship with their father were 82 % and 50 %, respectively. Consistent with these findings, we found that medical students who perceived a satisfactory childhood relationship with their mother rated their general health more positively and reported more resilience in appraising stressful life events (Hojat, 1996).

Individuals' perceptions of their early relationships with parents generally are positively associated with personality attributes that are conducive to interpersonal relationships (Hojat, Borenstein, & Shapurian, 1990). In our study of 422 medical students, we examined the differential effects of satisfactory early relationships with the mother and father and found that higher scores on the Jefferson Scale of Empathy (see Chap. 7) were significantly associated with students' retrospective reports concerning the level of satisfaction with the early relationship with their mother (Hojat et al., 2005). Such an association was not found regarding the students' perceived relationship with their father (Hojat et al., 2005).

These findings are consistent with those in another study in which undergraduates reported that their mothers, more than fathers, spent more time with them, were more affectionate with them, and expressed more empathy toward them (Barnett, Howard, King, & Dino, 1980). The undergraduates' scores on Mehrabian and Epstein's Emotional Empathy Scale (1972) (see Chap. 5) showed stronger association with their interactions with their mothers than with their fathers.

In another study, medical students' retrospective perceptions of a satisfactory relationship with the mother were significantly associated with a positive personality profile, such as higher self-esteem and more satisfactory relationships with peers (Hojat, 1998). In the same study, perceptions of satisfactory relationships with the mother were inversely associated with personality attributes that are detrimental to interpersonal relationships, such as depression, anxiety, and loneliness. Such patterns of significant associations were not observed for students' perceptions of their early relationships with the father. Also, the students' perceptions of the availability of the mother in childhood were significantly associated with higher scores on self-esteem and lower scores on depression and loneliness (Hojat, 1996).

In a study with kindergarten children and their mothers, a substantial correlation was observed in the empathy between mother and child (Trommsdorff, 1991). One explanation is that empathic mothers are likely to engage in empathic exchanges with their children, and empirical research supports this speculation. For example, Wiesenfeld, Whitman, and Malatesta (1984) observed that the mothers' scores on Mehrabian and Epstein's Emotional Empathy Scale (see Chap. 5) predicted their empathic responses to their infant's emotional distress and their desire to pick up the baby when baby was in distress. Other researchers found that mothers with high scores on the empathy scale were less disturbed by their infant's cry and rated the crying as less irritating than low-empathy scored mothers (Lounsburg & Bates, 1982). Conversely, a link was reported between mothers' low levels of empathy and maternal child abuse. For example, Letourneau (1981) reported that scores on Hogan's Empathy Scale and Mehrabian and Epstein's Emotional Empathy Scale could differentiate abusive and nonabusive mothers better than a measure of stressful life events. In a study of 177 adolescents and their mothers, Soenens et al. (2007) found that maternal support served as a mediator of the intergenerational transmission of empathy and quality of friendship. Moreover, it has been reported that a child who never developed the capacity for empathy will become an ineffective parent (Tucker, Luu, & Derryberry, 2005).

Why do mothers have a more crucial role in the development of their children's prosocial and empathic behavior? Nature has bestowed them with some unique privileges that enable them to perform their caregiving role. Some of these privileges are described here.

The Infant's Preference for the Mother's Voice and Face

Under normal circumstances, the voice the developing fetus hears most often is the voice of the expectant mother, who talks, may sing, shouts, laughs, and cries. Thus, the onset of interpersonal connection is with the mother's voice. Although the fetus is unable to respond, it is able to hear the mother's voice again and again and again. Her voice is different from the low-frequency rhythmic sound of her heartbeat, which probably has a calming effect.

Because the mother's voice is the most intense acoustical signal in the amniotic environment of the uterus, the newborn infant shows a clear preference for the sound of her voice within the first 3 days after birth (DeCasper & Fifer, 1980; Fifer & Moon, 1994). Fifer and Moon (1994) suggested that early experiences with the mother's voice have an enduring influence on the development of the infant's brain. In addition, the specific tone and range of pitch that mothers use to get the attention of preverbal infants have been described as the universal "maternal melodies" that serve as a potent mediator of affective communication (Papousek, Papousek, & Symmes, 1991).

By using a non-nutritive nipple attached to an electronic recorder that monitored the rate and amplitude of the infant's sucking pattern, DeCasper and Fifer (1980) found that newborn infants changed their sucking pattern when they heard a recording of their own mother's voice, but no such change was recorded for other female voices. Their sucking pattern also did not change when they heard a recording of their own father's voice (DeCasper & Prescott, 1984). DeCasper and Fifer (1980) suggested that the infant's preference for its mother's voice is important for initiating bonding with the mother. Thus, it appears that the biological mother has a unique advantage that is not shared by any other caregiver—the ability to establish the early attachment relationship with her newborn infant through the newborn's recognition of her voice. The onset of empathy can be traced back to this kind of early exchange between mother and child (Burlingham, 1967).

Preference for the maternal voice can lead the child to prefer the mother's face. Indeed, empirical data suggest that neonates quickly learn to recognize their mother's face. The infant not only shows a preference for her voice but pays particular attention to her varying facial expressions as well. Pascalis, DeSchonen, Morton, Deruella, and Fabre-Grenet (1995) reported that the 4-day-old neonate looks longer at its mother's face than at a stranger's face.

The Mother's Investment in Child-Rearing

Trivers (1972) pointed out that in all mammalian species, the mother is usually more involved in child-rearing than any other caregiver, including the father. The following factors contribute to greater investment on the mother's part: scarcity of gametes and maternal certainty; the psychology of pregnancy; the neurochemistry of motherhood; lactation and breast-feeding; and the mother–child attachment.

The Scarcity of Gametes and Maternal Certainty

Evolutionary scholars have proposed two reasons for more maternal than paternal investment in child care. First, women have far fewer gametes than men do—usually one ovum every 4 weeks during the limited period of fertility versus millions of sperm per ejaculation. This scarcity of gametes leads to the mother's greater protection of offspring and consequently to her greater investment in their care (Bjorklund & Kipp, 1996; Buss & Schmitt, 1993). Second, because of internal gestation and childbirth, maternal certainty (the mother's confidence that she is the biological mother) has historically been much greater than paternal certainty (the father's confidence that he is the biological father), which has resulted in greater maternal investment in preserving one's own genes (Bjorklund & Kipp, 1996; Buss, 2003; Buss & Schmitt, 1993; Trivers, 1972).

The Psychology of Pregnancy and the Neurochemistry of Motherhood

The psychology of internal gestation leads to a fundamentally unique maternal experience of bringing new life into the world (Ballou, 1978). Early in her pregnancy, the mother perceives the child as a developing part of herself. The initial attachment begins to develop at this stage. Nine months of carrying the fetus, the subsequent experience of childbirth, and a long period of breast-feeding and nourishing the infant provide a sense of emotional investment that is a unique experience for the expectant mother and no one else.

The neurochemistry of motherhood is unique to the biological mother, including hormonal changes during pregnancy, after birth, and during lactation. For example, levels of oxytocin increase drastically in human mothers around the time of childbirth. These high concentrations of oxytocin are believed to serve as the thread that weaves the ties between mother and child (Lewis et al., 2000), ties that Freud (1964, p. 188) described as "unique, without parallel, established unalterably for a whole lifetime as the first and the strongest love-object and as the prototype of all later love relations—for both sexes."

Oxytocin can influence the activation of dopamine-producing neurons (Insel, 2000; Oliver, 1939), which makes motherhood more pleasurable under normal circumstances. Studies have shown that increased oxytocin can induce maternal behavior in nonpregnant rats (Pedersen, Ascher, Monroe, & Prange, 1982; Pedersen & Prange, 1979). Conversely, other studies have shown that reduced binding of oxytocin in the brain inhibits the onset of maternal behavior (Fahrbach, Morrell, & Pfaff, 1985; Insel, 2000).

Lactation and Breast-Feeding

Oxytocin prepares the biological mother to feed her newborn by stimulating the release of prolactin and thus lactation (Mori, Vigh, Miayata, & Yoshihara, 1990). Breast-feeding is another physiological privilege that nature has bestowed only on the biological mother. In addition, providing nutritious mother's milk, contributes to the enhancement of the infant's immunocompetence and neurological development, breast-feeding is the first human interactive experience that satisfies the newborn's physiological and psychological needs. Winnicott (1987, p. 79) described the infant's breast-feeding experience as a means of communication that "sings a song without words." It paves the road to empathy.

The sequence of breast-feeding activities, such as proximity seeking toward the nipple; rhythmic movement of the head, mouth, and tongue; sucking that stimulates secretion of milk; ingestion of milk; and withdrawal and disengagement from the nipple, provides a unique opportunity for the behavioral and physiological regulation that develops in the mother–infant dyad (Smotherman & Robinson, 1994). Nursing at the breast is physiologically pleasurable for both mother and infant. The female physiological responses during coitus and lactation have been reported to be similar. For example, uterine contractions, nipple erection, and ejection of milk can occur during both sexual intercourse and breast-feeding (Newton & Newton, 1967). Breast-feeding not only has a calming effect on the human infant, mediated by activation of the opioid system (Smotherman & Robinson, 1994) but also serves as a thermoregulatory mechanism for the exchange of body warmth between mother and infant. During sucking, uterine contractions and increased skin temperature occur that are pleasurable to the lactating mother (Newton, Feeler, & Rawlins, 1968). The gratifying sensation mothers experience when breast-feeding their infants serves as a positive reinforcement of mother–child bonding. The seeds of empathy grow in the ecstasy of such loving interactions.

The universal synchronicity observed between mother and infant during breast-feeding (e.g., the holding position, visual gazes, and vocal exchanges) is, in itself, a unique model of human communication. According to Schore (1996), empathy is rooted in this early psychobiological attunement between mother and child. Isabella and Belsky (1991) reported that synchronous interactions between mother and infant open the highway to a secure attachment between them. All these early experiences affect the infant's growing brain by altering the strength of the synaptic connections that contribute to affective and cognitive behavior later in life.

These early physiological and psychological exchanges between the newborn child and the lactating mother can alter the trajectories of neural development and later interpersonal behavior. The attachment between mother and child that is strengthened by these exchanges between the two can be viewed as a prototypical example of an empathic engagement.

The Attachment Relationship

The bonding between a mother and her child strengthens at the moment of birth during skin-to-skin contact between the mother and her newborn baby (Klaus et al., 1972; Klaus & Kennell, 1970). John Bowlby (1973, 1980, 1982) elegantly described the dynamics and consequences involved in the infant's repeated encounters with the primary caregiver in his attachment theory, which he systematically formulated, advanced, and elaborated in the widely cited trilogy of books. The theory not only was conceived as a general theory of psychosocial development but also was viewed specifically as a framework for later interpersonal and social relationships. According to the tenets of the theory, a lovingly responsive mother serves as a secure base that allows the child to explore the world comfortably with no fear.

The mother's presence (or absence), her attentiveness and loving responses (or her inattentiveness or lack of appropriate responses) to her baby's signals, and her provision (or lack of provision) of physical and emotional nourishment gradually become a fact of life for the growing child. The formation of a secure mother–child attachment is most likely to occur in the presence of a lovingly responsive mother, whereas the opposite (an insecure attachment) is likely to occur if the mother is physically or emotionally unavailable (Bowlby, 1988). (For a review, see Hojat, 1995, 1996, 1998.) A strong mother–child attachment is a major antecedent of early interest in others and is a necessary condition for the development of the capacity for empathy (Mussen & Eisenberg-Berg, 1977).

The quality of the mother–child attachment relationship is assessed by the Strange Situation Procedures, a frequently used test developed by Ainsworth, Blehar, Waters, and Wall (1978). Individual differences among infants and toddlers concerning the quality of attachment with their primary caregiver can be measured with this controlled laboratory procedure, which takes approximately 20 min and includes the following seven episodes, each lasting 3 min or less: (1) an infant or a toddler (usually aged 12–18 months) and its mother are brought into a laboratory room containing some toys; (2) a stranger (usually a woman) enters the room, sits down, and talks to the mother and child; (3) the mother then leaves the room while the stranger stays in the room; (4) the mother then returns and the stranger leaves the room; (5) again, the mother leaves the room, leaving the child alone; (6) the stranger returns; (7) finally the mother returns.

According to Ainsworth and her colleagues, the reaction of the child, particularly in the two episodes of mother–child reunion in this procedure (Episodes 4 and 7) reflected the nature and quality of the mother–child attachment. Originally, the researchers identified three types of mother–child attachment. Briefly, if the child explored and played with the toys when the mother was present, expressed less interest in the toys when she left the room, and sought to be near her and initiate positive expression with her when she returned, the attachment was classified as a *secure* attachment (Ainsworth, 1985b). However, if the child continued to explore the toys during all seven episodes, exhibited no distress when the mother left the room, and avoided her when she returned, the child's attachment was classified as *avoidant*. Finally, if the child tended to be wary of the stranger, became intensely upset when the mother left, and exhibited ambivalent behavior when she returned (wanting to approach her and simultaneously being angry and avoiding being near her, thus difficult to soothe), attachment was classified as *ambivalent*. Main and Solomon (1990) introduced a new category of attachment, the "disorganized attachment," in an attempt to explain the situation when none of the other three patterns of attachment applied.

The type of attachment developed in early childhood is likely to endure throughout life (Ainsworth, 1985a, 1985b). Research has shown that securely attached children develop a sense of trust with caregivers who respond to them empathically and therefore develop the capacity to respond sensitively and empathically toward others in later relationships (Kestenbaum, Farber, & Sroufe, 1989). Furthermore, research has shown that the lack of a secure attachment with the mother can result in aggressive and noncompliant behaviors in later years that are not conducive to empathic engagement (Belsky, 1988; Karen, 1994) (for a review, see Hojat, 1995).

In a study of preschool children, Kestenbaum et al. (1989) observed a continuity between the quality of a child's early relationship with the primary caregiver and the child's capacity to respond empathically later. This observation confirmed the notion that "it is with the aid of modified mother–child signals that we establish and maintain friendly contact with our fellow men" (Eibel-Eibesfeldt, 1979, p. 230). Severe abnormalities in interpersonal relationships have been observed in infants, such as Romanian orphans, who have been deprived of maternal love (Konner, 2004). The abnormality in connecting to others, known as "reactive attachment disorder," is another testimony to the importance of the quality of early attachment to later empathic behavior or the lack thereof.

According to Bowlby (1988, p. 82), the need for a secure attachment remains "from cradle to grave." More important, as Bowlby pointed out, the quality of the child's early relationship with the mother will lead to the development of cognitive schemata regarding the world that reside deep in the child's mind and "tend to persist and are so taken for granted that they come to operate at an unconscious level" (p. 130). In other words, the prototypical model of the world as friendly and caring or as hostile and uncaring becomes an influential property of the child's cognitive structure, serving primarily as an unconscious motivational force that significantly influences the adult's interpersonal relationships and the capacity for empathic engagement (Ainsworth, 1985a, 1985b).

The nature and quality of the child's early interpersonal experiences with the primary caregiver and the positive or negative outcomes engrave relatively permanent cognitive images on the mind that attachment scholars describe as "internal working models" (Bretherton, 1987). This mental representation of the world, or the psychological "script," becomes a major motivational factor in empathic relationships later in life (Nathanson, 1996; Tomkins, 1987). The assertion that attachment relationships in childhood can influence interpersonal behavior across the life span has broad implications for developmental, social, and clinical psychology.

Also, it has been reported that relationships with family members, peers, and others are influenced by early attachment experiences (Bartholomew & Horowitz, 1991). Shaver and Hazan (1989) reported that adult love relationships share similarities with, and are rooted in the early attachment experiences with a primary caregiver. It has also been reported that attachment history can predict medical students' specialty preferences. For example, students with a secure attachment history are more likely to choose specialties that require more interaction with patients (Ciechanowski, Russo, Katon, & Walker, 2004). Early attachment experiences also can influence the style of clinical practice. For example, clinical psychologists with an insecure attachment history who reported less empathic parental responses were more in need of support and more vulnerable to work stress (Leiper & Casares, 2000).

The child's attachment behavior in all cultures becomes extremely strong in the second year of life, when major pathways of the limbic system become encased in myelin. According to Konner (2004), the aforementioned phenomenon improves the function of the subcortical circuits that process emotions and social behavior. Therefore, the quality of the mother–child attachment exerts a lasting influence on the development of the brain and prosocial behavior as well.

Because the capacity for empathy is deeply rooted in the early attachment relationship with a primary caregiver, a number of empirical studies have addressed the link between empathy and relationships with one's parents. The outcomes of these studies generally confirm a significant relationship between scores on empathy and the nature and quality of the early relationship with the primary caregiver and the rearing environment.

Kestenbaum et al. (1989) reported that children aged 12–18 months with a secure attachment to their mothers grew up to be more empathic to others and exhibited more prosocial behavior. Zahn-Waxler, Radke-Yarrow, and King (1979) reported that empathic caregiving (determined by whether mothers responded promptly to their child's call for help, anticipated dangers, and provided nurturing caregiving) was significantly associated with greater prosocial and altruistic behavior in the children.

Stern and Cassidy (2018) reviewed the research on mother–child attachment and empathy from infancy through adolescence. They reported that in childhood, low empathy was predictive of poor peer relationships, hostility, bullying, aggression, and antisocial behavior. Also, they found that low empathy in adulthood was associated with child abuse, violence, noncompliance behavior, and psychopathy. Consistent with these findings, we have found that high scores on our measure of clinical empathy (the Jefferson scale of Empathy, see Chap. 7) were associated with higher marks on personal qualities that were conducive to relationship building; and conversely, higher scores on our clinical empathy measure were inversely associated with qualities that were detrimental to relationship building (see Chap. 7).

The aforementioned theoretical perspectives and empirical findings suggest that the seeds of empathy are sown by the same hand that rocks the cradle. Stern and her colleagues (in press), in their longitudinal study of three generations, reported that attachment relationship and empathy can be transmitted across generations, and quality of mother–child attachment is a factor in the transmission (Also see Stern, Costello, Kansky, et al., 2021). Because of the importance of the quality of mother–child attachment in the development of children's capacity for empathy, Goldstein and Michaels (1985) proposed a series of training programs to enhance empathic communication between mothers and their children.

There are resemblances between the mother–child attachment and the clinician–patient relationship. The child needs the mother's help and protection to survive, and the attachment behavior (e.g., proximity seeking) intensifies when the child is in distress or pain. Similarly, patients have a natural tendency to bond with a caring figure (the clinician) to maintain their health during a time of pain and suffering. Therefore, clinician–patient bonding is associated, though unconsciously, with the early attachment relationship. One can speculate that people with a history of a secure attachment are more likely to form stronger empathic relationships quickly than are those with a history of ambivalent or avoidant attachment. This behavioral tendency also should be true for both clinician and patient.

Other Factors that Contribute to the Development of Empathy in Childhood

The following factors feed the development of empathy and social behavior in children.

Facial Imitation and Motor Mimicry

Nature has bestowed human infants with the gift of an imitative brain, which allows them not only to understand others' affective state of mind but to learn from the emotions of others as well. As was mentioned in Chap. 3, Meltzoff and Moore (1977, 1983) found that infants only 12–21 days old could imitate human facial gestures, such as protruding their tongue or lips and opening their mouth—an ability conceptualized as a type of primitive empathy (Bavelas, Black, Lemery, & Mullett, 1986) (see Meltzoff & Moore, 1977, for photos showing infants imitating facial expressions made by Dr. Meltzoff, or click on the following link: https://baillement.com/meltzoff.html). Early in life, the infant pays attention to expressions of emotion on the human face. The infant's attention to facial expressions and its apparent responses are described as "telepathic" exchanges that lay the foundation for empathic communications (Burlingham, 1967). Understanding one's own emotions and those of others emerges from these exchanges (Ickes, 1997). According to Decety and Jackson (2004), one adaptive advantage of mimicry is that it connects people together and fosters empathy.

Motor mimicry (e.g., wincing when a person or an animal is injured, mimicking a facial expression similar to the expression of another person who is in pain) is indeed a nonverbal mode of communication based on observing another person's affect. This phenomenon, which has been observed in children and adults alike, supports the notion that individuals are intricately and visibly connected in their interpersonal interactions (Bavelas et al., 1986). According to Decety and Jackson (2006), people can "catch" the emotional states of others as a result of motor mimicry. Bush, Barr, McHugo, and Lanzetta (1989) suggested that an observer's mimetic facial responses may play an important role in the development of empathic responses.

The "Still-Face" Experiments

Additional evidence supporting the infant's capacity to understand other people's emotions is provided by the "still-face" procedure developed by Tronick, Als, Adamson, Wise, and Brazelton (1978). In this procedure, the mother is instructed to distort her affective feedback to her one-year old infant by assuming an expressionless face (a still face) after a period of normal playful exchanges with her child. The child first becomes unpleasantly surprised to observe the mother's emotionless expression; the child then attempts to get her attention in an effort to restore affect to her emotionally blank face. When these efforts fail, the child becomes overtly uncomfortable, distressed, and anxious. Finally, when the mother's face does not change, the child becomes indifferent, detached, and apathetic. Most infants react physiologically to the mother's still face with an increased heart rate, which Weinberg and Tronik (1996) attributed to disruption of the infant's goal of relating to others. The still-face experiments with infants indicate that although the infant has not developed language to facilitate verbal communication, the face-to-face interactions between a mother and her child is a goal-directed, reciprocal system of communication that serves as a regulator of emotions in social relationships and a primary step toward the development of empathic capacity.

The "Visual Cliff" Experiments

Young children's understanding of others' emotions was also demonstrated in experiments involving the "visual cliff" apparatus (Gibson & Walk, 1960). This apparatus consisted of a sheet of heavy glass supported approximately one foot off the floor by a table-like frame. Patterned material in the open space under the glass looked to the infant like a bottomless crevasse. The baby was placed on one side of the frame and the mother stood on the other side and encouraged the child to come to her by crawling over the glass. Human infants can recognize depth as soon as they are old enough to crawl; the infants refused to crawl over the glass.

Sorce, Emde, Campos, and Klinnert (1985) demonstrated that by 12 months of age, children were more likely to feel confident enough to cross over the visual abyss when their mothers looked joyful or assumed a positive facial expression. However, when the mother adopted a negative facial expression, such as fear or anger, the children hesitated to cross over the glass. These findings suggest that young children not only can recognize the mother's emotional expressions but also can be encouraged by her positive look to risk crossing the cliff. The relevance of these findings to empathy was described by Campos and Sternberg (1981), who suggested that one developmental root of empathic understanding is a form of emotional communication known as "social referencing," through which children attempt to infer emotional information from interactions with others to adjust their own behavior accordingly.

Infants' ability to imitate facial expressions and mimic motor activities and to understand emotions indicates that infants possess a remarkable innate ability to establish social connections in the early days of life. Nurturing this ability lays the foundation for the development of a capacity to understand other people's positive and negative emotional states (Stern, 1985). Such understanding is the royal road to empathy.

The Theory of Mind

The capacity to represent the mental states of others is described in the theory of mind (Fonagy & Target, 1996; Wellman, 1991) as part of the human being's cognitive-emotional development. Empathy is linked to the theory of mind, because both are involved with the capacity to stand in another person's *mental shoes* (Gallese, 2001). Perspective-taking ability, a major feature of empathy, according to Eslinger (1998), is also a feature of the theory of mind. In contrast to Jean Piaget's proposition (1967) that children between the ages of 2 and 7 years are primarily egocentric and unable to stand in another person's shoes, subsequent research demonstrated that young children are aware of other people's emotions and therefore are capable of responding empathically to other people's feelings (Borke, 1971). Research in the theory of mind found that children often in the fourth year of life develop the ability to understand the other's mental states (Lieberman, 2007). The mechanisms involved in the human neonate's ability to understand and imitate facial gestures provide the foundation for understanding other people which is precursor to the theory of mind, a key ingredient in the conceptualization of empathy (see Chap. 1).

The theory describes meta-cognitive abilities that make a distinction between thoughts, desires, and intentions of self and others, which are among the ingredients of interpersonal relationships. Mentalization is a feature of the theory of mind which refers to the process of making inferences of another's mental states. It has been demonstrated that in the mentalization process, brain activities in the medial prefrontal cortex are involved (Lieberman, 2007). The same brain area is also implicated in empathic responses (see Chap. 13).

Regulation of Emotions

According to Marx, Heidt, and Gold (2005), regulation of emotions is defined as the process that enables individuals to control the quality, frequency, intensity, or duration of their emotional responses. It is reported that regulation of emotion is positively linked to an important aspect of empathy: namely, being concerned for others (Decety & Jackson, 2004). One mechanism for linking caregivers' behavior to the development of empathy in children can be explained by the process of regulation of emotions, which plays an important role in organizing, motivating, and sustaining social behavior and attributing meaning to experiences (Nathanson, 1996). Human infants are well-equipped for socialization because they are endowed with a system of affect that can be regulated and therefore lays the foundation for a key ingredient in the development of interpersonal relationships.

Some developmental scholars have proposed that regulation of emotions begins extremely early—from the face-to-face interactions with the primary caregiver (as attested to by infants' reactions in the "still-face" and "visual cliff" experiments) and from the quality of the mother–child attachment (as attested to by the experiments regarding secure and insecure attachment).

Regulation of emotions develops as a result of emotional attunement between mother and child (Black, 2004) and involves a process in which people recognize and express their emotions (Archer, 2004). Regulation of emotions is a necessary condition for demonstrating prosocial behavior, and it functions as a mechanism to achieve an internal state that is optimal for social relationships. Regulation of emotions plays an important role in maintaining a boundary between the self and others (Decety & Jackson, 2006), which is an important aspect of empathic engagement in patient care.

Although emotions play an important role in social behavior, their regulation also is believed to play an essential role in empathic relationships (Demos, 1988). The infant's emotional response depends on his or her regulatory capacities and the regulatory scaffolding provided by the mother (Weinberg, Tronick, & Cohn, 1999). Thus, the mother is the most important first regulator of emotions because she provides a supplementary context for the development of her infant's social behavior (Lott, 1998). The self-regulated behavior is a function of the quality of interactions with a primary caregiver during the formative period of brain development (Nathanson, 1996). Together, the mother and infant are a regulatory unit, and the mother's role in the regulatory exchanges is influenced by her own early attachment relationships (Mays et al., 1991).

The nature and quality of the neonate, infant, or young child's interaction with the mother set the stage for the development of a psychological script (Nathanson, 1996; Tomkins, 1962, 1963), an internal working model (Ainsworth, 1985a, 1985b; Bretherton, 1987), and an emotional regulatory system (Lott, 1998; Weinberg et al., 1999) that will serve as a guiding force for empathic behavior during the rest of one's life. The implicit memories of the early warm relationship with the primary caregiver lead to the development of an enduring neural structure that influences self-regulatory behavior reflected in interpersonal relationships (Amini et al., 1996). The emotional arousal generated by feelings of other people's pain and suffering needs regulation and control for empathic understanding (Decety & Jackson, 2004). According to Watson (2002), a propensity to regulate emotions in clinical encounters can enhance empathic engagement and improve patient outcomes.

Recapitulation

Evidence suggests that infants are endowed with a capacity to understand and respond to emotions. Empathy is nurtured in a facilitative family environment where opportunities are provided for forming secure attachment relationships with a primary caregiver (usually the mother). The motivation for prosocial behavior and the capacity for empathic relationships are the outcomes of early social–emotional exchanges that lead to the development of an internal working model, a mental script, and an emotional regulatory system that guide interpersonal responses from the cradle to the grave.

Chapter 5
Measurement of Empathy in the General Population

If you cannot measure it, you cannot improve it.
—(Lord William Thompson Kelvin, 1824–1907)

Abstract

- Some of the instruments that have been developed to measure empathy in children and adults, and used by researchers other than their own authors, are briefly described.
- The three that have been used most often in medical education and health care research are Hogan's Empathy Scale; Mehrabian and Epstein's Emotional Empathy Scale; and Davis's Interpersonal Reactivity Index. These instruments were developed for administration to the general population; therefore, their relevance to the context of health professions education and patient care is limited for two reasons. First, they are not framed in the context of physician–patient (clinician–client) relationships. Thus, the validity of their use in the context of health professions education and patient care is questionable. Second, these instruments were not developed specifically to address the cognitively defined concept of clinical empathy, a conceptualization that is more relevant to clinical empathy.
- The biotechnological advancements in functional brain imaging and the discovery of the mirror neuron system have opened up a new window for assessing empathy that is extremely promising.
- Given the findings that empathy tends to erode during medical and other health professions education, and in an era of changes in the health care system that hamper the clinician–patient relationship, a psychometrically sound instrument for measuring empathy in the context of health professions education and patient care is in high demand.

M. Hojat, *Clinical Empathy*, https://doi.org/10.1007/978-3-031-87413-0_5

Introduction

In Chap. 1, I indicated that one reason for the dearth of empirical research on empathy in the health professions was the lack of a psychometrically sound instrument that can be used to measure the concept of clinical empathy in health professions education and patient care. This chapter briefly describes some of the instruments that have been used most often to measure empathy in the general population and presents sample items enabling us to judge their *face validity* in the context of patient care. Although a detailed analysis of the psychometric properties of these scales can be informative, such a technical discussion is beyond the scope of this book. However, in Chap. 7, I will describe in detail the step-by-step development and psychometric properties of the Jefferson Scale of Empathy (JSE), which was specifically designed to measure empathy in medical and other health professions students, practicing physicians, and other health professionals.

In general, an instrument serves not only as a device for measurement but also as the basis of a common language that researchers use to communicate their empirical findings. Therefore, familiarity with the instruments and the scores they generate is necessary to comprehend and compare the results of research. For that purpose, I have selected a few research instruments designed to measure empathy in child and adult populations and described these in the following sections.

Measurement of Empathy in Children and Adolescents

Reflexive or Reactive Crying

Simner (1971) systematically investigated newborn infants' reactive crying and reported that newborns who heard another newborn crying cried significantly more often in response (reflexive crying) than they did to any other nonstartling noise. These findings were later replicated in other studies (Martin & Clark, 1982; Sagi & Hoffman, 1976). It is interesting to note that the newborns did not respond to their own cries (Martin & Clark, 1982), suggesting that infants are capable of distinguishing between self and others early in life (Decety & Jackson, 2004). The reaction of one infant to another infant's crying has been used as an indicator of empathy in infants based on the assumption that an infant crying in response to another infant's distress is a reflection of an empathic response (Eisenberg & Lennon, 1983). Eisenberg (1989) suggested that the capacity to respond to cues of another person's distress in childhood is a primitive precursor of more mature empathic sensibilities that develop later. However, the assumption that reflexive crying in infants is an indicator of empathy needs to be verified empirically in longitudinal studies.

According to Eisenberg and Lennon (1983), no convincing evidence is available to confirm that reflexive crying necessarily implies an empathic response. Martin and Clark (1982) reported that children of both sexes cried more in response to a male newborn's crying than to a female newborn's crying. These reports raise questions about the validity of reflexive crying as an indicator of empathic capacity.

The Picture or Story Methods

One popular method of measuring empathy in young children, developed by Eisenberg and Lennon (1983), has been to expose children to another person's distress by showing them pictures or telling them stories depicting hypothetical situations. The children are subsequently asked to describe their own feelings about the story's protagonist either verbally or by choosing an image from a set of pictures representing a variety of faces exhibiting various expressions, such as a happy or sad face. A match between the child's feelings and the protagonist's feelings is considered to be an indication of empathic understanding. The difficulty of differentiating empathy from sympathy when using picture or story methods of assessment raised concern about the validity of this method. Also, the predictive validity of this method awaits empirical verification.

The Feshbach Affective Situations Test of Empathy

The Feshbach Affective Situations Test of Empathy (FASTE), published by Feshbach and Roe (1968), is a widely used variation of the picture or story method of measuring empathy in children. Children (usually aged 6 or 7 years) are shown cartoons on a series of slides accompanied by hypothetical stories depicting children in different affectively charged conditions (happiness, sadness, fear, and anger). The children are then asked to describe their own feelings and emotions about the picture or story either verbally or by choosing a response from a set of facial expressions depicting different emotions. For example, a theme for happiness is a picture of a birthday party, a theme for sadness is a lost dog, a theme for fear is a frightening dog, and a theme for anger is a false accusation. The child's capacity for empathy is determined by a match between the child's expressed feeling and the theme depicted in the picture or story. The FASTE has been modified to accommodate studies by different researchers (Zhou, Valiente, & Eisenberg, 2003).

Some have criticized the FASTE because of its weak psychometric support, its suggestive test instructions (e.g., instructions designed in a way that elicits the desired behavior), and a lack of clarity in scoring (Eisenberg & Lennon, 1983; Eisenberg-Berg & Lennon, 1980; Hoffman, 1982; Zhou et al., 2003). Concern also has been raised about the confounding effect of the "demand characteristic" in children's responses (Goldstein & Michaels, 1985). This phenomenon makes the respondents modify their responses to what they believe the testing situation demands. The demand characteristic (e.g., a tendency to respond in a certain way that can undermine the validity of the results) is inherent in children's self-reports when an adult constantly asks them about their feelings. Another concern is the confounding effect of the experimenter's gender on the results of the FASTE, because research indicated that when the experimenter was a woman, girls scored higher than boys did (Levine & Hoffman, 1975; Roe, 1977).

The Index of Empathy

The self-report Index of Empathy, developed by Bryant (1982), consists of 22 items designed to measure empathy in children and adolescents. The measure is comparable to Mehrabian and Epstein's Emotional Empathy Scale, which was developed to measure empathy in the adult population (this scale will be described later in this chapter). The author of the Index of Empathy indicated that these comparable instruments can be useful for exploring changes in empathy at different ages. A sample item is, "I really like to watch people open presents, even when I don't get a present myself." The internal consistency reliability coefficients of this measure were reported to be 0.54 for first graders, 0.68 for fourth graders, and 0.79 for seventh graders (Bryant, 1982; Zhou et al., 2003).

Although the abovementioned methods of measuring empathy in children and adolescents seem to be useful for measuring reactions to affective situations, no convincing evidence is available in support of the instrument's predictive validity as indicators of the capacity for empathy.

Measurement of Empathy in Adults

The Most Frequently Used Instruments

The first three self-report measures of empathy discussed in this section—Hogan's Empathy Scale; Mehrabian and Epstein's Emotional Empathy Scale; and Davis's Interpersonal Reactivity Index—have been the most frequently used instruments in empathy research. Although they were developed for use in the general population, rather than with health professions students and practitioners, they have also been used in healthcare research. These measures are briefly described in the order in which they were originally published. Although other instruments have been designed to measure empathy, they have not received widespread attention. Some of them will be briefly described later in this chapter.

The Empathy Scale

Published by Robert Hogan (1969) and based on his doctoral dissertation at the University of California at Berkeley, the Empathy Scale includes 64 true-false items adopted from the California Psychological Inventory (CPI), the Minnesota Multiphasic Personality Inventory (MMPI), and other tests used at the Institute of Personality Assessment and Research. The scale was developed within the framework of the theory of moral development. A typical item is, "I have seen some things so sad that I almost felt like crying."

Evidence in support of the scale's validity was provided by showing that high scorers were more likely than low scorers to be socially acute and sensitive to nuances in interpersonal relationships, and low scorers were more likely to be hostile, cold, and insensitive to the feelings of others (Hogan, 1969). Also, in a group of medical students, Hogan found a significant and positive correlation between scores on this scale and a criterion measure of sociability on the CPI ($r = 0.58$); and a significant negative correlation with social introversion on the MMPI ($r = -0.65$) (Hogan, 1969). Factor analysis of the Empathy Scale across different studies resulted in an inconsistent factor structure. For example, Greif and Hogan (1973) reported the following factors: "even-tempered disposition," "social ascendancy," and "humanistic sociopolitical attitudes"; and Johnson, Cheek, and Smither (1983) reported "social self-confidence," "even-temperedness," "sensitivity," and "nonconformity." These inconsistent findings raised questions about the scale's construct validity. Based on the factor analytic findings, it is suggested that the entire scale may not capture the essence of empathy (Baron-Cohen & Wheelwright, 2004). The scale's reliability has also been questioned (Cross & Sharpley, 1982).

The Emotional Empathy Scale

This instrument was developed by Albert Mehrabian and Norman Epstein (Mehrabian & Epstein, 1972) and includes 33 items intended to measure emotional empathy. "It makes me sad to see a lonely stranger in a group" is a typical item. The title of the measure and the contents of the items pertain to susceptibility to emotional contagion (Zhou et al., 2003), indicating that the authors used an affective conceptualization of empathy when developing the scale (Davis, 1994). This conceptualization conflicts with the definition of empathy as a primarily cognitive concept in the context of patient care that was adopted in this book (see Chap. 6).

Items are answered on a 9-point Likert-type scale (Very Strongly Agree = +4, Very Strongly Disagree = −4). The split-half reliability of this scale was reported to be 0.84, and the internal consistency reliability was 0.79 (Zhou et al., 2003). The validity of this scale was determined by using an experimental paradigm similar to Milgram's experiments (1963, 1968) in which high scorers on this scale were less likely than low scorers to administer electric shocks to the experimental subjects (Mehrabian & Epstein, 1972) (see Chap. 8 for a description of Milgram's experimental paradigm). On the basis of their subjective view, Mehrabian and Epstein reported that the scale included the following components and identified the items that measured each of these components: extreme emotional responsiveness, appreciation of the feelings of unfamiliar and distant others, tendency to be moved by others' emotional experiences, and tendency to be sympathetic. A study by Dillard and Hunter (1989) failed to support the aforementioned multidimensional components.

Later, Mehrabian, Young, and Sato (1988) changed the scale's name to the Emotional Empathic Tendency Scale. Subsequently, Mehrabian introduced a new instrument, the Balanced Emotional Empathy Scale (BEES), to measure vicarious empathy (Mehrabian, 1996), which is similar in content to the Emotional Empathy Scale. It contains 30 items, each answered on a 9-point Likert scale (4 = Very Strongly Agree, −4 = Very Strongly Disagree). A sample item is, "Unhappy movie endings haunt me for hours afterward." Information about the scale is posted on Mehrabian's personal website, and to the best of my knowledge, no empirical study has been published to specifically address psychometrics of the BEES. In a study of empathy and aggression, a Cronbach's alpha coefficient of 0.87 was reported for this scale (Mehrabian, 1997).

The Interpersonal Reactivity Index

As part of his doctoral dissertation at the University of Texas at Austin, Mark Davis developed the Interpersonal Reactivity Index (IRI) (Davis, 1983) to measure individual differences in empathy. The instrument includes 28 items tapping four components of empathy in the cognitive and emotional domains. These four components are reflected in four subscales (Perspective Taking, Empathic Concern, Fantasy, and Personal Distress), each of which includes seven items answered on a 5-point scale ranging from 0 (Does not describe me well) to 4 (Describes me very well). These components were originally determined by subjective judgment without statistical support. However, confirmatory factor analysis provided mixed results concerning the existence of the four subscales (Cliffordson, 2002; Litvack-Miller, McDougall, & Romney, 1997). Costa, de Carvalho-Filip and colleagues (2017) examined the underlying constructs of the IRI, and generally reaffirmed the four components (subscales) of the IRI in a factor analytic study of medical students in five countries.

The Perspective Taking subscale measures the tendency to adopt the views of others spontaneously. "I sometimes try to understand my friends better by imagining how things look from their perspective" is a typical item. The Empathic Concern subscale measures a tendency to experience the feelings of others and to feel sympathy and compassion for unfortunate people. A typical item is "I often have tender, concerned feelings for people less fortunate than me." The Fantasy subscale measures a tendency to imagine oneself in a fictional situation. A typical item is "After seeing a play or movie, I have felt as though I were one of the characters." The

Personal Distress subscale taps a tendency to experience distress in others. "When I see someone who badly needs help in an emergency, I go to pieces" is a representative item. According to Davis, the Perspective Taking subscale is more likely to measure cognitive empathy, whereas the Empathic Concern and Personal Distress subscales are more likely to assess emotional empathy (Davis, 1983, p. 114).

The internal consistency reliability coefficients ranged from 0.71 to 0.77 for the four subscales, and their test–retest reliabilities ranged from 0.62 to 0.71 (Davis, 1983). The test–retest reliabilities in an adolescent sample over a 2-year period ranged from 0.50 to 0.62 (Davis & Franzoi, 1991; Zhou et al., 2003). In correlating the IRI subscale scores with scores on Hogan's Empathy Scale, the highest positive correlation was found for the Perspective Taking subscale ($r = 0.40$) and the highest negative correlation was found for the Personal Distress subscale ($r = -0.33$) (Davis, 1983). The Perspective Taking subscale of the IRI yielded the lowest correlation with the scores of Mehrabian and Epstein's Emotional Empathy Scale ($r = 0.24$), and the Fantasy and Empathic Concern subscales yielded the highest correlations (0.52 and 0.60, respectively) (Davis, 1983). This pattern of correlations confirms Davis's claim about the cognitive nature of the Perspective Taking subscale.

In 1994, Davis stated that convincing evidence existed in support of some psychometric aspects of the IRI, although no satisfactory statistical evidence has been presented to confirm the stability of the four components of the index. In a study with physicians and undergraduate psychology students, Yarnold, Bryant, Nightingale, and Martin (1996) discovered an additional component called "involvement" in their statistical analysis of the IRI. The findings that scores on the Personal Distress subscale of the IRI were negatively correlated with scores on the Perspective Taking subscale raise a serious question about the validity of scoring the IRI by summing up the scores of all its subscales, including the Personal Distress subscale. According to D'Orazio (2004), summing up the scores of all four subscales of the IRI would not be meaningful because of the negative correlation between the Personal Distress and Perspective Taking subscales and because high scores on Personal Distress are associated with dysfunctional interpersonal relationships.

Other Instruments

Several other instruments for measuring empathy in the adult population are described here in chronological order. Kerr developed a test of empathy with the intention of measuring respondents' ability to "anticipate" certain typical reactions, feelings, and behavior of other people (Kerr, 1947). The test consists of three sections which require respondents to rank the popularity of 15 types of music, the national circulation of 15 magazines, and the prevalence of 10 types of annoyances for a particular group of people (Chlopan, McCain, Carbonell, & Hagen, 1985). The respondent's rankings are compared to the empirical data to assess their accuracy. This test seems to be a measure of general information, rather than a measure of empathy. Nevertheless, Kerr and Speroff (1954) claimed that the test was an indicator of empathic understanding and that it could predict a person's popularity, feelings for others, leadership, and sales records.

A measure of insight and empathy was introduced by Dymond (1949, 1950). This measure was based on the conceptualization of empathy as the imaginative transposing of oneself into another person's thinking, feeling, and acting. In Dymond's Rating Test (of empathic ability), respondents rate themselves and one another on a 5-point scale on six attributes such as "superior–inferior," "friendly–unfriendly," "leader–follower," "self-confidence," "selfish–unselfish," and "sense of humor." The concordance between individuals' ratings of themselves and their predictions of how others would rate them was considered as a measure of empathic ability. High scorers on the Dymond's Rating Test were classified as empathizers by analyses of their responses to the Thematic Apperception Test (TAT) (Dymond, 1949). Although no satisfactory evidence is available to confirm the instrument's validity as a measure of empathy, some preliminary data on its psychometric characteristics were presented by Chlopan et al. (1985). However, those investigators raised concerns about the measure's lack of easy administration and scoring procedures.

Barrett-Lennard (1962) developed an instrument called the Relationship Inventory, which was designed to investigate changes in the clinician–client relationship in the psychotherapeutic context. The instrument can be completed by either the clinician or the client. The original inventory included 92 items. However, one revised version consists of 64 items divided into four subjectively determined subtests of interpersonal relationships: (1) Empathic Understanding, described as the extent to which one person is conscious of the awareness of another person; (2) Level of Regard, the affective aspect of one person's response to another; (3) Unconditionality of Regard, the degree of constancy of regard one person feels for another person; and (4) Congruence, the degree to which one person is functionally integrated in the context of his or her relationship with another person (Barrett-Lennard, 1986). The "Willingness To Be Known" subtest included in the original version of the Relationship Inventory was defined as the degree to which a person wants to be known as a person by another person. This subtest was dropped in the revised version because of its nonsignificant predictive validity concerning therapeutic outcomes (Barrett-Lennard, 1986). Subsequent versions of the Relationship Inventory have been developed for use in nonclinical situations involving family, friendship, coworker, and teacher–pupil relationships (Bennett, 1995).

A 16-item subtest of this instrument called Empathic Understanding contains such items as "The [clinician/client] understands me." Items are answered on a Likert-type scale ranging from −3 ("No," as strongly felt disagreement) to +3 ("Yes," as strongly felt agreement). A negligible clinician–client correlation of 0.09 was reported for the Empathic Understanding subtest (Barrett-Lennard, 1962).

Truax and Carkhuff (1967) developed the 141-item Relationship Questionnaire to measure clients' perceptions of psychologists or counselors in psychological counseling and psychotherapy. Forty-six of the 141 items of the Relationship Questionnaire form a subscale called the Accurate Empathy Scale, which consists of such items as

"He [she] sometimes completely understands me so that he knows what I am feeling even when I am hiding my feelings." A number of questions have been raised about the validity, reliability, and score stability of the Accurate Empathy Scale (Beutler, Johnson, Neville, & Workman, 1973; Blass & Hech, 1975; Chinsky & Rappaport, 1970).

Carkhuff (1969) developed the Empathic Understanding in Interpersonal Processes Scale. This single-item instrument gives clinicians an overall empathy score based on five levels of empathic behavior, as judged by observers. Clinicians who score at Level 1 are judged as unable to express any awareness of even the most obvious of a client's feelings, whereas those who score at Level 5 are judged to be fully aware of and able to respond accurately to all of the client's feelings. Because an observer rates clinicians' empathic global behavior on a single item, the validity of this instrument is questionable (LaMonica, 1981).

The Fantasy-Empathy (F-E) Scale, developed by Stotland, Mathews, Sherman, Hansson (1978), measures the tendency to respond emotionally to situations. The scale contains three items answered on a 5-point scale: for example, "When I watch a good movie, I can very easily put myself in the place of a leading character." Some psychometric data on this brief scale have been reported (Stotland, 1978). For instance, a correlation of 0.44 was reported between scores of the F-E Scale and Mehrabian and Epstein's Emotional Empathy Scale (Williams, 1989).

Layton (1979) developed the Empathy Test, a two-part 48-item instrument, as part of a research project designed to teach empathy to nursing students. The purpose of this measure was to evaluate whether empathy can be learned by observing models of empathic behavior. Each part of the Empathy Test consists of 12 true-false items and 12 multiple-choice items. According to Layton's reports, the reliability coefficients for the measure are unacceptably low (in the 0.20s), and no significant correlations were found between this measure and the Empathic Understanding subtest of Barrett-Lennard's Relationship Inventory and Carkhuff's Empathic Understanding in Interpersonal Processes Scale (Carkhuff, 1969).

Another instrument for measuring empathy is the Empathy Construct Rating Scale developed by LaMonica (1981). The instrument consists of 84 items about the respondent's feelings or actions toward another person, answered on a 6-point Likert-type scale (−3, Extremely Unlike; +3, Extremely Like). A typical item is, "Seems to understand another person's state of being." The bipolar grand factor of this scale includes the notion of "well-developed empathy" (e.g., "Shows consideration for a person's feelings and reactions") at one pole and "lack of empathy" (e.g., "Does not listen to what the other person is saying") at the opposite pole.

A 15-item unidimensional instrument (The Emotional Contagion Scale) was developed by Doherty (1997) to measure emotional empathy. Each item is answered on a 5-point Likert-type scale. A sample item is, "I cry at sad movies." A Cronbach's alpha coefficient of 0.90 is reported for the scale. Higher correlation was found between scores of this scale and those of the Empathic Concern scale ($r = 0.37$) than scores of the Perspective Taking scale of the IRI ($r = 0.14$).

A measuring instrument—the Empathy Quotient (EQ)—was developed in England by Baron-Cohen and Wheelwright (2004) and contains 40 empathy items plus 20 filler items to distract the participants from relentless focus on empathy

(Lawrence, Shaw, Baker, Baron-Cohen, & David, 2004). Each item is answered on a 4-point Likert-type scale from Strongly Agree to Strongly Disagree. Although the authors claim that the EQ was explicitly designed to have clinical applications, the contents of most of the items do not support such an application. Sample items are "I really enjoy caring for other people" and "I tend to get emotionally involved with a friend's problems." A test–retest reliability of 0.83 is reported for the EQ. Three factors, Cognitive Empathy, Emotional Reactivity, and Social Skills, emerged from factor analyses of the EQ. With the exception of the Cognitive Empathy factor, which was not correlated with any subscales of the IRI, the EQ yielded moderate correlations with the Empathic Concern and Perspective Taking subscales of the IRI and a negligible negative correlation with the Personal Distress subscale (Lawrence et al., 2004).

Another empathy-measuring instrument for the general population is the Toronto Empathy Questionnaire (TEQ) for measuring emotional empathy (Spreng, McKinnon, Mar & Levine, 2009). This instrument contains 16 questions. A sample item is, "I become irritated when someone cries." Some psychometric data exist in support of the validity and reliability of the TEQ in a study by its authors (Spreng et al., 2009).

A 31-item instrument introduced by Reniers, Corcoran, Drake, Shryane, and Vollm (2011) is the "Questionnaire of Cognitive and Affective Empathy (QCAE). Items in this instrument were derived from four other instruments. Authors describe it as measuring both cognitive and affective (emotional) dimensions of empathy based on the results of exploratory and confirmatory factor analysis. Items are answered on a 4-point Likert scale (from Strongly Agree to Strongly Disagree). A sample item from cognitive empathy is: "I am good at predicting how someone will feel" and a sample item from affective/emotional empathy is: "I am happy when I am with a cheerful group and sad when the others are glum."

The Adolescent Measure of Empathy and Sympathy (AMES) was developed by Vossen, Piotrowski, and Valkenburg (2015) to measure cognitive empathy, affective empathy, and sympathy (12 items, 4 items per subtest) in adolescents. A sample item for measuring cognitive empathy is: "I can easily tell how others are feeling." A sample item for measuring affective empathy is: "when a friend is scared, I feel afraid." A sample item for measuring sympathy is: "I feel sorry for someone who is treated unfairly."

Mercer and colleagues (Mercer, 2004; Mercer, Maxwell, Heaney, and Watt, 2004; Mercer, McConnachie, Maxwell, Heaney, and Watt, 2005) developed the Consultation and Relational Empathy (CARE) instrument for administration to patients to assess their doctors' or health care providers' empathic engagement in clinical encounters. This instrument includes 10 items; each is answered on a 5-point Likert scale (1 = Poor, 5 = Excellent). A sample item is, "How good was the doctor at being interested in you as a whole person." Data in support of validity of the instrument and a Cronbach's alpha coefficient of 0.92 have been reported by the test's authors (Mercer, Maxwell, Heaney, & Watt (2004). We developed an instrument for measuring perception of patients of their clinician empathy (The Jefferson Scale of Patient Perception of Physician Empathy [JSPPPE]) that will be described in Chap. 7.

There are a few review articles about empathy-measuring instruments. For example, Yu and Kirk (2009) identified 20 empathy measures used in nursing research and concluded that none of the reviewed measures was psychometrically robust. Hemmerdinger, Stoddart, and Lilford (2007), based on their systematic review of the literature, identified 36 empathy-measuring instruments, but only eight demonstrated evidence in support of their validity, internal consistency, and reliability. To assess the psychometric qualities of empathy-measuring instruments that were developed for administration to the general population, Lima and Osorio (2021) reviewed 50 studies in which 23 such empathy-measuring instruments were used (including the EQ, IRI, Questionnaire of Cognitive and Affective Empathy, and TEQ). They concluded that the instruments have limitations, especially in terms of validity. Thus, none can be nominated as a gold-standard instrument. There are other instruments, described by their authors as measures of empathy; however, either no convincing evidence has been presented to support their psychometrics, or they have not been used by other researchers except their own authors.

Physiological and Neurological Indicators of Empathy

Some social psychologists have studied empathy by using physiological measures, such as heart rate, skin conductance, palmar sweating, and vasoconstriction, as indicators of understanding other people's distress (Goldstein & Michaels, 1985; Stotland et al., 1978). Although most of these physiological measures are likely to be free of a social desirability response bias, they seem to be indicative of a person's emotional reaction to another person's distress. Such physiological reactions are more likely to be akin to sympathy than to empathy. Correspondingly, they may not be appropriate for the measurement of cognitively defined empathy in patient care.

Recently, functional brain imaging methods (e.g., fMRIs and PET scans) have been used as indicators of brain activity in individuals experiencing empathy (Carr, Iacoboni, Dubeau, Mazziotta, & Lenzi, 2003; Wicker et al., 2003). In addition to advancements in functional brain imaging, the discovery of the mirror neuron system activated by observing another person in pain or performing an act (see Chap. 13) is, I believe, the beginning of a promising approach to quantifying neurophysiological manifestations of empathy in future research (see Chap. 13 for more detailed discussion).

Relationships Among Measures of Empathy

The results of studies attempting to determine correlations among different measures of empathy have not been encouraging. For example, Jarski, Gjerde, Bratton, Brown, and Matthes (1985) tested a group of medical students and found no significant correlations among the Empathy Scale (Hogan, 1969), the Empathic Understanding subtest of the Relationship Inventory (Barrett-Lennard, 1962), or the Empathic Understanding in Interpersonal Processes Scale (Carkhuff, 1969).

Another study with registered nurses examined correlations among four measures of empathy (Layton & Wykle, 1990). The results showed that Carkhuff's Empathic Understanding in Interpersonal Processes Scale was moderately correlated ($r = 0.25$) with Layton's Empathy Test but was not correlated with the Empathic Understanding subtest of Barrett-Lennard's Relationship Inventory. In addition, LaMonica's Empathy Construct Rating Scale was not correlated with Layton's Empathy Test but was moderately correlated ($r = 0.37$) with Carkhuff's Empathic Understanding in Interpersonal Processes Scale and highly correlated ($r = 0.78$) with the Barrett-Lennard's Empathic Understanding subtest of the Relationship Inventory.

In a review article, Chlopan et al. (1985) reported the findings of studies on the validity and reliability of several measures of empathy, including Mehrabian and Epstein's Emotional Empathy Scale and Hogan's Empathy Scale. They argued that both of these scales seem to measure two different aspects of empathy. As its name indicates, the Emotional Empathy Scale is more likely to measure the affective aspects of empathy, or general emotional arousability (Mehrabian et al., 1988), whereas the Empathy Scale is more likely to measure role-taking ability, a cognitive aspect of empathy. Chlopan and colleagues also reported that the subscales of the IRI seem to tap both the emotional (e.g., Personal Distress subscale) and the cognitive (Perspective Taking subscale) aspects of empathy.

The intercorrelations among these empathy measures are often weak and inconsistent and, in most cases, nonsignificant or negligible (Bohart, Elliot, Greenberg, & Watson, 2002; Gladstein & Associates, 1987). One reason for these inconsistent findings is that different instruments tap different aspects of empathy based on different definitions of the concept. Although these instruments can have potential value in particular situations, none can be recommended as the best for all patient-care situations (Bennett, 1995). With the exception of the Perspective Taking subscale of the IRI, the contents of the other instruments described in this chapter do not reflect the cognitive conceptualization of empathy adopted in this book (see Chap. 6). Thus, their face validity (and content validity) would be questionable when empathy is conceptualized as a predominantly cognitive attribute in the context of patient care advocated for in this book.

A Need for an Instrument Specifically Designed to Measure Empathy in Patient Care

A measure that assesses empathy in patient care—particularly in medical and surgical treatment—needs to be more specific than the instruments I have described in this chapter so far. Because of the findings on the decline of empathy during health professions education (see Appendix A), and changes evolving in the market-driven health care systems that hamper clinician–patient relationships, the empirical study of empathy in health care education and practice is both important and timely. Among prerequisites to empirical research on empathy in the health professions education and the practice of patient care are (1) an operational definition of the concept (see Chaps. 1 and 6), and (2) a psychometrically sound instrument for quantifying the concept of clinical empathy in the context of health professions education and patient care. In 2000, in response to a need for a psychometrically sound instrument to measure empathy in the context of patient care, our research team in the Asano-Gonnella Center for Research in Medical Education and Health Care at Jefferson (now Sidney Kimmel) Medical College developed an instrument specifically designed to measure clinical empathy among students and practitioners in the health care professions. This scale will be described in detail in Chap. 7.

Recapitulation

Several instruments exist that claim to measure empathy in children and adults. The three frequently used instruments intended to measure empathy in adults—Hogan's Empathy Scale, Mehrabian and Epstein's Emotional Empathy Scale, and Davis's IRI—were developed for administration to the general population. The examination of their contents suggests that they do not tap the essence of clinical empathy in the context of health professions education and patient care. In other words, their face and content validities are questionable in the context of health professions education and patient care. Recently, functional brain imaging technology that has been used to address brain activities in interpersonal relationships has emerged as a promising path for measuring empathic engagement. I suspect that the findings of most of the studies in which the instruments described in this chapter were used are questionable in addressing empathy issues in the context of patient care. The reason is that the content of most of the items in the self-reported instruments, described in this chapter, taps on feeling the pain and suffering of others (described as emotional or affective empathy, synonymous to sympathy and arousability) rather than empathic understanding in patient care (e.g., cognitive/clinical empathy, respectively) which has a different consequence in patient care (see Chaps. 1 and 6). Thus, there was a need for an instrument specifically developed to measure clinical empathy in the context of patient care which will be described in Chap. 7.

Part II
Empathy in Health Professions Education and Patient Care

Chapter 6
A Definition and Key Features of Clinical Empathy in Patient Care

Clinical study amounts to the study of one person by another, and dialogue and relationship are its indispensable tools.

—(George L. Engel, 1990, p. 15)

Abstract

- Clinical empathy in the context of health professions education and patient care is addressed in this chapter with regard to the World Health Organization's (WHO) definition of health, consistent with the notion of a biopsychosocial paradigm of health and illness.
- Clinical empathy is defined as a predominantly cognitive attribute that involves an understanding of the patient's experiences, concerns, pain and suffering, and perspectives, combined with a capacity to communicate this understanding and an intention to help. The four key features used in the definition of clinical empathy (i.e., cognition, understanding, communication, and an intention to help) are elaborated, and a suggestion is made to make a distinction between cognition and emotion, between understanding and feeling, and between empathy and sympathy because of their different consequences in patient outcomes.
- An abundance of cognitively defined empathic engagement, because of its cognitive nature, is always beneficial in the context of patient care, whereas excessive sympathetic involvement (akin to emotional empathy), because of its affective nature, can be detrimental to both the clinician and the patient, leading to exhaustion and burnout in clinician and dependency in patient.
- In the context of patient care, clinical empathy bonds the patient and the health care provider together, whereas emotional empathy (synonymous with sympathy) blinds them to objectivity and reason. Thus, efforts should be made to maximize

M. Hojat, *Clinical Empathy*, https://doi.org/10.1007/978-3-031-87413-0_6

clinical empathy and regulate emotional empathy or sympathy for optimal patient outcomes.
- To achieve optimal patient outcomes, communication of understanding in empathic engagement between clinician and patient must be reciprocal, confirming the patient's significant role in empathic engagement and in the outcomes of patient care.

Introduction

We cannot scientifically study empathy in patient care unless an agreement exists concerning its definition and unless a psychometrically sound instrument is available to measure the defined concept. The descriptions of empathy presented in Chap. 1 provide a framework for the definition and conceptualization of clinical empathy in the context of health professions education and patient care. I begin in this chapter by describing the definition of health proposed by the WHO and briefly describe the biopsychosocial paradigm of health and illness. Then I offer a definition of clinical empathy in patient care and elaborate on the definition's key features and their implications for patient outcomes.

The World Health Organization's Definition of Health and a Biopsychosocial Paradigm

The constitution of the WHO (1948, p. 1) defines health as, "*a state of complete physical, mental, and social well-being, and not merely an absence of disease or infirmity.*" This definition is consistent with the biopsychosocial paradigm of illness in medicine (Engel, 1977, 1990; Hojat, Samuel, & Thompson, 1995). Generally, human infirmity can be viewed from two different perspectives: biomedical and biopsychosocial.

The *biomedical* paradigm of disease, postulated by the German physician Robert Koch and the French scholar Louis Pasteur, although still valid for some diseases, presents an incomplete picture of infirmity suffered by humankind. This "microbe hunting" model of disease (DeKruif., 1926) has a more limited scope than the triangular *biopsychosocial* paradigm of illness (Engel, 1977, 1990; Hojat et al., 1995; Ray, 2004). In the biopsychosocial paradigm, the targeted treatment of an affected organ is replaced by curing the whole patient, who is viewed as a system of being, always in relation to the biological, psychological, and social elements interacting closely with one another in a functional system (see Chap. 14 for a discussion of the systems theory). Because of its limited scope, the biomedical model can neither describe the underlying interpersonal reasons for the victories in overcoming human illnesses (Frenk, 1998; McKinlay & McKinlay, 1981) nor explain the health-promoting effects of human connections, including empathic physician–patient engagement in health and illness.

In addition to considering the importance of pathophysiological determinants of infirmity, in the biopsychosocial paradigm of health and illness, psychological, social, and interpersonal factors are taken into consideration as well (Engel, 1977, 1990). This paradigm of health and illness attests that curing occurs when the science of medicine (the biomedical and pathophysiological aspects of disease) and the art of medicine (the psychological, social, and interpersonal aspects of illness) merge into one unified system of patient care. Empathy is a key element in the systemic holistic care.

The art of medicine, according to Blumgart (1964), consists of skillfully applying the science of medicine in the context of human relationships to maintain health and ameliorate illness. The unit of observation in the art of medicine is the individual person in relation to psychological, social, and cultural factors, whereas the unit of observation in the science of medicine is the affected organ or the pathophysiology of disease. Empirical evidence is available to support the art and science of medicine dichotomy in clinical competence (Hojat, Paskin et al., 2007).

The science of medicine in the treatment of diseases and the art of medicine in the curing of illnesses are not independent entities; they supplement one another (Peabody, 1984). As Peabody (1984, p. 814) pointed out, "Treatment of disease may be entirely impersonal, but the care of the patient must be completely personal." Considering that the clinician–patient relationship is an indispensable tool in clinical situations to achieve better patient outcomes (Engel, 1990), health care professionals should pay attention not only to the biomedical aspects of disease but to the psychosocial factors of illness as well (Spiro, 1992). Treating pathophysiological indicators of disease may not necessarily require as much empathy as is required in curing the biopsychosocial factors of a patient's illness in a holistic approach (Novack, 1987; Novack, Epstein, & Paulsen, 1999).

Definition and Key Features of Clinical Empathy in Patient Care

Empathy in patient care has been characterized as arising "out of a natural desire to care about others" (Baron-Cohen, 2003, p. 2). Gianakos (1996, p. 135) referred to empathy in patient care as "the ability of physicians to imagine that they are the patient who has come to them for help." Greenson (1967, p. 367) described empathy in patient care as follows: "I have to let a part of me become the patient, and I have to go through her [his] experience *as if* I were the patient." (Remember the "as if" condition in Rogers's definition of empathy described in Chap. 1.)

The notion of an empathic relationship with the patient was elegantly described in a statement attributed to Sir William Osler (1932): "It is as important to know what kind of man [sic] has the disease, as it is to know what kind of disease has the man." This quotation is often attributed to Osler, as cited in White, 1991, p. 74; it also is attributed to Hippocrates, as cited by Ray, 2004, p. 30.) In any case, this statement best describes the biopsychosocial paradigm in which science and the art of medicine are complementary. To Larson and Yao (2005, p. 1105) empathy is the royal road to treatment and "a symbol of the health care profession." Engaging in empathic relationships makes physicians/clinicians more effective healers and makes their careers more satisfying. Freud (1958a) suggested that empathy is not only a factor in enhancing the clinician–patient relationship; it also provides a condition for correct interpretation of the patient's problems. Therefore, empathy is valuable both in making accurate diagnoses and in achieving more desirable treatment outcomes. Both the patient and the physician benefit from empathic engagement. This topic will be discussed in more detail in Chap. 8.

Definitions of the key concepts in research serve as a common language to understand the nature of the concepts under study. Although not all experts may agree on all aspects of any definition, at least some agreement should exist on the key features of a definition; otherwise, research based on a vague concept obviously will prove to be fruitless. By considering the various descriptions and features of empathy that were described in Chap. 1 and by taking into account the specific nature of clinical empathy in the context of patient care and its implications for optimal patient outcomes, we proposed the following definition of clinical empathy in the context of patient care (Hojat, 2016; Hojat et al., 2001, 2002, 2009; Hojat, Erdmann, & Gonnella, 2014; Hojat, Spandorfer, Louis, & Gonnella, 2011):

> Empathy in the context of patient care is a predominantly *cognitive* (rather than an affective or emotional) response that involves an *understanding* (rather than feeling) of pain and suffering, experiences, concerns and perspectives of the patient, combined with a capacity to *communicate* this understanding, and an *intention to help*.

The four key terms in this definition are printed in *italics* to underscore their significance in the construct of empathy in the context of patient care. We developed this definition after a comprehensive review of the literature (Hojat et al., 2001, 2002) and a careful consideration of the factors that contribute to positive patient outcomes. Our original intention was to present a working definition that would clarify the key ingredients we believed were conceptually relevant to empathy in the health professions education and in patient care to provide a framework for quantifying the defined concept by developing an instrument with which to measure empathy in the context of the health professions education and patient care (the instrument will be described in detail in the next chapter). Also, in our definition we intended to make a distinction between empathy and sympathy in the context of patient care. Our deliberate choice of the four key ingredients in the definition of empathy—*cognition*, *understanding*, *communication,* and *intention to help*—needs some elaboration.

Mercer et al. (2004, p. 700) suggested a somewhat similar characterization of empathy in clinical context that "involves an ability (i) to understand the patient's situation, perspective and feelings (and their attached meanings); (ii) to communicate that understanding and check its accuracy; and (iii) to act on that understanding with patients in a helpful (therapeutic) way."

Cognition

Our research team viewed empathy as a predominantly cognitive (rather than an emotional) attribute based on a belief that in patient care situations, empathy emerges as a result of mental activities that are facets of cognitive information processing (described in Chap. 1). Such facets include reasoning and appraisal, which are the basis of clinical judgment. Although cognitive mental processing (a key feature of empathy) can lead to positive patient outcomes, overwhelming emotion (a key feature of sympathy, see Chap. 1) can impede the optimal outcomes by obscuring objectivity in clinical judgments.

Cognition and emotion, although seemingly related, have different qualities independent of their joint appearance (Lazarus, 1982). Experienced therapists tend to respond to patients' distress with cognitive rather than emotional feedback. For example, an analysis of the interpersonal responses between Carl Rogers and his patients showed that approximately two-thirds of his responses were referred to as cognitive as opposed to emotional reactions (Tausch, 1988).

The distinction between cognition and emotion (and correspondingly, between empathy and sympathy) may not seem as important in situations where patient care is not a primary consideration. In the context of patient care, however, such a distinction must be made in clinical encounters because of the different implications and consequences in patient outcomes. Clinicians should feel their patients' feelings only to the extent necessary to improve their understanding of the patients without impeding their professional judgment (Starcevic & Piontek, 1997). It is not essential for clinicians to experience their patients' feelings, pain, and suffering to an overwhelming degree. Emotional overinvolvement is a feature of sympathy, not empathy (Olinick, 1984). However, for the purpose of more accurate diagnoses, it is essential for physicians to understand (as opposed to feel), as much as possible, their patients' feelings and concerns.

The notions of "detached concern," "compassionate detachment," "affective distance," "exhaustion," and "professional burnout" have been mistakenly used to describe the limits of empathic engagement in clinician–patient relationships (Blumgart, 1964; Halpern, 2001; Jensen, 1994; Lief et al., 1963). However, linking those notions to empathy is a grave mistake. They are indeed most relevant to sympathetic involvement (not empathic engagement) in patient care, based on the definitions of empathy and sympathy (see Chap. 1).

Ayra (1993) suggested that physicians' dissociation from patients' emotions can help them to retain their mental balance. Farber, Novack, and O'Brien (1997) reported that although medicine is a profession characterized by caring and empathy, it has also been characterized throughout history as aspiring to "objective detachment." This is possible when emotional involvement in clinician–patient encounters is restrained. However, *complete* emotional detachment has its own perils in the context of patient care (Friedman, 1990). As described in Chap. 1, emotion is acceptable to some extent, and sometimes it is difficult to distinguish when emotion ends and cognition begins in the context of patient care. The controversy about "detached concern" in clinician–patient encounters arises from confusion about the nature and meaning of empathy and sympathy. Maintaining an affective distance to avoid emotional overinvolvement (a feature of sympathy) makes the physician's clinical judgment more objective, but cognitive overindulgence (a feature of empathy) can always lead to a more accurate judgment. Objectivity when making clinical decisions can be better achieved by avoiding emotional overinvolvement, which clouds clinical judgment (Koenig, 2002).

It is difficult to be highly emotional and objective at the same time (Wispe, 1986) because excessive emotion in patient care can interfere with the principle of objectivity when making diagnostic decisions and choosing treatments (Blumgart, 1964; Gladstein, 1977; Spiro, 1992). Perhaps one reason why physicians are advised not to treat close family members who have serious health problems is the notion that excessively sympathetic feelings toward close family members can impede clinical objectivity (Aring, 1958). Indeed, the professional guidelines on the treatment of immediate family members in the American Medical Association's Code of Ethics (Section E-8.19) state that "Professional objectivity may be compromised when an immediate family member of the physician is the patient; the physician's personal feelings may unduly influence his or her professional medical judgment, thereby interfering with the care being delivered."

Borgenicht (1984) suggested that in performing certain procedures, physicians must maintain a certain degree of emotional distance from the patient because overwhelming emotional involvement may prevent them from making objective decisions at times of crisis. Too much affect impedes effective communication between physician and patient, whereas an abundance of understanding facilitates it. Brody (1997) suggested that the real danger to the physician's effectiveness lies in sympathetic overengagement with the patient. Issues such as dependency, exhaustion, burnout, compassion fatigue, and vicarious traumatization (Figley, 1995; Linley & Joseph, 2007), which are often mistakenly attributed to empathic engagement in patient care, are indeed the results of sympathetic over engagement, which is overwhelming to the health care providers and their patients. This speculation was confirmed in a large-scale study of board-certified practicing physicians in Argentina (Gleichgerrcht & Decety, 2013) that found compassion fatigue, burnout, and secondary traumatic job-related stress were closely associated with personal distress (which is a feature of emotional empathy, analogous to sympathy). In a study of 562 physicians in China (Ye, Zhong, Hua, & Li, 2024), it is reported that "empathic fatigue" (measured from a quality of life instrument) can lead to physicians' considering resigning. However, in Chaps. 6 and 14 I have indicated that compassion (empathy) fatigue could be the results of emotional empathy (analogous to sympathy) not cognitive (clinical) empathic engagement with patients. To the best of my knowledge, no credible empirical study has confirmed a positive correlation between a validated measure of clinical empathy (e.g., JSE) and burnout or exhaustion. The issue needs further empirical scrutiny.

Lief and Fox (1963) introduced the concept of "detached concern" in the medical education literature to prevent emotional overengagement (certainly different from empathic engagement) between physicians and patients. In contrast, no one has ever expressed concern about excess in understanding (or empathic understanding). An "affective distance" between physician and patient is desirable not only to avoid an intense emotional involvement, which can jeopardize the principle of clinical neutrality, but also to maintain the physician's personal durability (Jensen, 1994). Empirical evidence suggests that physicians who had difficulty regulating their emotions were likely to experience more exhaustion and a lower sense of accomplishment (Gleichgerrcht & Decety, 2013). Bloom (2016), without acknowledging the consequential outcomes, asserts that "empathy is a negative in human affairs" (p. 13). Because excessive emotions (different from cognition and understanding) can obscure the physician's judgment concerning the patient's predicament, Freud (1958b) proposed that to achieve better therapeutic outcomes, clinicians must put aside all of their human sympathies (not empathies).

For practical reasons, a distinction between cognition (a major ingredient of empathy) and emotion (a major ingredient of sympathy) is important; it has implications for determining the contents of the items in instruments intended to measure empathy in the context of patient care (see Chap. 7) and for developing educational programs to regulate sympathy, maximize empathy, and assess their consequences in clinical outcomes. The amenability to change will vary for cognitive and emotional behaviors. Cognitive attributes (e.g., empathy) are more prone to change as a result of educational programs than are emotional responses (e.g., sympathy).

Understanding

Understanding others' feelings and behaviors is central to human survival (Keysers & Perrett, 2004) and a key ingredient of empathic engagement in the clinician–patient relationship (Levinson, 1994). Patients' perception of being understood, according to Suchman, Markakis, Beckman, and Frankel (1997), is intrinsically therapeutic because it helps to restore a sense of connectedness and support. Empathy in patient care is built on the central notion of connection and understanding (Hudson, 1993; Sutherland, 1993). Because being understood is a basic human need, the physician's understanding of the patient's physical, mental, and social needs, in itself, can fulfill that need. Accordingly, we proposed elsewhere that "when an empathic relationship is established, a basic human need is fulfilled" (Hojat, Gonnella, Mangione, Nasca, & Magee, 2003, p. 27).

According to Schneiderman (2002, p. 627), "the better we understand them [the patients], the closer we come to discovering the true state of affairs, and the more likely we will be able to diagnose and treat correctly." Understanding of the patient's perspective was considered an essential element of physician–patient communication by a group of medical education experts in a Kalamazoo, Michigan, conference held in 1999 (Makoul, 2001). A specific feature of understanding in the physician–patient relationship is the ability to stand in a patient's shoes (knowing that the shoes belong to someone else) and to view the world from the patient's perspective without losing sight of one's own personal role and professional responsibilities. With this background in mind, we decided to consider "understanding" (rather than "feeling") as a keyword in the definition of empathy in the context of patient care.

Accuracy of understanding is another topic of discussion in clinical empathy research. As Rogers (1975, p. 4) advised clinicians, "perhaps if we wish to become a better therapist, we should let our clients tell us whether we are understanding them accurately." In general, the accuracy of understanding depends on the strength of the empathic relationship and the feedback mechanisms. Because the accuracy of understanding is an issue that may be a subject of debate, clinicians should occasionally verify the degree to which their understanding is accurate by *communicating* with the patient—another essential ingredient of empathy in patient care that will be discussed in the following section.

Communication of Understanding

Communication of understanding is indeed a behavioral aspect of empathic engagement in patient care. According to Carkhuff (1969) and Chessick (1992), the central curative aspect of clinician–patient relationships rests not only on the clinician's ability to understand the patient but also on his or her ability to communicate this understanding back to the patient. Reynolds (2000), and Diseker and Michielutte (1981) included communication of understanding as a feature of empathy in clinician–patient relationships. Carkhuff (1969, p. 315) indicated that "[empathy is] the ability to recognize, sense, and understand the feelings that another person has associated with his (her) behavioral and verbal expressions and to accurately communicate this understanding to him or her." Similarly, Reynolds (2000, p. 13) defined empathy as "an accurate perception of the client's world and an ability to communicate this understanding to the client."

Communication of understanding also is a key feature in LaMonica's description of empathy: "Empathy…involves accurate perception of the client's world by the helper, communicating this understanding to the client, and the client's perception of the helper's understanding" (LaMonica, 1981, p. 398). Truax and Carkhuff (1967, p. 40) described empathy as involving the ability to sense the client's "private world" and to communicate this understanding in "a language attuned to the client's current feelings." A physician who has an empathic understanding of the patient but does not communicate such an understanding would not be perceived as an empathic physician (Bylund & Makoul, 2005). According to Branch and Malik (1993), there are windows of opportunities in clinical encounters for expressing mutual understanding when patients describe emotional, personal, and family concerns. Physicians must capture these moments of "potential empathic opportunities" (Suchman et al., 1997) to express their understanding of patients' concerns.

An important aspect of communication in patient care is the notion of "reciprocity" or "mutuality" (Makoul, 1998; Miller, 2002; Raudonis, 1993). Although the idea that empathy involves mutual understanding is not widely discussed in empathy research (Bennett, 2001), it must be regarded as an essential ingredient of empathic engagement in patient care. Mutual understanding generates a dynamic feedback loop that is helpful not only in strengthening empathic engagement but also in making a more accurate diagnosis and thus providing better treatment. It is important to note that mutual understanding and reciprocal feedback during verbal and nonverbal exchanges indicate that both clinician and patient must play an active role to enhance empathic engagement. Without such features, empathic engagement cannot fully develop.

Physicians should let their patients know that their health problems and their psychosocial concerns are fully understood. It is also desirable for a patient to confirm the physician's understanding. By using a coding system (Empathic Communication Coding System), Bylund and Makoul (2005) reported that most patients do provide physicians with potential empathic opportunities. Applying their coding system, physicians' reactions to these potential opportunities were recorded on a 7-point scale (0 = physician ignores the empathic opportunity, 6 = physician makes an explicit statement to express understanding of the patient's concerns). They found that more than 80 % of physicians could detect the opportunities and reacted either by confirmation, acknowledgment, or pursuing or elaborating the issues of concern. The patient's belief concerning the physician's understanding reinforces the empathic engagement between the two. The following statements represent some simple approaches to the communication of empathic understanding: "I understand your feelings. You have gone through a lot of difficulties"; "I can see how being in a cast would make you helpless" (the expression of empathic understanding approach); "I can understand why this problem is so difficult for you" (the validation approach); "I understand your problem very well because I went through a similar situation" (the self-disclosure approach); "I want to make sure that I understand your concern. Let me rephrase it this way …" (the rephrasing approach); "It is saddening to have that kind of feeling" (sympathy); or "This reminds me of the story of …" (the metaphorical approach) (Matthews, Suchman & Branch, 1993; Mayerson, 1976).

Mutuality generates a belief in the patient that not only enhances the empathic relationship but also has a mysteriously beneficial effect on clinical outcomes (Hudson, 1993). Although the mechanism of the positive effect of mutuality in understanding is not well understood, one could speculate that the beneficial outcomes are attributable to greater satisfaction with the health care provider, to better compliance with treatment, or to such psychological factors as reduced anxiety, enhanced optimism, and perceptions of social support, which are activated in mutually understood interpersonal relationships. The reciprocal communication can help to remove the constraints of physician–patient relationships because, as a golden rule in interpersonal relationships, when constraints diminish, people begin to reveal their secrets.

Intention to Help

Intention to help is another specific feature of empathic engagement in patient care. Decety and Jackson (2006) described empathy as the capacity to understand and respond to the needs of others. Understanding in itself does not necessarily imply that the individual is compelled to help. However, readiness to respond to another person's call for help is indeed synonymous with the intention to help. Such intention in patient care often derives from altruistic motivation, making it different from the empathy of, for example, a sales agent, whose understanding of potential consumers often rests on egoistic motivation for personal gain. This feature of empathic engagement in patient care is consistent with the golden ethical principle of medical practice that the best interest of the patient must be of primary consideration.

Empathy Versus Sympathy in Patient Care

A large number of empathy researchers have failed to make a distinction between empathy and sympathy and used the terms interchangeably. A clear distinction between these two terms, as indicated before, is utterly important in patient care. The conceptual confusion and interchangeable use of "empathy" and "sympathy" may not cause a serious problem in social psychology, but separating the two in the context of patient care is important. In social psychology, both empathy and sympathy can lead to a similar outcome (e.g., prosocial behavior), albeit for different behavioral motivations.

A prosocial behavior induced by empathic understanding is more likely to be elicited by a sense of altruism (Hojat, Spandorfer et al, 2011). A prosocial behavior prompted by sympathetic feelings, however, is more likely to be triggered by a self-serving motivation to reduce the observer's personal distress. In patient care, the two constructs must be distinguished because, in that context, they lead to different outcomes. For example, Nightingale, Yarnold, and Greenberg (1991) showed that in simulated conditions empathic physicians, compared with their sympathetic counterparts, used resources appropriately by ordering fewer laboratory tests, had less preference for unwarranted patient intubation, and did not perform cardiopulmonary resuscitation for an excessively long time. In an empirical study, we showed that it is possible to differentiate empathic and sympathetic responses to patient care and test the validity of such responses (Hojat, Spandorfer et al., 2011).

Empathy Bonds, Sympathy Blinds

Our definition of clinical empathy in the context of patient care as a predominantly *cognitive* attribute implies that it involves understanding another person's concerns. Sympathy as an *emotional* reaction implies that it involves feeling another person's pain and suffering. Some researchers have described two types of empathy: "cognitive empathy" and "emotional empathy" (e.g., Davis, 1983). Davis (1994) described cognitive empathy as "attempts to entertain the perspective of others" (p. 17) and "the capacity for role taking" (p. 29). However, he described emotional empathy (synonymous to sympathy) as "a tendency to react emotionally to the observed experiences of others" (Davis, 1994, p. 55). Others have also described emotional empathy in terms of vicarious empathy (Mehrabian & Epstein, 1972).

To understand the operational definition of a concept, researchers must not only describe specific features of the concept but also take into consideration the clinical relevance of the features (Morse & Mitcham, 1997). Our definition of clinical empathy in the context of patient care is close to Davis's description of cognitive empathy, whereas our conceptualization of sympathy is somewhat similar to Davis's description of emotional empathy and analogous to Mehrabian and Epstein's (1972) vicarious empathy. The distinction between cognitively defined empathy and affectively defined empathy (or sympathy) has important implications for both health professions education and health care research. As I discussed before, it can be speculated that, in the context of patient care, cognitively defined empathy almost always leads to positive clinical outcomes, whereas sympathy in excess, due to its emotional nature, can be detrimental to objectivity in clinical decision making. In addition, clinical empathy can lead to professional growth, career satisfaction, and optimal clinical outcomes, whereas sympathy can lead to unhealthy patient–physician dependency, professional burnout, compassion fatigue (Figley, 1995), exhaustion, and vicarious traumatization (Linley & Joseph, 2007). These speculations await empirical verifications.

If my assumptions (see Chap. 1) that (1) the relationship between clinical empathy and positive clinical outcomes is linear (that is, the outcomes progressively become better as a function of an increase in empathic engagement), and (2) the relationship between sympathy and clinical outcomes resembles an inverted *U* shape (similar to that between anxiety and performance in which performance can enhance by a limited degree of anxiety, but decline by excessive anxiety) are confirmed, then the following outcomes would be expected. (1) Abundance of empathy is always beneficial in patient care; (2) sympathy—to a limited extent—is beneficial, but excessive sympathy is detrimental to patient outcomes. In other words, for more optimal patient outcomes, empathy must be maximized, but sympathy must be optimized or regulated.

Soenens, Duriez, Vansteenkiste, and Goossens (2007) confirmed that past studies generally ignored the distinction between empathy and sympathy (or cognitive and emotional empathy, respectively). I agree, and take it as a justification for my repeated reminder of differences between empathy and sympathy throughout this book, which may seem redundant. However, I have deliberately placed the emphasis on this distinction in several pertinent occasions, because I believe that such differentiation is extremely important in clinical empathy research and in the context of patient care, but has been benignly neglected in that context. This failure is certainly not inconsequential in empathy research outcomes in patient care (see Chaps. 1 and 3) and particularly for exploring the neurological underpinnings of empathy as a separate entity from sympathy (see Chap. 13).

In summary, the distinction made by Solomon (1976) between the wisdom of "understanding" against the treachery of "emotion" with regard to the differences between empathic and sympathetic engagements in clinician–patient relationships can be translated into the following statement that "*empathy bonds, sympathy blinds!*"

Recapitulation

The triangular biopsychosocial paradigm of health and illness, consistent with the definition of health in the WHO's constitution, suggests that empathic engagement in clinician–patient encounters should lead to improvement in physical, mental, and social well-being. The distinction between cognition and emotion/affect and their corresponding features in empathy and sympathy has important implications for the health professions education, effects on patient outcomes, and explorations of their neurological roots. Empathy, due to its cognitive nature, is always beneficial to patient outcomes; thus, attempts must be made to maximize empathic engagement in patient care. However, sympathy in excess, because of its emotional nature, can be detrimental to the patient and health care provider; thus, it is desirable to regulate or optimize sympathy to prevent dependency, exhaustion, and professional burnout.

Chapter 7
The Jefferson Scale of Empathy: A Unique Instrument for Measuring Clinical Empathy

If anything exists, it exists in some amount,
If it exists in some amount, it can be measured.

—(E. L. Thorndike, 1926, p. 38)

Abstract

- To measure clinical empathy in the context of health professions education and patient care, we developed an instrument, known as the *Jefferson Scale of Empathy* (JSE), based on the belief that empathy-measuring instruments which were developed for the general population could not embrace the essence of clinical empathy.
- This chapter describes the steps taken in the development and psychometrics of the JSE. The evidence is presented in support of the JSE's validity (face, content, construct, criterion-related, predictive, convergent, and discriminant) and reliability (Cronbach's alpha coefficient in support of internal consistency and test–retest reliability in support of score stability).
- The significant relationships observed between JSE scores, clinical competence, and patient outcomes demonstrate the efficacy of this psychometrically sound instrument for measuring clinical empathy in the context of health professions education and patient care.
- The general findings on the JSE's psychometrics and measurement properties in samples of students and practitioners in a variety of health professions disciplines and in multiple countries with differing education systems and cultures suggest that the instrument can serve as a sound measure of clinical empathy among medical students (S-Version), students in the other health professions (HPS-Version), and practitioners in the health professions including physicians (HP-Version).

M. Hojat, *Clinical Empathy*, https://doi.org/10.1007/978-3-031-87413-0_7

- The JSE has a broad international reputation, having been translated into 63 languages and used in over 93 countries. It remains the only psychometrically sound instrument developed specifically for administration to health professions students and practitioners with strong psychometric support provided by both its author and a large group of national and international researchers.
- Further research is needed to continue investigating the relationship between scores on the JSE and pertinent outcomes such as clinical competence, accuracy of diagnosis, patient compliance, reduced risk of malpractice claims, and patient outcomes in various settings, health professions disciplines, and cultures. Further research should be undertaken to develop national norms and cutoff scores on the JSE to identify high and marginal scorers in health professions students and practitioners of different disciplines in different countries.

Introduction

Historic Background

The *Jefferson Empathy Project*, initiated at the turn of this century, is indeed an offshoot of the *Jefferson Longitudinal Study of Medical Education* (Gonnella, Callahan, Veloski, DeSantis & Hojat, 2022), which is the most comprehensive, extensive, and uninterrupted longitudinal study of medical students and graduates maintained in a single medical school for more than half a century. The Jefferson Empathy Project was initially supported, in part, by a grant from Pfizer Medical Humanities Initiative to study personal qualities of physicians-in-training and in-practice that are associated with clinical competence.

At the initiation of the Jefferson Empathy Project, professionalism in medicine was emerging as a hot topic in medical education and patient care. Several factors contributed to the shift of attention toward professionalism in medical education and patient care. For example, a concern was growing about overreliance on computer-based diagnostic and therapeutic technology that could limit students' and practitioners' vision of the importance of the human factor in patient care. This chain of events led to a trend that prompted a paradigm shift in health professions education and patient care. Training empathic physicians/clinicians has gained momentum in pursuit of reclaiming the altruistic image of caring doctors/healthcare providers of bygone days and regaining the reputation of medicine as providing caring services.

An extensive review of the literature did not uncover a workable definition of professionalism in medicine; thus, we conceptualized professionalism as arrays of personal qualities—beyond acquisition of factual and medical knowledge, and different from procedural skills that contribute to clinician competence and patient outcomes (Veloski & Hojat, 2006). Also, in our literature search, as we learned more about professionalism in medicine, we noticed that empathy was a frequently mentioned core element of professionalism (Veloski & Hojat, 2006). However, we were unable to find a workable definition of clinical empathy in the context of patient care. In addition, we could not find a content-specific and context-relevant instrument to measure clinical empathy. Obviously, no credible empirical research could be undertaken without an operational definition of the concept and a psychometrically sound instrument to measure it. The historical ambiguity associated with the term clinical empathy (see Chaps. 1 and 6), the lack of a valid and reliable instrument to measure it (see Chap. 5), and the dearth of empirical research on the topic prompted me to embark on a journey to an uncharted terrain of clinical empathy.

Although empathy has been described in the literature as the most frequently mentioned attribute of humanistic care (Linn, DiMatteo, Cope, & Robbins, 1987), the available empathy-measuring instruments, which were mostly developed for administration to the general population, did not adequately grasp the essence of the construct of clinical empathy (Evans, Stanley, & Burrows, 1993). Thus, no psychometrically sound instrument was available to specifically measure clinical empathy among health professions students and clinicians. None of the instruments described in Chap. 5 were specific enough to capture the essence of clinical empathy. In more technical terms, none of those instruments had "face" and "content" validity in the context of health professions education and patient care.

Given the aforementioned limitations, more than two decades ago our research team at Jefferson, now Sidney Kimmel Medical College, recognized the need for an instrument that could enable researchers to undertake empirical research to assess clinical empathy in professional development of students and practitioners. It also needed to enable researchers to investigate changes in clinical empathy, study group differences, and examine correlates, antecedents, development, and outcomes of clinical empathy in different stages of training, different health professions disciplines, and various practices. In response to this need, we developed our clinical empathy-measuring instrument. Originally designed for administration to medical students and physicians (Hojat, Mangione, Nasca et al., 2001) and entitled the *Jefferson Scale of Physician Empathy* (JSPE), it was subsequently modified (partly in respond to demands from potential users) to be applicable to not only medical students and physicians, but also to a broader population of health professionals-in-training and in-practice (Hojat, Gonnella, Nasca, Mangione, Vergare, & Magee, 2002). Thus, it was renamed the *Jefferson Scale of Empathy* (JSE). A brief description of the steps taken in developing and modifying the JSE is presented in the following sections.

Development of a Framework

To construct a test requires developing a framework for understanding the concept and its related elements that one intends to measure. This begins with a comprehensive review of the literature to explore conceptual frameworks, theoretical views, and empirical research on the topic and to identify behaviors that are relevant to the concept in question. To guide us in drafting items for the preliminary version of the instrument, in 1999, we began to search the Medline database for all studies published beginning in 1966 (the starting date in the Medline database) that would identify contexts and contents for assessing clinical empathy. Using "empathy" as a keyword in our search, we found 3541 published sources in English. Cross-searching with the terms "empathy" and "physician/medical student" resulted in 107 published entries. A review of these and other relevant references, most of which were cited in the original 107 entries, provided us with some ideas about what the contents of items in the preliminary version of the instrument should be to measure clinical empathy among health professions students and practitioners.

Drafting Preliminary Items Focusing on the Face Validity

The second step, subsequent to the review of the literature, was to draft preliminary items and examine the face validity of the drafted items. Face validity involves subjective judgments, usually by nonexperts, about the relevance of the content of the items to the concept being measured. We drafted 90 items for the preliminary version of the JSE that appeared to be relevant to clinical empathy in patient care and, therefore, seemed to have face validity.

The items in the preliminary version covered broad areas, such as understanding subjective experiences of the patients and their families; interpersonal relationships with the patients; attention to verbal and nonverbal signals in physician–patient communications; humor; appreciation of art, poetry, and literature; narrative skills; absorption in stories, music, plays, and movies; cognitive and affective sensitivities; emotional closeness and affective distance between physician and patient; objectivity in clinical decision making; clinical neutrality; clinicians' emotional expression and regulation of emotions; sentiments; imagination; tactfulness; perspective taking; role playing; and cues in verbal and nonverbal communications.

It is important to notice that during the process of examining the face validity of the items, a particular item may seem, at first glance, to be irrelevant to the topic. Consequently, including such an item must be justified. A convincing argument should support the inclusion of every item, in case a question is raised concerning the item's relevance to clinical empathy. We used the rational scale method of theory-based item selection (Reiter-Palmon & Connelly, 2000) for that purpose. For example, we included items related to an interest in literature and the arts based on the theoretical view that studying literature and the arts can improve a person's understanding of human pain and suffering (Herman, 2000; McLellan & Husdon Jones, 1996; Montgomery Hunter et al., 1995). Therefore, such an interest would be relevant to the capacity for clinical empathy. Another example was inclusion of an item about humor, based on the assumption that a clinician's sense of humor can reduce the stress perceived by the patient, thus contributing to an improved clinician–patient relationship (Yates, 2001). According to Martin (2007, p. xv), "humor is a ubiquitous human activity that occurs in all types of social interaction." Humor generally can reduce the harmful impact of stressful experiences (Martin & Lefcourt, 1983). Additional theoretical support for this proposition is based on observations that humor can reduce the restraints in clinician–patient relationships by relieving tension and reducing inhibitions (Lief & Fox, 1963). Also, a sense of humor has been listed as an element of professionalism in medicine (Duff, 2002). According to Golden (2002), humor is a "magical force" that detaches patients from their pain and suffering through the healing power of laughter. A popular movie based on the true story of the life of doctor Patch Adams beautifully depicted the role of humor in medical care. Thus, we included an item about sense of humor in the instrument.

In addition, we made every effort to incorporate components that were consistent with our conceptualization and definition of clinical empathy (see Chaps. 1 and 6). For example, because "understanding" is a key component of our definition, the word appears in approximately one-third of the items (seven items) in the final scale.

Examination of the Content Validity

In addition to face validity, examining the content validity of a new instrument is another important step in its development. Content validity involves the systematic examination of the instrument's contents, usually by experts, to confirm the relevance and representativeness of the items in covering the domains of behavior the instrument intends to measure (Anastasi, 1976). We probed the instrument's content validity to ensure that the instrument included a representative sample of the behaviors expected to fit within the framework of clinical empathy.

To examine the content validity of the preliminary version of the JSE, we used a version of the Delphi technique (Cyphert & Gant, 1970), which is usually used to obtain systematic and independent judgments from a group of experts. We mailed the preliminary version of the instrument to 100 full-time clinicians and academic physicians. A cover letter described the purpose of our study as the development of an instrument to measure clinical empathy among health professionals, such as physicians. The letter briefly described clinical empathy as an "understanding" of patients' experiences, emotions, pain, and feelings as opposed to sympathy, which was described as "feeling" of patients' pain, suffering, and emotions.

Respondents were asked to cross out any item they considered to be irrelevant to the measurement of clinical empathy, as described in the aforementioned brief definition. They were also asked to edit the remaining items for simplicity and clarity and to add new items they regarded as important to include in an instrument intended to measure clinical empathy in the context of patient care. The 55 physicians who responded offered suggestions, made editorial improvements, and provided additional comments. They also made recommendations about revisions, additions, and deletions.

During this stage of the study, we excluded all items from the preliminary version that five or more physicians had crossed out. We also incorporated appropriate editorial suggestions the respondents had made. After several iterations and revisions to ensure that the items reflected distinct and relevant aspects of clinical empathy in patient-care situations, 45 of the original 90 items were retained (Hojat, Mangione, Nasca, et al., 2001). It was this 45-item version of the instrument that was used in the next stage of development in preliminary psychometric analyses.

Preliminary Psychometric Analyses

For the purpose of a preliminary psychometric study, the 45-item instrument was administered to 223 third-year students at Jefferson (193 completed the instrument, an 86% response rate). Also, a group of 41 residents in the internal medicine program at Thomas Jefferson University Hospital and its affiliated hospitals completed the instrument.

Likert-Type Scaling

A 7-point Likert-type scale (1 = Strongly disagree, 7 = Strongly agree) was used to respond to each item in the 45-item instrument. We chose a Likert-type scale rather than a simple, dichotomous (Agree/Disagree, Yes/No) response format because Likert-type scales (Likert, 1932) provide a wider range of item scores, which allows for more variation and thus more precise discriminatory power (Oppenheim, 1992). Furthermore, a Likert scale usually yields a distribution that resembles a normal distribution (Likert, 1932) and results in numeric scores that can be treated as an interval scale of measurement. The underlying assumptions for using more powerful parametric statistical techniques would not be violated by the presence of a distribution approaching a normal distribution and an interval scale of measurement. We also chose a 7-point Likert-type scale, rather than the more common 5-point scale, because the two additional points could reduce respondents' tendency to consistently use the extreme points of the scale (Polgar & Thomas, 1988; Reynolds, 2000).

Factor Analysis to Retain the Best Items

Exploratory factor analysis (EFA) is a statistical method used to explore the underlying constructs associated with a set of items. Items that are highly correlated with one another would emerge under one factor (or a hypothetical construct). In addition, factor analysis can be used to reduce the length of an instrument by providing information to retain the items that have relatively high factor loadings (e.g., greater than |0.30|) under the important and meaningful factors (Gorsuch, 1974). Another type of factor analysis is used to test if the empirical relationships among a set of items (or variables) can be efficiently summarized by a theoretical model (a confirmatory factor analysis [CFA]).

To screen for the best items to include in the next version and thus reduce the length of the preliminary instrument, we used EFA with the data collected from 193 medical students for the 45-item instrument. We used principal component factor extraction (the most frequently used factor extraction method), followed by orthogonal varimax rotation. This type of mathematical rotation is frequently used to obtain a simpler factor structure and to produce independent (uncorrelated) factors.

The "Generic Version" of the Instrument

On the basis of the results of the EFA, we retained 20 of the 45 items in the generic (45-item) version of the instrument; the JSPE was later renamed the *Jefferson Scale of Empathy* (JSE) subsequent to making some slight modifications in the content for administration of the instrument to medical as well as other health professions students, and all practicing health professionals. Those 20 items had the highest factor structure coefficients (greater than 0.40) on the first extracted factor (grand factor). The eigenvalue (latent root) of this grand factor was 10.64, which was much higher than the eigenvalue for the next factor, 3.45. Eigenvalues indicate the importance of extracted factors in terms of the proportion of variance accounted for. A relatively large eigenvalue for the first factor is indicative of the factor's importance. A sudden drop in the magnitude of the eigenvalue and no significant decrease in the eigenvalues of subsequent factors are used to retain the substantial factors and disregard the trivial ones. This guideline is known as the "scree test" (Cattle, 1966). Because the sample size of 41 residents was insufficient (e.g., the ratio of the size of the sample of medical residents to the number of variables was less than 10; Baggaley, 1983), we did not perform a factor analysis for that sample. However, an examination of the patterns of inter-item correlations showed considerable similarities between medical students and residents (Hojat, Mangione, Nasca et al., 2001).

The item with the highest factor structure coefficient on the grand factor was "I believe that empathy is an important therapeutic factor in medical and surgical treatment." This item was regarded as an "anchor" with which to evaluate the other items by examining the magnitude and direction of correlations between the anchor item and the other items. In the generic version of the scale, 17 items with positive factor structure coefficients and positive and statistically significant correlations with the "anchor" item were directly scored on the 7-point Likert-type scale (e.g., 1 = Strongly disagree; 7 = Strongly agree). The other three items, which had negative factor

Table 7.1 Descriptive statistics for the generic version of the JSE

Statistics	Residents (n = 41)	Medical students (n = 193)
Mean	118	118
Standard deviation	12	11
Median (50th percentile)	119	117
Mode	119	112
25th percentile	110	111
75th percentile	126	126
Possible range[a]	20–140	20–140
Actual range[b]	88–140	87–139
Alpha reliability estimate	0.87	0.89

[a]The minimum and maximum possible scores

[b]The lowest and highest scores obtained by the samples

structure coefficients on the grand factor and also yielded negative correlations with the "anchor" item, were reverse scored (1 = Strongly agree, 7 = Strongly disagree). The descriptive statistics for the generic version of the two preliminary study samples of medical students and residents are reported in Table 7.1.

Construct Validity of the Generic Version

Construct validity refers to the extent to which a test measures the theoretical constructs of the attribute that it purports to measure (Anastasi, 1976). Factor analysis helps to determine whether the scale's dimensions (underlying factors) are consistent with the theoretical constructs of the concept one intends to measure. Therefore, using factor analysis to examine construct validity can reveal the major dimensions that characterize the test scores (Anastasi, 1976).

To investigate the underlying structure of the generic version, data collected from the medical students were subjected to principal component factoring with orthogonal varimax rotation. Four factors emerged, each with an eigenvalue greater than 1. An eigenvalue equal to or greater than 1 known, as the Kaiser's criterion (Kaiser, 1960), is often used to retain the most important factors. The four extracted factors accounted for 56% of the total variance. Ten items had factor coefficients greater than 0.40 on the first factor (eigenvalue = 7.56, accounting for 38% of the variance). We chose the magnitude of 0.40 as the minimum salient factor loading needed to assume a meaningful relationship between the item and the relevant factor (Gorsuch, 1974).

Assigning a title to a factor in factor analytic studies is a subjective judgment made according to the contents of the items with higher factor coefficients under the corresponding factor. Based on the contents of the ten items with the highest factor coefficients, the first factor was called a construct of “the physician’s view of patient’s perspective” (perspective taking). Five items had a factor coefficient greater than 0.40 on the second factor, which accounted for 7% of the variance (eigenvalue = 1.30). Based on the contents of items with high factor coefficients, this factor was entitled “feeling patient’s experiences” (compassionate care). Two reverse-scored items had factor coefficients greater than 0.40 on the third factor (eigenvalue = 1.14, accounting for 6% of the variance), which was entitled “ignoring emotions in patient care.” (This is the opposite pole of standing in a patient’s shoes.) Finally, two items had factor coefficients greater than 0.40 on the fourth factor (eigenvalue = 1.01, accounting for 5% of the variance), which was entitled “thinking like the patient.” According to Velicer and Fava (1998), a minimum number of three items per factor is required for a stable factor pattern. According to this criterion, the last two factors may not be as stable as the first two (residual factors).

Also, a relatively considerable change in the magnitude of the pre-rotational eigenvalue after extracting the first factor suggests that the first factor is the most salient and reliable among all other extracted factors. The factor structure of the generic version of the JSE is consistent with the multifaceted concept of empathy reported in the literature (Spiro, McCrea Curnen, Peschel, & St. James, 1993). Details regarding the factor analysis of the generic version of the JSE and a table of factor structure coefficients are reported elsewhere (Hojat, Mangione, Nasca et al., 2001).

Criterion-Related Validity of the Generic Version

Criterion-related validity involves an examination of the correlations between the test scores and selected criterion measures. One approach to criterion-related validation is to demonstrate significant correlations between scores on the instrument and conceptually relevant variables (convergent validity) accompanied by nonsignificant correlations with conceptually irrelevant measures (discriminant validity). Convergent and discriminant validities are concepts derived from the method introduced by Campbell and Fiske (1959), which was initially used in their analysis of the multitrait–multimethod matrix of correlations to describe a pattern of higher relationships among conceptually more relevant variables (convergent validity) than among conceptually less relevant variables (discriminant validity) in different methods of assessment.

We included the criterion measures listed in Box 7.1 in a questionnaire to examine the criterion-related validity of the generic version of the instrument. Criterion measures 1–6 were available for both samples of medical students and residents. The remaining 10 measures of personal attributes (items 7–16 in Box 7.1) were defined on the questionnaire and were answered on a 100-point scale. These criterion measures were available for the sample of students only. Respondents were asked to place a mark on the scale to identify the extent to which they perceived themselves as having each of those particular personal attributes. We also used scores of three subscales (Perspective Taking, Empathic Concern, and Fantasy of the Interpersonal Reactivity Index (IRI, Davis, 1983) described in Chap. 5). We did not use the Personal Distress scale of the IRI for two reasons: We wanted to reduce the length of the questionnaire and increase the response rate, and we thought that the Personal Distress scale was less germane to patient-care situations. The Pearson correlation coefficients between scores of the generic version of the instrument and all 16 criterion measures (in Box 7.1) are reported in Table 7.2. The correlations with the scores of the three scales of the IRI were statistically significant but moderate in magnitude.

Table 7.2 Correlations of scores of the generic version of the JSE with criterion measures

Criterion measures	Residents ($n = 41$)	Medical students ($n = 193$)
IRI subscales[a]		
Empathic concern	NA	0.41**
Perspective taking	NA	0.29**
Fantasy	NA	0.24**
Self-report (7-point scale)[b]		
Compassion	0.56**	0.48**
Sympathy	0.27***	0.33**
NEO PI-R personality facets[c]		
Warmth[c]	NA	0.33**
Dutifulness[c]	NA	0.24**
Faith-in-people (misanthropy)[d]	NA	0.12***
Self-report (100-point scale)[e]		
Empathy	NA	0.45**
Compassion	NA	0.31**
Trust	NA	0.27**
Sympathy	NA	0.26**
Tolerance	NA	0.25**
Personal growth	NA	0.15*
Communication	NA	0.13***
Self-protection	NA	0.11
Humor	NA	0.05
Clinical neutrality	NA	−0.05

* $p < 0.05$; ** $p < 0.01$; *** $p < 0.10$.

NA data were not available

[a]Subscales from the Interpersonal Reactivity Index (Davis, 1983)

[b]Single items

[c]Personality facets from the NEO PI-R (Costa Jr. & McCrea, 1992)

[d]Faith-in-People Scale (Rosenberg, 1957, 1965)

[e]Self-reported personal attributes on a 100-point scale

Box 7.1 Criterion Measures Used For The Validity Study

1. *Empathic concern*. A subscale of the IRI (Davis, 1983) (see Chap. 5).
2. *Perspective taking*. A subscale of the IRI.
3. *Fantasy scale*. A subscale of the IRI.
4. *Warmth*. A facet of personality (eight items) from the revised version of the NEO Personality Inventory (NEO PI-R©), a widely used instrument measuring the big five personality factors and their facets (Costa Jr. & McCrea, 1992). The inventory has been used in the USA with samples of both physicians and members of the general population. Physicians scored higher than the general population on Warmth (Hojat, Glaser, Xu, Veloski, & Christian, 1999). Also, positive female role models in medicine scored higher than the general population on this facet of personality (Magee & Hojat, 1998).
5. *Dutifulness*. A facet of personality from the NEO PI-R © (eight items). Both male and female positive role models in medicine scored higher than the general population on this facet (Magee & Hojat, 1998).
6. *Faith-in-people scale*. This scale was developed by Rosenberg (1957, 1965) and contains five items measuring one's degree of confidence in the trustworthiness of people (Robinson, 1978). A typical item is "Most people are inclined to help others."
7. *Global empathy*. Defined as "Standing in the patient's shoes in the experience of the illness."
8. *Global sympathy*. Defined as "Developing feelings for the patient's sufferings."
9. *Global compassion*. Defined as "Sympathy for the patient combined with the intention of doing good and a desire to help."
10. *Trust*. Defined as "Belief that patients report their illness experience honestly."
11. *Tolerance*. Defined as "The ability to evaluate a patient who shows offensive and self-destructive behavior without becoming judgmental or losing interest in helping."
12. *Personal growth (through interaction with the patient)*. Defined as "Learning and gaining reward through emotionally intense (either positive or negative) interactions with patients."
13. *Communication (of the understanding)*. Defined as "The capacity to reflect patients' emotions by providing some statements which validate the patient's feelings."
14. *Self-protection*. Defined as "Protecting one's self from being overwhelmed by patients' emotions and/or suffering."
15. *Humor*. Defined as "Ability to laugh with the patients about human foibles and absurdities related to their illness and treatment, as well as to offer appropriate jokes and lighter topics unrelated to illness."
16. *Clinical neutrality*. Defined as "Controlling expressions of emotional reactions to patients, whether their reactions are positive or negative."

Although statistically significant, the correlations between scores of the generic version and conceptually relevant variables—such as compassion, warmth, dutifulness, faith-in-people, trust, tolerance, personal growth, and communication—were not large in magnitude, possibly the result of the low reliability of the single items used as criteria. However, the fact that all these conceptually relevant criteria yielded positive and statistically significant correlations is consistent with our expectations, thus providing support for the "convergent" validity. Conversely, a lack of significant relationships between scores on the JSE and on personal attributes that seemed conceptually less relevant to empathy (e.g., self-protection and clinical neutrality) supported "discriminant" validity.

Sympathy overlapped with scores of the instrument to a limited degree, with correlations ranging from 0.27 to 0.33 (see Table 7.2). Self-reported empathy and compassion yielded the highest correlations with the scores of the generic version, with correlations ranging from 0.31 to 0.56 (see Table 7.2). These correlations provide evidence supporting the criterion-related validity of the generic instrument. (Details of these findings are reported elsewhere; Hojat, Mangione, Nasca et al., 2001).

The moderate magnitude of the correlations with the criterion measures suggests that empathy, as measured by the generic version of the instrument, can be regarded as a distinct personal attribute with a statistically significant but practically limited overlap with compassion, concern, sympathy, perspective taking, imagination, warmth, dutifulness, tolerance, personal growth, trust, and communication.

As shown in Table 7.2, the highest validity coefficients (> 0.40) were obtained for criterion measures of Empathic Concern (of the IRI), Compassion, and a single-item self-reported empathy (an indication of convergent validity), while the lowest nonsignificant validity coefficient (0.11) was obtained for the self-protection criterion measure (an indication of discriminant validity).

Internal Consistency Reliability of the Generic Version

The reliability of an instrument is an indication of the score precision in a single testing situation (internal consistency) or score stability in multiple testing situations. We studied the internal consistency aspect of the reliability by calculating Cronbach's alpha coefficient (Cronbach, 1951). The coefficient obtained was 0.89 for the sample of medical students and 0.87 for the sample of residents (Hojat, Mangione, Nasca et al., 2001). Reliability coefficients of these magnitudes are desirable for educational and psychological instruments (Anastasi, 1976).

Revisions to Develop Three Versions of the Jefferson Scale of Empathy

The generic version of the instrument was originally developed to measure medical students' orientations or attitudes toward empathic relationships in the context of patient care. However, there was a demand to use the instrument for administration not only to medical students, but also to physicians, other health professionals involved in patient care, and all health professions students other than medical students. Thus, we decided to slightly modify the content of the generic instrument so that three versions would be available: one version for administration to medical students (the S-Version, see Appendix B); a second version for administration to physicians and other practicing health professionals (the HP-Version; see Appendix C); and the third version for administration to students in all health professions disciplines other than medicine (the HPS-Version; see Appendix D).

The HP-Version was to be geared more toward the clinician's empathic behavior in patient encounters; the S-Version and HPS-Version were to reflect students' orientation or attitudes toward empathy in patient care. The content in the three versions was very similar with only minor modifications to make the items appropriate for the target groups. For example, the item in the S-Version that reads: "It is difficult for a physician to view things from patients' perspectives" was modified in the HP-Version to read as: "It is difficult for me to view things from my patients' perspectives," and it was modified as follows in the HPS-Version: "It is difficult for a health care provider to view things from patients' perspectives."

Revisions to Balance Positively and Negatively Worded Items

There were only three negatively worded (reverse-scored) items in the generic version of the instrument. Reverse-scored items are used in personality tests to disrupt aberrant responses (Paulhus, 1991; Weijters, Baumgartner, & Schillewaert, 2013) and to reduce the confounding effects of those unusual responses. The following three mechanisms often lead to invalid responses: (1) the "acquiescence response style" defined as a tendency to agree or disagree constantly with the test items (in the sociopolitical context, these individuals are called "yeasayers" or "naysayers"); (2) "careless responding" refers to random or inattentive responses to the test items regardless of their content; (3) "confirmation bias," a tendency to express beliefs that are consistent with the way in which the question is stated (Davies, 2003). For example, when a question is about extraversion, respondents tend to think about situations in which they are extraverted, and when the question is about introversion, respondents tend to think about situations in which they are introverted (Weijters, Baumgartner, & Schillewaert, 2013).

In the modified versions, a balance was maintained by making 10 items positively worded and the other 10 negatively worded. The positively worded items were directly scored according to their Likert weights (1 = Strongly disagree, 7 = Strongly agree), whereas the negatively worded items were reverse scored (1 = Strongly agree, 7 = Strongly disagree).

Revisions to Improve Clarity for an International Audience

Minor revisions also were made in the wording of a few items to improve their clarity for international audiences. For example, while researchers in Italy and Mexico were translating the instrument into Italian and Spanish, a question arose about the verbatim translation of the verb "touch" in the following item: "I do not allow myself to be touched by intense emotional relationships between my patients and their family members" (a negatively worded item). The symbolic meaning of "to be touched by" (to be affected or influenced by) was not apparent in the translated versions. Therefore, we revised this item by substituting "to be influenced" for "to be touched" to avoid confusion in translations in foreign languages.

Comparisons of the Generic and the Revised Versions

To study the effects of our modifications and revisions to the JSE, we administered the generic version (JSPE) and the JSE HP-Version to a group of 42 residents in internal medicine by using a crossover design; half the residents completed the HP-Version first and then the generic version, and the other half completed the two versions in the reverse order. The correlation between scores on the two versions was 0.85 ($p < 0.01$). We noticed an extremely slight nonsignificant trend toward improvement in the Cronbach's alpha coefficient reliability estimate of the HP-Version (an increase from 0.81 to 0.85). No significant change occurred in the descriptive statistics of the two versions. For example, the mean score on the generic version was 120.9 ($SD = 10.1$), and it was 120.2 ($SD = 10.7$) for the HP-Version. Data collected from medical students using the JSE S-Version showed descriptive statistics that were similar to those reported in Table 7.1 on medical students who completed the generic version. Similar data on the HPS-Version of the JSE have also been reported in nursing students (Fields, Mahan, Hojat, Tillman, & Maxwell, 2011) and pharmacy students (Fjortoft, Van Winkle, & Hojat, 2011) (see Appendix A).

We conducted studies to examine the psychometric characteristics of different versions of the JSE. For example, in the following study, we examined the psychometric properties of the HP-Version in a relatively large sample of practicing physicians. In the second study, we investigated the psychometric properties of the S-Version using a large sample of medical students.

Psychometrics of the JSE HP-Version

To study the psychometric and other aspects of the HP-Version, we mailed the JSE to 1007 physicians in the Jefferson Health System, affiliated with the Thomas Jefferson University Hospital in the greater Philadelphia area (postage-paid return envelopes were provided). After two follow-up reminders, 704 physicians completed and returned the questionnaire, a response rate of 70% (Hojat, Gonnella, Nasca, Mangione, Vergare, & Magee, 2002). A response rate of 70% is considerably higher than the typical rate of 52% reported for surveys mailed to physicians (Cummings, Savitz, & Konrad, 2001). However, some researchers have suggested that a response rate of at least 75% should be achieved for surveys mailed to professionals to ensure the representativeness of the sample (Gough & Hall, 1977). A comparison of respondents and nonrespondents failed to show any significant differences between the two groups with regard to the distribution of their specialties, providing support for the representativeness of the study sample regarding their specialties (Hojat, Gonnella, Nasca, Mangione, Vergare, & Magee, 2002).

To study the stability of scores on the HP-Version over time (test–retest reliability), 100 physicians who had completed the HP-Version were selected at random to receive a second copy of the instrument plus a letter thanking them for their participation and requesting that they complete the second copy of the scale to help us establish the scale's reliability. Of these, 71 physicians responded, and their scores on the two tests were correlated. The exact time interval between completion of the two tests could not be determined accurately because we did not ask physicians to specify the date on which they completed the survey. However, by examining the postmarks, we were able to reach a rough estimate of approximately 3–4 months as the testing interval. The test–retest reliability was 0.65 ($p < 0.01$) (Hojat, Gonnella, Nasca, Mangione, Vergare, & Magee, 2002).

Underlying Components (Factors) of the JSE HP-Version

We conducted an EFA to investigate the underlying components of the HP-Version. Three factors with eigenvalues greater than one emerged (4.2, 1.5, and 1.3) accounting for 21%, 8%, and 7% of the total variance, respectively (Hojat, Gonnella, Nasca, Mangione, Vergare, & Magee, 2002). The factor coefficients, the magnitudes of eigenvalues, and the proportions of variance are reported in Table 7.3. The 10 positively worded items had factor coefficients of at least 0.45 on factor 1 (shown in bold). This factor can be regarded as the grand component of the instrument, as the magnitude of its eigenvalue indicates. On the basis of the contents of items with high factor coefficients, the first factor can be titled "perspective taking," a component of the JSE that has been described as the core cognitive ingredient of empathy (Davis, 1994; Spiro et al., 1993) and as the stepping stone in empathic engagement (Jackson, Brunet, Meltzoff, & Decety, 2006; Jackson, Rainville, & Decety, 2006).

Table 7.3 Rotated factor loadings of items in the JSE HP-Version[a]

Items	Factors 1	2	3
1. An important component of the relationship with my patients is my understanding of their emotional status as well as that of their families	**0.70**	0.21	−0.08
2. I try to understand what is going on in my patients' minds by paying attention to their nonverbal cues and body language	**0.62**	0.06	0.23
3. I believe that empathy is an important therapeutic factor in medical and surgical treatment	**0.60**	0.28	−0.25
4. Empathy is a therapeutic skill without which my success in treatment would be limited	**0.58**	0.22	−0.16
5. My patients value my understanding of their feelings which is therapeutic in its own right	**0.58**	0.32	0.03
6. My patients feel better when I understand their feelings	**0.50**	−0.02	0.16
7. I consider understanding my patients' body language as important as verbal communication in caregiver–patient relationships	**0.48**	−0.18	0.30
8. I try to imagine myself in my patients' shoes when providing care to them	**0.46**	0.29	0.28
9. I have a good sense of humor that I think contributes to a better clinical outcome	**0.45**	−0.02	0.14
10. I try to think like my patients in order to render better care	**0.46**	0.20	0.25
11. Patients' illnesses can be cured only by medical treatment; therefore, affectional ties to my patients cannot have a significant influence on medical or surgical outcomes	0.17	**0.60**	−0.01
12. Attentiveness to my patients' personal experiences does not influence treatment outcomes	0.07	**0.59**	0.07
13. I try not to pay attention to my patients' emotions in history taking or asking about their physical health	0.02	**0.54**	0.02
14. I believe that emotion has no place in the treatment of medical illness	0.22	**0.50**	−0.03
15. I do not allow myself to be touched by intense emotional relationships between my patients and their family members	0.13	**0.44**	0.26
16. My understanding of how my patients and their families feel does not influence medical or surgical treatment	−0.03	**0.43**	0.14
17. I do not enjoy reading nonmedical literature or the arts	0.05	**0.37**	0.13
18. Asking patients about what is happening in their lives in not helpful in understanding their physical complaints	0.10	**0.37**	−0.12
19. It is difficult for me to view things from my patients' perspectives	0.10	0.05	**0.74**
20. Because people are different, it is difficult for me to see things from my patients' perspectives	0.17	0.20	**0.66**
Eigenvalues	4.2	1.5	1.3
Variance (%)	21	8	7

Responses were based on a 7-point Likert-type scale. Responses were reverse scored on items 11–20 (strongly agree = 1, strongly disagree = 7); otherwise, items were directly scored (strongly agree = 7, strongly disagree = 1)

[a]Items are listed based on the descending order of the magnitude of the factor structure coefficients within each factor. Values greater than 0.36 are in boldface

This major component is similar to the grand factor of "physician's view of the patient's perspective" that emerged in the generic version.

Factor 2 included eight of the negatively worded items with factor coefficients of at least 0.37. This factor can be regarded as a construct involving "compassionate care" according to the contents of the items (the positive pole of the contents of the items that were negatively worded but reverse scored). Conceptually, this construct is similar to the two factors that emerged in the generic version: "emotions in patient care" and "feeling patient's experiences." Finally, factor 3 included two other negatively worded items with high factor coefficients ($\geq$0.66) that can be called "standing in the patient's shoes" (the positive pole of the contents of the negatively worded but reverse-scored items). This is a trivial component that is similar to the factor "thinking like the patient," which emerged in the generic version.

These findings suggest that the factor structure of the JSE is consistent with the notion of the multidimensionality of empathy (Davis, 1983, 1994; Kunyk & Olson, 2001). In addition, the stability and the similarity between the factor structure and components across different samples (medical students and physicians) and across different versions (generic and revised) provide further support for the JSE's construct validity. A similar pattern of the factor structure was found by some other national and international researchers (see Appendix A).

Item Characteristics and the Corrected Item-Total Score Correlations of the HP-Version

The means of item scores on the HP-Version ranged from a low of 4.8 to a high of 6.5 on the 7-point scale (Hojat, Gonnella, Nasca, Mangione, Vergare, & Magee, 2002). This finding suggests that the physicians' responses to the items tended to be skewed toward the upper tail of the scale, although the distribution of their responses showed that the physicians actually used the full range of possible responses on all items. The standard deviations for the items ranged from 0.9 to 1.6 (Hojat, Gonnella, Nasca, Mangione, Vergare, & Magee, 2002). The corrected item-total score correlations were all positive and statistically significant ($p < 0.01$), ranging from 0.30 to 0.60 with a median correlation of 0.43. A similar pattern of findings was found by some other researchers (see Appendix A).

Descriptive Statistics and Reliability of the HP-Version

The descriptive statistics and the distribution of scores for the HP-Version are reported in Table 7.4. Also, the internal consistency aspect of reliability (Cronbach's alpha coefficient) was 0.81 for the sample of physicians, and the test–retest reliability coefficient was 0.65 (Hojat, Gonnella, Nasca, Mangione, Vergare, & Magee, 2002).

Table 7.4 Score distributions, percentiles, and descriptive statistics for the JSE HP-Version ($n = 704$ physicians)

Score interval	Frequency	Cumulative frequency	Cumulative percentage
≤75	3	3	<1
76–80	3	6	1
81–85	2	8	1
86–90	3	11	2
91–95	13	24	3
96–100	21	45	6
101–105	31	76	11
106–110	57	133	19
111–115	97	230	33
116–120	111	341	48
121–125	114	455	65
126–130	126	581	83
131–135	85	666	95
136–140	38	704	100
Mean		120	
Standard deviation		11.9	
25th percentile		113	
50th percentile (median)		121	
75th percentile		128	
Possible range		20–140	
Actual range		50–140	
Alpha reliability estimate		0.81	
Test–retest reliability[a]		0.65	

[a]Test–retest reliability is calculated for 71 physicians within an interval of approximately 3–4 months between testing

The reliability coefficients indicate that the HP-Version is internally consistent and its scores are relatively stable over time (see Table 7.4). A similar pattern of findings was reported by some other national and international researchers (see Appendix A).

Desirability of National Norms and Cutoff Scores

It would be desirable to develop norms based on representative national samples of physicians for comparative purposes or for evaluation of each individual physician's score (e.g., a female physician practicing family medicine) against the norm (e.g., percentile ranks) derived from a corresponding national sample (e.g., a national sample of female physicians in family medicine). Also, determining cutoff scores to identify those with marginal JSE scores could be helpful for assessment purposes. Obviously, the data reported in Table 7.4 cannot serve those purposes.

Psychometric Properties of the JSE S-Version

To examine the psychometrics and other measurement properties of the S-Version, we collected data from 2637 students who matriculated at Jefferson between 2002 and 2012 and completed the JSE S-Version at the beginning of medical school (orientation day, before they were exposed to formal medical education). There were 1336 (51%) women and 1301 (49%) men in this sample, which represented 94% of all matriculants during the 11-year study period ($n = 2802$). Frequency and percent distributions of the study sample by matriculation year and gender are reported in Table 7.5. Although the proportion of women varied from 46% (in year 2002) to 57% (in year 2006), no significant difference was found in gender composition in different matriculation years ($\chi^2_{(10)} = 9.8$, $p = 0.45$) (for more detailed report of this study, see Hojat & Gonnella, 2015).

Descriptive Statistics of the JSE S-Version

Means, standard deviations, medians, score ranges, skewness, and kurtosis indices for the entire sample and for matriculants of each year are presented in Table 7.6. As shown in the table, the JSE (S-Version) mean score for the entire sample was 114.3 ($SD = 10.4$), which varied from a low of 113.2 ($SD = 11.3$) for matriculants of 2009 to a high of 115.9 ($SD = 9.8$) for matriculants of 2004. Analysis of variance was used to test the significance of differences in mean scores of matriculants in different years. No statistically significant difference was observed ($F_{(10,2626)} = 1.2$, $p = 0.29$), meaning that students during the 11 years of this study period had similar

Table 7.5 Frequency and percent distributions of the study sample (2637 medical students) by matriculation year and gender

Matriculation year	Men, *n* (%)	Women, *n* (%)	Total, *n* (%)
2002	120 (54 %)	101 (46 %)	221 (100 %)
2003	105 (48 %)	113 (52 %)	218 (100 %)
2004	103 (46 %)	121 (54 %)	224 (100 %)
2005	126 (51 %)	121 (49 %)	247 (100 %)
2006	107 (43 %)	140 (57 %)	247 (100 %)
2007	132 (53 %)	116 (47 %)	248 (100 %)
2008	120 (51 %)	117 (49 %)	237 (100 %)
2009	111 (46 %)	128 (54 %)	239 (100 %)
2010	124 (49 %)	128 (51 %)	252 (100 %)
2011	125 (50 %)	127 (50 %)	252 (100 %)
2012	128 (51 %)	124 (49 %)	252 (100 %)
Total	1301 (49 %)	1336 (51 %)	2637 (100 %)

$\chi^2_{(10)} = 9.8$, $p = 0.45$ (nonsignificant)

Table 7.6 Means, standard deviations, range, skewness and kurtosis indices, and reliability coefficients (Cronbach's α coefficient) of the JSE S-Version by matriculating classes and summary results of statistical analysis

Matriculating class	*n*	Mean	SD	Median	Range	Skewness	Kurtosis	Cronbach α
2002	221	114.1	9.9	114	81–137	−0.24	0.04	0.80
2003	218	113.9	10.0	115	75–140	−0.44	0.52	0.79
2004	224	115.9	9.8	117	82–140	−0.35	0.12	0.78
2005	247	114.5	9.7	116	82–133	−0.66	0.46	0.78
2006	247	114.8	9.4	115	86–135	−0.46	0.19	0.75
2007	248	114.6	10.6	114	71–136	−0.47	0.74	0.81
2008	237	113.5	12.1	114	52–140	−0.92	2.66	0.84
2009	239	113.2	11.3	113	73–140	−0.28	0.05	0.84
2010	252	113.8	10.7	114	70–140	−0.62	0.88	0.81
2011	252	114.1	10.1	116	76–140	−0.57	0.79	0.79
2012	252	114.8	10.6	116	79–140	−0.65	0.90	0.81
Total	2637	114.3	10.4	115	52–140	−0.56	0.92	0.80

$F_{(10,2626)} = 1.2, p = 0.29$ (nonsignificant)

empathy scores at the beginning of medical school. These descriptive statistics are somewhat similar to most of those reported for medical students in the USA by other researchers (see Appendix A).

Skewness index is a measure of symmetry in score distribution. In a perfectly normal distribution, the skewness is close to zero. As shown in Table 7.6, the skewness index was negative for the entire sample (−0.56) and for each matriculating year (ranging from −0.92 for matriculants of 2008 to −0.24 for matriculants of 2002, with a median of −0.53). Negative skewness indicates that the peak of JSE score distributions tended to be to the right side of the distribution (bulk of data to the side of higher scores). However, the magnitudes of the skewness indices suggest that distributions were just moderately skewed (distributions with skewedness indices out of the −1 to +1 range are considered highly skewed).

Kurtosis is an index of the peak of score distribution. Higher values indicate a higher peak and lower values a flatter peak. Normal distributions have a kurtosis index close to three (mesokurtic); those greater than three are high-peaked distributions (leptokurtic), and those with kurtosis less than three are flatter peaked (platykurtic). The kurtosis for the entire sample was 0.93, ranging from a low of 0.04 (for matriculants of 2002) to 2.66 (for matriculants of 2008) with a median of 0.52 (Table 7.6). These findings indicate that the distributions of the JSE scores tend to be platykurtic (Hojat & Gonnella, 2015). Similar findings have been reported in other studies with medical and other health professions students (see Appendix A). Also, in a nationwide project in osteopathic medical education and empathy, we found similar descriptive statistics for a national sample of osteopathic medical students in the USA who completed the JSE S-Version at the beginning of medical school education (see Chap. 14; and Hojat, DeSantis, Shannon et al., 2018).

Internal Consistency Reliability of the JSE S-Version

We calculated Cronbach's α coefficient for the entire sample of medical students, which was 0.80, ranging from a low of 0.75 (for matriculants of 2006) to a high of 0.84 (for matriculants of 2008 and 2009) with a median of 0.80 (Table 7.6). These reliability coefficients were in the range of most JSE studies by other national and international researchers (see Appendix A). We found similar results in a national sample of osteopathic medical students in the USA who completed the JSE S-Version at the beginning of medical school education (see Chap. 14, and Hojat, DeSantis, Shannon et al., 2018).

Score Distributions and Percentile Ranks of the JSE S-Version

Frequency distributions of the JSE scores and percentile ranks for men, women, and the entire sample are presented in Table 7.7. As shown in the table, the mean, median, and standard deviation for the entire sample were 114.3, 115, and 10.4, respectively. Because we found significant gender differences on the JSE scores, we examined the score distributions for men and women separately (Hojat & Gonnella, 2015). Later in this chapter, I will discuss how the data reported in Table 7.7 can be used as "proxy" norms and for determining "tentative" cutoff scores.

Item Statistics of the JSE S-Version

Respondents used the full range of possible answers (1–7) for each item. Item mean scores ranged from a low of 3.6 (SD = 1.4) for this item: "Physicians should not allow themselves to be influenced by strong personal bonds between their patients and their family members" to a high of 6.5 (SD = 0.8) for this item: "Patients feel better when their physicians understand their feelings."

The corrected item-total score correlations ranged from a low of 0.13 (for the aforementioned item with the lowest mean score) to a high of 0.61 (for this item: "Physicians' understanding of the emotional status of their patients, as well as that of their families, is one important component of the physician–patient relationship"). The median item-total score correlation was 0.44. All correlations were positive and statistically significant ($p < 0.01$), which indicates that all items contributed positively and significantly to the total score of the JSE scale (for more detailed information, see Hojat & LaNoue, 2014). Item-total score correlations are reported in Table 7.8. A similar pattern of findings was observed in a nationwide project in osteopathic medical education and empathy, with large samples of osteopathic medical students in the USA (see Chap. 14; and Hojat, DeSantis, Shannon et al., 2018).

To address the discrimination power of each item, we calculated an item discrimination effect size index. For that purpose, we divided the total sample into two

Table 7.7 Frequency and percent distributions and descriptive statistics of scores on the JSE S-Version by gender

Score interval	Men ($n = 1301$)			Women ($n = 1336$)			Total ($n = 2637$)		
	Freq.	Cumulative freq.	Percentile ranks (%)	Freq.	Cumulative freq.	Cumulative %	Freq.	Cumulative freq.	Percentile ranks (%)
≤80	11	11	1	5	5	<1	16	16	<1
81–85	8	19	1	2	7	<1	10	26	1
86–90	22	41	2–3	1	8	1	23	49	2
91–95	48	89	4–7	21	29	2	69	118	3–4
96–100	87	176	8–13	56	85	3–6	143	261	5–10
101–105	136	312	14–24	89	174	7–13	225	486	11–18
106–110	214	526	25–40	165	339	14–25	379	865	19–33
111–115	252	778	41–60	258	597	26–45	510	1375	34–52
116–120	232	1010	61–78	279	876	46–65	511	1886	53–71
121–125	159	1169	79–90	221	1097	66–82	380	2266	72–86
126–130	91	1260	91–97	171	1268	83–95	262	2528	87–96
131–135	34	1294	98–99	56	1324	96–99	90	2618	97–99
>135	7	1301	100	12	1336	100	19	2637	100
Descriptive statistics									
Mean[a]		112.3			116.2		114.3		
Median		113			117		115		
Standard deviation		10.8			9.7		10.4		
Possible range		20–140			20–140		20–140		
Actual range		70–140			52–140		52–140		

[a] $t_{(2635)} = 9.9$, $p < 0.01$ for testing the null hypotheses that JSE mean scores for men and women are not different

Table 7.8 Rotated factor pattern for the JSE S-Version[a], item-total score correlations, and effect size estimates of item discrimination indices

Items[b]	Factors			Item-total score correlation*[c]	Discrimination index effect size[c]
	Factor 1	Factor 2	Factor 3		
• Patients value a physician's understanding of their feelings which is therapeutic in its own right (10)	**0.66**	0.02	0.01	0.55	1.3
• Physicians should try to stand in their patients' shoes when providing care to them (9)	**0.64**	−0.05	0.02	0.50	1.2
• Physicians should try to think like their patients in order to render better care (17)	**0.61**	−0.16	0.00	0.37	1.0
• Physicians' understanding of the emotional status of their patients, as well as that of their families is one important component of the physician–patient relationship (16)	**0.46**	**0.29**	0.00	0.61	1.4
• I believe that empathy is an important therapeutic factor in medical treatment (20)	**0.44**	**0.26**	−0.02	0.59	1.3
• Patients feel better when their physicians understand their feelings (2)	**0.44**	0.00	0.03	0.41	0.89
• Physicians should try to understand what is going on in their patients' minds by paying attention to their nonverbal cues and body language (13)	**0.40**	0.17	0.04	0.49	1.2
• Empathy is a therapeutic skill without which the physician's success is limited (15)	**0.36**	0.20	−0.04	0.44	1.2
• Understanding body language is as important as verbal communication in physician–patient relationships (4)	**0.30**	0.09	0.08	0.35	0.88
• A physician's sense of humor contributes to a better clinical outcome (5)	**0.29**	0.03	0.00	0.26	0.79
• Patients' illnesses can be cured only by medical or surgical treatment; therefore, physicians' emotional ties with their patients do not have a significant influence in medical or surgical treatment (11)	0.03	**0.59**	0.01	0.52	1.2

(*continued*)

Table 7.8 (continued)

Items[b]	Factors			Item-total score correlation[*c]	Discrimination index effect size[c]
	Factor 1	Factor 2	Factor 3		
• I believe that emotion has no place in the treatment of medical illness (14)	0.23	**0.54**	0.04	0.46	1.0
• Attentiveness to patients' personal experiences does not influence treatment outcomes (8)	0.01	**0.52**	0.05	0.48	1.1
• Asking patients about what is happening in their personal lives is not helpful in understanding their physical complaints (12)	0.03	**0.49**	0.00	0.44	1.0
• Physicians' understanding of their patients' feelings and the feelings of their • Patients' families do not influence medical or surgical treatment (1)	0.04	**0.49**	−0.09	0.35	0.94
• Attention to patients' emotions is not important in history taking (7)	0.01	**0.48**	0.09	0.43	1.0
• I do not enjoy reading nonmedical literature or the arts (19)	0.00	**0.25**	0.00	0.20	0.62
• Physicians should not allow themselves to be influenced by strong personal bonds between their patients and their family members (18)	−0.02	0.21	0.01	0.13	0.50
• Because people are different, it is difficult to see things from patients' perspectives (6)	−0.05	0.06	**0.75**	0.15	0.59
• It is difficult for a physician to view things from patients' perspectives (3)	0.06	−0.06	**0.68**	0.14	0.57

$^{*}p < 0.01$ for all of the reported correlations

[a]Principal component factor extraction with oblique rotation was used for approximately half of the sample ($n = 1380$) in the EFA, and the other half of the sample was used for the CFA to examine the three-factor model

[b]Items are listed by the order of magnitude of factor loadings within each extracted factor. Factor loadings equal to or greater than 0.25 are in bold. Numbers in parentheses represent the sequence of the items in the actual scale. Items were scored using a 7-point Likert-type scale. Half of the items are reverse scored

[c]These are partial correlations between score of each item and total JSE score by excluding the corresponding item score from the total score. Item-total score correlations and discrimination indices were calculated based on data for the entire sample ($n = 2612$). For calculation of the effect size estimates of discrimination indices, the item mean score for JSE high scorers (top 33%) was subtracted from the item mean score for JSE low scorers (bottom 33%), divided by the pooled standard deviation of the corresponding item

groups of approximately top-third high scorers on the JSE (score > 119, n = 835) and bottom-third low scorers (JSE score < 111, n = 857). For each item, we calculated the mean score difference between the top-third and bottom-third JSE scoring groups, divided by the pooled standard deviation of the item to calculate the item discrimination effect size index, similar to the Cohen's d (item discrimination effect size index = $M_{\text{top-third}} - M_{\text{bottom-third}}$)/pooled SD) (Hojat & LaNoue, 2014). The item discrimination effect size indices ranged from a low of 0.50 for the aforementioned item which showed the lowest item-total score correlation to a high of 1.4 for the abovementioned item with the highest item-total score correlation. The median effect size was 1.2 (see Table 7.8). Cohen (1987) suggests that the effect size values around 0.30 or lower are considered negligible, around 0.50 are moderate, and around 0.70 and higher are large and practically important. According to these operational definitions, the item discrimination effect size indices were all substantial and practically (clinically) important (Hojat & Xu, 2004). We found a similar pattern of findings in a national sample of osteopathic medical students in the USA who completed the JSE S-Version at the beginning of medical school education (see Chap. 14, and Hojat, DeSantis, Shannon et al., 2018).

Underlying Components of the JSE S-Version

For factor analytic studies we divided the medical student sample into two groups: (1) matriculants between 2002 and 2007 (n = 1380) whose data were used for EFA; and (2) matriculants between 2008 and 2012 (n = 1232) whose data were used for CFA. We used principal component factor extraction with oblique rotation in our EFA to reexamine the underlying components of the JSE. CFA was performed by using structural equation modeling (SEM), and several measures of model fit were evaluated, including root mean square error of approximation (RMSEA) (Arbuckle & Wothke, 1999) to confirm the latent variable structure of the JSE S-Version.

In almost all of the factor analytic studies of the JSE, orthogonal (varimax) rotation was used to obtain independent factors. In the present study, we used oblique rotation (promax) to allow correlations among the extracted factors and examine if the previously reported factor pattern in our study of physicians for the JSE HP-Version (Hojat et al., 2002c) would remain unchanged. We also limited the number of retained factors to three to make the findings comparable to the previously reported factor analytic study with physicians (Hojat et al., 2002c). Indeed, the scree test, used to determine the appropriate number of factors to retain before rotation, showed that the plot of the eigenvalues leveled off after the extraction of the third factor, supporting our decision to retain three factors for rotation. The Kaiser-Meyer-Olkin measure for sampling adequacy (MSA) was used prior to factor extraction, which resulted in an overall index of 0.86, supporting the adequacy of data for factor analysis. Also, the Bartlett's test for sphericity showed that the intercorrelation matrix was factorable ($\chi^2_{(190)} = 5332.5$, $p < 0.0001$).

The eigenvalues for the first, second, and third retained factors were 4.7, 1.6, and 1.4, respectively. The first factor, "Perspective Taking," included 10 items with relatively high factor coefficients of at least 0.28, accounting for 23% of the total variance. A sample item (with the highest factor coefficient) is "Patients value a physician's understanding of their feelings which is therapeutic in its own right." The Cronbach's alpha coefficient for items under this factor was 0.79.

The second factor, "Compassionate Care," included seven items with relatively high factor coefficients (>0.25), accounting for 8% of the total variance. A sample item is "Patients' illnesses can be cured only by medical or surgical treatment; therefore, physicians' emotional ties with their patients do not have a significant influence on medical or surgical treatment." This is a negatively worded item which is reverse scored. The Cronbach's alpha coefficient for items under this factor was 0.69.

The third factor, "Standing in the Patient's Shoes," included only two items with factor coefficients greater than 0.67, accounting for 7% of the total variance. A sample item is "Because people are different, it is difficult to see things from patients' perspectives" (reverse scored). The Cronbach's alpha coefficient for items under this factor was 0.68. One item had a low factor coefficient (0.21) on Factor 2. However, this item showed a significant item discrimination effect size index and yielded a statistically significant (but low in magnitude) item-total score correlation.

Summary results of the EFA are reported in Table 7.8. The general pattern of findings is similar to that in most other studies in the USA and abroad. For example, similarities in the factor pattern are observed in studies reported for physicians (Hojat, Gonnella, Nasca, Mangione, Vergare, & Magee, 2002) and nurses (Ward et al., 2009) in the USA; for samples of physicians in Italy (DiLillo, Cicchetti, Lo Scalzo, Taroni, & Hojat, 2009); and medical students in Iran (Shariat & Habibi, 2013), Korea (Roh, Hahm, Lee, & Suh, 2010), Japan (Kataoka, Koide, Ochi, Hojat, & Gonnella, 2009), Mexico (Alcorta-Garza, Gonzalez-Guerrero, Tavitas-Herrera, Rodrigues-Lara, & Hojat, 2005), South Africa (Vallabh, 2011), mainland China (Wen, Ma, Li, Liu, Xian, & Liu, 2013; Wen, Ma, Li, & Xian, 2013), Taiwan (Hsiao, Tsai, & Kao, 2012), Brazil (Paro, Daud-Gallotti, Tiberio, Pinto, & Martins, 2012), Austria (Preusche & Wagner-Menghin, 2013), and England (Tavakol, Dennick, & Tavakol, 2011a, 2011b). The two factors of "Perspective Taking" and "Compassionate Care" emerged in almost all factor analytic studies of the JSE. We found a similar pattern of the factor structure in a national sample of osteopathic medical students in the USA who completed the JSE S-Version at the beginning of medical school education (see Chap. 14; and Hojat, DeSantis, Shannon et al., 2018).

Confirming the Latent Variable Structure of the JSE S-Version

In CFA, all 20 items were modeled as functions of three underlying latent variables which emerged in the EFA and have been widely reported (see Appendix A). Maximum likelihood (ML) estimation was used. The regression coefficient for one item-to-latent variable path for each latent variable was set to 1.0 to scale the latent variable. Additionally, the variance of one error term (that is corresponding to item 6) was set to 0.0 to facilitate convergence of the ML estimation. Without this constraint, the model was inadmissible due to the negative error variance of item 3 (Kolenikov & Bollen, 2012).

We also evaluated a two-factor model, one which omitted the two items which comprise factor 3, "Standing in the Patient's Shoes." This was done because of the failure of the maximum likelihood of CFA to converge without constraining one error variance, which can indicate a mis-specified model (Kolenikov & Bollen, 2012), and the other CFA studies of the scale which modeled only two factors (Tavakol et al., 2011a, 2011b; Williams, Boyle, & Earl, 2013; Williams, Brown, Boyle, & Dousek, 2013 ; Williams, Brown, & McKenna, 2013). We compared the fit of this two-factor model to the fit of the three-factor model (Hojat & LaNoue, 2014).

Assessment of model fit was made through the use of several well-accepted metrics in structural equation modeling (SEM). First, the χ^2 test for the model was reviewed. In SEM, it is a measure of fit, rather than a test statistic, and desired values are small and nonsignificant. However, since χ^2 is sensitive to sample size, it is possible to obtain a large and significant value even when the fit of the model to the data is acceptable. To address this, a widely used "rule of thumb" was also evaluated—the ratio of the χ^2 to its degrees of freedom, which is suggested to reflect good fit at values <4.0 (Joreskog, 1993).

We also evaluated the adjusted "goodness-of-fit" index (AGFI), which indexes the proportion of the observed covariance matrix that is explained by the model-implied covariance matrix (Kline, 1998). The Tucker-Lewis Index (TLI) was used to compare the fitted model to a null model. Hu and Bentler (1998) recommend values > 0.95. Finally, the RMSEA for the structural model was evaluated. Hu and Bentler (1998) showed that a cutoff of 0.06 for RMSEA indicates a good model fit.

For model comparisons, an additional fit and incremental fit improvement metrics were used. The models were first compared to each other through the use of the χ^2 test for the significance of the difference in fit. The non-normed fit index (NNFI; also known as the TLI) was used to assess improvements in fit from model to model. The TLI normally results from SEM output as a comparison to a "null" model, but a version can be calculated for the improvement in fit between any two competing models. Hu and Bentler (1998) suggested that improvements in the TLI greater than 0.02 are of "substantive interest." See Fig. 7.1 for the measurement model structure of 20 variables and three correlated factors.

The two-factor solution did not indicate a good fit (RMSEA = .07, AGFI = 0.88); however, the three-factor CFA yielded a marginally good fit to the data; RMSEA = 0.05 and AGFI greater than 0.90. Both the χ^2 difference test and the TLI suggest that the three-factor model is a better fit than the two-factor model. Summary results for fit statistics are shown in Table 7.9.

Results of CFA support the three-factor model of the JSE and are in agreement with those reported in Iranian medical students (Shariat & Habibi, 2013) and British medical students (Tavakol et al., 2011a, 2011b). A satisfactory three-factor model fit was also achieved in Portuguese medical students after relaxing model restrictions

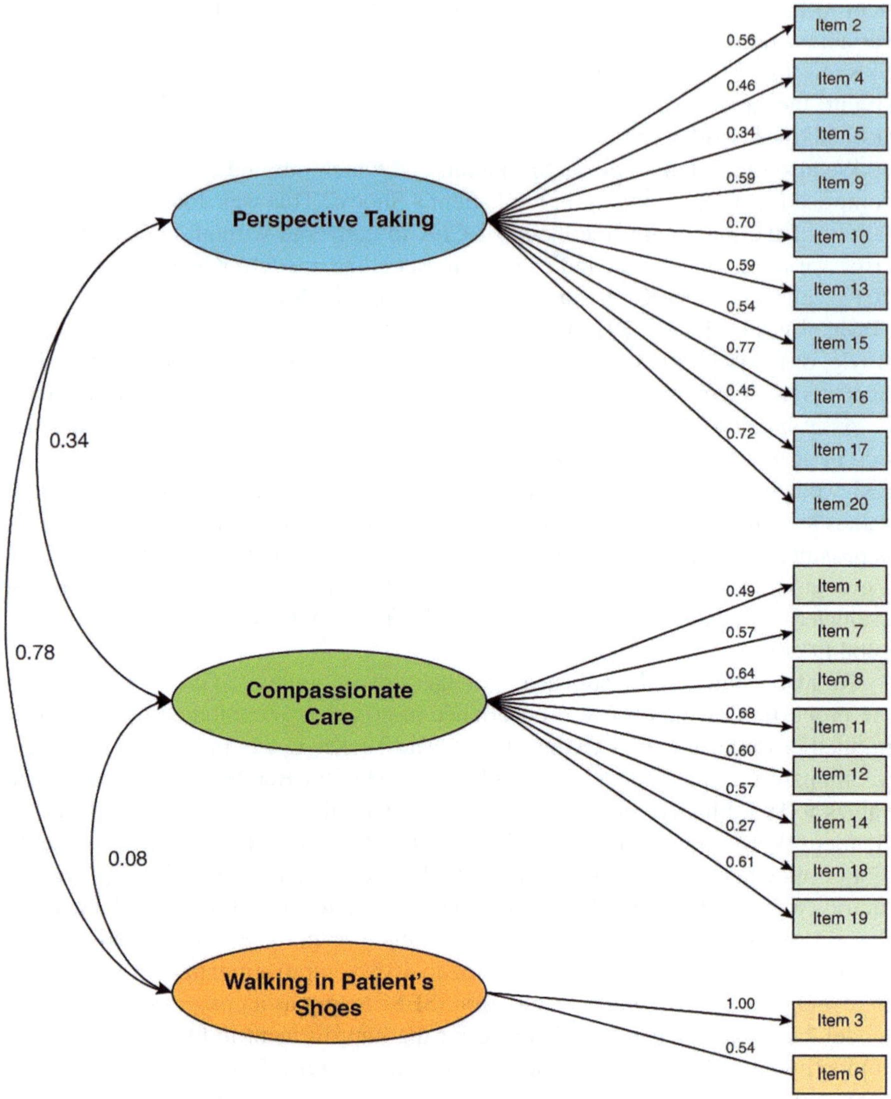

Fig. 7.1 Three-factor model (latent variable structure) of the Jefferson Scale of Empathy ($n = 1232$). 2014 *International Journal of Medical Education*. Reproduced with permission (Hojat & Lanoue, 2014)

(Magalhäes, Salgueira, Costa, & Costa, 2011). The two-factor model ("Perspective Taking" and "Compassionate Care") in Australian paramedic students (Williams, Boyle, & Earl, 2013; Williams, Brown, Boyle, & Dousek, 2013; Williams, Brown, & McKenna, 2013) partly resembles findings of the present study. Although we acknowledge that these findings overall are not definitive with regard to the structure of the instrument, we do not agree with suggestions made by some that a few JSE items should be excluded for a better latent variable structure model (Williams,

Table 7.9 Summary results of confirmatory factor analysis fit statistics ($n = 1232$)

Model	Parameters estimated	χ^2	*df*	χ^2/df	AGFI	TLI	RMSEA	AIC
Fitted three-factor model	42	887.87	168	5.28	0.93	0.89	0.05	971.87
Fitted two-factor model	36	984.51	135	7.29	0.88	0.843	0.071	
Difference		205.65	33*			0.47[a]		
Null model (one factor model)	20	6469.32	190	34.05	0.39	0.00	0.16	7468.25

* $p < 0.05$

[a]Calculated as recommended in Hu and Bentler (1998), this value represents a significant improvement in fit over the two-factor model

Boyle, & Earl, 2013; Williams, Brown, Boyle, & Dousek, 2013; Williams, Brown, & McKenna, 2013). First, deletion of items can cause an incompatibility problem in comparative research. Second, in most of the psychometric studies of the JSE (including our own study), significant item-total score correlations have been reported, suggesting that each item contributes significantly to the total score of the JSE. In addition, we showed that each item can discriminate substantially between high and low scorers of the JSE (Hojat & LaNoue, 2014).

Data in our study with 11 classes of allopathic medical students supported the previously reported findings on the reliability (Cronbach's α coefficient), underlying constructs, and confirmation of the latent variable structure of the JSE S-Version. In a national project with osteopathic medical students, we found similar patterns of results (see Chap. 14; and Hojat, DeSantis, Shannon et al., 2018). Also, similar results are reported in other studies with medical and other health professions students in the USA and abroad (see Appendix A).

Similarities in factor patterns of the JSE in different samples and countries indicate that the underlying components of the scale are relatively stable, regardless of variation in medical education system and culture. The three components of "Perspective Taking," "Compassionate Care," and "Standing in the Patient's Shoes," which emerged in our study and some other factor analytic studies of the JSE are consistent with the ingredients of empathy often reported in the literature. These underlying factors are also supportive of the pillars of empathic engagement in patient care, namely seeing with the mind's eye (e.g., Perspective Taking and Walking in Patient's Shoes) and listening with the third ear (e.g., Compassionate Care). Based on the findings from our own (Hojat & LaNoue, 2014; Hojat, DeSantis, Shannon, et al., 2018) and other CFA studies (Magalhäes et al., 2011; Shariat & Habibi, 2013; Tavakol et al., 2011a, 2011b), we recommend retaining all 20 items for comparability of the findings.

The psychometric properties of a complex attribute, such as clinical empathy, can be a function of several factors, including sociocultural, educational, and environmental factors. These necessitate a continued effort to examine psychometrics of the JSE in different sociocultural environments, populations, and translated versions of the instrument to ensure that the psychometric soundness of the JSE can be retained in a variety of settings. Such broad psychometric support would further add to the credibility of the JSE and increase the confidence of its users wherever it is applied.

Proxy Norm Data for the JSE S-Version

Data for a large sample of medical students from a single medical school ($n = 2637$) presented an opportunity for exploring the possibility of providing norm data and cutoff scores (Hojat & Gonnella, 2015). Because of the large sample from a large allopathic medical school—which is similar to other large medical schools in the USA with regard to its 4-year medical education curriculum, composition of student body, attrition rate, and career choices—the statistics reported in Table 7.7 can serve as proxy norm data for matriculating students in other US allopathic medical schools under the condition that descriptive statistics and score distributions of the JSE in those medical schools are not substantially different from data reported in Table 7.7. For example, a score of 120 on the JSE obtained by a male matriculant would place him in the 78th percentile, and the same score obtained by a female matriculant would place her in the top 65th percentile of the score distributions.

The score distributions and percentile ranks reported in Table 7.7 can be used as proxy norms for the purpose of comparing the relative rank of JSE scores of a medical student at matriculation (assuming that the score distributions and descriptive statistics of the medical school from which the JSE score is being compared are not substantially different from data reported in Table 7.7). For example, the JSE score of a male first-year matriculant to medical school "X" who falls between 131 and 135 would place him in the top 98–99 percentile, and a score of a female first-year matriculant from the same school who falls between 126 and 130 would place her in the 83–95 percentile (assuming similarities in descriptive statistics and score distribution of the JSE in medical school "X" with those reported in Table 7.7).

In a nationwide project in osteopathic medical education and empathy, we similarly developed national norms for osteopathic medical students who completed the JSE S-Version at the beginning of medical school education and at the end of each year of medical school (Hojat, Shannon, DeSantis, Speicher et al., 2019) (described briefly in Chap. 14).

Tentative Cutoff Scores for the JSE S-Version

To determine tentative cutoff scores of the JSE for the purpose of identifying high and low scorers among the entering medical students participating in the 11-year study (Hojat & Gonnella, 2015), we arbitrarily chose two points on the score distributions: one point was 1.5 standard deviations above the mean score (to identify the high scorers), and another point was 1.5 standard deviations below the mean score (to identify the low scorers). These cutoff points were separately calculated for men and women. Thus, the cutoff scores for identifying low and high scorers for men were ≤ 96 and ≥ 127; and ≤ 102 and ≥ 129 for women, respectively. These cutoff scores include approximately 7% of top scorers and 7% of bottom scorers in both men's and women's score distributions (Hojat & Gonnella, 2015).

We used a similar approach to identify high and low scorers in our nationwide project in osteopathic medical education and empathy for new matriculating students. The corresponding cutoff scores for low and high scorers were ≤ 96 and ≥ 131 for men, and ≤ 104 and ≥ 131 for women (Hojat, DeSantis, Shannon et al., 2018).

In our 11-year study of allopathic medical students (Hojat & Gonnella, 2015), we compared performance measures among high, moderate, and low JSE scorers by using the aforementioned cutoff scores. Results showed a consistent pattern of findings that the low JSE scorers, as compared to the moderate and high scorers, received lower average ratings on clinical competence in six third-year core clerkships in medical school (family medicine, internal medicine, obstetrics/gynecology, pediatrics, psychiatry, and surgery); and also on the residency program directors' ratings on the factors of the "art" and the "science" of medicine (Hojat, Paskin et al., 2007) given at the end of the first postgraduate training year. However, the results of analysis of variance indicated that the differences, while in the expected direction, were marginally significant for the ratings of clinical competence in the six third-year core clerkships ($F_{(2,2284)} = 2.57$, $p < 0.07$) (Hojat & Gonnella, 2015).

The tentative cutoff scores suggested in both allopathic and osteopathic samples are not definitive. We need data on well-validated criterion measures to examine the predictive validity of the cutoff scores. In particular, we also need more data from representative samples of allopathic medical schools at the national level to develop national norm tables (we have already undertaken such a nationwide project in osteopathic medical education and empathy in the USA, see Chap. 14; Hojat, DeSantis, Shannon et al., 2018; Hojat, Shannon, DeSantis et al., 2019), and to determine cutoff scores for male and female matriculants and students. Using a similar approach, national norm tables can also be developed in different countries; in different medical education systems; for students in other health profession schools; for male and female students; for physicians in different specialties; for the assessment of clinical empathy of applicants; for practicing clinicians; and for the development of professionalism. These ideas set an agenda for future research.

Additional Indicators of Validity of the JSE

The "Contrasted Groups" Method

Other indicators that support the validity of the JSE are based on the notion that a measuring instrument is valid when it can demonstrate group differences or relationships in the expected direction. The expectations are based on previous research, theories, and behavioral tendencies described in the literature. This approach, in which different groups are compared to examine whether the differences in their scores in clinical empathy are in the expected direction, is known as validation by the method of "contrasted groups" (Anastasi, 1976).

Expectation of Gender Difference on the JSE Scores in Favor of Women

In a majority of studies, women scored higher than men on measures of empathy in general and clinical empathy in particular (see Chap. 10, and Appendix A). Some authors have suggested that women's behavioral style is generally more "empathizing" than men's style (Baron-Cohen, 2003). Thus, we expected to find gender differences in favor of women on the JSE scores. Empirical confirmation of this expectation could be regarded as an indicator of the JSE's validity. Consistent with our expectation, in most studies in which the JSE was used, female health professions students and practicing health professionals obtained significantly higher JSE mean scores than their male counterparts. This pattern of gender difference in the JSE scores in favor of women has also been reported in most national and international studies (see Appendix A).

In our study of 11 entering classes (between 2002 and 2012) of Jefferson (described before in this chapter), we reexamined gender differences on the JSE for each entering class (Hojat & Gonnella, 2015). As reported previously, there were 1336 women (51%) and 1301 (49%) men in this sample (see Table 7.5). With one exception, women obtained substantially higher mean empathy scores than men in all of our comparisons for different matriculating classes, and the differences were statistically significant ($p < 0.01$ by *t*-test). The exception was the matriculating class of 2008 in which women's higher JSE mean score ($M = 114.8$, $SD = 12.3$) was not significantly different from that for men ($M = 112.2$, $SD = 11.9$) at the conventional level of statistical significance ($t_{(235)} = 1.6$, $p < 0.10$). This is consistent with the previous findings in which the JSE was used (Alcorta-Garza et al., 2005; Fjortoft et al., 2011; Hojat, Gonnella, Nasca, Mangione, Vergare, & Magee, 2002; Hojat, Mangione, Nasca et al., 2001). The effect size estimates of gender differences varied for different matriculating classes, ranging from a low of 0.21 (for the matriculating class of 2008) to a high of 0.57 (for the matriculating class of 2009). For the entire sample, the effect size estimate was 0.40 (Hojat & Gonnella, 2015). Means and standard deviations of the JSE scores by matriculation year and gender are reported in Table 7.10. Gender differences in favor of women have been reported in many national and international studies (see Appendix A). Also, in a nationwide study of clinical empathy among osteopathic medical students in the USA, female students, consistent with our expectation, obtained significantly higher mean scores on the JSE than their male counterparts (see Chap. 14; and Hojat, DeSantis, Shannon et al., 2018; Hojat Shannon, DeSantis, Speicher et al, 2019; Hojat, DeSantis, Shannon, Speicher et al., 2020).

Table 7.10 Gender differences on the JSE S-Version scores by matriculating classes

	Men		Women			
Matriculating class	*n*	*M* (SD)	*n*	*M* (SD)	*t*	Effect size[a]
2002	120	112.3 (10.1)	101	116.3 (9.3)	3.1**	0.41
2003	105	111.5 (10.8)	113	116.1 (8.6)	3.4**	0.46
2004	103	113.7 (9.6)	121	117.7 (9.6)	3.1**	0.43
2005	126	112.1 (10.2)	121	117.0 (8.6)	4.1**	0.52
2006	107	112.8 (9.2)	140	116.3 (9.3)	3.0**	0.37
2007	132	112.8 (11.7)	116	116.6 (8.6)	2.7**	0.40
2008	120	112.2 (11.9)	117	114.8 (12.3)	1.6***	0.21
2009	111	109.8 (11.5)	128	116.1 (10.3)	4.5**	0.57
2010	124	111.7 (10.8)	128	115.8 (10.4)	3.1**	0.38
2011	125	112.6 (11.0)	127	115.6 (9.0)	2.4*	0.30
2012	128	113.4 (10.9)	124	116.4 (10.2)	2.3*	0.28
Total	1301	112.3 (10.8)	1336	116.2 (9.7)	9.9*	0.40

Note: ** $p < 0.01$, * $p < 0.05$, *** $p = 0.10$

[a]Cohen's effect size estimate

Several plausible explanations have been given for gender differences in empathy, including social learning, genetic predisposition, evolutionary underpinnings, and other factors (Hojat, Mangione, Nasca et al., 2001; Hojat et al., 2002a, 2002b) (see Chap. 10 for more detailed explanations for gender differences on empathy).

Specialty Interest

Although clinical empathy is the backbone of the patient–clinician relationship in all specialties, there are some specialties that require a higher degree of empathic engagement because of the frequency of clinical encounters, broader consultations, and the provision of continuous care. Based on this, some medical education researchers have classified specialties into two broad categories of "people-oriented" and "technology- or procedure-oriented" specialties (Lieu, Schroeder, & Altman, 1989). The so-called people-oriented specialties often require long-term patient–physician relationship with continuous care. The patient–physician relationship (in people-oriented" specialties) often begins as office-based first-encounter health or illness appraisals; and includes preventive education or interventions; episodic and long-term comprehensive care of a wide variety of medical problems (e.g., family medicine, general internal medicine, pediatrics, plus obstetrics and gynecology, and psychiatry). The so-called "technology- or procedure-oriented" specialties do not often require long-term continuous care. They primarily involve specialized diagnostic or technical computer-based procedures (e.g., primarily hospital-based specialties such as anesthesiology, pathology, and radiology) and may include specialties that require performing highly skilled and specialized therapeutic techniques or procedures (e.g., surgery and surgical subspecialties), or providing episodic or long-term care of a limited number of medical problems that may include instrumentation and technical interventions with a mix of ambulatory and hospital-based practice (e.g., medical subspecialties such as cardiology, gastroenterology, and other nonprimary care specialties).

Due to the nature of the patient–physician interpersonal relationship, we expected that those physicians-in-training and in-practice interested in "people-oriented" specialties would outscore in clinical empathy those interested in "technology- or procedure-oriented" specialties. Out of 2637 entering medical students in our study sample, 75% (n = 1979) specified the specialty they planned to pursue after graduation from medical school (965 were interested in "people-oriented", 590 in "technology- or procedure-oriented," and 424 in other specialties). We compared the JSE scores of the three groups by using analysis of covariance to partial out the effect of gender (men = 0, women = 1). Summary results of statistical analysis are reported in Table 7.11.

Consistent with our expectation, those who were interested in pursuing "people-oriented" specialties obtained a significantly higher JSE mean score (M = 115.35) than their classmates who were interested in "technology- or procedure-oriented" (M = 112.34) and other specialties (M = 114.51) (adjusted $F_{(2,1973)} = 16.25, p < 0.001$). It is important to notice that the differences observed in this sample of entering medical students who completed the JSE prior to their formal medical education cannot be attributed to their exposure to medical education experiences and training. Instead, the baseline differences can be attributed to a personality attribute developed prior to medical school that prompted some to express interest in different specialties, even though some of these students might change their specialty choice during medical school (Forouzan & Hojat, 1993). The findings regarding higher JSE in those interested in "people-oriented" compared to those interested in "technology/procedure-oriented" specialties are in agreement with our previous research findings (Hojat et al., 2002b; Hojat, Zuckerman et al., 2005) and findings reported by others in the USA and abroad (Chen, Lew, Hershman, & Orlander,

Table 7.11 Means and standard deviations of the JSE S-Version by specialty and summary results of analysis of covariance

Specialty	n	M (SD)	F-ratio[a]	p
People oriented[b]	965	115.35 (9.9)	Adjusted $F_{(2,1975)} = 5.79$	<0.001
Technology oriented[c]	590	112.34 (11.02)	Unadjusted $F_{(2,1973)} = 16.25$	<0.01
Other[d]	424	114.51 (10.20)		

[a]Effect of gender was controlled by entering gender as a covariate in statistical analysis. Post hoc mean comparisons showed that technology-oriented < people-oriented; and technology-oriented < other specialties

[b]People-oriented specialties included family medicine, general internal medicine, general pediatrics, obstetrics and gynecology, and psychiatry

[c]Technology-oriented specialties included anesthesiology, pathology, radiology, surgery, and surgical specialties

[d]Other specialties included medical subspecialties, dermatology, emergency medicine, etc

2007; Chen, Kirshenbaum, Yan, Kirshenbaum, & Aseltine, 2012; Cheng et al., 2007; Kataoka et al., 2012; Voinescu, Szentagotai, & Coogan, 2009). These findings confirmed our expectation on specialty differences which provide support for the validity of the JSE.

It might be argued that differences in JSE scores at the beginning of medical school could be due to prior undergraduate education. However, in his master's thesis, Smolarz (2005) did not find a significant difference in the JSE scores among first-year medical students who majored in science and non-science disciplines as undergraduates. In other studies with nursing students (Fields et al., 2011; Ward et al., 2009), academic major prior to nursing school did not predict JSE scores in nursing school. Thus, it seems that undergraduate education has no significant link to clinical empathy in health professions students. However, in a large-scale study of osteopathic medical students in the USA, we observed that undergraduate background (majors) could have a significant effect of scores on the JSE only in preclinical components (the first two years) of medical school education (see Chap. 14, and Hojat, DeSantis, Shannon, Speicher et al., 2020).

Relationships with Pertinent Measures (Criterion-Related Validity)

Additional data in support of the criterion-related validity of the JSE include positive and significant correlations between scores of the JSE and measures of variables that are conceptually relevant to clinical empathy, no correlation with measures irrelevant to clinical empathy, and negative correlations with measures of attributes that are conceptually detrimental to empathic engagement in patient care. Numerous empirical studies have reported associations between scores of the JSE and several pertinent variables, including personal qualities.

Variables Conducive to Relationship Building

Empirical evidence showed that a number of personality attributes that are conducive to relationship building, thus relevant to clinical empathy, have been positively correlated with JSE scores, including: sociability (Hojat, Zuckerman et al., 2005); personality facets of Warmth and Dutifulness of the NEO PI-R (Costa Jr. & McCrea, 1992) reported by Hojat, Mangione, Nasca, and colleagues (2001); agreeableness, conscientiousness, extraversion, and openness to experience of the "big five" personality factors (Costa, Alves, Neto et al., 2014); emotional intelligence (Arora et al., 2010; Austin, Evans, Goldwater, & Potter, 2005; Kliszcz, Nowicka-Sauer, Trzeciak, Nowak, & Sadowska, 2006); cooperation (Hong, Bahn, Lee & Moon, 2011); attitudes toward teamwork and collaboration (Calabrese, Bianco, Mann,

Massello, & Hojat, 2013; Hojat, Spandorfer, Isenberg et al., 2012; Hojat, DeSantis, Cain et al., 2021a; Van Winkle, Fjortoft, & Hojat, 2012; Ward et al., 2009); desirable professional behavior (Brazeau, Schroeder, Rovi, & Boyd, 2010); therapists' psychological growth (Brockhouse, Msetfi, Cohen, & Joseph, 2011); psychological well-being and satisfaction with psychosocial needs (Cho & Jeon, 2019); optimism and personal accomplishment (Hojat, Vergare, Isenberg et al., 2015); orientation toward integrative patient care (Hojat, Bianco et al., 2015; Hojat, DeSantis, Cain et al., 2021a); positive social influence (Hojat, Michalec et al., 2015); peer nomination in clinical and humanistic excellence in medical school (Pohl, Hojat, & Arnold, 2011); patient-centered care (Beattie, Durham, Harvey, Steele, & McHanwell, 2012); and a friendly and relaxed style of communication (Brown et al., 2011).

Also, empirical research indicates that positive social influence (measured by peer nomination of students who were recognized by their classmates as having positive influence on them) scored significantly higher on the JSE (Hojat, Michalec, Veloski, & Tykocinski, 2015); and students who were recognized by their classmates as being excellent in clinical skills and humanistic qualities obtained significantly higher JSE mean scores than others without such recognition (Pohl, Hojat, & Arnold, 2011). Moreover, the peer nomination used in the aforementioned studies is a robust method of assessment of personal qualities that is free from social desirability response bias, a limitation of most self-reported personality tests.

The JSE scores of medical students who volunteered to participate in a student-run free clinic to provide healthcare services to indigent and underserved patients were compared with their non-volunteering classmates. Findings showed that the JSE scores of non-volunteers tend to decline in medical school, but no such erosion in clinical empathy was observed in the volunteer group (Modi, Fascelli, Daitch & Hojat, 2017). Another study found that medical students who volunteered to participate in a program, called "No One Dies Alone" (in which volunteer students provided compassionate companionship at the bedside of lonely dying patients by simply sitting at the patients' bedside; holding patients' hands; rendering therapeutic touch; playing music; and reading books, stories, and poetry), obtained significantly higher JSE mean scores (administered prior to the experiment) than their non-volunteer classmates, showing that those who volunteered to participate in the program, regardless of whether they had the opportunity to visit a dying patient or not (due to scheduling conflict such as unavailability of patients in students' free time) obtained higher mean scores on the JSE than their non-volunteering classmates (Hojat, DeSantis, Ney, & DeCleene, 2021b). This suggests that willingness to render compassionate care to terminally ill patients, in itself, is an indication of students' empathic inclination in patient care.

In a study with 1805 new matriculants at Jefferson, a computerized form of linguistic content analysis was applied to medical school admissions essays (Yaden, Yaden, Buffone et al., 2020). The purpose was to identify the words that were frequently used by medical students in their admissions essays and to examine their associations with students' scores on the JSE administered at the beginning of medical school education. Results showed that the top three words most frequently chosen by high scorers on the JSE were "health," "patient," and "care." The extracted topics from linguistic content analysis were: "empathy," "understanding," "compassion," "caring," "perspective," and "trust" (Yaden, Yaden, Buffone et al., 2020), which are among key feature of clinical empathy.

In a national sample of osteopathic medical students, we found that scores on the JSE were significantly and positively correlated with higher scores on measures of attitudes toward interprofessional collaboration and teamwork, orientation toward lifelong learning, emotional empathy, and attitudes toward integrative and holistic care (see Chap. 14; Hojat, DeSantis, Cain, Speicher et al., 2021).

In a sample of dental students at the University of Washington School of Dentistry, Sherman and Cramer (2005) found positive and significant correlations between scores on the JSE and ratings on 18 of 26 questions measuring attitudes toward clinical competence. The highest correlation was found between JSE scores and ratings of the following clinical competency: "application of the principles of behavioral sciences that pertain to patient-centered oral health care" ($r = 0.52$).

Furthermore, consistent with views on the effects of early interpersonal relationship experiences on the development of empathy (see Chap. 4) we observed that higher levels of self-reported satisfaction with the early maternal relationship (an indication of a secure mother–child attachment) and satisfactory peer relationships in school (an indication of social skills) were significantly associated with higher scores on the JSE (Hojat, Zuckerman et al., 2005).

Variables Detrimental to Relationship Building

Conversely, scores of the JSE yielded negative correlations with personality attributes that are detrimental to interpersonal relationships, such as measures of aggression-hostility (Hasan, Babar, Chen, Ahmed, & Mitha, 2013; Hojat & Zuckerman, 2005); indicators of burnout such as depersonalization and exhaustion (Hojat, Vergare, Isenberg, Cohen, & Spandorfer, 2015; Lamothe, Boujut, Zenasni, & Sultan, 2014); burnout experiences (see Chap. 14); and harm and avoidance (Hong et al., 2011). In his doctoral dissertation, Reisetter (2003) reported significant correlations between JSE factor scores and subscale scores of the Physician Belief Scale (PBS) (Ashworth, Williamson, & Montano, 1984; McLellan, Jansen-McWilliams, Comer, Gardner, & Kelleher, 1999). For example, a negative correlation ($r = -0.30$) was found between the JSE "Standing in the Patient's Shoes" factor scores and the PBS "Burden" subscale scores. However, in this study, the correlation between the "Compassionate Care" factor scores of the JSE and the "Belief and Feeling" subscale of the PBS was significant and positive ($r = 0.50$). In a national study of osteopathic medical students in the USA, we found a negative correlation between students' scores of the JSE and students' self-reported burnout experiences (see Chap. 14).

Correlations Between Scores on the JSE and the IRI

In a study involving 93 residents in internal medicine at Thomas Jefferson University Hospital (Hojat, Mangione, Kane, & Gonnella, 2005), we examined the relationships between total scores and factor scores (Perspective Taking, Compassionate Care, and Standing in the Patient's Shoes) on the HP-Version and the IRI (see Chap. 5) and four subscale scores (Perspective Taking, Empathic Concern, Fantasy, and Personal Distress). A study by Yarnold, Bryant, Nightingale, and Martin (1996) found that the Perspective Taking and Empathic Concern scales of the IRI were likely to measure empathy, whereas the Personal Distress and Fantasy subscales were likely to measure sympathy. We assumed that the IRI's Perspective Taking and Empathic Concern scales were more relevant to the clinician–patient relationship than were the Personal Distress and Fantasy scales. Therefore, we expected significant but moderate correlations between the JSE total and factor scores and scores on the IRI's Perspective Taking and Empathic Concern subscale scores. Conversely, we expected to obtain trivial correlations between scores on the JSE (and its factors) and scores on the IRI's Personal Distress and Fantasy subscale scores. A summary of the results is reported in Table 7.12.

As expected, the correlations between scores on the IRI Personal Distress subscale, and the JSE total and factor scores, were all nonsignificant. Scores on the IRI Fantasy scale yielded modest correlations with scores on the JSE's Perspective Taking and Compassionate Care subscales ($r = 0.24$, $p < 0.05$, and $r = 0.37$, $p < 0.01$, respectively). The highest correlations were found between the scores on the IRI Empathic Concern scale and the JSE Compassionate Care and Perspective Taking factors ($r = 0.41$, $p < 0.01$, and $r = 0.40$, $p < 0.01$, respectively). The correlation between the scores on the perspective taking dimensions of both instruments was $r = 0.35$ ($p < 0.01$).

Table 7.12 Correlations between scores on the JSE and the IRI ($N = 93$ first-year internal medicine residents)

	JSE factors			
IRI subscales	Perspective taking	Compassionate care	Standing in patient's shoes	Total score
Perspective taking	0.35**	0.31**	0.17	0.40**
Empathic concern	0.40**	0.41**	0.16	0.48**
Fantasy	0.24*	0.37**	0.12	0.35**
Personal distress	0.01	0.02	0.13	0.02
Total score	0.34**	0.40**	0.22*	0.45**

* $p < 0.05$; ** $p < 0.01$

Therefore, our expectation was confirmed regarding significant correlations of moderate magnitude between total and factor scores on the JSE and scores on the Perspective Taking and Empathic Concern subscales of the IRI. Furthermore, our prediction about the lack of relationship between the scores on the JSE and the scores on the IRI Personal Distress subscale was correct (Hojat, Mangione, et al., 2005). In a national study with osteopathic medical students in the USA, we found modest associations between scores on the JSE and two subscales of the IRI (namely Empathic Concern and Personal Distress) that are indicators of emotional empathy (see Chap. 14; see Hojat, DeSantis, Cain et al., 2021a).

Scores on the JSE, Academic Performance, and Clinical Competence

We expected to find a positive and significant relationship between medical students' scores on the S-Version of the JSE and global ratings of their clinical competence in core clinical clerkships given by medical school faculty. The reason for this expectation was that an ability to communicate with patients and understand their concerns is often considered when assessing global clinical competence. Our expectation was confirmed in a study with third-year medical students in which we found that students with higher scores on the JSE S-Version obtained better ratings of clinical competence than did classmates with lower JSE scores (Hojat, Gonnella, Mangione, Nasca, Veloski et al., 2002).

Regarding performance on tests of acquisition of knowledge, the lack of convincing evidence precluded a hypothesis that performance on objective (multiple-choice) tests should be associated with empathy scores. Therefore, we did not expect such an association and, indeed, did not find one (Hojat, Gonnella, Mangione, Nasca, Veloski et al., 2002). Our findings were consistent with those of other researchers (Diseker & Michielutte, 1981; Hornblow, Kidson, & Jones, 1977; Kupfer, Drew, Curtis, & Rubinstein, 1978).

A Litmus Test of Predictive Validity: Patient Outcomes

Because the ultimate purpose of medical and all other health professions education is optimal patient outcome, the ultimate criterion measure for the validity of any measure of empathy in patient care should include tangible patient outcomes, independent of patients' subjective judgment. In two studies that I will describe in more detail in Chap. 11, we found significant associations between physicians' scores on the JSE and clinical outcomes in diabetic patients. In the first study in the USA (Hojat, Louis, Markham et al., 2011) we showed that physicians with higher

JSE scores, compared to their counterparts with lower JSE scores, had a higher proportion of patients whose disease was under control (evident by the results of laboratory tests such as A1c < 7.0 %, and LDL-C < 100, extracted from patients' electronic records). In another study in Italy (Del Canale et al., 2012), statistically significant associations were found between physicians' scores on the JSE and rates of hospitalization due to metabolic complications (e.g., diabetic ketoacidosis, coma, and hyperosmolar). Findings of these two studies provide undeniable evidence in support of validity of the JSE in predicting clinical outcomes.

In a study in China, Yang and colleagues (2018), studying patients with advanced prostate cancer, reported that urologists' clinical empathy (measured by the JSE) negatively correlated with patients' anxiety and stigma and positively correlated with patients' self-efficacy and with the natural killer cells' activities. It was concluded that physicians' empathy contributed to improvement of patients' immune cellular function (i.e., natural killer cells' activities) through mediating roles of patients' anxiety, stigma, and self-efficacy.

Administration and Scoring

All three versions of the JSE can be administered either individually or in groups. Half of the items are directly scored according to their Likert weights (1 = Strongly disagree, 7 = Strongly agree) and the other half are reverse scored (1 = Strongly agree, 7 = Strongly disagree). We recommend handling missing data by using the following guidelines: if a respondent fails to answer more than 20% (four) of the items, the scale should be regarded as incomplete and be excluded from the data analysis. In the case of a respondent with four or fewer unanswered items, we recommend replacing each missing value with the mean item score, calculated from items completed by the respondent. The scale is "untimed" and takes approximately 5–10 min to complete. We do not recommend a strict time limit for completing the instrument.

The total score of the JSE is calculated by summing the item scores (directly and reversed scored items) possible total score range is 20–140). Factor scores (for US samples) can also be calculated by using the following instructions:

- Score for the "Perspective Taking" factor: sum of scores of the following 10 items: 2, 4, 5, 9, 10, 13,15, 16, 17, and 20.
- Score for the "Compassionate Care" factor: sum of scores of the following 8 items: 1,7, 8, 11, 12, 14, 18, and 19.
- Score for the "Standing in the Patient's Shoes" factor: sum of scores of the following 2 items: 3 and 6.

To ensure integrity in scoring and statistical analyses, we have developed scoring instructions that we share with JSE users. We strongly encourage them to follow the instructions; use the text and the order of appearance of the items as provided without any modification; and use the 7-point Likert scale for meaningful comparisons of the findings. Also, scannable forms of the three versions of the JSE have been developed and used by researchers and can be processed at Thomas Jefferson University. Web-based administration of the scale is also available.

A Brief Instrument to Measure Patient Perceptions of Physician Empathy

To investigate the relationship between physicians' self-reported scores on the JSE and their patients' perceptions, we developed a brief instrument to measure patients' perceptions of physicians' empathic orientation and behavior. Patients complete the *Jefferson Scale of Patient Perceptions of Physician Empathy* (JSPPPE) (Appendix E) to assess their physician's empathy.

The JSPPPE is a brief scale, containing five Likert-type items that patients can answer in a few minutes after an encounter with a physician or a healthcare professional. For example, a physician's concern regarding a patient and the patient's family is reflected in the following item: "This physician seems concerned about me and my family." The physician's perspective taking is reflected by the following item: "This physician can view things from my perspective (see things as I see them)." In a study conducted by Kane, Gotto, Mangione, West, and Hojat (2007) with residents in an internal medicine program, and in another study by Glaser and colleagues with residents in a family medicine program (Glaser et al., 2007), scores on the JSPPPE correlated significantly with selected items from the Physicians' Humanistic Behaviors Questionnaire (developed by Weaver, Ow, Walker, and Degenhardt, 1993). Also, scores on the JSPPPE correlated significantly with scores on selected items from a questionnaire measuring patients' appraisal of physicians' performance that was developed by Matthews and Feinstein (1989).

The two aforementioned studies of the JSPPPE conducted at Thomas Jefferson University Hospital used data from 225 encounters between patients and resident physicians in the internal medicine residency program (Kane et al., 2007) and 90 encounters between patients and residents in the family medicine residency program (Glaser, Markham, Adler, McManus, & Hojat, 2007). Item-total score correlations of the JSPPPE were statistically significant in both departments (median correlations were 0.78 for family medicine and 0.81 for internal medicine). The item and total scores on the JSPPPE in the Department of Internal Medicine study also yielded significant correlations with scores obtained from a rating form for patients developed by the American Board of Internal Medicine to assess physicians' communicative skills, humanistic qualities, and professionalism (Lipner, Blank, Leas, & Fortna, 2002). The median correlation between the two instruments was 0.64. The internal consistency reliabilities (coefficient alphas) of the patient perceptions scale were in the lower range (0.50s), partially due to the brevity of the instrument.

In a study with 535 outpatients treated by family physicians (Hojat, Louis et al., 2010), we found that the JSPPPE is a unidimensional instrument based on the results of EFA, a finding that was previously reported (Kane et al., 2007). Corrected item-total score correlations of the JSPPPE ranged from 0.88 to 0.94 (see Table 7.13). Cronbach's alpha coefficient ranged from 0.97 to 0.99 for the total sample and for patients in different gender and age groups (Hojat, Louis et al., 2010). Scores on the JSPPPE were highly correlated with measures of physician–patient trusting relationships ($r > 0.73$). Also, the correlation between scores of the JSPPPE and a measure of patient overall satisfaction with the primary care physician (Hojat, Louis et al., 2010) was 0.93 (see Table 7.14).

In addition, we found that higher scores on the JSPPPE were predictive of patients' compliance with their physicians' recommendations (compliance rates >80%) for preventive care (e.g., colonoscopy for male and female patients, mammogram for female patients, and PSA for male patients) (Hojat, Louis et al., 2010).

Table 7.13 Factor coefficients of the Jefferson Scale of Patient Perceptions of Physician Empathy, item-total score correlations, and correlations of each item with scores of patient satisfaction and recommendation ($n = 535$)

Items	Factor coefficients[a]	Item-total score[b]	Patient satisfaction[c]	Recommendation[d]
1. My doctor understands my emotions, feelings, and concerns	0.93	0.94	0.87	0.80
2. My doctor is an understanding doctor	0.92	0.93	0.95	0.89
3. My doctor seems concerned about me and my family	0.92	0.93	0.87	0.82
4. My doctor asks about what is happening in my daily life	0.88	0.91	0.80	0.73
5. My doctor can view things from my perspective (see things as I see them)	0.84	0.88	0.79	0.74

[a]Items are reported by descending order of factor coefficients

[b]Correlation between scores of the item and the rest of the scale

[c]Correlation between scores of the item and scores on the Jefferson Scale of Patient Overall Satisfaction (Hojat, Louis et al., 2010)

[d]Correlation between scores of the item and responses to this anchor item: "I would recommend my doctor to my family and friends"

Table 7.14 Concurrent validity coefficients of the Jefferson Scale of Patient Perceptions of Physician Empathy and criterion measures of patient–physician interpersonal trust by patients' gender and age

	Gender		Age		
Criterion measures	Men (n = 174)	Women (n = 355)	<56 (n = 266)	≥56 (n = 269)	Total (n = 535)
Patient overall satisfaction with physician[a]	0.94	0.93	0.96	0.90	0.93
I would recommend my doctor to my family and friends	0.88	0.86	0.91	0.80	0.87
My doctor listens carefully to me	0.88	0.91	0.96	0.84	0.91
My doctor spends sufficient time with me	0.79	0.80	0.85	0.75	0.80
My doctor really cares about me as a person	0.93	0.85	0.89	0.87	0.88
I would like my doctor to be present in any medical emergency situation	0.73	0.78	0.80	0.73	0.77
I am satisfied that my doctor has been taking care of me	0.86	0.86	0.90	0.83	0.87

[a]Scores on the Jefferson Scale of Patient Overall Satisfaction with Primary Care physician

The correlation coefficient between patients' ratings of their physicians on the patient perceptions scale and the residents' self-reported empathy (JSE scores) was 0.48 ($p < 0.05$) in the family medicine study (Glaser et al., 2007), but it was only 0.24 (nonsignificant) in the internal medicine study (Kane et al., 2007). Further inspection of data for the Department of Internal Medicine showed that the majority of patients (78%) gave the highest possible scores to the residents, leading to a highly skewed JSPPPE score distribution with a restricted range of scores. This "ceiling effect" would not allow the correlation between residents' self-reported empathy and patients' perceptions of residents' empathy to be fully captured.

In their study of orthopedic patients, Keulen and colleagues (2020) reported a significant correlation of 0.70 between scores of the JSPPPE and the Consultation and Relational Empathy measure (CARE, described in Chap. 5). In a study of psychiatry residents in Iran who completed the JSE and their standardized patients who completed the JSPPPE (Nasr Esfahani, Behzadipour, Nadoushan, & Shariat, 2014), a moderate correlation between the JSE and JSPPPE was observed ($r = 0.39$). This was not statistically significant, probably due to a small sample size, according to the study's authors. Consistent with these findings, it was also discovered that although the relationship between physicians' self-report measures of empathy (measured by the Hogan's Empathy Scale) and patients' evaluations was positive, it was statistically nonsignificant (Linn et al., 1987). It is interesting to note from the aforementioned findings that the associations between physicians' or medical students' self-reported empathy (JSE scores), and real or standardized patients' perceptions of clinicians' empathy (JSPPPE scores), were mostly moderate or negligible. However, correlations between patients' assessment of clinicians' empathy (JSPPPE scores) and patients' global assessments of clinicians' competence and empathy were found to be larger in magnitude (Grosseman, Hojat et al., 2014; Grosseman, Novack et al., 2014). A possibility exists that patients' views regarding their clinicians' empathic behavior may differ from the clinicians' views of their own empathy. Grosseman and her colleagues raised a question about some physicians' ability to gauge or to communicate their empathic engagement with patients. Further research is needed to explore these and other possibilities.

The link between physicians' self-reported empathy and patients' perceptions of their physicians' empathy could also be strengthened by physicians' efforts to communicate their understanding to their patients (Free, Green, Grace, Chernus, & Whitman, 1985). Measuring patients' perceptions is important because research has shown that their perceptions of clinicians' empathy yield the highest correlations with clinical outcomes; this is followed by observers' ratings of clinicians' empathy and, finally, by clinicians' self-reported empathy (Bohart, Elliot, Greenberg, & Watson, 2002). Because other factors can contribute to patients' perceptions of clinicians' empathy, including the degree to which patients can cope with their illnesses (Mercer, Watt, & Reilly, 2001), more studies are needed to examine the complex reasons for patients' and clinicians' concordant and discordant views on empathic engagement in clinical encounters.

The associations between clinicians' self-reported empathy and patients' perception of clinician empathy may be confounded by gender and ethnicity. For example, in a few studies, standardized patients assessed medical students' empathic engagement by completing the JSPPPE in Objective Structured Clinical Examination (OSCE) stations. Findings showed statistically significant associations between scores of the JSPPPE (completed by standardized patients) and scores of medical students' self-reported empathy (measured by the JSE) (Berg, Majdan, Berg, Veloski, & Hojat, 2011a, 2011b; Berg et al., 2015). However, we noticed that students' gender and ethnicity (Berg et al., 2011b) and their interactions could confound the relationships between self-reported empathy in medical students (measured by the JSE) and standardized patients' assessments of medical students' empathy as measured by the JSPPPE (Berg et al., 2015). We have reported a summary of evidence in support of the validity and reliability of the JSPPPE (Hojat, DeSantis & Gonnella, 2017).

Broad National and International Reputation of the JSE

Over the years, we have been receiving increasing requests from researchers in the USA and abroad for copies of the JSE and for permission to use it. The JSE has been described as "possibly the most researched and widely used instrument in medical education" (Colliver, Conlee, Verhulst, & Dorsey, 2010a, 2010b, p. 1813). As of this writing, we have received a large number of requests from the USA and other countries. The JSE has been translated into 63 languages and used in 93 countries (see Fig. 7.2 and Box 7.2) in which the JSE was used. To ensure the accuracy of translations, we have always strongly recommended using the back-translation procedure (Brislin, 1970; Geisinger, 1994; Guillemin, Bombardier, & Beaton, 1993) to all those who asked us to grant them permission to translate the JSE.

Box 7.2 List of the countries within each region corresponding to the numbers in Fig. 7.2

Africa:

1. Egypt
2. Ghana
3. Kenya
4. Malawi
5. Morocco
6. Nigeria
7. Rwanda
8. South Africa
9. Tunisia
10. Uganda

Asia:

11. Bangladesh
12. China
13. Georgia
14. Hong Kong
15. India
16. Indonesia
17. Japan
18. Malaysia
19. Mongolia
20. Nepal
21. The Philippines
22. Russia
23. Singapore
24. South Korea
25. Sri Lanka
26. Taiwan
27. Thailand
28. Uzbekistan

Europe:

29. Albania
30. Austria
31. Belgium
32. Bulgaria
33. Croatia
34. Czech Republic
35. Cyprus
36. Denmark
37. England
38. Estonia
39. Finland
40. France
41. Germany
42. Greece
43. Hungary
44. Ireland
45. Italy
46. Latvia
47. Lithuania
48. The Netherlands
49. Norway
50. Poland
51. Portugal
52. Romania
53. Scotland
54. Serbia
55. Slovenia
56. Spain
57. Sweden
58. Switzerland
59. Ukraine
60. United Kingdom

Middle East:

61. Iran
62. Iraq
63. Israel
64. Jordan
65. Kuwait
66. Oman
67. Lebanon
68. Pakistan
69. Qatar
70. Saudi Arabia
71. Turkey
72. United Arab Emirates

Oceania:

73. Australia
74. New Zealand

North & Central America:

75. Canada
76. Costa Rica
77. Guatamala
78. Dominican Republic
79. Haiti
80. Mexico
81. Panama
82. St. Maarten
83. Trinidad & Tobago
84. United States

South America:

85. Argentina
86. Brazil
87. Chile
88. Columbia
89. Ecuador
90. Paraguay
91. Peru
92. Uruguay
93. Venezuela

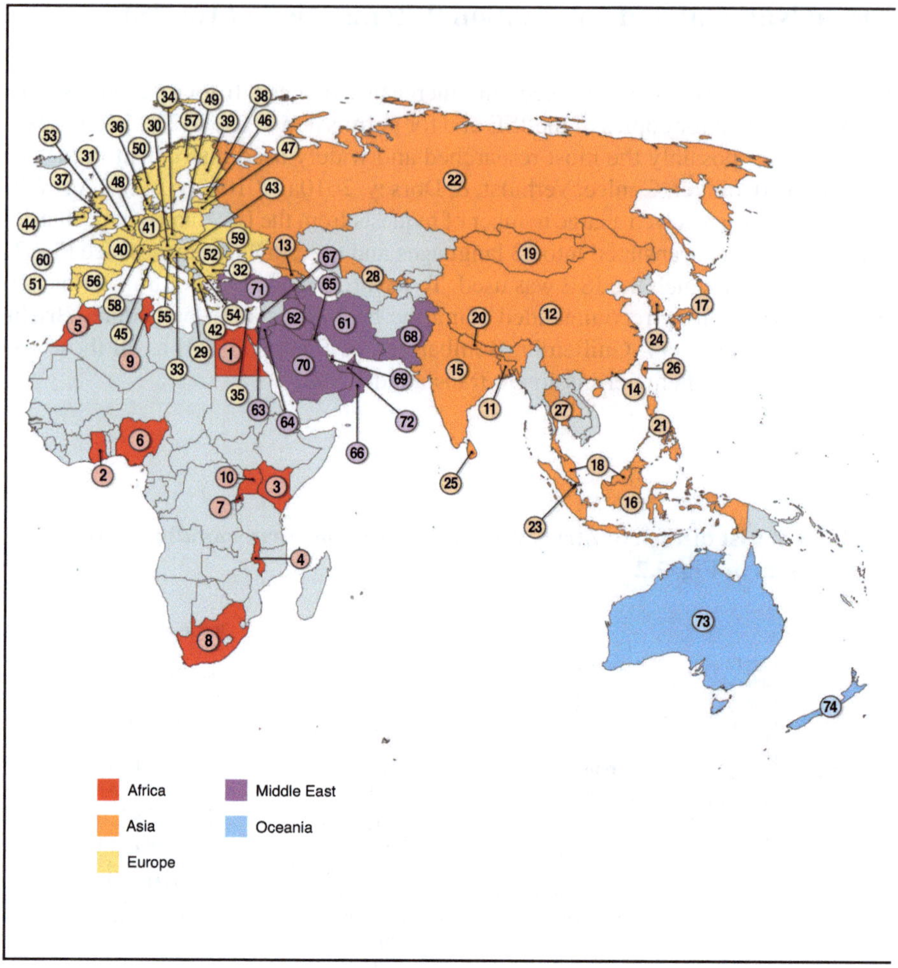

Fig. 7.2 Worldwide use of the Jefferson Scale of Empathy (See Box 7.2 for the list of countries corresponding to the numbers of this map within each region)

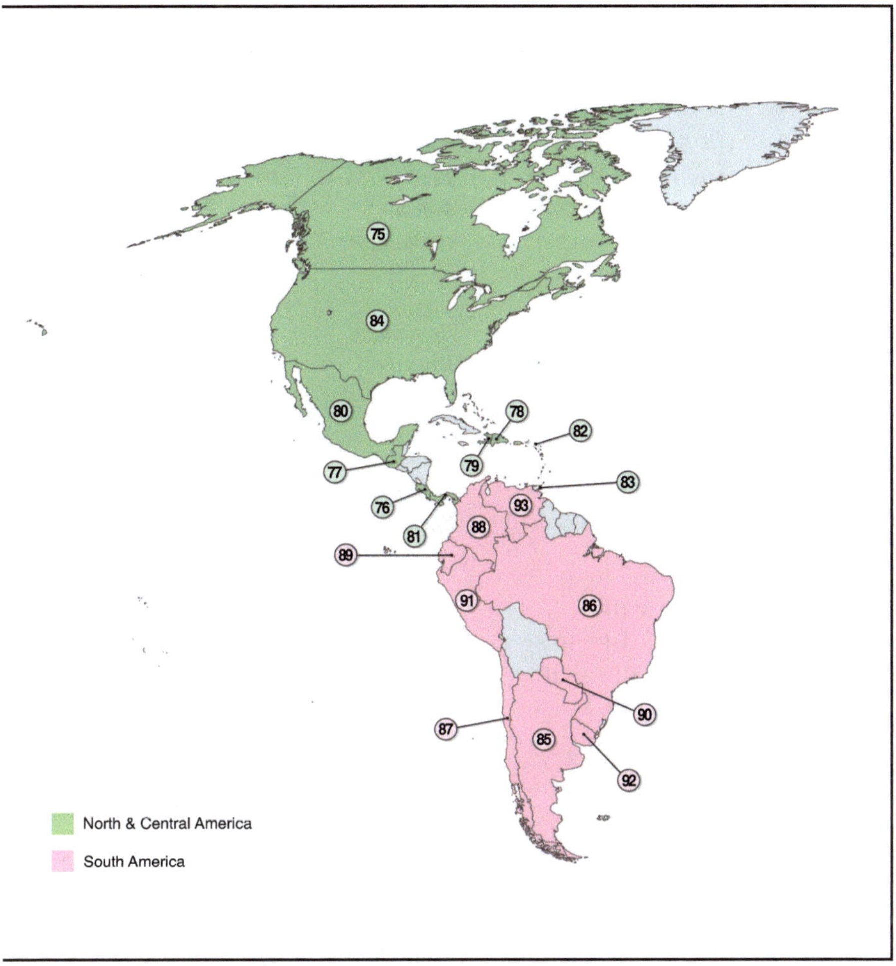
75
84
80
78
82
79
77
83
93
76
88
81
89
91
86
90
87
85
92
North & Central America
South America

Box 7.3 Translations of the Jefferson Scale of Empathy

Albanian	HPS*	***Malaysian Malaysian***	HPS*
Arabic	HP* & HPS*	***Norwegian***	HP*
Arabic	(Moroccan) HPS*	***Persian (Farsi)***	HP*, HPS* & S*
Bengali	S*	***Polish***	HP* & S*
Bulgarian	HP*	***Portuguese***	(Portugal), HP*, S* & HPS*
Chinese	(Simplified), HP*, HPS*		(Brazil), HP*, S* & HPS*
Chinese	(Mainland), HP* & S*	***Romanian***	HP*,HPS* & S*
	(Taiwan), HP*, S* & HPS*	***Russian***	HP* & S*
Croatian	HP*, S* & HPS*		(Uzbekistan) HP
Czech	HP* & S*	***Serbian***	HP*, S* & HPS*
Danish	HP* & S*	***Sinhalese***	(Sri Lanka) S*
Dutch	(Flemish, Belgium), S*	***Slovenian***	HP*, HPS* & S*
	(Dutch, Netherlands), HP* & S	***Spanish***	(Argentina) HP*
Estonian	HPS*		(Chile), HP*, S* & HPS*
Finnish	HP*, S* & HPS*		(Catalan), S*
French	(Belgium), HP*, HPS*		(Dominican Republic), S*
	(Canada), HP* & HPS*		(Mexico), HP*, S* & HPS
	(France), HP*, S*		(Panama), HP* & HPS*
	(Switzerland) S*		(Peru), HP*, HPS* & S*
German	HP* & S*		(Spain), HP*, S*, HPS*
Greek	HP* , HPS* & S*		(El Salvador), HP* & HPS*
Hebrew	S*	***Swedish***	HP*
Hindi	HP*	***Tagalog (Filipino)***	HP*, S
Hungarian	HP* HPS* & S*	***Tamil (India)***	HPS*
Indonesian	HP* HPS* & S*	***Tamil (Sri Lanka)***	S*
Italian	HP*, S* & HPS*	***Thai***	HP*& S*
Japanese	HP*, S* & HPS*	***Turkish***	HP*, S* & HPS*
Korean	HP* & S* & HPS*	***Ukrainian***	S*
Lithuanian	HP*, S*, HPS*	***Urdu (Pakistan)***	HP* & S*

HP=Health Professions/Physician Version, S=Student Version, HPS=Health Professions Student Version
** PDF available*

Findings from National and International Studies

Interestingly, our findings have been replicated by many other researchers. The patterns of findings of most of the studies in the USA and other countries are similar to those we have reported in our own studies (see Appendix A). The increasing national and international attention to the JSE is reflected in the "Annotated Bibliography on the Jefferson Scale of Empathy" (listed in Appendix A). An overall review of findings of the annotated studies in Appendix A provides strong evidence to support the psychometric soundness of the three versions of the JSE in different samples of health profession students and practitioners, in a variety of health professions disciplines, and in different countries with different medical education systems and cultural values. Most of the major findings in those studies are consistent. For example, in almost all of those studies, findings generally show that reliability coefficients of the JSE, reflected in the Cronbach's alpha coefficients, are in the 0.70s and 0.80s ($M = 0.78$), a well-acceptable range for psychological tests. Also, in most EFA studies of the JSE (Appendix A), three factors of "Perspective Taking," "Compassionate Care," and "Standing in the Patient's Shoes" have emerged, sometimes in different order; and the three-factor model has been confirmed in a number of the CFA studies.

In many of the studies reported in Appendix A, the mean scores of different versions of the JSE (when there is no remedial/education intervention) hover around 112 (standard deviations hover around 12); and in most of those studies, women outscored men in different versions of the JSE. In addition, in most of those studies with health professions students in the USA, a decline of empathy has been observed during the course of medical and health professions education, particularly at a point in training when curriculum shifts toward the clinical phase that involves patient contact—when empathy is most needed. Also, in most of the experimental programs which were developed to enhance clinical empathy, an increase in the JSE mean scores has been observed in the health professions students who were exposed to or participated in the targeted educational programs (see Appendix A). However, none of the studies with follow-up data reported that the enhanced empathy scores sustained for a longer time without additional reinforcement.

Information reported in Appendix A and further expansion of the scope of the studies in which the JSE has been used provide a unique opportunity for meta-analytic studies for graduate students' master's theses, doctoral dissertations, and researchers interested in the topic of clinical empathy in health professions education and in patient care. We hope that in the future, a large and valuable central data bank and a number of meta-analytic studies will be undertaken to summarize findings from different samples, professions, and countries on correlates of empathy in the context of health professions education and patient care. Further research is warranted to develop effective approaches to enhance and sustain empathy among health professions students and practitioners, examine group differences, and analyze changes in empathy as students progress through professional training, etc.

Two Caveats

Attitudes, Orientation, Capacity, and Behavior

When we submitted manuscripts describing the results of our empathy studies to peer-reviewed journals, a few reviewers expressed a legitimate concern about the link between physicians' scores on the JSE and their actual empathic behavior in patient care. If one assumes that the physicians' scores on the JSE indeed reflect their own attitude or orientation toward empathy in physician–patient relationships, and not necessarily their empathic behavior, a convincing argument plus empirical data are needed to establish a link between attitudes and behavior.

Although social psychologists have long debated the link between attitude and behavior, the issue has not been completely settled yet (for a meta-analytic review, see Wallace, Paulson, Lord, & Bond, 2005). When people have formed an attitude or an orientation toward a subject, they are no longer neutral about that subject. In other words, they are likely to take a stand or develop a behavioral tendency consistent with their attitude or orientation (Sherif, Sherif, & Nebergall, 1965). Attitude, orientation, and perception share common cognitive and neural elements that can activate relevant behavior (Prinz, 1997; Viviani, 2002). A concordance between an attitude and behavior is necessary to avoid an unpleasant psychological tension that resembles "cognitive dissonance" (Festinger, 1964), which occurs when a person is caught in a cognitive struggle between opposing motivational forces. Cognitive dissonance research has established that when individuals perform a behavior or make a choice that conflicts with a previously established attitude, the attitude tends to change in the direction that resolves the conflict with the behavior. This process appears to involve rationalization, whereby individuals strategically change their attitudes in order to avoid appearing inconsistent (Lieberman, 2007).

Attitudes often generate strong emotions (affective components) and form a cognitive orientation (cognitive components) leading to preferences that ultimately elicit actions (behavioral components) (Rosenberg & Hovland, 1960). Therefore, attitudes, orientations, beliefs, and intentions are all motivating forces that can elicit corresponding behaviors (Fishbein & Ajzen, 1975). For example, acculturation studies have reported that attitudinal changes, even in relation to deeply rooted social institutions, such as marriage and the family, can lead to tangible behavioral changes, such as increased rates of marital discord and divorce (Hojat, Shapurian et al., 1999, 2000). An abundance of empirical studies have been published about hostile or hateful behaviors resulting from prejudicial attitudes toward members of the opposite sex and toward racial, ethnic, and religious groups. For corroborative proof of such behaviors, one only needs to consult a daily newspaper.

In a recent meta-analysis of 797 studies (Wallace et al., 2005), it was found that the mean of attitude–behavior correlations was 0.41, but the magnitude of the relationship varied, depending on social pressure and perceived difficulty. Considering that the average effect of only 0.21 was found in an analysis of more than 25,000 studies of 8 million research participants in social psychology (Richard, Bond, &

Stokes-Zoota, 2003), the aforementioned attitude–behavior correlation ($r = 0.41$) seems impressive. These findings suggest that forming an empathic attitude, possessing the capacity to understand others, or developing a tendency or an orientation toward empathic relationships do not necessarily ensure empathic behavior. What is certain, however, is that a higher degree of empathic attitude, tendency, orientation, or capacity will increase the likelihood that these qualities will be manifested as empathic behavior under certain conditions. All measures of empathy, including the JSE, are at best a proxy of empathic behavior. Validity evidence would indicate the extent to which these measures are predictive of actual empathic behavior and optimal clinical outcomes.

Transparency and Social Desirability Response Bias

Respondents can always manipulate their answers on self-reported personality tests to produce a more socially desirable result. Edwards (1957), who was the first to systematically study the "social desirability phenomenon," believed that respondents were likely to be unaware of the tendency to show themselves in the most socially acceptable light.

Because most items in the JSE are transparent and thus susceptible to social desirability response bias, they can be answered in a way that is recognized as more socially acceptable. Constructing socially neutral items that measure personal attributes, such as empathy, is difficult and raises questions about not only the face and content validities of such items but the empirical validity of the test as well. For example, the relevance to empathy of nontransparent items, such as those about an interest in literature and the arts or a sense of humor (used in the JSE), is not necessarily apparent. Indeed, some peer reviewers who evaluated the manuscripts we submitted to professional journals questioned the reasons for including those items in the JSE. (The reasons for including those items were discussed earlier in this chapter.)

The degree to which socially desirable responses to items have a confounding effect on test scores could be a function of the test taker's belief in testing outcomes. For example, when testing is used to screen applicants for employment or college admission, test takers may be more inclined to provide socially acceptable answers to test items that will increase their advantage.

In response to concerns about the possible effect of socially desirable response bias in our clinical empathy studies, we offer three plausible explanations. First, the JSE has been administered in "nonpenalizing" situations where the purpose was described as research, not college admission or employment. Respondents were assured that their responses would be confidential and would be used only for research purposes approved by the Institutional Review Board's Research Ethics Committee. This assurance, in itself, could mitigate respondents' tendency to give socially desirable (faked) responses.

Second, the pattern of relationships in our validity studies, particularly the convergent and discriminant validities (described previously in this chapter), suggests that social desirability response bias, even if operative, did not substantially distort the expected relationships. For example, we observed that the magnitude of the correlation between the JSE scores and a more relevant concept, such as compassion, was twice the magnitude of the correlation between JSE scores and a less relevant concept, such as personal growth (see Table 7.2). Such a correlational pattern would be unlikely to emerge in the presence of the significant confounding effects of social desirability response bias.

Third, we conducted empirical studies to investigate the influence of faking "good impression" responses on the JSE scores. For example, in one study (Hojat, Zuckerman et al., 2005), we administered the JSE and other personality tests, including the Zuckerman-Kuhlman Personality Questionnaire (ZKPQ), to 422 first-year medical students who matriculated at Jefferson. The ZKPQ includes an "Infrequency" scale that was developed to detect intentionally false responses by identifying respondents with an invalid pattern of responses (Zuckerman, 2002). A sample item from the Infrequency scale is "I never saw a person I didn't like." Scores on this scale can be regarded as indicators of the degree of social desirability response bias. Attempts to give socially desirable responses were determined by a cutoff score of greater than three, which the test's author considered to indicate questionable for the record (Zuckerman, 2002, p. 383). An examination of the distribution of scores on this scale indicated that less than 5% of the respondents attempted to give "good impression" responses or to respond carelessly without regard for the truth (Zuckerman, 2002). The hypothesis that social desirability would not distort the validity of the JSE scores in nonpenalizing testing situations was tested and confirmed in our study (Hojat, Zuckerman et al., 2005).

We replicated that study by using a large sample ($n = 2637$) of first-year students who matriculated at Jefferson between 2002 and 2012 and completed the JSE and the ZKPQ. In this study (unpublished), we found that approximately 6% of respondents ($n = 169$) attempted to give "good impression" responses, determined by their score of 3 or higher on the Infrequency scale of the ZKPQ, which is close to the 5% figure found in our previous study (Hojat, Zuckerman et al., 2005). We used two approaches to examine the possible effects of social desirability response bias on the JSE in the outcomes of our research.

First, we conducted two different sets of statistical analyses. In one set, we included all students in the sample, and in another set we excluded those who, according to their scores (>3) on the Infrequency scale, attempted to give socially desirable or "good impression" responses. Analyses of data regarding the relationship between scores on the JSE and on scores of the five scales of the ZKPQ clearly demonstrated that research outcomes remained virtually unchanged whether or not respondents who showed a social desirability response bias were included or excluded in statistical analyses. This finding was expected because of the small proportion of respondents in the sample who scored above the cutoff score of the Infrequency scale (6%), suggesting that the magnitude of descriptive statistics as the mean and median is unlikely to be inflated as a result of the small proportion of respondents' faking in nonthreatening testing conditions.

Second, we used the analysis of covariance (ANCOVA) method to control for the effect of giving false responses on the research outcomes by using the "Infrequency" score as a covariate (JSE scores as the dependent variable; gender and scores on different personality measures from the ZKPQ as the independent variables). Again, we noted no substantial change in the general pattern of findings with or without statistical control for social desirability response bias.

Lastly, in a large-scale national project in osteopathic medical education and empathy (see Chap. 14; Hojat, DeSantis, Shannon, Mortensen et al., 2018; Hojat, DeSantis, Shannon Speicher et al., 2020; Hojat, Shannon, DeSantis, Speicher et al., 2020; Hojat, Shannon, DeSantis, Speicher et al., 2019; Hojat, DeSantis, Cain et al., 2021a), similar to the aforementioned study, we included the Infrequency scale of the ZKPQ in the study survey. In some of our statistical analyses, we excluded those respondents who scored > 3 on the Infrequency scale (indicating an attempt to give socially desirable responses). In some other statistical analyses, we used ANCOVA to statistically control for the effect of social desirability response bias on the JSE scores by using the Infrequency scores as covariate. Proportions of participating students who scored > 3 on the Infrequency scale in different study samples ranged from 2–3%. We found no significant changes in the patterns of findings, with or without control for the effect of social desirability response bias (or "good impression response"). These findings generally suggest that social desirability response bias did not distort the validity of the JSE scores, at least under nonthreatening testing conditions.

Our findings were consistent with the results of an earlier study on the heritability of empathy by Matthews, Batson, Horn, and Rosenman (1981), who reported that their derived index of empathy was not affected by social desirability response bias or by scores on a "good impression" scale. Two other studies reported no significant correlations between empathy scores obtained on the Emotional Empathy Scale and social desirability response bias (Mehrabian & Epstein, 1972; Mehrabian & O'Reilly, 1980). Despite these findings, the confounding effects of giving "good impression" responses and attempting to present a socially acceptable image in penalizing testing situations (e.g., by applicants for college admission or employment) need to be further addressed in future studies.

Why Is the JSE a Unique Instrument for Measuring Clinical Empathy?

As indicated in Chap. 5, the empathy-measuring instruments that were developed to measure empathy in the general population cannot capture the essence of clinical empathy in health professions students and clinicians. The JSE at the present time is the only psychometrically sound instrument that was developed to fill this gap. As described in this chapter, in the preliminary drafting of the items of the JSE, we attempted to focus on the "face" and "content" validities, and then in further assessments, we shifted our focus on examining "construct" validity of the instrument by exploring the underlying factors (constructs, latent variable structure) of the JSE. We also reported evidence on item-total score correlations, item discrimination indices, and the internal consistency aspect of reliability (Cronbach alpha coefficient), and stability of scores (test–retest reliability)—all supporting measurement properties and psychometrics of the JSE.

In addition, we provided empirical evidence (in this chapter and in Chaps. 9 and 11) in support of criterion-related validity by examining positive associations between scores of the JSE and pertinent personality variables that were conducive to relationships and negative associations between JSE scores with personal qualities that were detrimental to forming empathic connections (see also Appendix A).

More importantly, as described in this chapter and in Chap. 11 and elsewhere (Hojat & Gonnella, 2017), the litmus test for the validity and utility of a clinical empathy instrument is empirical evidence for its predictive validity by confirming significant links between scores on the instrument and tangible clinical outcomes. The JSE has already successfully passed this litmus test by showing significant associations between physicians' scores on the JSE scores and positive patient outcomes in diabetic patients (see Chap. 11; and Hojat, Louis, Markham et al., 2011; Del Canale, Louis, Maio et al., 2012). Also, as reported previously, evidence shows a significant link between medical students' scores on the JSE and their clinical competence in core clerkships, as assessed by medical school faculty (Hojat, Gonnella, Mangione et al., 2002).

Because of its features, the JSE is a unique instrument for measuring clinical empathy and has been recognized as the most frequently used instrument for measuring clinical empathy in medical students (Sulzer, 2016). Also, in a review of empathy research in healthcare, the JSE was described as the most frequently used measure of clinical empathy in healthcare research (Nembhard, David, Ezzaddeh, Betts, & Radin, 2023). Hong and Han (2020) reviewed a total of 11 empathy-measuring instruments used for care professionals from studies published between 1950 and 2018 to identify empathy-measuring instruments with the best psychometrics evidence. The JSE was identified as one of the instruments with the highest quality appraisal. Thus, the three versions of the JSE presently remain unique, without parallel, for quantifying clinical empathy in health professions students and practitioners.

Recapitulation

The JSE was developed in response to a need for a psychometrically sound instrument specifically designed to measure clinical empathy in the context of health professions education and patient care. Evidence reported in this chapter in support of the face, content, construct, criterion-related, and predictive validity and reliability of the JSE adds to researchers' confidence in using the JSE as a unique measure of clinical empathy, that is well-accepted by international researchers.

Chapter 8
The Interpersonal Dynamics in Clinician–Patient Relationships

It is difficult to hate the people with whom you empathize.

—(Walter Stephan & Krystina Finlay, 1999, p. 736)

By far, the most frequently used drug in general practice was the doctor. It was not only the bottle of medicine or the box of pills that mattered, but the way doctor gave them.

—(Michael Balint, 1957, p. 1)

Abstract

- Some factors that contribute to interpersonal dynamics in patient care are described, and it is proposed that patients as well as clinicians can benefit from empathic engagement.
- The curing versus caring models and the concept of disease versus illness contribute to the development of attitudes that influence empathic behavior in clinical encounters.
- Certain interpersonal dynamics operate in role expectations, the clinical environment, and clinician–patient encounters, including a tendency to bind with others for survival, comply with the orders of authority figures, and uncritically accept authority figures.
- Important facets of interpersonal psychodynamics and their impact on empathic understanding in clinical encounters are described; and the placebo effect of empathic relationships, cultural factors, personal space, and boundaries in clinician–patient encounters is also discussed.
- Emphasis is placed on how listening with the "third ear" and seeing with the "mind's eye" can enhance empathic understanding in the context of patient care.

M. Hojat, *Clinical Empathy*, https://doi.org/10.1007/978-3-031-87413-0_8

Introduction

In Chap. 4, in the general context of human relationships, I described factors that contribute to the development of empathic understanding. This chapter describes the interpersonal dynamics specifically involved in clinical encounters. The way a clinician encounters patients can make a significant difference in patient outcomes. In support of this, Houston (1938) indicated that physicians are themselves therapeutic agents through which cures are effected. The "goodness of the physician" was viewed as a therapeutic agent by Hippocrates, who suggested in the fourth century B.C. that "the patient, though conscious that his condition is perilous, may recover his health simply through his contentment with the goodness of the physician" (cited in DiMatteo, 1979, p. 14).

The moments of understanding and connectedness in clinical encounters, according to Matthews, Suchman, and Branch (1993, p. 973), "[are] often marked by physiological reactions such as gooseflesh or a chill; by an immediacy of awareness of the patient's situation (as if experiencing it from inside the patient's world), by a sense of being part of a larger whole; and by a lingering feeling of joy, peacefulness, or awe. Such moments seem to be therapeutic for the patient and the clinician alike."

Matthews et al. (1993) referred to this powerful interpersonal dynamic, which is beneficial for both clinician and patient, as a "connexion" ("co" for "being together" and "nexus" for "to form a whole") to indicate that the interpersonal dynamics in clinician–patient encounters generate a totality that is greater than the sum of its parts. The importance of empathic relationships in clinician–patient encounters has been discussed in the medical literature (Bylund & Makoul, 2002; Platt & Keller, 1994; Spiro, McCrea Curnen, Peschel, & St. James, 1993; Squier, 1990; Winefield & Chur-Hansen, 2000), and the positive effect of empathy in patient outcomes has been confirmed (see Chap. 11).

In antiquity, medicine was primarily a "craft" (Lewis, 1998), and it was an art when practiced by Greek healers (many of whom were unable to read and write). Medicine was not based on the sciences (mathematics and philosophy in those days); it was based on observation, insight, tradition, and, most importantly, interpersonal relationships (Lewis, 1998). As Rachel Lewinsohn (1998, p. 1268) rightly stated: "We cannot understand the disease without understanding the patient." The clinician cannot fully understand the patient without entering into the patient's world on the bridge of empathy. Empathy in patient care is bidirectional, affecting both the clinician and the patient. Because of the intrinsic reward associated with establishing a meaningful relationship with others, both clinician and patient can benefit from forming an empathic engagement. However, research attention on the beneficial effects of empathy has focused almost exclusively on the patient's side of the equation; the clinician's side has been the victim of benign neglect.

Benefits of Empathic Relationships for Clinicians

Medicine and other health care professions, although intrinsically self-rewarding, are stressful and often demand a lifestyle that restricts participation in social and family events. From the perspective of personal life, such restrictions can contribute to the discontent of healers who themselves need to be healed. Despite these problems, the good news is that clinicians' satisfaction with their relationships with patients can serve as a buffer against the professional stress, burnout, substance abuse, and even suicide attempts that are reported to be unusually high among health professionals (Sullivan, 1990).

Physicians are not invincible, and research indicates that they are vulnerable to a number of psychosocial problems. For example, physicians are more than twice as likely as the general population to commit suicide (Miller & McGowen, 2000), and divorce rates also are higher among physicians than they are in the general population (Sotile & Sotile, 1996). Research indicates that physicians often do not practice what they preach to their own patients and sometimes are reluctant to seek medical help (Forsythe, Calnan, & Wall, 1999). It is important to note that Miller and McGowen (2000) discovered that physicians who enjoyed the support of social networks (e.g., spouse, family, friends, and acquaintances) were less likely to abuse drugs or to suffer from burnout.

Because physicians often perceive empathic relationships with patients as meaningful interpersonal connections, those relationships can serve as a buffer against dissatisfaction with the health care system and professional burnout. Human life is lived in relationships (Lewis, 1998); thus, physician–patient relationships provide an intrinsically joyful reward that serves as a remedy for the stress of a demanding profession (Zuger, 2004). Empathy has been identified as a protective factor against the stress experienced by clinicians (Shamasundar, 1999) and as a potential factor for their well-being (Hyyppa, Kronholm, & Mattlar, 1991). In a number of studies it was found that clinicians' empathy scores were significantly associated with personality attributes that were conducive to positive interpersonal relationships (see Chaps. 7 and 9), confirming the beneficial effects of empathy in clinicians' well-being.

A study of physician executives, i.e., physicians with a management role, showed that those who treated patients expressed more satisfaction and happiness with their careers than did physician executives who did not have an opportunity to treat patients (O'Conner, Nash, Buehler, & Bard, 2002). However, it should be mentioned that the relationship between physicians' satisfaction and number of encounters with patients is not linear after a certain saturation point; too large a patient load was likely to result in distress (Dunstone & Reames, 2001). Nonetheless, satisfactory clinician–patient relationships, reinforced by empathy, can reduce professional stress and contribute positively to physicians' well-being.

Benefits of Empathic Relationships for Patients

Now let us shift our attention to the benefits that patients derive from empathic relationships with their clinicians. In clinical encounters, interpersonal communication is the primary tool for the exchange of information. A large volume of literature is devoted to the beneficial effects of clinician–patient relationships on patients' adherence to treatment regimens; satisfaction with the health care provider and the health care system; the recall and understanding of medical information; the ability to cope with the disease; improvement in quality of life; and physical, mental, and social well-being. Empirical research has shown that physicians' worried demeanor when communicating with patients resulted in the patients' recalling less of the information the physician attempted to convey and negatively influenced patients' perceptions of their serious health condition (Shapiro, Boggs, Melamed, & Graham-Pole, 1992).

In the practice of medicine, an empathic physician–patient relationship is regarded as the royal road to optimal care. Illness cannot be understood without understanding the patient, and healing begins not *when* medicine is administered, but with *how* it is administered. In addition to a physician's knowledge and clinical skills, effective delivery of health care depends on other factors, such as the quality of clinician–patient interactions (Beisecker & Beisecker, 1990; Di Blasi, Harkness, Ernst, Georgiou, & Kleijnen, 2001). Moreover, the nature of the physician–patient relationship varies in different clinical encounters. For example, unlike chronic illnesses, which require continuous care, emergency surgical encounters are brief and thus preclude firm establishment of an empathic engagement. As indicated by Mayerson (1976), it might be difficult for a physician in an emergency room to feel empathy for an injured drunken driver who has killed a number of people in a car accident. However, by focusing on the patient's immediate needs and asking what it would be like to be in that situation, the physician may find it easier to make an empathic connection (Mayerson, 1976). Empathic understanding, however, is an important interpersonal capacity of physicians (Squier, 1990), regardless of the duration or nature of clinical encounters. Empathic engagement, according to Spiro (1998), helps healing and improves the medical practice.

Curing Versus Caring, Disease Versus Illness

In rendering treatment, two models of patient care—curing and caring—have been identified (Baumann, Deber, Silverman, & Mallette, 1998; DeValck, Bensing, Bruynooghe, & Batenburg, 2001; Spiro, 1986). In the "curing" model, the emphasis is placed on the biomedical paradigm of disease (see Chap. 6) in identifying the pathophysiology of the disease with the aim of treating the symptoms. In the "caring" model, the emphasis is placed on the biopsychosocial paradigm; the patient is viewed as a whole by focusing on the treatment of illness, not just on removal of the symptoms of disease. A disease can be detected by objective laboratory tests and microscopic examinations (as in the curing model), but detection of illness requires more than that. It is suggested that "cure is directed at disease, and care at patients" (Spiro, 1998, p. 2). The treatment of disease, according to Dr. Francis Peabody (1984), can be entirely impersonal, but curing the illness requires interpersonal attention and empathy.

Some investigators have argued that medical education and practice traditionally lean toward the curing model, whereas nursing education and practice emphasize the caring model (Baumann et al., 1998; Linn, 1974, 1975; Webb, 1996). Support for this argument is provided in a study in which nursing students were found to be twice as likely as medical students (67% versus 33%) to agree that patients' recovery alone should not be the focal point of patient care. Significant differences in rates of agreement were also found between nursing and medical school faculty (89% and 51%, respectively) (Linn, 1975). Despite the heavy training of nurse practitioners in diagnostic and treatment procedures, their orientation toward the caring model was close to the nurses' (Linn, 1974). It seems that in medical education, more learning opportunities are provided for curing than the caring aspect of patient care. According to Spiro (1998, p. 2) "physicians learn how to *cure* but little about how to *care*."

The notion of professionalism in medical education and practice that places emphasis on the enhancement of empathy and compassionate care in the delivery of health care suggests that the curing and caring models must be integrated in the education of health professionals. Incorporating some of the educational concepts of the caring model from the nursing discipline into the curing model in medical education curricula could help to improve empathy in patient care.

For a better understanding of the nature of the curing and caring models, it is useful to distinguish between "disease" and "illness." A disease is a result of a malfunction or maladaptation of biological and pathophysiological processes that cause organ pathology, whereas an illness represents a personal reaction to the disease (Kleinman, Eisenberg, & Good, 1978; Spiro, 1986). Illness can be experienced in the absence of disease, as indicated by findings that approximately half of all visits to physicians are based on complaints that lack an ascertainable biological reason. These complaints are known as somatization disorders (Hojat, Samuel, & Thompson, 1995; Kleinman et al., 1978), and patients with these disorders turn repeatedly to one physician after another, a phenomenon called "doctor shopping" (Ketterer & Buckholtz, 1989) or "doctor hopping" (Smith, 1991), because they do not experience empathic understanding from their physicians. In a survey of patients in California, 85% reported that they had changed their physicians in the past 5 years or were thinking of changing their physicians for reasons such as poor communication skills, the physician's inability to inspire confidence in the patient, and so forth (Moser, 1984).

It is argued that empathy in clinical encounters is cost effective because it leads to more accurate and early diagnosis, better compliance, and more efficient treatment planning, thereby avoiding doctor shopping and spiraling costs of unnecessary medical tests and hospitalizations (Bellet & Maloney, 1991; Book, 1991). In addition, a study of patients in primary care and surgical settings showed that the physician–patient visits tended to be more time consuming when physicians did not demonstrate understanding and empathy (Levinson, Gorawara-Bhat, & Lamb, 2000). Thus, an empathic physician–patient engagement can lead to the development of trust, which in turn will lead to better management of illness and containment of costs by preventing doctor shopping or hopping.

Uniqueness of Clinician–Patient Empathic Relationships

The encounter between clinician and patient is a purposeful interpersonal event, and its effectiveness in yielding positive clinical outcomes depends heavily on the clinician's skills in forming an empathic relationship, thus earning the patient's trust. A more positive patient outcome is achieved in a caring model in which clinician and patient establish a mutual understanding about the patient's health problem (Starfield et al., 1981), which has been identified as an important element of patient satisfaction with medical care (Kenny, 1995).

Being empathic is among the ingredients of the ethics of caring (Branch, 2000). The American Medical Association's first Code of Ethics, published in 1847, included the following: "The life of a sick person can be shortened not only by the acts, but also by the words or the manner of a physician. It is, therefore, a sacred duty to guard himself [or herself] carefully in this respect, and to avoid all things which can have a tendency to discourage the patient and to depress his [or her] spirit" (cited in Katz, 1984, p. 20).

An empathic relationship develops when the clinician avoids being arrogant and curbs the sense of superiority and instead becomes friendly, confident, relaxed, unhurried, and capable of communicating his or her empathic understanding and genuine concerns to the patient as well as to the patient's family. Rosenow (1999) argued that physicians who are arrogant in interpersonal contacts are committing a sin that is worse than the sin of greed because arrogance interferes with the development of empathy.

The clinician–patient relationship is unique compared to any other kind of human connection when you consider the combination of the patient's need to survive; the unequal positions of the clinician and patient in clinical encounters; the atmosphere of patient care; the psychodynamics of interpersonal exchanges in seeking and giving help; and cultural factors and boundaries in patient care. The following studies provide support for the uniqueness of the clinician–patient relationship.

Bonding for Survival (the Stockholm Syndrome)

In 1973, during a bank robbery in Stockholm, Sweden, two robbers held four people hostage for 6 days. During the ordeal, the hostages developed an attachment to their captors, coming to believe that their captors were protecting them from harm by the police. After the hostages were released and the ordeal was over, one of the hostages began raising funds for the robbers' legal defense! The phenomenon of bonding with captors to reduce the fear of death is known as the "Stockholm syndrome." Although this syndrome may seem to have no relevance to clinician–patient encounters, some psychological factors are common to both situations.

First, bonding occurs in situations where a person's survival depends on the mercy of another person. Second, bonding occurs when a person perceives that the other person is not ignorant and therefore pays some attention to the person. Third, bonding occurs when a person feels isolated from other people. Fourth, bonding occurs when a person perceives that he or she is unable to escape without the help of another person.

If some or all of the psychological factors underlying the Stockholm syndrome are present when a fearful patient consults a physician (for treatment, possible hospitalization, and possible surgery), then the similarity between psychological factors characterizing the syndrome and the physician–patient encounter becomes apparent.

The Clinician as an Authority Figure

In rendering help, the clinician is often perceived by the patient as an authority figure. This inequality in relation to power makes the patient more vulnerable to the clinician's influence (Koenig, 2002), which can be strengthened in the presence of empathic understanding.

Obedience to Authority (the Milgram Study)

In a well-known study of obedience conducted at Yale University, Stanley Milgram (1968) used an experimental paradigm to determine if people would be willing to comply with an authority figure's order even when compliance could have painful consequences. The study participants (who played the role of "teachers") were told that they were participating in an experiment to improve learning and memory. Their task was to teach another group of participants (who played the role of "learners") a list of paired associations. The learners were supposed to recall the associated words. The teachers were instructed to administer an electric shock every time a learner made a mistake and were told that the voltage would increase with each subsequent shock. The experimenter ordered the teachers to increase the intensity of the shock until a learner demanded to terminate the experiment or to continue delivering shocks as long as they liked regardless of the learner's protests. Therefore, the teachers could either comply with the experimenter's orders or refuse to comply and heed the learner's pleas.

The experiment was carried out under three different conditions: (1) the teacher and learner were in adjacent rooms, and the teacher could not hear the learner's reactions to the shocks unless the learner expressed distress by pounding on the wall; (2) the teacher and learner were in adjacent rooms, but the teacher could hear the learner's reactions; and (3) the teacher and learner were in the same room. In reality, there were no actual electric shocks, and the experimenter had instructed the learners to pretend that they were experiencing increased pain with each subsequent shock.

Milgram's results showed that approximately two-thirds of the teachers complied with the experimenter's orders and continued to deliver shocks up to the maximum levels, although complying was stressful for them and seemingly painful for the learners! The results also indicated that teachers who could hear the learners' screams or see the learners' reactions stopped delivering shocks earlier than did the teachers who were unaware of the learners' reactions. Milgram concluded that visual and auditory cues provided a more complete picture of another person's pain and suffering and thus could increase empathic responses.

Forty-five years after the original Milgram experiment, Burger (2009) conducted a partial replication of the study by limiting the maximum shock level to 150 V (rather than 450 V in the original experiment). It was found that obedience rates were only slightly lower than the original study. Burger (2009) found some evidence that scores on the Empathic Concern subscale of the IRI affected participants' responses. Although Milgram's research on obedience has been criticized on a number of ethical grounds, it continues to be viewed as a powerful demonstration of compliance with authority. Mehrabian and Epstein (1972) used Milgram's experimental paradigm to examine the construct validity of their Emotional Empathy Scale (see Chap. 5).

Assuming that the physician performs the role of the experimenter in Milgram's study and the patient performs the role of the research participant, the patient is psychologically set to comply with the physician's orders. As an authority figure, the physician has a profound influence on the patient's compliance with the treatment regimen even if the treatment is painful. More important, Milgram's finding that a suffering person's visual and auditory cues can enhance the empathic response in another person suggests that face-to-face clinician–patient encounters have an important advantage that cannot be replaced by any approach to patient care that precludes direct observation of the patient (e.g., computerized medical care, long-distance consultations).

The Milgram's well-known social psychology study has important implications for understanding factors that contribute to turning good people to evil (see the "Lucifer effect" described in the following section on the Stanford Prison Experiment). Could the inconceivable events such as atrocities committed in the Holocaust and brutality of beheading and burning humans by those so-called Islamic State militants be linked to the notion of obedience to authority?

Uncritical Acceptance of Authority (the Doctor Fox Lecture)

An experiment conducted by medical education researchers confirmed the influence that authority figures exerted, even on experts. Naftulin, Ware, and Donnelly (1973) hired a professional actor to deliver a lecture to an audience of 55 physicians, psychologists, social workers, educators, and medical school administrators attending a professional meeting. Introduced as "Dr. Myron L. Fox, a distinguished speaker and an authority on the application of mathematics to human performance," the actor delivered a lecture titled "Mathematical Game Theory as Applied to Physical Education."

The actor knew nothing about the subject. However, the researchers coached him on how to deliver the lecture and conduct the question-and-answer session with excessive use of double-talk, neologisms, and contradictory statements interspersed with humor and meaningless references to unrelated materials. When the researchers subsequently asked members of the audience to assess "Dr. Fox's" presentation, a large number of them highly praised the presentation!

This experiment has relevance to patients' adherence to physicians' orders and supports the notion that a physician's statements are likely to be accepted uncritically by patients, even by medically knowledgeable patients. Some have suggested that the experts' positive assessment of Dr. Fox's presentation was the result, in part, of the professional actor's nonverbal expressions when communicating information (Friedman, Prince, Riggio, & DiMatteo, 1980). This interpretation provides support for the importance of nonverbal communication in enhancing patients' trust in clinical encounters (see Chap. 3).

Role Expectations (the Stanford Prison Experiment)

The expectations of both clinician and patient can influence the process and outcome of their relationship to a significant degree. Role expectations, defined as "patterns of behavior viewed as appropriate or expected of a person who occupies a particular position" (Arnkoff, Glass, & Shapiro, 2002, p. 336), are a result of social learning and cultural factors. The interpersonal dynamics involved in role expectations were examined in a well-known social psychology experiment conducted by Philip Zimbardo and his colleagues at Stanford University in 1971 (Haney, Banks, & Zimbardo, 1973). Although the primary purpose of the experiment was to assess the power of social forces on individuals' behavior, the findings are relevant to clinician–patient encounters.

Twenty-one young healthy male college students were recruited to participate in the Stanford experiment in exchange for receiving money for each day they participated. Ten students were randomly assigned to play the role of prisoners and 11 were assigned the role of prison guards. The participants were told that the purpose was to study a simulated prison.

The mock prison was set up in a basement corridor in the university's psychology building. The prisoners and guards were dressed in different-colored uniforms to distinguish between the two groups. The researchers noticed immediately that the "prisoners" had adopted a generally passive role, and the "guards" had assumed an active role in their interactions with the prisoners.

It was made clear to the participants before the experiment began that no verbal abuse or physical violence would be allowed; however, the situation became so tense because of the guards' increasingly aggressive behavior and the prisoners' suffering that the experiment, designed to last for 2 weeks, had to be terminated prematurely after only 6 days. Five prisoners suffered from extreme depression, crying, rage, or acute anxiety disorder. When the experiment had to be terminated prematurely because of the aforementioned problems, all the prisoners were delighted, but most of the guards seemed reluctant to give up their role of controlling the prisoners. Although the researchers observed individual differences in the prisoners' coping behaviors and the guards' aggressive behavior, the findings generally suggest that role expectations were the determining factor in eliciting typical behaviors. An interesting observation was that the prisoners with higher empathy scores (a combined score on measures of helpfulness, sympathy, and generosity used in the study) were more resilient than other prisoners during the adversity.

The transformation of good people turning bad due to environmental demands and role expectations has been called the "Lucifer effect" by Zimbardo (2007) (Lucifer is a fallen angel who turned to Satan). Because of the notoriety of the Stanford prison experiment, a commercial movie was made about the entire experiment. The movie benefitted from input and consultation by the experimenter Philip Zimbardo (Chamberlin, 2015).

The relevance of the Stanford experiment to clinical encounters is that physicians and patients have different roles that lead to different behavioral expectations. As an expert, the physician is often expected to play an active role; and the patient, as a person in need of help, usually plays a submissive role by complying with the physician's orders. It is interesting to note that even physicians who consult a colleague as patients are likely to adopt the patients' role by becoming more passive and less assertive. The role expectations in clinician–patient encounters are determining factors in patient outcomes (Shapiro & Shapiro, 1984; Turner, Deyo, Loeser, von Korff, & Fordyce, 1994). Needless to say, an empathic clinician–patient engagement can lead to more productive expectations.

The Effect of Environment (the Rosenhan Study)

The results of an experiment titled, "On Being Sane in Insane Places," conducted by Rosenhan (1973), suggest that the environment in which a clinician encounters a patient creates specific expectations in the minds of both that influence their behavior. Rosenhan instructed a group of eight sane people (three psychologists, a psychiatrist, a pediatrician, a graduate student, a housewife, and a painter) to make appointments with physicians in different hospitals in five different states on the East and West coasts complaining that they were hearing unfamiliar voices in their heads.

All these "patients" used false names and were admitted to the hospitals' psychiatric wards. Upon admission, all the patients behaved normally but were diagnosed by hospital experts as schizophrenics "in remission" and were kept in the hospital for an average of 19 days. Interestingly, many of the hospitals' real patients were able to recognize that nothing was wrong with the study participants, telling them: "You are not crazy" or "You are a journalist or professor" (referring to the fact that the research participants were taking notes).

Rosenhan (1973) reported another experiment that was conducted at a research and teaching hospital whose staffs had been aware of Rosenhan's original study and doubted that such an error could occur in their hospital. The hospital staff was informed that during the next 3 months, one or more pseudopatients would attempt to be admitted to the psychiatric ward. Staff members were asked to specify their level of confidence concerning their judgment regarding whether each patient admitted during the study period was one of the pseudopatients. Among 193 patients admitted during the period, 41 were judged to be pseudopatients with a high level of certainty by at least one staff member, and 23 patients were considered to be suspect by at least one psychiatrist. In reality, no pseudopatients were sent to the hospital during the study! Rosenhan's findings suggest that the patient-care environment creates specific expectations that may influence the dynamics of interpersonal relationships, leading to an exaggerated account of illness or an incorrect diagnosis. Needless to say, an empathic understanding is a useful defense against situational misunderstandings and can lead to more accurate diagnoses and to decisions more consistent with reality.

The Kitty Genovese Tragedy

In March 13, 1964, 3 h after midnight, a young and physically petite New York City woman (Catherine "Kitty" Genovese) who was coming back from her work (a bar manager) was brutally attacked on the street near her home by a merciless rapist. She was stabbed repeatedly and viciously, screaming in despair: "Oh my God, he stabbed me! Help me!" She cried for help repeatedly, to no avail. Thirty-eight neighbors heard or watched from their windows as a killer stabbed the tiny woman to death; none called the police during the assault, nor did anything to prevent the crime. The attacker ran away when hearing one neighbor shouting "Leave that girl alone!" The attacker came back to finish his evil intent when no one showed up to help the victim. Only one witness called the police after the woman was dead. When the killer after apprehension was asked how he dared to attack a woman in a crowded neighborhood, he replied: "I knew they wouldn't do anything, people never do." (Takooshian, 2014).

The tragedy of Kitty Genovese, raped and killed in two subsequent attacks over a half-hour witnessed by 38 neighbors, has attracted the attention of social psychologists, not only because of its haunting image, but also for defying the well-known "bystander's effect," indicating that in the case of emergency, bystanders are likely to show apathy when other people are present to help. However, in the case of Kitty Genovese, no bystander offered help to engender apathy in other witnesses. The entire incident reminded me of the statement attributed to Edmund Burke: "The only thing necessary for the triumph of the evil is for good men to do nothing" (cited in Manning, Levine, & Collins, 2007, p. 561). If only one of those neighbors had had an empathic understanding of that terrified and helpless victim, the evil could have been defeated and Kitty Genovese's tragic story would not have been told here in a discussion of empathic understanding.

The Psychodynamics of Clinical Encounters

In addition to altruistic and egoistic motivational factors (Chap. 3), other psychological mechanisms can be involved in clinician–patient encounters. Because the psychological mechanisms involved in any interpersonal communication are complex, scrutinizing the psychodynamics involved in clinician–patient encounters is important to gaining a better understanding of the underlying mechanisms that can enhance or impede the relationship. A few of the psychological mechanisms that function in clinical encounters are described in the following sections.

Identification

Among psychological defense mechanisms, identification is commonly associated with empathy (Berger, 1987). Freud (1955, p. 110) referred to the link, "from identification by way of imitation to empathy" (cited in Szalita, 1976, p. 147). Identification is an unconscious mental process in which an individual attempts to satisfy some unmet needs by becoming like another person (Moore & Fine, 1968). To form an empathic relationship, the clinician should experience a sense of temporary oneness with the patient through a transient identification followed by a sense of separateness (Jaffe, 1986). In other words, the clinician should first think *with* the patient (identification, oneness) and then think *about* the patient (empathic separation) (Jaffe, 1986). According to Fenichel (1945), empathy consists of two acts: identification and awareness. Clinicians use the mechanism of identification to understand patients' concerns better while simultaneously becoming aware of their own feelings as well as their patients' feelings. Schwaber (1981) believed that identifying with the patient is a way of truly experiencing the patient's inner world and argued that empathy, although not equivalent to identification, occurs as an outcome of identification.

Identification may sometimes blur the boundaries between clinician and patient (Watson, 2002). Beres and Arlow (1974) proposed that empathy may involve a transient identification with another person's mental activities. In addition, they believed that empathy was mediated by communication of unconscious fantasies shared by the patient and the clinician through both verbal and nonverbal cues emanating from words, gestures, and behaviors. The clinician's understanding of the mechanism of identification can facilitate forming empathic engagement with the patient.

The "Wounded Healer" Effect

Similar to the mechanism of identification, feeling similar to and sharing common characteristics with the patient can influence the empathic engagement between clinician and patient. According to Decety and Jackson (2004, p. 73), the sense of "self-other overlap" between the helper and the person in need of help can contribute to the enhancement of empathic understanding. Further, people who were led to believe that their personality and values were more like those of a "performer" empathized more with the performer who appeared to experience pleasure and pain (Krebs, 1975).

The tendency of health professionals to help those with whom they share common characteristics is described as the "wounded healer" effect (Jackson, 2001). For example, studies have shown that the therapists' own illness can constitute a source of cure for their patients (Cristy, 2001; Holmes, 1992). The notion is that a wounded healer can better understand the experiences of another wounded person by sharing common experiences, by reflection, and by validation of feelings (Laskowski & Pellicore, 2002). For example, I came to grasp analogous pain to that of delivering a child after I painfully passed a kidney stone! I could then recognize, with more empathic understanding, the pain I observed my wife suffer in the delivery room.

Gustafson (1986) suggested that clinicians who have experienced pain are better able to understand the pain of others and to respond more appropriately. The successful resolution of psychological pain, according to Fussel and Bonney (1990), engenders empathy in the psychotherapist and influences the therapeutic process in a positive manner. Common wounds, according to Means (2002), provide a foundation for shared life experience and contribute to better understanding of patient's concerns, thus connecting clinicians with their patients. The philosophy underlying self-help programs, such as Alcoholics Anonymous (AA), is based on the wounded healer concept from common problems and experiences among participants. It is interesting to note that although perceived similarities between clinician and patient promote empathic understanding, patients' familiarity with their physicians does not predict empathic engagement (Makoul & Strauss, 2003). The fact that familiarity is not an important factor in empathic engagement in clinical situations suggests the unique nature of empathy in clinical encounters.

Transference

In his analysis of psychological illness, Freud (1958) noticed that two psychological phenomena could occur during clinician–patient encounters. One occurred in the patient (transference); the other occurred in the clinician (countertransference). These two phenomena are universal and can shape the nature of clinician–patient relationships (Goldberg, 2000). The transference often develops in the patient in relation to the clinician in ways that mimic an important relationship with a significant other (usually a primary caregiver, a parent, or even a lover) in the patient's past. Transference can be viewed as a repetition of an infantile object relationship that causes the patient to resist the treatment unless the resistance is countered appropriately by the clinician (Gabbard, 1994). Empathy plays an important role in the emergence of transference and in the development of the therapeutic alliance (Book, 1988). The importance of transference in the context of medical care, particularly in the primary care setting, has been discussed by Zinn (1990).

Because the patient unconsciously identifies the clinician with the former significant other, the patient is likely to behave *as if* the clinician is the significant other. The patient's need for understanding and reassurance, especially when experiencing illness and pain, triggers the unconscious tendency to view the clinician as an authoritative parental figure (Novack, 1987), thus increasing the likelihood of transference. The clinician is viewed in the patient's mind as the former significant other, which prompts the patient to reexperience the intense emotions associated with the relationship with the significant other in the past. According to Kohut (1959), this complex phenomenon, called transference in the psychoanalytic literature, plays an active role in the development of empathic engagement in the context of patient care. Awareness of the patient's inner world is possible not only through the senses (hearing, seeing, smelling, and touching) but also through understanding and analysis of the transference phenomenon. Empathic understanding can be enhanced if the clinician handles the phenomenon by an appropriate countertransference.

Countertransference

Transference is by no means confined to the patient. The clinician may, in response, develop mixed feelings toward a patient. The way a clinician handles the patient's transference is called countertransference. Lending oneself to becoming a wise figure to resolve the patient's past frustrations and conflicts is an example of an appropriate countertransference, which would lead to a positive patient outcome. In contrast, a clinician who projects his or her irrationalities and past unresolved conflicts onto the patient's transference relationship is an example of an inappropriate countertransference, which would lead to a negative patient outcome (Katz, 1984). According to Book (1988), difficulties in countertransference arise when the clinician uses empathy defensively to gratify his or her own psychological needs.

According to Zinn (1990, p. 293), physicians bring their own "biases and emotional needs to the encounter, resulting in a dynamic interaction that ultimately shapes the outcome of the relationship." Clinicians' awareness of the transference phenomenon and their skill in handling it can empower them to make their interventions more effective even in ambulatory practice settings (Schmidt & Baker, 1986).

By handling the patient's transference properly, the clinician paves the way for an empathic engagement and becomes a secure base the patient can use to resolve past frustrations and explore options for a healthy personal and social life. Although the transference and countertransference phenomena are believed to occur in intense psychoanalytic relationships, their presence in medical consultations cannot be ruled out (Zinn, 1990).

Medical students and physicians tend to eschew probing for psychological factors during interviews with patients, probably for fear of being unable to handle such factors properly (Smith, 1984). The presence of this fear was confirmed in a study with medical students in which it was found that a great majority of them expressed feelings of being unable to handle talking with patients about fears associated with cancer and death because they were afraid of harming the patients (Smith, 1984). Medical educators should pay more attention to teaching medical students and residents the psychodynamics of interpersonal encounters, including transference and countertransference (briefly described in this Chapter), to improve their understanding of the peculiarities of clinical encounters and to enhance their capacity for empathic engagement with their patients suffering from psychosocial problems.

Empathy-Enhancing Factors in Clinician–Patient Encounters

A number of factors contribute to the quality of relationships between clinician and patient. Some of the factors that are more relevant to the enhancement of empathy are discussed briefly in the following sections.

The Placebo Effect

White (1991) proposed that once an empathic clinician–patient relationship is formed, the clinician becomes a powerful placebo-like agent, an "X" factor in healing, that has a tangible positive influence on patient outcomes. It was further suggested that the placebo effect of the clinician–patient relationship is independent from any other placebo-like intervention (Hróbjartsson & Gøtzsche, 2001).

The placebo effect, defined as an intervention that simulates medical treatment but is not believed to be a specific treatment for the target condition (Brody, 1985), has a long history in medicine. The existence of the placebo effect is, in itself, a testimony to the notion that psychosocial factors have a tangible influence on the pathophysiology of disease (Spiro, 1986). The reported rate of response to placebos ranges from 15% to 58% (Turner et al., 1994). However, the notion that a placebo may be an effective treatment in one-third of cases remains the standard in clinical research (Hróbjartsson & Gøtzsche, 2001) (This rate was first suggested about half a century ago by Beecher, 1955.) Although no convincing evidence exists concerning the underlying mechanisms of the placebo effect, some authors have speculated that expectation, reduced anxiety, learning, and an endorphin-mediating effect may explain the placebo response (Turner et al., 1994). Research suggests that the placebo effect is more pronounced when patients comply with clinician's orders (Turner et al., 1994). Better compliance is a function of clinician–patient empathic engagement (Pumilia, 2002). Thus, through leading to better compliance, the empathic relationship can prompt a more positive placebo effect and a better patient outcome.

Recognition of Nonverbal Cues

In clinician–patient encounters, recognition of nonverbal cues and explicit acknowledgment of patients' feelings, concerns, and experiences are important to establish "rapport" (Matthews et al., 1993), which is the essential element of empathic relationships. Rapport can also be strengthened by physicians' ability to decode and encode nonverbal messages and convey their understanding of those messages to their patients (DiMatteo, 1979). Some nonverbal behaviors that are said to promote rapport include clinicians' efforts to match patients' postures, gestures, respiration rates, tempo and pitch of speech, and language patterns (Matthews et al., 1993). Other important nonverbal cues in clinical encounters are tone of voice, gaze, aversion of gaze, posture, silence, laughter, teary eyes, facial expression, hand and body movements, trembling, touch, physical distance, leaning forward or backward, sighs, sweating, and other signs of distress or comfort (Fretz, 1966; Wolfgang, 1979) (see Chap. 3 for a detailed discussion about nonverbal communication in a general context).

Physicians' ability to decode nonverbal cues is an important component in forming empathic relationships with their patients (DiMatteo, 1979). Using the Profile of Nonverbal Sensitivity Test (PONS Test) (Rosenthal, Hall, DiMatteo, Rogers, & Archer, 1979), DiMatteo and associates found that a patient's perception that the physician listened was predicted by the physician's ability to decode nonverbal cues, such as smiles, grimaces, finger tapping, and a high-pitched voice (DiMatteo, Taranta, Friedman, & Prince, 1980).

Other authors have pointed out that leaning forward during interpersonal interactions is perceived as an indication of a warm, intimate, attentive, and empathic relationship (Fretz, 1966; Harrigan & Rosenthal, 1983; Hasse & Tepper, 1972; Trout & Rosenfeld, 1980). Authors have also reported that postural congruency (positioning one's head, hands, and legs in a corresponding manner when interacting with another person) is an indication of nonverbal social rapport among friends, colleagues, and those engaged in conversation with a common goal (Buchheimer, 1963; Trout & Rosenfeld, 1980). Postural congruency may be a remnant of synchronized behavior between mother and child (Chap. 4), a reflection of the understanding and sharing that are important in empathic relationships.

Other components of nonverbal behavior can influence patients' perceptions of rapport during encounters with physicians. For example, physicians who nod their heads (indicating agreement and approval), lean toward the patient (indicating attentiveness, accessibility, closeness, and empathic concern), and sit with their hands resting on their laps (indicating openness, confidence in their abilities, and readiness to respond), rather than folding their arms across their chests (indicating defensiveness), convey a positive rapport that opens the gate to more empathic exchanges (Harrigan & Rosenthal, 1983). Arms and legs in the open position convey less defensiveness and a more positive attitude than closed arm and leg positions do (Mehrabian, 1969).

In addition, the degree of eye contact can indicate the nature of clinician–patient empathic engagement. For example, Mehrabian (1969) reported that a higher degree of eye contact is maintained when the interacting pair like, rather than dislike, one another. However, cultural and sex factors help to determine the desirable degree of eye contact in clinician–patient encounters. For example, Mehrabian (1969) indicated that in American culture, people tend to maintain more eye contact when they are dealing with high-status individuals. In some non-Western cultures described as collectivistic (as opposed to individualistic) (Triandis, 1995), direct eye contact between people of the opposite sex or of different status is avoided.

The face is recognized as a primary channel for affective communication (Ekman & Friesen, 1974). Changes in facial expression (e.g., expressions conveying pain) are often accompanied by parallel changes in autonomic arousal and subjective feelings (Vaughan & Lanzetta, 1981). Facial expressions and nonverbal cues often "leak" unconscious messages (DiMatteo et al., 1980). However, when assessing nonverbal cues and detecting deception, one may make more accurate judgments by observing the body rather than the face (Ekman & Friesen, 1974). In psychoanalytic interviews, the psychoanalyst sits behind the patient, who is lying on the couch, to prevent the patient from viewing the analyst's facial expressions and emotional reactions (Slipp, 2000). Hearing hidden messages beyond spoken words with "the third ear" and seeing nonverbal cues emitted often beyond conscious behavior with "the mind's eye" pave the road for empathic engagement in encounters between clinician and patient.

The "Third Ear" and the "Mind's Eye"

For a better understanding of interpersonal dynamics in clinical encounters, clinicians must learn to hear their patients not only with their anatomical ears but also with their "third ear" to get beyond the spoken words. In addition, to enhance their empathic understanding, clinicians must view their patients' inner worlds not only with their anatomical eyes but also with their "mind's eye." The rapport between clinician and patient will be stronger and the empathic understanding between them will become deeper if the clinician listens to the patient's narrative account of illness with the third ear and sees the personal, psychological, social, and cultural factors involved in the patient's interpersonal relationships with the mind's eye. The more that is said, the more that is heard, and the more that is understood, the deeper the relationship becomes (Jackson, 1992). The seeds of empathy are sown by listening with the third ear and seeing with the mind's eye.

During the nineteenth century, seeing was more prominent than hearing in the realms of sickness and healing (Jackson, 1992). As a result, observation of nonverbal cues was given an important place in the diagnosis and treatment of illness. Waisman (1966) suggested that in clinical medicine, physicians needed to look at the hidden aspects of a patient's illness not only by observation (seeing with the mind's eye) but also by listening with their third ear.

In the therapeutic relationship, listening is a crucial method for acquiring information from the help seeker, for understanding the problem, and for bringing about the help seeker's healing (Jackson, 1992). This tradition is attributed to William Osler, who said: "Listen to the patient, he is telling you the diagnosis" (cited in Jackson, 1992, p. 1630). According to Samuel Coleridge (1802), to submerge ourselves in the thoughts of another being, we must have "the eye of a North American Indian" tracking the footsteps of the enemy upon the leaves that strew the forest, "the ear of a wild Arab" listening to the silent desert, and "the touch of a blind man" feeling the face of a darling child. In the context of patient care, these qualities translate into a clinician's ability to listen with the third ear, to see with the mind's eye, and to possess the capacity for empathy to understand the patient beyond spoken words and observable behavior.

Listening from the "outside" only with one's anatomical ears is insufficient in these encounters. According to Greenson (1960), clinicians must shift their attention to listening and feeling from the "inside." As Jackson (1992) pointed out, such listening can be initiated from an empathically attuned position. Research has demonstrated that teachers who attempt to listen to their students with a third ear by using an empathic response were better able to help them with academic and behavioral problems (Cleghorn, 1978).

Empathy, according to Schwaber (1981), is a "mode of analytic" listening. Similarly, Theodore Reik (1948) pointed out that a clinician must hear not only what the patient's words do say but what the words do not say as well. To achieve that goal, Reik emphasized that the clinician "must learn to listen with the third ear" (p. 144). By listening with the third ear, clinicians can catch what other people feel and think but do not say. Therefore, they need to learn how one person's mind "speaks" to another person in silence. To form an empathic relationship with patients to provide them with optimal care, clinicians must tune in and listen with the third ear to understand what the patients intend to say beyond the spoken word (Good, 1972).

Listening with a third ear can be accomplished by becoming more vigilant during verbal communication with patients, and seeing with the mind's eye can be accomplished better by becoming more observant of nonverbal clues in clinician–patient encounters. Spoken language is more than a vehicle for the transfer of information; it can influence thoughts as well (Hunt & Agnoli, 1991). In a broader context, Lee Whorf (1956) said back in the mid-nineteenth century that language can convey more than perspectives and feelings; it can shape the thoughts of a culture as well. Therefore, in the context of patient care, the voice that can be heard by the anatomical ear can have a more powerful meaning when processed with the third ear. Charles Darwin (1965, p. 354) proposed that the "force of language is much aided by the expressive movements of face and body." Thus, important information about a person's cognitive and affective states can be communicated through nonverbal cues (Lanzetta & Kleck, 1970) that show a wider picture through the mind's eye. Empathic understanding can be enhanced by recognizing hidden and unspoken messages by decoding nonverbal cues with the mind's eye.

Cultural Factors

Culture, defined as "the set of attitudes, values, beliefs, and behaviors shared by a group of people, communicated from one generation to the next" (Sternberg, 2004, p. 325), determines how people connect with one another. People in different cultures have strikingly different views of self and others (Markus & Kitayama, 1991) that can influence their help-seeking and help-giving behaviors. Cultural norms, racial or ethnic differences, religious beliefs, sex stereotyping, and other embodied sources of identity can influence empathic engagement in the context of patient care. Comas-Diaz and Jacobsen (1991) postulated that ethnocultural factors can not only influence the individual's presentations and interpretations in clinical encounters, but they can also significantly affect the process and outcomes of patient care.

For a better understanding of interpersonal dynamics of care-seeking and care-giving behaviors, these behaviors must be examined in the cultural context, because culture is inextricably interlinked to any kind of behavior. For example, in a cross-cultural study of care-seeking attitudes, it was found that a Belgian sample expressed more cure-oriented than care-oriented attitudes toward health care (DeValck et al., 2001). A study by Nelson and Baumgarte (2004) showed that unfamiliarity with cultural norms of others reduces empathic understanding mediated by a lack of perspective taking on the part of the observer. Thus, the clinician's familiarity with the patient's culture is another factor that must be considered when studying empathic engagement in patient care. However, little empirical research has been conducted on this topic. Although similarities have been noted in Western and non-Western (e.g., Japanese) cultures with regard to physician–patient communication and patient satisfaction (Ishikawa, Takayama, Yamazaki, Skei, & Katsumata, 2002), it is crucial to recognize that clinician–patient encounters are determined by cultural factors that bring cognitive and affective content as well as therapeutic values, expectations, and goals to the relationship (Kleinman et al., 1978).

Despite the importance of cultural awareness in clinical encounters, a study showed that only 8% of the medical schools in the USA and no medical school in Canada offered formal courses about cultural issues in patient care (Flores, Gee, & Kastner, 2000). In another study on cross-cultural medical education among a national sample of residents in different specialties in the USA, it was found that although 96% of the residents indicated that it was important to understand cultural issues when providing care, two-thirds reported that no evaluation was made with regard to their skills in the cross-cultural aspects of communication with patients (Weisman et al., 2005).

Cultural differences can influence the clinician–patient empathic engagement as well as the outcomes of patient care to a significant degree (Hall, Roter, & Katz, 1988; Hooper, Comstock, Goodwin, & Goodwin, 1982; Kleinman et al., 1978; Waxler-Morrison, Anderson, & Richardson, 1990). Cultural differences have been observed in physicians' behavior when revealing cancer diagnoses to patients (Holland, Geary, Marchini, & Tross, 1987). For example, in some cultures, the diagnosis of terminal illnesses is withheld from patients based on the assumption that disclosure may generate such fear that progression of the disease will accelerate (Adib & Hamadeh, 1999; Surbone, 1992; Zahedi, 2011). Evidence suggests that this assumption may not be entirely baseless because increased fear has been reported to be a major factor in "voodoo death" (Cannon, 1957) that is believed in some primitive societies to be caused by strong fear and necromancy (communication with dead people, witchcraft). The power of suggestion often observed in research imagery is a testimony to the belief that disclosing a serious illness to some patients may result in making their situation worse rather than better.

Hopelessness generated by revealing a fatal diagnosis can cause sudden death among some patients (Richter, 1957). Revealing the diagnosis of a terminal disease is viewed as cruel, inhumane, and unempathic in some cultures but as ethical and empathic in other cultures (Holland et al., 1987). An international survey of oncologists from 20 countries revealed that fewer than 40% of physicians in Africa, Hungary, Iran, Panama, Portugal, and Spain would disclose a cancer diagnosis to patients, whereas greater than 80% of physicians in Austria, Denmark, Finland, the Netherlands, New Zealand, Norway, Switzerland, and Sweden would reveal the diagnosis (Holland et al., 1987). Clinical realities are culturally constituted, and the nature of physician–patient relationships varies in different cultures and in different ethnic groups within a culture (Kleinman et al., 1978). Clearly, culture can exert an important influence on the nature and contents of clinician–patient communication. However, empathic understanding is always beneficial in clinical encounters regardless of cultural peculiarities.

Furthermore, despite the highly recommended advice that physicians must share their treatment decisions with patients to obtain the patients' input and compliance, such is not the case in the training and practice of physicians in all cultures. In a study by Ali, Khalil, and Yousef (1993) in which American and Egyptian cancer patients were compared, it was found that Egyptian patients preferred not to be involved in decision making; instead, family had an important role in making decisions. Disclosure of a serious diagnosis was socially unacceptable. Emotional support was considered to be the responsibility of the family, not of the health care provider (Ali et al., 1993). Many Moslem patients, for example, believe in the doctrine of predestination, fatalism, and stoicism. With this group of patients, empathic physician–patient relationships can be better formed when physicians convey to them that it is God's will that provided the opportunity for the patient–physician encounter.

In some cultures, physicians are paternal figures who have absolute authority to dictate any treatment they deem necessary regardless of the patient's input. In those authoritarian cultures, the patient-centered approach to medical care is likely to convey a physician's lack of determination and competence! Therefore, because empathic concern has a different connotation in different cultures, clinicians' awareness of their patients' cultural peculiarities can enhance empathic understanding. For this reason, cultural issues must receive serious attention in undergraduate, graduate, and continuing medical education programs.

Personal Space

Everyone knows that most animals display territoriality by marking off certain areas as their own space. Human beings exhibit a similar tendency by establishing an invisible bubble around themselves called "personal space" (Hall, 1966; Sommer, 1969). The boundaries of that space determine the distance individuals need to preserve their privacy. Overcrowding that interferes with one's personal space (or territory) can lead to aggressive behavior (Calhoun, 1962). It is interesting to note that the boundaries of personal space are reduced to a minimum in intimate and empathic relationships (Hall, 1966). Shamasundar (1999) postulated that interpersonal interactions represent an enmeshment of personal spaces in exchange for affective and cognitive information that results in empathic understanding. Sharing of personal spaces is the essence of an empathic relationship—the more desirable overlap in personal spaces, the deeper the empathic understanding.

The nature of the relationship, gender, personality, and cultural factors determine the desirable amount of personal distance. People who are emotionally disturbed or have low self-esteem tend to maintain more personal space (Shamasundar, 1999). Furthermore, the desirable amount of personal space varies in different individuals and in different cultures. For example, in the USA, a maximum of 18 inches of personal space was observed in most intimate encounters (e.g., romantic relations), and a personal space ranging from one to four feet was considered a desirable distance between friends and acquaintances (Hall, 1966). People who like each other and form empathic relationships with one another tend to maintain less personal space between themselves when conversing than strangers do (Mehrabian, 1969).

Encroaching on a person's personal space can elicit negative attitudes if the relationship is not empathic (Mehrabian, 1969). For example, violation of an individual's personal space can lead to anxiety or irritability and, sometimes, to increased aggression and the breakdown of interpersonal communication. One study found that people sit closer when expecting approval and sit farther away when expecting disapproval (Rosenfeld, 1965). In the context of clinician–patient encounters, a desirable degree of personal space should be maintained to facilitate empathic interpersonal exchanges.

Boundaries

On the basis of Carl Rogers's description of empathic relationships in clinical encounters (Rogers, 1959), one can perceive another person's internal frame of reference "as if" one were the other person. If the "as if" condition is lost, a sense of profound emotional involvement (sympathy) in the clinician–patient relationship can develop, leading to potential risks (see Chap. 1), including the clinician's increased susceptibility to the patient's pain and suffering, on the one hand, and the patient's dependence on the clinician, on the other hand (Chaps. 1 and 3).

In clinician–patient relationships, sharing of emotions always necessitates setting limits or boundaries regarding affective involvement. Although boundaries in clinician–patient encounters are often unspoken and unwritten, they are mutually understood (Gabbard & Nadelson, 1995). Boundaries imply the refraining from intense emotional and erotic involvements. Some boundaries are spelled out in codes of professional ethics. Clinicians violate boundaries when they purposefully exploit the patient's trust and dependency and respond unprofessionally to the patient's desires and expectations. Frequently reported violations of boundaries include sexual relationships, dual relationships, receiving inappropriate gifts or services, bartering, unusual time and duration of visits, use of seductive and erotic language, excessive self-disclosure, and inappropriate physical contact (Gabbard & Nadelson, 1995). All the aforementioned violations can sabotage the development of an empathic clinician–patient relationship.

The extent of intimacy in clinician–patient relationships is defined by boundaries that prevent the exploitation of both parties (Farber, Novack, & O'Brien, 1997). On the one hand, patients who seek help are vulnerable and tend to form a secure attachment to the clinician, who is viewed as an omnipotent authority figure resembling a wise parent (e.g., through the transference mechanism). On the other hand, being human beings, too, and thus vulnerable, clinicians must be vigilant about not bonding with a patient as a result of a strong emotional involvement (e.g., an inability to deal with the patient's transference).

Because "to err is human," errors can be made in clinician–patient relationships (Kohn, Corrigan, & Donaldson, 2000). However, education and the guidelines of professional ethics can minimize the violation of boundaries during encounters with patients (Sage, 2002). Several factors contribute to the maintenance or violation of boundaries in clinician–patient relationships: age, sex, ethnicity, culture, attitudes, developmental and family background, personality, education, and the capacity for empathic understanding.

Transgression of boundaries can occur in all specialties, but the likelihood of transgression is greater in psychological and psychiatric consultations because of the transference arising from the intense emotions generated in such consultations (Gabbard, 1994). Transgressions involving sexual issues are often initiated by patients (Gartrell, Herman, Olarte, Feldstein, & Localio, 1986). The oldest skill in medicine, as Thomas (1985) pointed out, is the physician's laying hands on the patient. Therefore, touching during physical examinations has traditionally been regarded as the opening gate to the diagnosis and sometimes to therapeutic benefits. Touching is not only a reminiscent of maternal stroking that generates a feeling of security but also conveys affection and empathic support (Mayerson, 1976). However, the inappropriate use of touch is certainly a transgression of boundaries that diminishes trust and ruins the empathic relationship.

When medical students and physicians are insufficiently trained with regard to potential transgressions of interpersonal boundaries, medical education is often blamed (Gartrell et al., 1986); but the problem is that the "rules of engagement" concerning identification of boundary transgressions are vague and therefore not easy to teach. Needless to say, empathic engagement in clinician–patient relationships can help to avoid the transgression of boundaries.

Recapitulation

Empathic engagement in the context of patient care is a complex phenomenon driven by many factors operating in the dynamics of the clinician–patient relationship. Factors that bind clinicians and their patients together include the need for human connection, particularly at times of crisis; the need for survival; the clinician's position as an authority figure; role expectations in the patient-care environment; psychological dynamics of clinical encounters; and clinicians' ability to understand patients by listening with the third ear and seeing with the mind's eye. Empathic engagement in patient care can also be influenced by cultural factors, personal space, and boundaries. When two people are empathically connected, many factors beyond spoken words and observable behavior provide the glue for binding them together. Because of the importance of understanding psychodynamics of interpersonal relationships in general, and their implications in clinical encounters, it would be highly desirable to include the topic of interpersonal dynamics in the educational curriculum of any health professions education.

Chapter 9
Clinical Empathy as Related to Personal Qualities, Career Choice, Acquisition of Knowledge, and Clinical Competence

Man is essentially a bulb with many thousands of roots.

—(George Christoph Lichtenberg, 1742–1799; cited in Strauss, 1968, p. 285)

Abstract

- The link between clinical empathy, personality, selected psychosocial variables, career choice, specialty interest, clinical competence, and patient outcomes is described.
- Empirical research suggests that empathy correlates positively with prosocial and altruistic behaviors and with a number of desirable personal qualities that are conducive to relationship building, including sociability, social skills, likeability, flexibility, tolerance, emotional intelligence, moral judgment, sense of humor, conscientiousness, agreeableness, openness to experiences, positive social influence, personal accomplishment, teamwork, and interprofessional collaboration.
- A number of undesirable personal attributes that are detrimental to positive interpersonal relationships correlate negatively with empathy, including aggression, hostility, externalization, antisocial behaviors, depersonalization, depression, anxiety, conduct disorders, neurotic or psychotic disturbances, lying, stealing, physical abuse, and dogmatism. Also linked to clinical empathy are factors such as satisfaction with early maternal relationships, selection of a career in medicine for humanistic reasons, and attention to psychosocial issues in medicine.
- Empirical findings suggest that scores on clinical empathy are associated with indicators of clinical competence and career choice. Health professions students and practitioners who choose the so-called "people-oriented" specialties are more likely to obtain higher average scores on clinical empathy than those interested in the "procedure- or technology-oriented" specialties.

M. Hojat, *Clinical Empathy*, https://doi.org/10.1007/978-3-031-87413-0_9

Introduction

Empathy, like any other personality attribute, varies among individuals with different constitutional, developmental, experiential, and educational backgrounds. This chapter reviews findings regarding the link between clinical empathy, personal qualities, academic attainment, clinical competence, career choice, and tangible patient outcomes.

Psychosocial Correlates of Clinical Empathy

Prosocial Behaviors

Prosocial behavior has been defined as a person's voluntary act that can benefit another person (Eisenberg & Miller, 1987). The notion that empathy is a determining factor in altruism and prosocial behavior has been widely discussed and accepted (Aronfreed, 1970; Batson & Coke, 1981; Eisenberg & Miller, 1987; Hoffman, 1981; Staub, 1978).

Some argue that prosocial behavior can be initiated by an egoistic motivation (e.g., the expectation of a reward, an attempt to avoid aversive stimuli or punishment, or an attempt to reduce personal distress by helping others). Others suggest that prosocial behavior can be evoked by an altruistic motivation (e.g., the act of helping to reduce other people's distress, without expecting any reward, even if the act is harmful to oneself). One study found that people who were more empathic behaved more altruistically: that is, they were willing to help others, even when their own welfare was jeopardized (Krebs, 1975). In another study, teachers' ratings indicated that children's empathy was associated with their helpful behavior (Litvack-Miller, McDougall, & Romney, 1997).

Some authors have argued that empathy-induced helping behavior can be the result of merging the self with others. In certain circumstances, feelings of oneness emerge so that human beings experience others as "we," rather than as "they" (Hornstein, 1978). In these circumstances, we may be psychologically indistinguishable from others and may understand their experiences better. And when this feeling of oneness emerges, the two shall become one, and, as reported by Lerner and Meindl (1981, p. 227): "If the empathic tie is dominant, it would be natural for us to engage in acts which we or others might label as self-sacrifice or martyrdom." In summarizing their research findings, Batson and Sager et al. (1997, p. 508) reported that "empathy evokes concern for the other, distinct from oneself, that is beyond self-interest."

Prosocial behavior initiated by altruism has been studied in relation to empathy (Eisenberg & Miller, 1987). However, in an earlier meta-analytic review of 11 studies, most of which involved children, the investigators found no consistent link between empathy and prosocial behavior (Underwood & Moore, 1982). This unexpected result can be explained by the finding that the evaluation of empathy in children could be confounded by such factors as validity issues regarding measurements of empathy and the evaluators' gender (Chap. 5). In addition, Eisenberg and Miller (1987) proposed that the association between empathy and prosocial behavior is weaker among children than among adults because emotional or cognitive responses and prosocial behavior become more integrated with age. In a later meta-analytic study of a larger number of research articles involving adults in which empirical studies and doctoral dissertations were reviewed, Eisenberg (1983) reported a significant link between empathy and prosocial behavior.

Individuals with high scores on Mehrabian and Epstein's Emotional Empathy Scale (Chap. 5) were more likely to demonstrate helping behavior than were individuals with low-empathy scores (Barnett, Howard, King, & Dino, 1980; Rushton, Chrisjohn, & Fekker, 1981). Cohen and Hoffner (2013) found that empathic concern (measured by the IRI, see Chap. 5) predicted organ donation willingness. In a review of studies on empathy and individual differences, scores on the Emotional Empathy Scale (see Chap. 5) were not only significantly correlated with altruistic behavior but also with greater physiological arousability (greater skin conductance and increased heart rate), more emotionality (a greater tendency to weep), spending more time with and displaying more affection to children, higher moral judgment, more volunteerism, and less aggressive behavior (Mehrabian, Young, & Sato, 1988). It is also reported that empathy leads to moral behavior, justice, and preference for fairness (Decety & Cowell, 2015).

Prosocial behaviors such as willingness to render compassionate care to terminally ill patients were associated with high scores on the JSE in medical students. For example, we found that students who volunteered to participate in student-run free clinics to provide healthcare services to indigent and underserved patients scored significantly higher on the JSE-S version than their non-volunteering classmates, prior to participating in the student-run free clinics program (Modi, Fascelli, Daitch, & Hojat, 2017). In another study, medical students who volunteered to participate in a program, called "No One Dies Alone" to provide compassionate companionship at the bedside of lonely dying patients by simply sitting at the patients' bedside; holding patients' hands; rendering therapeutic touch; playing music; and reading books, stories, poetry aloud, obtained a significantly higher average score on the JSE than their non-volunteer classmates in the pretest (administered prior to participation in the program) (Hojat, DeSantis, Ney, & DeCleene-Do, 2021).

College students who scored higher on empathy were more eager than low-scoring students to help neurologically handicapped children who could benefit from a volunteer's efforts (Barnett, Feighny, & Esper, 1983). College students who were members of help-oriented groups, such as those helping the underprivileged, scored higher on the Emotional Empathy Scale than did students who were members of self-interest organizations, such as the biology honors fraternity (Van Orum, Foley, Burns, DeWolfe, & Kennedy, 1981). In a study with prison inmates, the investigators observed that the inmates who volunteered to help disadvantaged individuals in the prison scored higher on Hogan's Empathy Scale than non-volunteers (Gendreau, Burke, & Grant, 1980).

Personal Qualities

A number of empirical studies have addressed the relationships between empathy, personality, and psychosocial measures. In an earlier empirical study (Kerr & Speroff, 1954), significant correlations were reported between students' scores on a measure of empathy (developed by the study authors) and scores of popularity and likeability measured by a sociometric method developed by Moreno (1934). Also, empathy scores in that study were correlated with the smiles observed at a commencement exercise and with understanding emotions of others. Kerr and Speroff (1954) reported a positive link between empathy scores and automobile salesmen's sales records and their merit rankings. However, a later study by Lamont and Lundstrom (1977) found that the performance of successful industrial salesmen was negatively correlated with scores on Hogan's Empathy Scale but was positively related to a measure of endurance.

Hogan and colleagues conducted several studies comparing scores on Hogan's Empathy Scale with scores obtained on other measures of personal qualities. For example, Hogan and Mankin (1970) reported a significant correlation between scores on the Empathy Scale and those on a measure of likeability. Two years later, Hogan and Dickstein (1972) found a significant correlation between empathy and mature moral judgment. A year later, Greif and Hogan (1973) reported a significant link between college students' scores on the Empathy Scale and a personality factor called "person-orientation" they derived from the California Psychological Inventory (Gough, 1987). This finding is consistent with the significant link observed between clinical empathy (measured by the JSE) and "people-oriented" versus "technology- or procedure-oriented" specialty interest in physicians-in-training and in-practice that will be described later in this chapter.

Medical students' scores on Hogan's Empathy Scale were positively and significantly correlated with measures of intellectual efficiency, flexibility, tolerance, good impression, and extraversion, and were significantly but negatively correlated with depression, anxiety, and introversion (Hogan, 1969). The following adjectives had the highest positive correlations with scores on Hogan's Empathy Scale: pleasant, charming, friendly, dreamy, cheerful, sociable, sentimental, imaginative, discreet, and tactful. In contrast, the following adjectives correlated most highly but negatively with scores on Hogan's Empathy Scale: cruel, cold, quarrelsome, hostile, bitter, unemotional, unkind, hard-hearted, argumentative, and opinionated (Hogan, 1969). Hogan's findings paint a picture of an empathic person as one who is emotionally stable and socially mature—that is, a person who possesses the major attributes described as emotional intelligence (Goleman, 1995; Salovey & Mayer, 1990). Indeed, the link between empathy and emotional intelligence has been confirmed in some empirical studies. For example, it has been reported that scores on a measure of emotional intelligence were positively correlated with empathic perspective taking (Schutte et al., 2001). The positive relationship between empathy (measured by the JSE) and emotional intelligence has been confirmed in studies with health profession students (Arora et al., 2010; Austin, Evans, Goldwater, & Potter, 2005; Kliszcz, Nowicka-Sauer, Trzeciak, Nowak, & Sadowska, 2006).

Moral judgment and helping behavior were significantly correlated with scores on Mehrabian and Epstein's Emotional Empathy Scale (Eisenberg-Berg & Mussen, 1978). Students who scored higher on a modified version of the Emotional Empathy Scale were more assertive, less narcissistic, more sensitive, less self-focused, and more concerned about a healthy lifestyle (Kalliopuska, 1992a). It was also reported that people living in the countryside obtained a higher average score on the Emotional Empathy Scale than did those living in towns (Kalliopuska, 1994). In a study with female Japanese physicians, it was found that those who reported living with their parents in an extended family or living close to their parents scored higher on the JSE than those who were living alone or in a small nuclear family (Kataoka, Koide, Hojat, & Gonnella, 2012).

Significant and positive correlations have been observed between scores on the IRI and measures of hypnotic susceptibility and self-absorption (Wickramasekera & Szylk, 2003). Among nurses, effective leadership has been linked to scores on the IRI (Mansen, 1993). In a meta-analytic study it was found that empathy was negatively related to aggressive, antisocial, and externalizing behaviors, such as conduct disorders, lying, and stealing, as well as to physical abuse (Miller & Eisenberg, 1988). Physically and emotionally abusive parents scored significantly lower than a comparison group of foster parents on the Perspective Taking, Empathic Concern, and Personal Distress subscales of Davis's IRI (Wiehe, 2003). When Hogan's Empathy Scale was administered to incarcerated child molesters, their scores showed deficits in empathy (Marshall & Maric, 1996). The findings in these studies reveal that individuals who are deficient in empathy naturally possess less capacity to understand and respond to the needs of others, including their own children (Stern, Baily, Castello, et al., 2024).

Negative relationships were reported between scores on Hogan's Empathy Scale and measures of anxiety, phobia, obsession, and depression (Kupfer, Drew, Curtis, & Rubinstein, 1978), and indicators of neurotic and psychotic disturbances (Hekmat, Khajavi, & Mehryar, 1974, 1975). Scores on Mehrabian and Epstein's Emotional Empathy Scale were inversely related to a measure of psychopathic personality (Sandoval, Hancock, Poythress, Edens, & Lilienfeld, 2000). In addition, negative correlations were reported between scores on Hogan's Empathy Scale and measures of state and trait anxiety (Deardroff, Kendall, Finch, & Sitartz, 1977). Also, scores on the Emotional Empathy Scale were negatively correlated with a measure of narcissism among undergraduate students (Watson, Grisham, Trotter, & Biderman, 1984) and among young baseball players in Finland (Kalliopuska, 1992b).

Symptoms of depression and dogmatism among medical students were negatively correlated with scores on Hogan's Empathy Scale (Streit-Forest, 1982). In a study of medical students at the Louisiana State University Medical Center, perceptions of changes in empathy during medical school (measured by a single item) were strongly associated with students' perceptions of changes in their sensitivity, helpfulness, and concern for patients (Wolf, Balson, Faucett, & Randall, 1989).

In an attempt to validate Hogan's Empathy Scale for medical students at Monash University in Australia, researchers found a significant correlation between students' scores on Hogan's scale and the ratings of peers on students' social skills, sense of humor, and awareness of the impression they made on others (Hornblow, Kidson, & Jones, 1977). Furthermore, medical students in that study obtained higher average empathy scores than did psychiatric patients diagnosed with a personality disorder.

Streit-Forest (1982) studied first-year medical students at the University of Montreal and found that students with a more positive attitude toward the physician–patient relationship and students who chose medicine for humanistic reasons scored highest on Hogan's Empathy Scale. The author also noted that the students who were more likely to watch television in their leisure time scored lower on empathy than did classmates who were more likely to spend their leisure time on a hobby.

In a study with medical students in Canada (Streit, 1980), significant and positive correlations were observed between scores on Hogan's Empathy Scale and scores on the following subtests of the Attitudes Toward Psychosocial Issues in Medicine (Parlow & Rothman, 1974): Doctor–Patient Relations (recognition of the importance of interpersonal clinician–patient relationships in effective patient care), Social Factors (recognition of the importance of social factors as determinants of health and illness), General Liberalism (open-mindedness about social issues outside of medicine), Preventive Medicine (recognition of medicine's role in maintaining health), and Government Role (endorsement of government's involvement in regulating health care costs). In a study with dental students, Sherman and Cramer (2005) found that empathy (measured by the JSE) yielded a statistically significant correlation with students' ratings on willingness to apply the principles of behavioral sciences to oral health care.

In a study with medical students, scores on the Empathic Concern and Perspective Taking subscales of the IRI were correlated with a measure of femininity that included such qualities as gentleness, warmth, helpfulness, kindness, understanding emotions, devotion to others, and awareness of other people's feelings (Zeldow & Daugherty, 1987). In another study with medical students, empathy was correlated with a measure of androgyny (Yarnold, Martin, & Soltysik, 1993).

In a study with nurses, social workers, and teachers (Williams, 1989), the respondents' scores on the Emotional Empathy Scale were significantly and positively correlated with both emotional exhaustion and personal accomplishment (measured by the Maslach Burnout Inventory, MBI, 1993). The investigator suggested that high emotional empathy—as opposed to cognitive empathy—may predispose helping professionals to emotional exhaustion that must be mediated by personal accomplishment to avoid depersonalization and burnout (Williams, 1989) (see Chaps. 1 and 6 for the distinction between cognitive and emotional empathy). In a study with medical students, Brazeau, Schroeder, Rovi, and Boyd (2010) reported significant and positive correlation between scores of a measure of cognitive empathy (the JSE) and scores on the Personal Accomplishment scale of the MBI ($r = 0.41$), but negative correlation with scores of the Emotional Exhaustion

($r = -0.30$) and Depersonalization ($r = -0.41$) scales of the MBI. Similar patterns of findings were reported in medical students (Hojat, Vergare, Isenberg, Cohen, & Spandorfer, 2015b; Lamothe, Boujut, Zenasni, & Sultan, 2014), and by Zenasni et al. (2012) in samples of French general practitioners.

By imagining how other people feel when watching someone whose hand was painfully caught in a machine, Stotland (1969) demonstrated that perspective taking was a major mechanism that generated empathy. In a later study, Stotland (1978) reported that scores on the Fantasy-Empathy Scale (see Chap. 5) were correlated with altruism, more palmar sweat, and more vasoconstriction while study participants were observing others in pain. Stotland attributed this finding to the tendency of more empathic individuals to understand and feel another person's experiences.

Hogan (1969) reported that young delinquents and prison inmates scored approximately one standard deviation lower on the Hogan's Empathy Scale than college students. Hogan (1976) also reported that inmates scored lower on the empathy scale than Air Force officers. Furthermore, incarcerated delinquents scored lower on the Empathy Scale than nondelinquent undergraduate students (Kurtines & Hogan, 1972). Individuals with low scores on the scale were more likely to be deficient in morality. A group of repeat offenders scored lower on Hogan's Empathy Scale than did first-time offenders and research participants from the general public (Deardroff, Finch, Kendall, Liran, & Indrisano, 1975). Also, men with high scores on the Emotional Empathy Scale were influenced to a significantly lesser degree by a female potential coworker's physical attractiveness than were men with low scores (Crouse & Mehrabian, 1977).

Mehrabian, Young and Sato (1988) found that empathy measured with the Emotional Empathy Scale was associated with emotional arousability, explained as the degree to which a person's emotions are influenced by events. Similarly, emotional empathy can lead to an individual's tendency to be affected by other people's emotional experiences. Therefore, it followed that scores on emotional empathy (which was viewed as analogous to sympathy in Chap. 1) would be positively linked to arousability. However, arousability has not been associated with cognitive (clinical) empathy.

In our study of 422 first-year medical students (Hojat, Zuckerman et al., 2005), we found that higher scores on the JSE were associated with higher scores on Sociability and lower scores on Aggression-Hostility scales of the short version of the Zuckerman–Kuhlman Personality Questionnaire (ZKPQ) (Zuckerman, 2002). Similar findings were reported by Beven, O'Brien-Malone, and Hall (2004), who found a positive correlation between empathy measured by the Perspective Taking subscale of the IRI and a measure of socialization; but they found a negative correlation with a measure of impulsivity in a sample of violent offenders. However, in a study with medical students in Kuwait (Hasan, Al-Sharqawi et al., 2013), no significant correlation was found between clinical empathy (measured by the JSE) and scores of the five personality scales of the ZKPQ (Sociability, Neuroticism-Anxiety, Impulsive Sensation Seeking, Aggression-Hostility, Activity), but authors reported a negative trend toward an inverse association between empathy and Aggression-Hostility scale scores. In some other studies, clinical empathy, measured by the JSE, has been linked to the "big five" personality factors such as Agreeableness, Openness to Experience, Conscientiousness, and Extraversion in a sample of 472 medical students in Portugal (Costa et al., 2014).

It is also reported that clinical empathy (measured by the JSE) could positively predict therapists' psychological growth (Brockhouse, Msetfi, Cohen, & Joseph, 2011). Significant associations were found between empathy in patient care and a friendly and relaxed style of communication in 860 undergraduate health science students in Australia (Brown et al., 2011). Also, significantly positive associations were reported in a sample of Korean residents in psychiatry (Hong, Bahn, Lee, & Moon, 2011) between clinical empathy (the JSE scores) and measures of Cooperativeness, Persistence, Self-Directedness, and Reward Dependence, measured by the Cloninger's Temperament and Character Inventory (Cloninger, Svrakic, & Przybeck, 1993). In a study with 229 Chinese nursing students (Xia, Hongyu, & Xinwei, 2011), an inverse relationship was found between clinical empathy (JSE scores) and the Neuroticism scale of the Eysenck Personality Questionnaire (Eysenck & Eysenck, 1975).

Furthermore, our study of medical students (Hojat, Zuckerman et al., 2005) showed that higher scores on the JSE were associated with higher levels of self-reported satisfaction with early maternal relationships, but not with the paternal relationships. Similar findings have also been reported by Hasan and Al-Sharqawi et al. (2013b). These results were consistent with our earlier findings (Hojat, 1998) that medical students' perceptions of satisfaction with the early relationship with their mother were predictors of higher self-esteem; better peer relationships; less loneliness, depression, and anxiety; and more resilience when faced with stressful life events. We did not find such associations with students' perceptions of their early relationship with their father (Hojat, 1998).

In a study of physicians in postgraduate training, we found a significant link between the physicians' perceptions of their early relationship with their mother and their clinical competence in their interpersonal skills and attitudes, as assessed by the directors of the training programs (Hojat, Glaser, & Veloski, 1996). Again, this link was not observed in relation to the physicians' perceptions of their early relationship with their father. These findings provide support for the developmental aspect of empathy (discussed in Chap. 4) and that the quality of the relationship with a primary caregiver (usually the mother) early in life can be a precursor of empathy in adulthood.

At the conceptual level, clinical empathy and interprofessional collaboration have been described as important elements of professionalism in the provision of health care (Veloski & Hojat, 2006). At the empirical level, clinical empathy (measured by JSE scores) has been found to be significantly associated with orientation toward teamwork and interprofessional collaboration. For example, in a study with 373 osteopathic medical students (Calabrese et al., 2013), statistically significant correlation was found between scores of the JSE and those of the Jefferson Scale of Attitudes Toward Physician-Nurse Collaboration (Hojat et al., 1997; Hojat, Gonnella, Nasca et al., 2003; Hojat, Nasca et al., 2001). In a nationwide study of osteopathic medical students in the USA, we found that scores on the JSE were positively and significantly correlated with measures of interprofessional collaboration and teamwork, and orientation toward lifelong learning, but scores of the JSE were negatively correlated with burnout experiences (see Chap. 14, Tables 14.31 and 14.32).

Also, in nursing students a statistically significant correlation was observed between scores of the JSE and attitudes toward physician–nurse collaboration (Ward et al., 2009). Similarly, a statistically significant correlation was found in pharmacy and medical students (Hojat, Spandorfer, Isenberg, Vergare, & Fassihi, 2012; Van Winkle, Bjork et al., 2012) between scores of the JSE and the Scale of Attitudes Toward Physician-Pharmacist Collaboration (Hojat, Gonnella, Nasca et al., 2003a; Van Winkle et al., 2011).

Peer nominations on positive social influence have been found to be associated with empathy in the context of patient care. For example, 630 fourth-year medical students were asked to nominate classmates who had significant positive influences in their professional and personal development. Students who were nominated most were compared to the rest on the JSE. Those nominated the most (top 10%) obtained a significantly higher JSE mean score (Michalec, Veloski, Hojat, & Tykocinski, 2015). In another study (Hojat, Michalec, Veloski, & Tykocinski, 2015), it was found that the top positive social influencers (nominated by their peers at the completion of medical school) scored higher than the rest of their peers on the JSE and on measures of Sociability and Activity (measured by the ZKPQ), but scored lower on experiences of loneliness, measured by a brief version of the UCLA Loneliness Scale (Russell, Peplau, & Cutrona, 1980). These positive social influencers were considered potential leaders in medicine. In a sample of 255 third-year medical students, it was found that students who were nominated by their classmates in six areas of clinical and humanistic excellence obtained a significantly higher JSE mean score than other classmates who were not nominated (Pohl, Hojat, & Arnold, 2011).

Empathy and Age

The link between empathy and age has been studied with some inconsistent results. For example, younger nurses with a moderate amount of professional experiences expressed more empathy toward elderly patients than older nurses (Pennington & Pierce, 1985). Similarly, younger, less experienced physicians showed more empathic concern for their patients than did older, more experienced physicians (Hall & Dornan, 1988); and in another study, younger Iranian medical students obtained higher JSE scores than their older counterparts (Khademalhosseini, Khademalhosseini, & Mahmoodian, 2014).

On the contrary, older health profession students in Australia demonstrated higher empathy (measured by the JSE) than younger students (Williams, Brown, Boyle et al., 2014; Williams, Brown, McKenna et al., 2014). Similarly, in other studies in which the JSE was used, no significant association was found between empathy and age in nursing students (McKenna et al., 2012), Korean medical students (Park, Roh, Suh, & Hojat, 2015), Iranian residents (Shariat & Kaykhavoni, 2010), Australian occupational therapy students (Brown et al., 2010), Malaysian pharmacy students (Hasan, Babar et al., 2013), and Italian residents in hygiene and public health (Soncini et al., 2013). In a recent study with a national sample of students in the osteopathic medical colleges in the USA (Hojat, DeSantis, Shannon, Speicher et al., 2020), no significant association was found between scores of the JSE and students' age (see Chap. 14). Findings on most of these studies are limited because of the restriction of range of age in samples of young students. To overcome that limitation, more research is needed to capture the true relationship between empathy and age by using samples with a wider range of ages.

Clinical Empathy and Academic Background

In a recent nationwide cross-sectional study of osteopathic medical students in the USA (Hojat, DeSantis, Shannon, Speicher et al., 2020), we found that scores on the JSE were associated with medical students' undergraduate background (undergraduate major/degree). Those with an undergraduate background in arts and humanities and those with a background in social and behavioral sciences scored significantly higher on the JSE than their counterparts with undergraduate backgrounds in chemical and physical sciences. We noticed the differences on JSE scores among students with different undergraduate backgrounds became less pronounced and practically unimportant in later years of medical school education, (also see Chap. 14). It is desirable to undertake a longitudinal study for better understanding of changes in a study cohort as students progress through medical school and explore the reasons for changes.

Clinical Empathy and Career Choice

A student's choice of a career and interest in a particular specialty can be influenced by a number of variables, including constitutional factors, aptitudes, personality, skills, social trends, role models, cultural factors, market forces, and developmental and educational experiences (Bland, Meurer, & Maldonado, 1995; Christodoulou, Lykousras, Mountaokalakis, Voulgari, & Stefanis, 1995; Kassebaum & Szenas, 1994; Richard, Nakamoto, & Lockwood, 2001; Sierles, Vergare, Hojat, & Gonnella, 2004; Weissman, Haynes, Killan, & Robinowitz, 1994). Some empirical studies have reported a link between empathy and career interest. For example, Hogan (1969) reported that college students majoring in psychology, education, and medicine obtained the highest scores on his Empathy Scale, while engineering and architecture students and military officers obtained the lowest scores. Rovezzi-Carroll and Fitz (1984) found that students majoring in physical therapy scored high on Hogan's Empathy Scale and were more people-oriented while those majoring in medical technology were more task-oriented and low in empathy.

Studies with Medical Students

Medical students in Israel scored higher on a Hebrew version of Mehrabian and Epstein's Emotional Empathy Scale than did college students majoring in psychology, social work, economics, physics, and chemistry (Elizur & Rosenheim, 1982). However, the investigators found that the medical students unexpectedly scored lower than the other students in their attention to psychosocial areas related to health and illness. They interpreted this unexpected finding as an indication that medical schools overemphasize achievement in the sciences and fail to devote adequate attention to understanding of psychosocial aspects of disease and infirmity. In a Canadian study, medical students who had high scores on Hogan's Empathy Scale had chosen medicine for humanistic reasons, whereas the students who had low scores had chosen medicine for scientific reasons (Streit-Forest, 1982).

A study at Baylor College of Medicine found that medical students interested in family medicine, general internal medicine, and pediatrics obtained the highest mean scores on humanistic attributes (measured by ratings given by standardized patients during the clerkship's Objective Structured Clinical Examinations), whereas students interested in anesthesiology, pathology, radiology, emergency medicine, and physical medicine and rehabilitation obtained the lowest mean score (Coutts-van Dijk, Bray, Moore, & Rogers, 1997). Using the Physician Belief Scale (Ashworth, Williamson, & Montano, 1984), which is a measure of psychosocial orientation in patient care, the researchers found a significant association with empathy scores. A study with medical students at the University of Washington, School of Medicine, found that among the major factors that prompted students to choose primary care as their specialty was interaction with patients, a reflection of empathic engagement (Burack et al., 1997).

Although Harsch (1989) observed no relationship between medical students' scores on Hogan's Empathy Scale and the specialties they were interested in, a later study with medical students contradicted that report. The researchers who conducted the later study reported that after the effect of gender was controlled in the statistical analyses, the students who expressed interest in pursuing "core" specialties, such as family medicine or pediatrics, scored significantly higher on the Emotional Empathy Scale than did students who were interested in pursuing "noncore" specialties, such as radiology or pathology (Newton et al., 2000). In her doctoral dissertation, Bailey (2001) reported that medical students who planned to pursue a career in specialties requiring extensive and prolonged encounters with patients received significantly higher average scores on the IRI than did their counterparts who planned to pursue procedure-oriented specialties.

A large number of the aforementioned studies did not use a validated measure of clinical empathy in the context of patient care. However, there are a number of studies in which the JSE was used to examine associations between medical students' clinical empathic orientation and their academic background and specialty interests. For example, in a study with first-year medical students at Jefferson, the JSE was administered on orientation day at the beginning of medical school education, before students were exposed to formal medical education (Hojat, Zuckerman et al., 2005). Significant association was found between JSE scores and specialty interest in favor of those planning to pursue "people-oriented" specialties (also see Chaps. 7 and 14).

The finding of significantly higher JSE mean score being obtained by students who planned to pursue "people-oriented" specialties (compared to those planned to pursue "technology- or procedure-oriented" specialties) was confirmed in another study of 685 medical students at Boston University School of Medicine (Chen, Lew, Hershman, & Orlander, 2007). However, such association was not observed in a study with 476 health sciences students in Portugal (Magalhäes, Salgueira, Costa, & Costa, 2011). In another study with osteopathic medical students in the USA (Calabrese, Bianco, Mann, Massello, & Hojat, 2013), no statistically significant association was found between empathy (JSE scores) and students' interest in specialty. In his doctoral dissertation research, McTighe (2014) did not find a significant link between scores of the JSE and specialty interest in 717 osteopathic medical students. In another study with 255 third-year medical students at Jefferson (Pohl et al., 2011), students who were nominated by their peers as being excellent in clinical skills and humanistic attributes expressed more interest in pursuing "people-oriented" rather than "technology- or procedure-oriented" specialties.

To address the issue of whether the differences in empathy among students interested in different specialties can be detected when students enter medical school (empathy attributed to personal qualities before being exposed to formal medical education) or after they have been exposed to medical training (empathy attributed to medical education), we administered the JSE to 422 students on orientation day, before they were exposed to the medical school curriculum (Hojat, Zuckerman et al., 2005). We also asked the new students about the medical specialty they planned to pursue after graduating from school. Because some students may have lacked a clear plan regarding a choice of specialty, we presented them with the following four scenarios and asked them to choose the one they were most interested in at that moment:

1. Performing specialized diagnostic procedures or basic or applied laboratory research and major contact with colleagues, not patients: primarily hospital based (e.g., radiology, pathology).
2. Performing highly skilled and specialized therapeutic techniques or procedures; serving as an expert consultant: primarily hospital based, with some office activities (e.g., orthopedic surgery, neurosurgery).
3. Providing episodic or long-term care of a limited number of medical problems, and a mix of ambulatory and hospital-based practice (e.g., cardiology, gastroenterology, dermatology, emergency medicine, psychiatry, obstetrics, and gynecology).
4. Providing first-encounter health or illness appraisal, preventive education and intervention, and episodic and long-term comprehensive care of a wide variety of medical conditions: primarily office based (e.g., family medicine, general internal medicine, general pediatrics).

Our results indicated that students who were interested in Scenario 4 as a career choice obtained the highest mean score on the JSE, followed by students who were interested in Scenario 3, Scenario 2, and finally Scenario 1 (Hojat, Zuckerman et al., 2005). Inferential statistical analyses indicated that students who were interested in Scenario 4 (commonly considered primary care specialties) obtained a significantly higher JSE mean score than those who were interested in Scenarios 1 and 2 (technology- or procedure-oriented specialties).

These results suggest that some students often come to medical school with a preconceived idea about a career choice that is consistent with their already developed personality. However, the findings cannot eliminate the possibility that educational experiences or the interaction of personal qualities and educational experiences can also influence the choice of medical specialty. In our large-scale study of entering classes between 2002 and 2012 reported in Chap. 7, students' scores on the JSE (administered on the first day of medical school) were significantly associated with students' specialty interest (expressed at the beginning of medical school). As reported in Table 7.11 (Chap. 7), students who expressed an interest in pursuing "people-oriented" specialty after graduation from medical school obtained a significantly higher JSE mean score than others who were interested in pursuing "technology- or procedure-oriented" specialties. The effect of gender was statistically controlled in the aforementioned analyses (also see Table 14.13 in Chap. 14).

Studies with Physicians and Health Professionals

Truax, Altmann, and Millis (1974) compared the scores of general practitioners, other medical professionals (e.g., nurses), and nonmedical professionals (e.g., clergymen, lawyers) on the Accurate Empathy scale of Truax and Carkhuff's Relationship Questionnaire (see Chap. 5) and on measures of warmth and genuineness. They reported that the general practitioners received the highest scores. These results are consistent with the findings of another study that ongoing interpersonal relationships with patients and their families and interprofessional collaboration with colleagues in other specialties were among the features ascribed to primary care physicians (Hennen, 1975). In a 1983 study comparing physicians in family medicine, internal medicine, and surgery, the family physicians obtained the highest mean score on a humanism scale, the surgeons obtained the lowest mean score, and the mean score of the internists fell in between (Abbott, 1983).

In a survey of 327 physicians representing five graduating classes in the School of Medicine at the University of Missouri-Kansas City, views of a group of primary care physicians were compared with those of a group of nonprimary care physicians (Arnold, Calkins, & Willoughby, 1997). The results showed that the primary care physicians assigned significantly higher ratings to such professional qualities as a pleasant personality, the ability to relate to people, and the ability to empathize.

Among personal values, the primary care physicians also gave a higher rating to empathy and a lower rating to competition than did the other group.

In one of our studies involving 704 physicians, we noticed that psychiatrists obtained the highest mean score on the JSE, followed by physicians in internal medicine, pediatrics, emergency medicine, and family medicine (Hojat, Gonnella, Nasca, Mangione, Vergare et al., 2002a). The lowest mean scores were obtained by anesthesiologists, orthopedic surgeons, neurosurgeons, and radiologists. When gender was controlled for, the differences in empathy scores among physicians specializing in psychiatry, internal medicine, pediatrics, emergency medicine, and family medicine did not reach the conventional level of statistical significance ($p < 0.05$). However, the psychiatrists' mean score was significantly higher than the mean scores of anesthesiologists, orthopedic surgeons, neurosurgeons, radiologists, cardiovascular surgeons, and obstetricians and gynecologists. A higher mean score by psychiatrists was expected because of their specific interpersonal training and findings that showed that they scored high on a measure of tolerance for ambiguity (Geller, Tambor, Chase, & Holtzman, 1993), which facilitates empathic engagement with patients.

In two other studies, we compared two groups of physicians (Hojat, Gonnella, Nasca, Mangione, Veloski et al., 2002b; Hojat, Gonnella, Nasca, Mangione, Vergare et al., 2002a). Group 1 included 462 physicians in "people-oriented" specialties, such as family medicine, general internal medicine, pediatrics, emergency medicine, psychiatry, and obstetrics and gynecology. Group 2 included 242 physicians in "technology- or procedure-oriented" practices, such as anesthesiology, radiology, pathology, surgery, and surgical subspecialties. The physicians in Group 1 outscored their counterparts in Group 2 not only on the total JSE scores, but on all 20 items of the JSE as well (Hojat, Gonnella, Nasca, Mangione, Veloski et al., 2002). However, the differences were statistically significant for only 11 of the 20 items. A similar pattern of findings was observed when medical students were compared on their JSE scores by their planned specialty choice after graduation from medical school (Hojat et al., 2002a).

In another study, we compared the JSE scores in three groups: female pediatricians, female physicians in hospital-based specialties (anesthesiology, pathology, and radiology), and female nurse practitioners (Hojat, Fields, & Gonnella et al., 2003). Physicians in the hospital-based specialties obtained a significantly lower JSE mean scorer than pediatricians and nurse practitioners. In a study with 285 female Japanese physicians, those in "people-oriented" specialties scored significantly higher on the JSE than their counterparts who were practicing "technology- or procedure-oriented" specialties (Kataoka et al., 2012). A study of 352 Italian resident physicians showed that physicians who had health care administrative experiences scored significantly higher on the JSE than those who were only involved in research with no administrative experience (Soncini et al., 2013).

Interestingly, the pattern of malpractice claims against physicians in different specialties has proven to be consistent with research findings on empathy among physicians practicing in different specialties. For example, in a large-scale study involving 12,829 physicians, the following specialists experienced the highest rates of malpractice claims: neurosurgeons, orthopedic surgeons, general surgeons, anesthesiologists, and obstetricians and gynecologists. The lowest rates occurred among specialists in psychiatry, pediatrics, and internal medicine (Taragin et al., 1994). The specialists who experienced low rates of malpractice claims in that study scored highest on the JSE in the aforementioned studies.

Clinical Importance of the Differences

Differences in clinical empathy among physicians in different specialties do not necessarily indicate a deficiency in empathy in the low-scoring groups. It is important to emphasize this point for two reasons.

First, according to the information available so far, almost all the statistically significant differences in empathy among medical students interested in or physicians practicing in different specialties appear to be moderate at best. Second, the duties involved in the technology- or procedure-oriented specialties obviously are primarily procedural and therefore may not demand a high degree of empathic engagement necessary in the people-oriented specialties. For example, empathic understanding of patients' experiences and emotions, although important in any patient–physician encounter, is more crucial for primary care physicians than for pathologists, radiologists, or anesthesiologists.

Contribution of Personality and Medical Education in Specialty Choice

The question of the unique and interaction effects of personality formed prior to medical school and educational experiences in medical school on specialty interest and empathy is important to be addressed. Our study with medical school matriculants who completed the JSE prior to the beginning of their formal medical education and expressed their specialty interest showed a significant association between JSE scores and specialty interest. This finding indicates that there might be baseline differences in career interests of medical students before they start medical school, prompting them to prefer one specialty over another, which can be reflected in their empathy scores.

Obviously, medical school curriculum, observations, and experiences in medical school can also influence specialty interest and empathic orientation toward patient care. For example, in some medical school clerkships and residency programs, such as family medicine, internal medicine, pediatrics, and psychiatry, more emphasis is placed on training in interpersonal skills and physician–patient relationships. Therefore, a stronger empathic orientation could be expected to develop among students or residents who are exposed to such training.

An important question is to tease out the relative contribution of personality formed prior to formal medical education, contribution of medical education, and their interaction in specialty interest and differences in empathic orientation among physicians in different specialties.

Clinical Empathy and Acquisition of Factual Knowledge

Few attempts have been made to examine relationships between measures of empathy and indicators of academic attainment. A consistent link between measures of knowledge acquisition and empathy has not been established. For example, a study by Hogan and Weiss (1974) showed a lack of correlation between empathy and academic performance. In another study, scores on a test of empathy developed by the investigators proved to be independent of intelligence, reading level, mechanical comprehension, spatial relations, or aptitude in chemistry and mathematics (Kerr & Speroff, 1954).

In the late 1970s, a study of five classes of medical students at the University of Pittsburgh School of Medicine found that scores on a brief version of Hogan's Empathy Scale and scores on the Medical College Admission Test (MCAT) were positively correlated in one class, negatively correlated in another class, and not correlated at all in the three remaining classes (Kupfer et al., 1978). At Wake Forest University's Bowman Gray School of Medicine, medical students' scores on Hogan's Empathy Scale were not correlated with either their scores on Parts 1 or 2 of the National Board of Medical Examiners (part of medical licensing examinations) nor with their grades on preclinical and clinical examinations (Diseker & Michielutte, 1981).

Furthermore, all correlations between the students' scores on Hogan's Empathy Scale and the Verbal, Quantitative, Science Problems, and General Information subtests of the MCAT were negative and negligible. In our own study of 371 third-year medical students (Hojat, Gonnella, Mangione et al., 2002), we found that the students' scores on the JSE were not significantly correlated with their performance on objective (e.g., multiple-choice) tests of acquisition of medical knowledge (e.g., examinations on sciences basic to medicine in the first 2 years of medical school); the MCAT's Biological Sciences, Physical Sciences, and Verbal Reasoning subtests; or Steps 1 and 2 of the United States Medical Licensing Examination.

Clinical Empathy and Clinical Competence

Significant relationships between empathy and indicators of clinical competence have been reported in some studies. For example, some of these studies involved assessments of medical students by standardized patients. In one study, Colliver, Willis, Robbs, Cohen, and Swartz (1998) reported that the patients' assessments of empathy among the fourth-year medical students were associated with indicators of better clinical performance. In another study, Coutts and Rogers (2000) found low correlations between medical students' scores on a measure of humanism in medicine and assessments of their academic performance in medical school. Among these low correlations, the highest one (r = 0.31) was obtained between the standardized patients' assessment of the students' history-taking skills and the students' "humanism" scores.

In a study with 284 medical students (Berg, Majdan, Berg, Veloski, & Hojat, 2011a), significant associations were observed between students' self-reported JSE scores and ratings of clinical competence given by standardized patients in ten Objective Structured Clinical Examination (OSCE) stations. The associations between measure of empathy and the patients' assessments of students' clinical competence were stronger when standardized patients assessed students' empathic engagement (measured by completion of the Jefferson Scale of Patient Perceptions of Physician Empathy (JSPPPE); see Chap. 7, and Appendix E), compared to students' self-reported empathy (measured by the JSE). This pattern of findings was observed in a few other studies, as well (Berg, Majdan, Berg, Veloski, & Hojat 2011b; Berg et al., 2015; Grosseman, Novack et al., 2014). The modest association between medical students' self-reported empathy and standardized patients' assessments of students' clinical skills has been partly attributed to confounding effects of gender and ethnicity of students and standardized patients (Berg, Majdan, Berg, Veloski, & Hojat, 2011b, 2015) and partly to students' inability to gauge the effectiveness of their empathic communications while playing the role of a clinician in simulated clinical encounters with standardized patients (Grosseman, Novack et al., 2014).

In a study with 371 third-year medical students (Hojat, Gonnella, Mangione et al., 2002), we observed a statistically significant link between the students' JSE scores and the faculty's global ratings of students' clinical competence in third-year core clerkships (family medicine, internal medicine, pediatrics, psychiatry, surgery, and obstetrics and gynecology). These results are in agreement with those reported by Colliver et al. (1998). This pattern of findings was expected because the students' understanding of patients' concerns and experiences, as measured by the JSE, could be reflected in their interpersonal communication with patients, a factor usually taken into consideration when assessing students' clinical competence. However, because such personal qualities cannot be measured with objective tests of medical or clinical knowledge, one may not expect to find a significant link between students' empathy scores and measures of knowledge acquisition.

Clinical Empathy and Patient Outcomes

Very important evidence in support of validity and utility of measures of empathy in the context of patient care is their ability to predict clinical or patient outcomes. Demonstrating that empathy in patient care is significantly associated with patient outcomes is utterly important because the ultimate goal of medical education and all other health professions is optimal clinical outcomes. We have shown in two empirical studies with diabetic patients in the USA and in Italy that physicians' empathy (measured by the JSE) could significantly predict positive patient outcomes, which are described in more detail in Chap. 11.

Recapitulation

Clinical empathy is associated with a number of psychosocial variables, clinical competence, and career interest. A large number of desirable personal qualities that are conducive to relationship building are positively correlated with our measure of clinical empathy (the JSE scores). Conversely, a number of undesirable personal attributes that are detrimental to positive relationships are negatively linked to scores of the JSE. Those with high clinical empathy scores demonstrate greater clinical competence and are more interested in people-oriented (mostly primary care) rather than technology- or procedure-oriented specialties (mostly hospital based and surgical). Also, physicians' scores on the JSE can significantly predict positive patient outcomes in their diabetic patients.

Chapter 10
Clinical Empathy and Gender: Are Men and Women Complementary or Opposite Sexes?

Then the Lord said: "It is not good for the man to be alone,
I will make him a helper who is just right for him."

—(Genesis 2:18)

Abstract

- Findings from a large number of gender studies indicate that women in the general population and in health professionals-in-training and in-practice often obtain higher scores than men on self-reported measures of empathy.
- There are some plausible explanations for gender differences in empathy. For example, women exhibit a greater capacity for social relationship than men, evident by the observations that at an early age they often begin showing more sensitivity to social stimuli and emotional signals and demonstrate more care-oriented qualities.
- Although social learning and cultural values have important roles in determining gender differences in social behavior and empathy, other factors also contribute to the differences, such as human evolution history (e.g., sexual selection, parental investment in child-rearing, and ancestral division of labor), constitutional dispositions, and hormonal and biophysiological factors.
- Evidence suggests that some of gender differences could be pre-wired beyond social or observational learning.
- Although in a broader context men and women are more similar than different, accumulated evidence continues to confirm that gender differences in some personal qualities and mental abilities should not be considered trivial or nonexistent.

M. Hojat, *Clinical Empathy*, https://doi.org/10.1007/978-3-031-87413-0_10

- The fact that some of the gender differences are in favor of women (e.g., "communal" inclination, verbal ability) and some in favor of men (e.g., "agentic" inclination, spatial ability) implies that in social skills and mental abilities, men and women should be viewed as "complementary" rather than "opposite" sexes.

Introduction

Differences in personal qualities between men and women have long been discussed, and the implications of those differences have been hotly debated. Although most gender differences have been attributed to social learning, role adaptation, and other sociocultural factors, studies on gender differences in infants and toddlers, before social learning takes place, suggest that some differences may be "pre-wired"—that is, apart from social learning and sociocultural factors (Cahill, 2005; Campbell, 2008; Carter, 2007; Hall, 1978, 1990; Hittelman & Dickes, 1979; Kimura, 1999; Singer et al., 2006; Van Honk et al., 2011). Any discussion of gender differences must include the role of sexual selection, parental investment, and division of labor during the history of human evolution, and the contribution of hormones and biophysiological functions in human behavior.

The issue of gender differences in social behavior and mental abilities is a sensitive topic. One reason for such sensitivity is that in an atmosphere of political correctness, there is a tendency to overlook gender differences for fear of inappropriate social implications and adverse reactions. However, the fact remains that despite many gender similarities, universal variations observed between men and women exist and are part of life.

Research Evidence in the General Population

In addition to the obvious gender differences in physical attributes and reproductive function, empirical evidence consistently indicates that men and women differ substantially from one another in social behavior and the capacity for empathy. Findings from a large volume of empirical research in the general population indicate that women often outscore men on measures of empathy (Davis, 1983; Eisenberg & Lennon, 1983; Hoffman, 1977; Hogan, 1969; Jose, 1989; Karniol, Gabay, Ochion, & Harari, 1998). Block (1976) reported that the results of most of the studies she examined favored women with regard to empathy. However, Eisenberg and Lennon (1983) reported a significant gender difference in empathy favoring women when the measures of empathy were self-reported inventories. But they noted no gender difference when the measures of empathy were either physiological or unobtrusive observations of behavior. Similarly, Michalska, Kinzler, and Decety (2013) reported gender difference in favor of women when comparisons were made on explicit self-ratings, but not when neurophysiological indicators of empathy were compared.

These controversial findings indicate that women may have an image of themselves as empathic that is reflected in their self-reported measures of empathy. Accordingly, some empathy scholars suggest that women's superiority on self-reported measures of empathy may be due in part to "demand characteristics" that prompt women to respond in a manner that confirms how the researcher expects them to respond (Eisenberg & Lennon, 1983; Ickes, Gesn, & Graham, 2000). However, there are a number of studies in which gender differences were noticed on objective measures, such as physiological reactions and brain activities.

Studies with adults indicate that women are more skillful than men at initiating empathic relationships. They typically exhibit "communal" behaviors (e.g., social sensitivity, caring attitudes, friendliness), whereas men tend to manifest "agentic" behaviors (e.g., controlling, independent, dominant) (Eagly, 1995). Also, Rokeach (1973) found that women place more emphasis on the emotional aspects of their interactions than do men, who instead place more emphasis on the rational aspects. Consistent with Rokeach's findings, a study of undergraduate students found that women differed significantly from men on emotional empathy (akin to sympathy) but not on the perspective taking aspect of cognitive empathy (Riggio, Tucker, & Coffaro, 1989).

Other authors have reported that women tend to adopt care-oriented moral perspective, whereas men tend to have a more justice-oriented moral view (Gilligan, 1982; Gilligan & Attanucci, 1988; Sochting, Skoe, & Marcia, 1994). In a meta-analytic study, Jaffee and Hyde (2000) reported that gender differences in the care-oriented morality favoring women and in justice-oriented mentality favoring men are consistent, but the effect size estimates of differences are not large (see Chap. 7 for a description of the effect size estimates). Gender difference in moral judgment is reflected in their choice in the "runaway trolley" ethical conundrum, which was introduced by Philippa Foot, the British social philosopher. When confronted with a dilemma to divert an out-of-control runaway trolley down to a side track by pulling a signal lever to save five people who are on the train but killing another person who is trapped on the side track (Edmonds, 2015), more men than women choose to pull the signal lever to save five lives, but killing one person. In a brain imaging study (Singer et al., 2006), men and women were engaged in a game in which two confederates who played fairly and unfairly received painful stimuli. Results of the functional magnetic resonance imaging (fMRI) showed that both men and women exhibit pain-related brain activities. However, empathy-related brain responses were significantly reduced in men when observing an unfair person receiving pain, accompanied by increased brain activation in reward-related brain areas, and correlated with an expressed desire for revenge. This pattern of brain activities was not observed in women.

These brain imaging findings suggest that men are more justice-oriented than women in perception of others' pain. In a brain activity experiment by Horton (1995), the hypotheses that men and women differ in their empathic responses and that the comforting substrate is located in the right parietal area of the brain were confirmed. Horton (1995) also concluded that the right-brain activities of the comforting substrate are more pronounced among women in general and among mothers in particular.

In a brain imaging study, it was noticed that men and women show different brain responses to an infant crying and laughing (Seifritz et al., 2003). Correct recognition of infant vocalization is crucial for offspring well-being and survival. Women, independent of their parental status, and mothers, in particular, were more sensitive to infant crying than laughing. The gender difference in vocalization recognition is attributed to the variation in biologically based emotional regulation in men and women (Decety & Jackson, 2004). In another study, it was found that at 30 days postpartum, 80% of mothers, compared to only 45% of fathers, were able to recognize their own infants' cries (Green & Gustafson, 1983).

In a study of nursing and medical students, the differences in judicial and moral considerations regarding patient care appeared to be explained by gender, rather than by differences in professional roles (Peter & Gallop, 1994). When the students were faced with a hypothetical clinical dilemma, female students, regardless of academic major, were more care-oriented than their male counterparts. Gender differences in empathy have been observed among various professionals. In a study of nurses, social workers, and teachers (Williams, 1989), women obtained significantly higher empathy scores than men did on Mehrabian and Epstein's Emotional Empathy Scale (Chap. 5).

Despite their advantage in interpersonal style and empathic capability, a study found women seemed to be more vulnerable than men when working under stressful conditions. This differential vulnerability to stress prompts women to appraise stressful events as being more overwhelming than men do (Barnett, Biener, & Baruch, 1987). In our study with medical students, we found that women were more sensitive than men to stressful life events and consequently appraised the same stressful events (e.g., change of health of a family member) as more disturbing than men (Hojat, Gonnella, Erdmann, & Vogel, 2003). These results indicate that although female health professionals have an advantage when it comes to establishing empathic engagement with their patients, vulnerability to professional stress puts them at a disadvantage.

It should also be noted that although empathy enhances patient outcomes (see Chap. 11) and is valued by both clinicians and patients, research shows that empathy is not associated with promotion (Carmel & Glick, 1996), and this may exert more effect on women than men in professional advancement. In one large-scale study involving 5314 medical students, we found that female medical students at the beginning of their medical education expected 23% less financial gain, on the average, from the practice of medicine than their male counterparts, regardless of their planned specialties (Hojat, Gonnella, Erdmann, Rattner et al., 2000). These findings are consistent with the notion that women are more likely than men to choose medicine for altruistic reasons (Gross, 1992) than for financial gain or promotion (Stamps & Boley Cruz, 1994).

Evidence in the Health Professions

In a study of 7746 foreign medical school graduate physicians in the USA, who were assessed by standardized patients, it was found that female physicians scored significantly higher than their male counterparts on indicators of empathic capacity (e.g., skills in interviewing and counseling, rapport, and personal manner conducive to empathic engagement) (Van Zanten, Boulet, Norcini, & McKinley, 2005). English proficiency of participating physicians was controlled in statistical analyses by their scores on the Test of English as a Foreign Language (TOEFL). In this study, patients also expressed more satisfaction with female than male physicians. In our own studies as well as others with physicians-in-training and in-practice and other health professions students and practitioners in different cultures, gender variations on the JSE scores in favor of women have been frequently observed (Hojat, Mangione, Nasca et al., 2001; Hojat, Gonnella, Mangione et al., 2002; Hojat, Gonnella, Nasca, Mangione, Veloski et al., 2002; Hojat, Gonnella, Nasca, Mangione, Vergare et al., 2002). Chen, Lew, Hershman, and Orlander (2007) and Michalec (2010) reported that female medical students and physicians in the USA, on average, outscored their male counterparts on the JSE.

This pattern of gender difference in the JSE has also been observed in osteopathic medical students (Calabrese, Bianco, Mann, Massello, & Hojat, 2013), nursing students (Fields, Mahan, Hojat, Tillman, & Maxwell, 2011; Ward et al., 2009), dental students (Sherman & Cramer, 2005), pharmacy students (Fjortoft, Van Winkle, & Hojat, 2011), and physician assistant students (Mandel & Schweinle, 2012) in the USA and abroad (see Appendix A).

Inconsistent with our findings, however, Kupfer, Drew, Curtis, and Rubinstein (1978) found no gender differences in medical students at the University of Pittsburgh School of Medicine on their scores on an abbreviated version of Hogan's Empathy Scale. In a study of positive role models in medicine, however, female physicians scored higher than their male counterparts on measures of personality facets that were conceptually relevant to empathy, such as openness to new experiences, aesthetics, and feelings (Magee & Hojat, 1998).

Women in other cultures outscored men on the JSE: for example, in Mexican medical students (Alcorta-Garza, Gonzalez-Guerrero, Tavitas-Herrera, Rodrigues-Lara, & Hojat, 2005), Italian medical students (Leombruni et al., 2014), Iranian medical students (Rahimi-Madiseh, Tavakol, Dennick, & Nasiri, 2010; Shariat & Habibi, 2013), Japanese medical students (Kataoka, Koide, Ochi, Hojat, & Gonnella, 2009), Chinese medical students (Wen, Ma, Li, Liu, Xian & Liu, 2013), Korean medical students (Park, Roh, Suh, & Hojat, 2015), medical students in Kuwait (Hasan, Al-Sharqawi et al., 2013; Hasan, Babar, Chen, Ahmed, & Mitha, 2013), Portuguese medical students (Gonçalves-Pereira, Trancas, Loureiro, Papoila, & Caldas-De-Almeida, 2013; Magalhäes, Salgueira, Costa, & Costa, 2011), medical students in South Africa (Vallabh, 2011), medical students in Thailand (Jumroonrojana, & Zartrungpak, 2012), medical students in Bangladesh (Mostafa, Hoque, Mosrafa, Rana, & Mostafa, 2014), Caribbean medical students (Youssef, Nunes, Sa, &

Williams, 2014), Malaysian pharmacy students (Hasan, Babar et al., 2013), Taiwanese nursing students (Hsiao, Tsai, & Kao, 2012), nursing students in Greece (Ouzouni & Nakakis, 2012), Australian health professions students (Boyle et al., 2009; Brown et al., 2011; Nunes, Williams, Sa, & Stevenson, 2011), Australian paramedic students (Williams, Boyle et al., 2015), and medical students in England (Austin, Evans, Magnus, & O'Hanlon, 2007).

Also, women obtained higher JSE scores than men in Korean physicians (Suh, Hong, Lee, Gonnella, & Hojat, 2012), Italian physicians (Soncini et al., 2013), and resident physicians in Romania (Voinescu, Szentagotai, & Coogan, 2009). There are a few other studies in which the gender difference on the JSE did not reach the accepted level of statistical significance ($p < 0.05$). For example, no statistically significant gender difference was found in Italian physicians (DiLillo, Cicchetti, Lo Scalzo, Taroni, & Hojat, 2009), dental students in the USA (Hsieh, Herzig, Gansky, & Danley, 2006), Polish medical students (Kliszcz, Nowicka-Sauer, Trzeciak, Nowak, & Sadowska, 2006), Czech medical students (Kožený, Tišanská, & Hoschl, 2013), Brazilian medical students (Paro, Daud-Gallotti, Tiberio, Pinto, & Martins, 2012), residents in internal medicine and family medicine in the USA (Grosseman, Hojat et al., 2014), Korean medical students (Hong et al., 2012), medical students in New Zealand (Lim et al., 2013), and nursing students in Australia (McKenna et al., 2012).

In a study with students in the first and final years of a medical school in Poland (Kliszcz, Hebanowski, & Rembowski, 1998), women scored higher than men on both the Emotional Empathy Scale and Davis's Interpersonal Reactivity Index (IRI) (see Chap. 5). A survey of physicians showed that the female physicians rated themselves as more empathic than their male counterparts (Barnsley, Williams, Cockerill, & Tanner, 1999). Similarly, female residents in internal medicine (Day, Norcini, Shea, & Benson, 1989) and family medicine (Abbott, 1983) outscored their male counterparts on a measure of humanism.

In our large-scale study of 2637 medical students (1301 men, 1336 women), described in Chap. 7 (also see Hojat & Gonnella, 2015), we examined stability of gender differences on the JSE during a period of 11 years for matriculating students between 2002 and 2012 at Jefferson, before students were exposed to formal medical education. Summary results of statistical analysis were presented in Chap. 7 (see Table 7.10). Consistent with these findings (also see Appendix A), women consistently obtained higher mean empathy scores than men in all of our comparisons in different matriculating classes Between 2002 and 2012). The gender differences in favor of women were all statistically significant, with the exception of only one matriculating class (overall Cohen's effect size = 0.40). These results agree with a great majority of empirical findings on gender difference in empathy in the general population and in health professions students and practitioners. The overwhelming evidence and consistent findings in observational, empirical, and experimental research on differences in empathy between men and women in different samples, settings, and cultures demand plausible explanations.

Plausible Explanations for Gender Differences

Because some of the gender differences are robust regardless of social and cultural differences, they prompt an intriguing question: How can those differences be explained? Debate about the reasons for gender differences can be summarized in terms of nature–nurture dichotomy (Eagly & Wood, 1999). Wood and Eagly (2002) suggested that gender differences derive from the interaction between nature and nurture factors, including, for example, physical differences, reproductive capacity, as well as the social and economic factors in societies. A large volume of studies, views, and reviews, particularly in social psychology literature, explain gender differences in terms of social learning, role expectations, and sociocultural factors (more relevant to the nurture aspects of gender differences). Detailed discussion of the contribution of social learning and other social and cultural factors in gender differences is beyond the scope of this book.

Therefore, this chapter will not focus on those findings or theories related to social learning and social-cultural factors that contribute to gender differences; instead, it briefly presents evidence in support of the notion that some aspects of gender differences may be pre-wired (more relevant to the nature aspects of the gender differences), independent from social learning. I will provide brief explanations for gender differences in terms of evolutionary history and hormonal and biophysiological factors. However, those explanations should not be viewed at all as an argument against the undeniable role of social learning and social-cultural contributions to gender differences.

Evolutionary Underpinnings

In Chap. 3, I indicated that human beings are evolved to make connection for survival purposes. Human beings are endowed with a capacity to understand and a need to be understood. Although manifestations of the aforementioned capacity and need might be different in men and women, evolutionary psychology suggests that men and women in the course of human evolutionary history developed some gender-specific characteristics for better adaptation to survival challenges (Buss, 1995; Tooby & Cosmides, 1990). According to this view, the evolved gender differences are indeed accommodations for survival in the living environment. I will discuss a few aspects of evolutionary theory of gender differences that are more relevant to social behavior and empathic orientation, such as mate selection, parental investment, and division of labor.

Mate Selection

The evolutionary explanation of gender differences in sexual selection was initially described by Darwin (1871/1981). There is a large volume of research showing that men and women have different preferences in mate selection for the purpose of survival of the genes (Buss & Schmitt, 1993). For example, studies on mate selection have shown that historically women have higher preference for a mate with higher social status, better access to resources (indicators of better earning potential and more security), and ambitiousness (an indicator of better prospect) (Feingold, 1992). Men, however, place more value on physical attractiveness and child-bearing capacity in searching for potential mates (Feingold, 1990). In a study of 37 cultures, Buss (1989) observed the aforementioned pattern of mate preferences in men and women across all of the studied cultures. These findings confirmed the views in the evolutionary theory that women evolved to prefer mates who are resource providers and men are evolved to prefer mates who are physically attractive (an indication of the women's health and younger age to bear and rear children).

Aspects of physical appearance such as smooth skin, muscle tone, lively gait, shiny and reddish lips, lustrous hair, curvy hip, and breast shape were proximate cues to a women's age and health that could increase reproduction success (Buss & Barnes, 1986) (at the time in which no birth certificate or medical tests were available to confirm a women's age or health status). Age in men, however, imposes less constraint for reproduction success; thus, preference for signs of younger age in men did not present a great advantage for mate selection. However, potential for earning and financial prospect remained a strong selection advantage for women's mate selection. Remnants of the aforementioned mate selection factors are still noticeable in most modern societies. For example, could women's inclination to use makeup, beauty parlors, cosmetic surgery, or seductive dressing be an evolutionary leftover of retaining physical appeal, an advantage in sexual selection? Or, could the preference for richer male mates with college educations or successful businesses, family fortune, or high ambitious be the remnants of human evolution history to indicate potential for higher social status and better resources, aimed for survival of genes? Eagly and Wood (2013) suggest that changes in romantic mate selection have occurred in some industrial societies as women have entered the labor force and increasingly engaged in paid employment. Gender differences in mate selection contributed to the development of gender-specific propensity for social skills and interpersonal behavior.

Maternal Investment

Chapter 4 reported that during the course of human evolution, mothers have usually been involved more than any other person (including the fathers) in taking care of their own children (Trivers, 1972). Several reasons were described for the unmatched maternal investment (as opposed to paternal investment) including gestation and pregnancy experiences and bearing, weaning, and rearing children (Buss, 2003; Isabella & Belsky, 1991; Smotherman & Robinson, 1994). Also, maternal certainty (as opposed to paternal certainty), scarcity of women's gametes (compared to the abundance of men's sperm), lactation, and breast-feeding prompt mothers to invest more than fathers in child care.

Maternal tender loving care and intimate experiences in raising their own child contributed to women's development of caring attitudes, reflected also in their interpersonal relationships and social behavior. This notion was confirmed in a meta-analytic study by Feingold (1994) in which it was found that women rated themselves as more nurturing than did men. Such unique caring experiences can naturally enhance women's ability in forming empathic engagement. According to Reverby (1987) and Trivers (1972), women's caring attitude toward their offspring, which can be generalized to other humans, has evolutionary roots. Women's caring attitude toward their children often takes precedence over other matters. For example, caring attitudes toward offspring can sometimes interfere with a woman's career advancement in ways that have nothing to do with the barrier known as the "glass ceiling" effect. In support of this notion, Carr, Ash, and Friedman (1998) reported that male and female faculty members of academic medical centers who did not have children showed equivalent career accomplishments, but female faculty members who had children progressed more slowly in their careers because of their involvement with raising children. This phenomenon is an indication of the intrinsic motivation that also prompts professional women to enter into "caring" careers, rather than the prospect of great financial gain. This, in turn, can contribute to gender differences in propensity for empathic engagement.

Division of Labor

Gender roles within the society are not chosen arbitrarily; they are firmly rooted in the human biology that laid the foundation for the genders' historical division of labor. The ancestral division of labor in men and women, determined by Mother Nature, can provide plausible explanation for the development of gender differences in social skills and interpersonal relationship as well as mental abilities. For example, because of women's advantage to bear and raise children, they naturally developed a propensity for nurturance. Men, because of their greater size, speed, and strength, naturally took the role of hunting, competing for resources, and protection of the family. The division of labor paved the road for gender differences, so that men took on the responsibilities for hunting and scavenging, defending the family against predators and enemies, and making and using weapons, while women took on the responsibilities of gathering and preparing food, making clothing, and caring for small children. The division of labor contributed to disparate development of specific areas of the brains of men and women, which were more often developed and activated by their gender-specific tasks during the course of human evolution.

Obviously, those routine and daily activities performed by men and women for a long ancestral history that consistently activated different areas of their brain contributed to pre-wiring their brains differently, providing them with a differing propensity for social behavior and mental abilities. The notion of "neurons that fire together wire together" (Doidge, 2007, p. 63) means that acts or experiences that are repeated enough become embedded in the brain neurons, which are activated together simultaneously by performing that act or experience. The set of brain network connections strengthen each time the act or experience is repeated. Hence, propensity for performing that act is "pre-wired" in the brain. On the contrary, lack of experience prevents cells to form a set of network. This notion is reflected in the statements that "neurons that fire apart wire apart" (Doidge, 2007, p. 64). That may explain why men acquired better spatial skills (acquired from hunting experiences) and women acquired superior skills in recognizing landmarks (required to locate a gathering spot and return to the correct place of living). These "pre-wired" gender differences in mental ability have been shown in large volumes of empirical gender studies (Eagly & Wood, 1999; Geary, 1995; Voyer, Voyer, & Bryden, 1995).

Men's "Agentic" and Women's "Communal" Characteristics

No doubt that the human evolutionary history has significantly contributed to the development of distinct psychological qualities in men and women, labeled by Eagly (1987) as the "agentic" personal qualities in men and "communal" personal characteristics in women. Bakan (1966), who coined the terms "agency" and "communion" in this respect, argues that agency is important for the existence of an individual, and communion is important for the existence of the group in which the individual is a member. According to Abele and Wojciszke (2007) agency characteristics emerged from striving to expand the self, which involves qualities such as dominance and ambition, while communion characteristics emerged from striving for integration in the group and involve qualities such as emotional expressiveness and cooperation. Thus, gender stereotypes are reflected in the two aforementioned agentic and communal characteristics (Abele & Wojciszke, 2007).

Women's historical role as domestic child-rearing individuals requires interpersonal skills that favor development of personality attributes that are linked to tender loving care and social skills, friendliness, concern, compassion, emotional expression, and empathic engagement, described as specific features of the "communal" personality (Eagly & Wood, 1999; Wood & Eagly, 2010). Men's instrumental roles in proving food and security which favor assertiveness and competition are described as specific features of the "agentic" personality (Eagly & Wood, 1999; Wood & Eagly, 2010). Women's communal attributes foster prosocial behavior such as caring for others, while men's agentic characteristics facilitate some other forms of prosocial behavior such as physical challenges, acts of rescuing, and chivalrous protection (Wood & Eagly, 2010). Women's communal characteristics inspire close relationship, friendliness, perspective taking, and empathy, which are indispensable for survival (Abele & Wojciszke, 2007). Findings from our own research and by other researchers have confirmed that female students and practitioners of health professions are significantly more likely than their male counterparts to obtain higher scores on clinical empathy (JSE) (see Chap. 7, and Appendix A).

The difference between men and women in communal and agentic attributes is reflected in the title of a meta-analytic article on gender differences, "Men and things, women and people" (Su, Rounds, & Armstrong, 2009). Tannen (1990) in her book, "You Just Don't Understand: Women and Men in Conversation," described the difference in interpersonal style in boys as often doing things together (a feature of agentic attribute), and in girls as often talking together (a feature of communal attribute). In his popular book, "Men Are from Mars, Women Are from Venus," Gray (1992) suggested that the difference in social behavior and communication between men and women is so wide that they seem to come from different planets!

In stressful situations, women would tend to express their emotions and talk about problems to acquire their mates' support (communal characteristic), but men often prefer not to talk but rather do something about problems (an agentic characteristic). According to Wood and Eagly (2010), women more often use communication to enhance interpersonal relationships due to their communal character. However, because of their agentic character, men use communication to achieve tangible outcomes and exert dominance.

Despite the aforementioned gender differences, I must caution that the above-mentioned evolutionary determinants of gender behaviors should not lead us to making the fundamental "attribution error." In judging the gender differences, this well-known error can be committed by incorrectly assuming from evolutionary history that gender roles have been fixed for good! In modern societies, women's domestic role and their maternal investment in nurturing their children on demand and men's role as the sole breadwinners for the family have changed to some extent. The evolutionary advantages in mate selection and division of labor have also been changing in most modern societies. These adjustments, in the long run, can insert their effects into the gender role equation formulated by evolutionary history and bring about some new gender roles suited to better survival in modern societies. Consistent with this, Zentner and Mitura (2012) studied a large sample of research participants in 10 nations and concluded that the historical gender differences in preference for mate selection declined proportionally in nations with a higher gender parity.

However, these findings have been challenged by others (Schmitt, 2012). Changes currently occurring in modern societies include women's out-of-home employment, provision of child care by nonparental sources, and reconstruction of the traditional family structure and function. Over a sufficiently long period of time, this progression may influence the trace of the old history of human evolution by the tracks of modern history, in a way that transforms current gender differences to something more beneficial to survival of the human race. But for now, the impact of evolutionary history on current social behavior of men and women should not be dismissed.

Hormonal and Biophysiological Differences

Exposure to various sex hormones from the time of conception plays an important role in gender differentiation. The starting point in gender differentiation is the presence of the "Y" chromosome at conception, which contributes to the development of testes and male gonads, and its absence, which leads to forming ovaries in women. Male hormones (e.g., androgens or testosterone, its chief derivative) produced by male testes will have permanent effects on the brain development from inception. Some hormones that are relevant to understanding gender differences include testosterone, oxytocin, and to some extent cortisol. These hormones act as chemical transmitters in the brain that contribute to performance in certain social behaviors.

Higher levels of testosterone, for example, are associated with dominance or behaviors that gain or maintain status, often entailing competition, risk taking, thrill seeking, and aggression (Booth, Granger, Mazur, & Kivlighan, 2006), which are consistent with men's agentic characteristic. It is reported that fathers as well as non-father men with lower levels of testosterone showed a higher need to respond and more empathic sensitivity to infant cries than fathers with higher testosterone levels (Fleming, Corter, Stallings, & Steiner, 2002). In contrast, higher levels of oxytocin (and low levels of testosterone) are associated with human bonding and attachment; affiliation and friend seeking; nurturance; intimacy; and a propensity for empathic engagement (Campbell, 2008), which are consistent with women's communal attribute.

Some authors have argued that the difference in levels of prenatal testosterone in male and female fetuses supports the notion that the hormone has an important role in forming sex-specific interpersonal styles and verbal ability (Baron-Cohen, 2003; Connellan, Baron-Cohen, Wheelwright, Batki, & Ahluwalia, 2000). For example, a study in which an inverse relationship was found between levels of fetal testosterone and size of the vocabulary in children at 18 and 24 months of age supported the importance of fetal testosterone levels in verbal ability in men and women (Lutchmaya, Baron-Cohen, & Raggatt, 2002).

It is well known that the hormone oxytocin rises in women during childbirth and is released during childbirth and lactation. It has also been shown that women with higher level of oxytocin in early pregnancy and postpartum engage in more intimate behaviors with their babies such as gazing, eye-to-eye contact, affectionate touching, and tender loving care (Feldman, Weller, Zagoor-Sharon, & Levine, 2007). Oxytocin is associated with pair bonding, sexual behavior, maternal care, social attachment, prosocial behavior, and trust in others (Chakrabarti & Baron-Cohen, 2006; Kosfeld, Heinrichs, Zak, Fischbacher, & Fehr, 2005). It is also reported that oxytocin improves the "mind-reading" ability and adeptness to infer the mental state of others from social cues of the eye region (Domes, Heinrichs, Michel, Berger, & Herpertz, 2007), measured by the Reading the Mind in the Eye Test (Baron-Cohen, Wheelwright, Hill, Raste, & Plumb, 2001), which can facilitate empathic engagement. Hurlemann et al. (2010) reported that oxytocin can enhance social learning and emotional empathy in humans.

Another sex-typed hormone, cortisol, is also implicated in initiation of the parental role and in gender differences. Hormonal changes have been linked to gender-typed behaviors. Such changes in mothers accompany childbirth and stimulate nursing (Fleming, Ruble, Krieger, & Wong, 1997). It has been observed that anticipation of becoming a father could lead to hormonal changes in men, parallel to the changes that occur in mothers. Such changes may include a decrease in testosterone (Berg & Wynne-Edwards, 2001). These changes can influence social behavior and empathic orientation.

Inborn Sensitivity to Social Stimuli and Propensity to Social Interaction

Inborn gender differences in responses to social stimuli, prior to any social learning, can be observed in children at an early age. For example, female newborns are more responsive than male newborns to auditory and social stimuli and are able to maintain eye contact for longer periods of time (Hittelman & Dickes, 1979; Osofsky & O'Connell, 1977). Infant's eye contact, recognized as an inducer of maternal caregiving (Hittelman & Dickes, 1979), is a social interaction which is under the control of the infant and occurs immediately after birth prior to any social learning. Female neonates also smile more and show less rapid buildup of arousal and excitement (Osofsky & O'Connell, 1977). A study of neonates (mean age 36.7 h) in which a human face and a mobile were presented simultaneously found that the female infants exhibited a stronger interest in the human face, whereas the male infants showed a greater interest in the mobile (Connellan et al., 2000).

Female newborns have shown less irritability than male newborns (Moss, 1967), and infant girls had less difficulty regulating emotions and displayed less irritation than infant boys when confronted with their mother's expressionless face (the still-face experiment described in Chap. 4) (Weinberg, Tronick, & Cohn, 1999). Obviously, these early differences that are precursors to social development cannot be attributed to socialization and adaptation to gender roles.

It has been reported that girls, compared to boys, show more concern for fairness (Charlesworth & Dzur, 1987) and respond more empathically to the stress of others (Hoffman, 1977). Also, at 1 year of age, girls can show their empathic concern through sad looks and sympathetic vocalization (Hoffman, 1977).

Perception of Emotions and Decoding of Emotional Signals

Empirical research suggests that from an early age, females seem to be more sensitive to emotional signals than males. For example, female infants exhibit more reactive crying when another crying infant is present than male infants (Sagi & Hoffman, 1976) (in Chap. 5, a reactive crying response was described as an indication of a primitive empathic response).

A significant difference has also been observed in favor of women regarding the transmission and detection of nonverbal emotional cues (Brown & Dunn, 1996; Buck, 1984; Buck, Savin, Miller, & Caul, 1972). In a meta-analytic study, effect sizes of gender differences in sensitivity to nonverbal cues were reported to be in a moderate range of 0.40–0.50 (Hall, 1998). Women's ability to understand emotional cues has been observed in a number of studies in both children and adults (Brown & Dunn, 1996; Davis, 1983, 1994; Eisenberg & Lennon, 1983; Eisenberg & Strayer, 1987; Feshbach, 1982; Hogan, 1969; Jose, 1989; Litvack-Miller, McDougall, & Romney, 1997).

The ability to perceive the emotions of another person and to "send" and "receive" nonverbal signals through facial expressions and body language (Hall, Carter, & Horgan, 2000; Hall & Gunnery, 2013) contributes significantly to empathic engagement. Yawning, for example, has been linked to empathic ability and social awareness, as described in Chap. 2. In a study of naturalistic observations, it was found that the rate of contagious yawning was significantly higher in women than men (Norsica, Demuru, & Palagi, 2016). Also, women are more receptive to emotional signals than men (Trivers, 1972) and are more perceptive about their meaning (Baron-Cohen, 2003; Bjorklund & Kipp, 1996; Buss & Schmitt, 1993).

Despite the fact that women are generally better at perceiving other people's emotions and are less socially constrained about expressing their emotions, they are not always superior to men in the expression of certain emotions (Brody & Hall, 2008). For example, although women generally are better at expressing fear, sadness, love, and happiness, men are better at expressing anger and hatred (Wagner, Buck, & Winterbotham, 1993), characteristics that are not conducive to empathy. Women have been stereotyped as nurturing and interpersonally oriented (Eisenberg & Lennon, 1983), characteristics that have been identified as central components of female identity (Jack, 1993) and that facilitate empathic engagement.

Research found women not only understand other people's facial expressions better than men, but they are also more facially expressive (Buck, Miller, & Caul, 1974). In one experiment, female pairs were more skillful than male pairs at understanding nonverbal emotional cues (by observing on closed-circuit television the facial expressions of a person who was watching slides with varied emotional content) (Buck et al., 1972). Hall's review (1978) of 75 studies on gender differences in the ability to decode other people's emotional states confirmed women's superiority in decoding visual and auditory cues. Another study (Zuckerman, DePauls, & Rosenthal, 1981) found that women could even detect negative aspects of interpersonal behavior, such as deception, better than men. Obviously, the ability to correctly interpret nonverbal cues and another person's state of mind is relevant to the capacity to form empathic relationships.

Women are more likely than men to exhibit comforting behavior, even to strangers in stress (Hoffman, 1977). Women value reciprocity in relationship and endorse cooperation more than men do, whereas men place more value on competition and power (Ahlgren & Johnson, 1979). These characteristics are conducive to empathic engagement in women.

Interpersonal Style, Verbal Ability, Aggressive Behavior, and Caring Attitudes

Men and women have different interpersonal styles. Research has shown that men are more likely to interrupt when women are talking with each other, whereas women are less likely to interrupt when men are talking with each other (McMillan, Clifton, McGrath, & Gale, 1977). In addition, a study found men tend to speak more assertively than women during verbal communication (Kramer, 1974). Taylor et al. (2000) reported that men and women often exhibit different biobehavioral responses to stressful events that reflect differences in their neuroendocrine and physiological systems. The authors suggested that men generally tend to react to stress with the "fight-or-flight" response, whereas women's response tends to be characterized as "tend-and-befriend" (Taylor et al., 2000), a pattern involving nurturing activities developed during human evolution to protect the self and offspring.

Taylor et al. (2000) suggested that the underlying biobehavioral mechanism responsible for this "tend-and-befriend" pattern might be set in motion by the attachment system described in Chap. 4, and by hormones such as oxytocin in conjunction with other female reproductive hormones, and the activities of endogenous opioid peptides. The "tend-and-befriend" approach of social behavior is reflected in typical acts such as talking on the phone for a longer period of time and simple social contacts such as asking for directions without hesitation when lost. Both of these examples are more typical characteristics of women than men. Obviously, these gender differences in interpersonal styles and biobehavioral responses can influence the formation of empathic relationships.

In interpersonal interactions, smiling is the best single predictor of warmth (Bayes, 1972) and an indicator of prosocial behavior and positive affect. Appropriate use of smiling serves as a positive signal in interpersonal communication. A meta-analytic study of gender differences with regard to smiling found that women and adolescent girls were significantly more likely to smile than men and adolescent boys (LaFrance, Hecht, & Paluck, 2003). Based on a meta-analytic study of 20 published articles on gender differences in smiling, Hall (1984) reported a relatively large effect size of 0.63 on gender differences in smiling. Research found women are generally more expressive and emotional than men (Briton & Hall, 1995; Kring

& Gordon, 1998). Women's higher rate of expressing emotion and smiles is an uncomplicated facial signal that can strengthen interpersonal relationships.

Also, women's superiority on tests of verbal ability has been documented in many empirical studies (e.g., see Maccoby & Jacklin, 1974). Girls often begin talking at an earlier age than boys, and they maintain their superior verbal ability thereafter (Rutter et al., 2005). In addition to verbal skills, women surpass men in sociability. For example, Hall (1984) reported that women make more eye contact during interpersonal interactions than age-matched men. Women also tend to understand the social context of certain matters better than men (Willingham & Cole, 1997). For example, female college students identified with story characters to a greater degree than the male students did. The researcher found that such identification correlated positively with scores on the Empathic Concern subscale (measure of emotional empathy or sympathy) of the IRI (Jose, 1989).

Women's typical characteristic of expressing their emotions (e.g., externalizing) and men's typical characteristic of concealing their emotions (e.g., internalizing) prompt the two sexes to reveal their emotions differently (Buck et al., 1972). An empirical study reported that the men and women who received higher femininity marks on the Gender Role Orientation Inventory (Bem, 1974) also had significantly higher empathy scores on the IRI (Karniol et al., 1998).

Although some gender differences in interpersonal styles and verbal skills can be attributed to socialization and learned sex roles (Eagly, 1995), evidence suggests that these differences may be partially biological in origin (Baron-Cohen, 2003). In a study by Singer et al. (2006) using fMRI, it was noticed that while both men and women exhibited empathy-related activation in areas that register pain (fronto-insular and anterior cingulated cortices), the empathy-related brain activities were significantly reduced in men when observing a cheater in pain, as described earlier in this chapter.

Although generally no consistent gender difference in anger has been reported, research indicates men often show physical aggression more than women, and women often show verbal aggression more than men (Archer, 2004). Verbal aggression and aggressive behavior reflect a negative affect, which interferes with the formation of empathic relationships. Women are generally less likely than men to exhibit aggressive behavior (for a meta-analytic study, see Eagly & Steffen, 1986). Gender differences in the expression of aggression may be attributable not only to hormonal differences but also to social learning and stereotypical sex roles that lead men to become tougher, more assertive, and more behaviorally aggressive than women. However, it is important to note that social learning explains only part of the picture, because research indicates that aggression is more observable and pronounced in male than in female children (Hyde, 1984).

Women express aggression in different ways than men and toward different targets. For example, a study showed women tend to direct their aggression toward other women, not men (Eagly & Steffen, 1986). Women are more likely than men to show "indirect" aggression often verbally, whereas men are likely to show "direct" physical aggression (e.g., pushing, punching) (Chakrabarti & Baron-Cohen, 2006). Indirect aggression requires regulation of emotion and better mind reading (Kosfeld et al., 2005), which are conducive to empathic engagement. Daly and Wilson (1988) studied data collected over 700 years on homicide and noticed that male-on-male rate of homicide was 30–40 times more than female-on-female homicide. Women often feel guilty to a greater degree than men about aggressive behavior, so that feeling guilty about aggressive behavior often prohibits women from expressing aggression (Frodi & Macauley, 1977). Control of aggression is a self-regulatory behavior that promotes empathic relationships. By using the "still-face" procedure (described in Chap. 4), male infants were observed to have greater difficulty than female infants in maintaining emotional regulation (Weinberg et al., 1999), suggesting that women may have more control over regulation of their emotions, which leads to better interpersonal interactions.

Social stereotypes often portray men who help others as heroic and chivalrous (e.g., those who risk their own life to save others from harm) and portray women as nurturing and caring (Eagly & Crowley, 1986). A meta-analytic review of the literature revealed that, in general, men were more likely than women to give help and women were more inclined to receive help (Eagly & Crowley, 1986). However, women historically have been more inclined than men to place the needs of others, especially those of their children, above their own (Chodorow, 1978) and are more oriented toward care giving (Gilligan, 1982). Charles Darwin also noticed this quality. In his seminal book, *The Descent of Man*, Darwin (1981) indicated that women exhibit greater tenderness in social relationships than men, and because of their maternal instincts, their tenderness toward their infants is likely to extend toward others.

Gender Differences in the Practice of Medicine

It seems reasonable to speculate that gender differences concerning empathy could influence male and female physicians' styles of practice and provision of patient care, and multiple empirical studies have confirmed this speculation (Bertakis, Helms, Callahan, Azari, & Robbins, 1995; Bylund & Makoul, 2002; Fruen, Rothman, & Steiner, 1974; Henderson & Weisman, 2001; Maheux, Duford, Beland, Jacques, & Levesque, 1990; Weisman & Teitlebaum, 1985). In examining factors that influence medical students' learning of psychopathology in a psychiatry clerkship, Fabrega, Ulrich, and Keshavan (1994) reported that female medical students showed better achievement due to gender-related factors such as students' ability to assimilate and cope with clinical experiences of the psychiatric clerkship.

Female physicians were more likely than male physicians to engage patients in positive talk; discuss psychological and social issues in health and illness; use more positive statements; engage in more verbal exchanges with patients; and spend a longer time with them (Cooper-Patrick, Gallo, & Gonzales, 1999; Hall, Irish, Roter, Ehrlic, & Miller, 1994; Meeuwesen, Schaap, & Van der Staak, 1991; Roter & Hall, 1997; Roter, Lipkin, & Korsgaard, 1991; Roter, Hall, & Aoki, 2002). On the average, female physicians spent three to four more minutes with their patients than their male counterparts, engaged in more humorous conversations with their patients, and shared more decision-making responsibility with them (Charon, Greene, & Adelman,

1994). Studies have also shown female physicians also are more prevention oriented than their male counterparts (Bertakis et al., 1995; Frank & Harvey, 1996; Maheux et al., 1990). Furthermore, they provide more screening and more preventive counseling about sensitive topics, particularly with female patients (Henderson & Weisman, 2001). These gender differences in practice style, according to Bylund and Makoul (2002), can be the result of the female physicians' tendency to communicate with their patients with a higher degree of empathy than their male counterparts.

Charon et al. (1994, p. 216) observed that female physicians acted as if they were alert to their patients' emotional and daily-life concerns—concerns that otherwise "tend to be muted in medical interactions." Their observation agreed with the idea posed by others that women, more than men, can bring empathy to the healing relationship (Bickel, 1994; Bylund & Makoul, 2002). Charon et al. also found that patients reacted to male and female physicians differently. Patients of both sexes reported that female physicians were more willing to discuss medical topics and probe about personal habits, such as smoking, alcohol, drug use, sex, sleep, psychological issues, finances, emotional problems, and family and work problems.

In a study of patients' satisfaction, both male and female patients gave more favorable ratings to the care they received from female residents than from male residents (Linn, Cope, & Leake, 1984). However, Howell, Gardiner, and Concato (2002) found that although a greater number of patients preferred female over male obstetricians, their satisfaction with medical care was unrelated to a physician's sex. With regard to medical malpractice claims, the fact that female physicians have a better record than male physicians is attributed more to better physician–patient relationships than to taking on less risky patients (Sloan, Mergenhagen, Burfield, Bovjerg, & Hassan, 1989). In the area of clinical competency, our study showed that directors of residency training programs rated female residents higher than their male counterparts on the "socioeconomic aspect of patient care" at the end of the first year of postgraduate medical education (Hojat et al., 1994). These findings suggest that female and male health care providers have different practice styles resulting from their differences in interpersonal style that is reflected in their empathic engagement with patients.

Complementary or Opposite Sexes?

Despite all gender differences I described in this chapter, a number of meta-analytic studies reported that gender similarities in social behavior are overwhelmingly higher than the overinflated claims of the differences (Eagly & Wood, 2013; Hyde, 2005; Spelke, 2005; Stewart-Williams & Thomas, 2013; Su et al., 2009; Twenge, 1997; Zell, Krizan, & Teener, 2015). Because men and women are similar in many psychosocial qualities, Zell et al. (2015) and Hyde (2005) suggested that in gender research, it would be more desirable to test hypotheses of gender similarities rather than differences. However, despite the fact that the effect size of gender differences is typically small, Zell et al. (2015) suggest that the small differences accumulate when summed across domains. Therefore, differences should not be necessarily considered negligible. Consistent trivial differences can have important consequences that need to be constantly explored. In her meta-analytic review of 46 studies on psychological and mental ability variables, Hyde (2005) advanced the idea of gender similarities rather than gender differences and concluded that men and women are alike on most, but not all, psychological and mental ability variables and declared that gender differences have been substantially overinflated.

The modest and sometimes negligible magnitude of gender differences does exist, observed consistently and universally in social skills, mental abilities, emotions, personality, interest, attitudes, and behaviors. However, such differences should not be considered as an argument for viewing men and women as "opposite" sexes; rather, they should be viewed as "complementary" genders. For example, women's superiority in communal and men's advantage in agentic characteristics can complement one another to make a better world. Together, men and women are like a completed jigsaw puzzle.

Recapitulation

A great majority of empirical studies in the general population and in health professions students and practitioners have reported that women outscore men in measures of interpersonal relationships and empathy. The differences in men and women in social behavior and empathy have often been attributed to social learning and sociocultural factors. In this chapter, I argued that while the contribution of social learning and cultural factors in gender differences cannot be ignored, there are other evolutionary factors and inborn characteristics that can provide plausible explanations for gender differences in social skills, beyond social learning, gender stereotypical role models, and social and cultural factors. Relying on the human evolutionary history, I proposed that ancestral history in preferred advantages in mate selection, parental investment in child care, division of labor, and hormonal and physiological factors have endowed women with a greater propensity for social skills and empathic engagement. However, some of the current gender differences may cease to exist in the future. Changes currently occurring in modern societies, if continuing over a sufficiently long period of time, require adjustments that can alter the effects of past evolution in gender differences and transform them into something else for better survival.

Chapter 11
Clinical Empathy and Patient Outcomes

The secret of the care of the patient is in caring for the patient.

—(Francis W. Peabody, 1927/1984, p. 818)

The failure to empathize is the basis of most of the unhappy doctor–patient relationships.

—(Harry A. Wilmer, 1968, p. 248)

Abstract

- The theoretical link between clinical empathy and positive patient outcomes is based on the following assumptions: When an empathic engagement is formed, then a trusting relationship will develop, the constraints of relationship will diminish, and this will lead to a more accurate diagnosis and greater compliance, and ultimately to desirable patient outcomes.
- In an empathic engagement, the patient perceives the clinician as a helping member of a social support system with all the beneficial health effects of human connection. All of these should theoretically contribute to optimal patient outcomes, including patients' greater satisfaction with their healthcare providers, a reduced likelihood of malpractice litigation, and more optimal clinical results.
- Research findings, showing significant associations between scores of a validated measure of clinical empathy (JSE) and tangible patient outcomes in diabetic patients (e.g., laboratory test results and hospitalization rate due to acute metabolic complications), present strong evidence in support of the link between the healthcare provider's empathy and clinical outcomes, independent of patients' subjective assessments.
- The psychosocial and biophysioneurological factors involved in interactions between a clinician and the patient are described as the plausible underlying mechanisms that can explain the link between clinician's empathy and patient outcomes.

M. Hojat, *Clinical Empathy*, https://doi.org/10.1007/978-3-031-87413-0_11

Introduction

In this chapter, I briefly discuss the link between clinical empathy and patient outcomes and present a theoretical framework and some empirical evidence in support of that link. Presumably, any factor that contributes to enhancement of the clinician–patient relationship, including clinical empathy, should in theory have a beneficial effect on patient outcomes (Mercer & Reynolds, 2002). Although the assumption that an empathic clinician–patient relationship will result in positive patient outcomes is theoretically sound, empirical evidence is needed to verify this assumption, and plausible explanations are required to clarify the underlying mechanisms that establish the link between empathic engagement in patient care and positive clinical outcomes.

A Theoretical Framework

The theoretical link between empathic clinician–patient engagement and positive patient outcomes is based on the assumptions that when an empathic relationship is formed between a clinician and a patient, trust will develop, the truth will emerge, and the result will be reflected in a more precise medical history and thus more accurate diagnostic information and greater compliance. Abundant evidence is available in support of this proposition (Hojat et al., 2013, 2023). In addition, in an empathic relationship, the patient perceives a clinician as a trustworthy attachment figure, an omnipotent person of authority similar to a protective wise parent. Therefore, the clinician becomes a secure base from which the patient can explore the unknowns of the illness and disclose real concerns without any constraints. Evidence in support of such beneficial effects of genuine human connection is plentiful, some of which was presented in Chap. 4. Also, when an empathic engagement is formed, patients view the clinician as a helpful member of a social support system with beneficial effects on their physical, mental, and social well-being. Ample evidence is available to support this claim as well, some of which was reported in Chap. 2.

On the basis of the assumptions just described, an empathic clinician–patient relationship paves the road to desirable patient outcomes. However, despite the abundance of reports in the medical, psychological, and sociological literature about these assumptions, empirical evidence supporting the direct link between clinical empathy and measurable patient outcomes in medical and surgical care is limited. As indicated in Chaps. 1 and 6, the dearth of empirical evidence in support of a direct link between empathy and patient outcomes can be attributed to two factors. First, the historical conceptual ambiguity regarding empathy in clinician–patient relationships has been an obstacle to the development of an operational definition of clinical empathy in patient care. A concept that is not well defined does not lend itself to empirical scrutiny. Second, until the development of the Jefferson Scale of Empathy (JSE), the lack of a psychometrically sound measure of clinical empathy designed specifically for use in the context of patient care had been an impediment to the empirical investigation of empathy and its outcomes in the context of the health professions education and patient care. However, because empathy is the backbone of clinician–patient relationships, we can safely assume that the majority of research findings about the effects of the quality of physician–patient "relationships" on patient outcomes could be generalizable or applicable to "empathic engagement" in patient care as well.

The Clinician–Patient Relationship and Patient Outcomes

A large volume of research has accumulated in support of the notion that the quality of the clinician–patient relationship can facilitate the process of patient care and thus have a positive influence on patient outcomes (Butow, Maclean, Dunn, Tattersall, & Boyer, 1997; Di Blasi, Harkness, Ernst, Georgiou, & Kleijnen, 2001; Neuwirth, 1997; Roghmann, Hengst, & Zastowny, 1979; Roter et al., 1998; Sanson-Fisher & Maguire, 1980; Staudenmayer & Lefkowitz, 1981; Stewart, 1996; Watts, 2012). The relevance of such research findings to the theme of empathy in patient care is evident if one assumes that empathic engagement is a core ingredient of positive clinician–patient relationships.

The medical literature contains abundant evidence in support of the idea that the quality of clinician–patient relationships has a significant effect on clinical outcomes. For example, a review of 21 published studies revealed that 16 (76%) of the articles reported a positive, statistically significant relationship between effective physician–patient communication and health outcomes (Stewart, 1996). Among the elements of effective communication were physicians' empathic engagement, supportive role, and concern about patients' feelings and experiences (Stewart, 1996).

The following sections present some empirical evidence from the medical literature in support of the notion that high-quality clinician–patient relationships positively influence patients' satisfaction and compliance and reduce the likelihood of malpractice litigation.

Patient Satisfaction

Patient satisfaction is a widely recognized outcome measure in healthcare research (Hall, Roter, & Katz, 1988). The relationship between patients' satisfaction with their healthcare providers and their recall of and compliance with the providers' medical advice suggests that satisfaction is an important determinant of the outcome of healthcare (Hall & Dornan, 1988).

Patients' overall satisfaction with their healthcare providers is often moderately high (in the 70 s or 80 s on a 100-point scale) (Hall & Dornan, 1988). Interpersonal exchanges between physician and patient have often proved to be significant predictors of patients' satisfaction (Butow et al., 1997). For example, a meta-analytic study found that such factors as nonverbal cues (e.g., touch, forward lean, closer distance, eye contact, nods, gestures), social-emotional conversation (about nonmedical issues), positive talk, and length of encounter contribute to the patients' satisfaction with their healthcare providers (Hall, Roter, Katz, 1988). Other determinants of patients' satisfaction were patients' participation in the therapeutic process (Speedling & Rose, 1985), commitment to the therapeutic relationship (i.e., willingness to return to the physician for care), the length of time the physicians spent with their patients, and the physicians' willingness to listen and be accessible when needed (DiMatteo, Prince, & Taranta, 1979).

Moreover, research has shown physicians' ability to communicate their concern, warmth, and interest to their patients also leads to patients' satisfaction (Speedling & Rose, 1985). Physicians' general sensitivity to patients' emotions and their ability to express feelings and understanding were associated with patients' satisfaction (DiMatteo, Taranta, Friedman, & Prince, 1980). All the qualities of physicians just described are among the ingredients of empathic engagement in patient care.

One can assume that the positive link between physicians' empathy and patient outcomes is the result of empathic engagement that can help patients formulate their health problems more clearly, thus leading to more accurate diagnoses, more acceptable solutions to their health problems, and firmer commitment to the treatment regimen (Stiles, Putman, Wolfe, & James, 1979). For example, patients infected with the human immunodeficiency virus (HIV) indicated that the quality of interpersonal relationships with medical staff was an important factor in their satisfaction with the care they received (Stein, Fleisman, Mor, & Dresser, 1993). In another study, patients' perceptions of their physicians' interpersonal and communication skills, rather than physicians' knowledge, contributed more to patients' satisfaction with clinical outcomes (Clearly & McNeil, 1988).

Investigators who conducted a study with residents in internal medicine and their patients noticed that patients' satisfaction was related more to interpersonal relationships reflected in physicians' courtesy and giving of information than to physicians' nonverbal behavior, such as eye contact and body posture (Comstockas, Hooper, Goodwin, & Goodwin, 1982).

An explanation for positive clinical outcomes of empathy in patient care may be found in reports that patients are generally more satisfied with an empathic health provider (Beckman & Frankel, 1984; Bertakis, Roter, & Putman, 1991; Francis & Morris, 1969; Korsch, Gozzi, & Francis, 1968; Zachariae et al., 2003) and comply more with physicians who understand them better (Blackwell, 1973; Davis, 1968; Hall et al., 1988; Squier, 1990; Stewart, 1996). Patients generally view physicians' conduct as a key determinant of their satisfaction with medical care (Moss, 1967). The finding that the physicians' understanding of their patients' perspective is related to the patients' perceptions of being helped (Eisenthal, Emery, Lazare, & Udin, 1979) provides additional support for the link between empathic understanding and improved patient empowerment (Street, Makoul, Arora, & Epstein, 2009). In a factor analytic study, 52% of the variance in patients' ratings of their satisfaction with medical care was accounted for by the physician's level of interpersonal warmth and respect (Kenny, 1995). In a study with diabetic patients, dieticians' empathic understanding was predictive of the patients' satisfaction and the success of consultations (Goodchild, Skinner, & Parkin, 2005). To summarize, the practice style reflected in a clinician's communication skills and empathic concern leads to more patient's satisfaction.

Adherence and Compliance

Adherence to and compliance with treatment regimens are recognized as predictors of clinical outcomes (Hall et al., 1988; Kim, Kaplowitz, & Johnston, 2004; Ong, DeHaes, Hoos, & Lammies, 1995; Roter et al., 1998; Sackett & Haynes, 1976; Stewart, 1996). Although the terms "adherence" and "compliance" are often used interchangeably in the literature, their meaning is not identical. For example, compliance reflects a biomedical paradigm of disease that reinforces passivity in patients (Roter et al., 1998) and refers to the patient's acceptance of the clinician's orders or advice without participating in the decision-making process (Kelman, 1958). However, when the patient follows the clinician's instructions as a participant in the process, adherence is the more appropriate term. Adherence implies a more active patient–clinician collaboration involving the patient's choice in planning the treatment (Eisenthal et al., 1979; Roter et al., 1998; Squier, 1990).

Abundant evidence suggests that positive patient–clinician relationships not only contribute to patients' satisfaction with their healthcare providers and adherence to the providers' advice but also lead to adequate disclosure of problems, all of which can have a significant impact on patient outcomes (Beckman & Frankel, 1984; Butow et al., 1997; Falvo & Tippy, 1988; Sanson-Fisher & Maguire, 1980). Physicians' understanding of their patients was found to be significantly correlated with patients' adhering to treatment and feeling better (Eisenthal et al., 1979). In a pediatric healthcare setting, investigators reported that mothers of sick children adhered more closely to the care provider's advice when they perceived that the provider attempted to understand their concerns (Francis & Morris, 1969; Korsch, Gozzi, & Francis, 1968). In another study, physicians' empathic understanding, reflected in their expression of positive affect, increased adherence to the physicians' advice among mothers after emergency visits to a children's hospital (Freemon, Negrete, Davis, & Korsch, 1971).

Patients' adherence to treatment reportedly varied from 25 to 94% depending on several factors, including interactions between physician and patient (Eisenthal et al., 1979). Despite the important benefits patients derived from following their physician's advice, a significant number of patients (30–60%) in two studies failed to follow that advice (Kaplan & Simon, 1990; Luscher & Vetter, 1990). This can be attributed to a lack of empathic engagement. Physicians' empathic skills and interpersonal style have been cited as crucial factors determining whether patients adhere to treatment regimens (DiMatteo et al., 1993). Indicators of a physician's empathy, such as sensitivity, decoding skills, tone of voice, and nonverbal communication, were related to patients' compliance with scheduled appointments (DiMatteo, Hays, & Prince, 1986). Furthermore, in situations where the physician failed to demonstrate empathic engagement, the patient easily forgot their advice and was likely to miss follow-up appointments (Falvo & Tippy, 1988). In addition, physicians who expressed willingness to answer patients' questions without being concerned about the time had a positive influence on patients' adherence to treatment (DiMatteo et al., 1993). These studies suggest that an interpersonal style that reflects a physician's empathic understanding of patients can enhance patients' adherence to treatment.

Malpractice Claims

Research indicates that a problematic physician–patient relationship can increase the likelihood that a patient will initiate a legal action against the physician. A physician's style of communication, in particular, is an important factor in a plaintiff's decision to take such an action (Beckman, Markakis, Suchman, & Frankel, 1994; Hickson, Clayton, Githens, & Sloan, 1992; Levinson, Roter, Mullooly, Dull, & Frankel, 1997; Meyers, 1987; Shapiro, Simpson, & Lawrence, 1989). Empirical evidence suggests that a positive physician–patient relationship reduces not only the actual malpractice claims but also patients' intention to take such action, regardless of the severity of the adverse medical outcomes (Moore, Adler, & Robertson, 2000). In a survey of malpractice attorneys, it was found that more than 80% of malpractice suits were based on unsatisfactory physician–patient relationships (Avery, 1985).

One study found that physicians who exhibited empathic concern for their patients were better diagnosticians and provided better treatments (Barsky, 1981). Conversely, poor communication skills on the physicians' part, which led to inadequate empathic engagement with patients, proved to be the most important factor prompting patients to file a lawsuit against a physician (Beckman et al., 1994).

In a study examining rates of malpractice claims for different medical specialties, Taragin et al. (1994) controlled for confounding factors (e.g., physicians' age, training, and certification status and the severity of the diseases they treated) and concluded that the variation in claim rates could not be explained by differences in the physicians' academic achievements. Consistent with these findings, researchers in another study found no relationship between malpractice claims against obstetricians and the technical quality of physician's care (Entman et al., 1994).

Among mothers of infants who had been permanently injured or had died, dissatisfaction with the obstetrician's interpersonal style (e.g., not listening, not talking openly, and not discussing long-term outcomes) was a major factor in determining whether the obstetrician was sued (Hickson et al., 1992). Compared with obstetricians who had been sued, those who had never been sued were viewed as concerned, accessible, and willing to talk (Hickson et al., 1994). Other studies have shown that the physician's communication skills and empathic concern are the factors that reduce the risk of malpractice litigation (Beckman et al., 1994; Levinson et al., 1997). A review of allegation transcripts revealed that physicians' failure to understand the perspectives of their patients or their patients' families—an indication of a lack of empathic engagement—was among the important factors that contributed to patients' decisions to sue (Beckman et al., 1994; Levinson et al., 1997).

Clinical Empathy and Clinical Outcomes

Some studies showed a link between empathic engagement and patient outcomes in the context of medical and surgical treatments (Luborsky, Chandler, Auerbach, Cohen, & Bacharach, 1971; Nightingale, Yarnold, & Greenberg, 1991; Lelorain, Bredart, Dolbeault, & Sultan, 2012). For example, in a review of 39 studies in cancer care, Leloriann et al. (2015) reported that clinicians' empathy is beneficially related to certain patient outcomes, such as patient satisfaction and psychological well-being. In a study by Licciardone and colleagues (Licciardone, Tran, Ngo, Toledo, 2024), associations between physician empathy, perception of pain, and health-related quality of life were examined in patients with low back pain. Findings suggest that greater patient's perception of physician empathy (measure by the Consultation and Relational Empathy instrument (see Chap. 5) was inversely associated with perception of pain intensity and pain-related disability. Empirical evidence in support of empathic engagement and patient outcomes has been reported more often in the context of psychotherapy (Free, Green, Grace, Chernus, & Whitman, 1985; Gladstein, 1977; Kurtz & Grummon, 1972; Moyers & Miller, 2013). For example, premature termination of therapy has been reported among clients who gave their therapists low ratings on a measure of empathy (Burns & Nolen-Hoeksema, 1992). It is also reported that the therapist's deficiency in empathy is "toxic" to patient outcomes because of its association with high dropout and relapse rates, weaker therapeutic alliance, and less positive change in patients (Moyers & Miller, 2013). Conversely, some reviews of the literature have linked the therapist's empathy, warmth, and genuineness to positive changes in clients (Patterson, 1984). Other reviews have reported positive patient outcomes resulting from empathic engagement between patients and nurses (Bennett, 1995).

Research on psychotherapeutic outcomes, for example, has reported a high level of empathic clinician–patient engagement as the most important factor in the reduction of symptoms (Rogers, Gendlin, Kiesler, & Truax, 1967). Also, therapists' scores on the Accurate Empathy Scale of Truax and Carkhuff's Relationship Questionnaire (see Chap. 5) were significantly higher in successful than in unsuccessful therapy cases. Bacharach (1976) reported that a therapist's empathy was consistently correlated with other qualities such as regard, genuineness, concreteness, and self-disclosure that are associated with treatment outcomes. Some studies have provided evidence supporting the causal role of empathy in psychotherapeutic outcomes (Burns & Nolen-Hoeksema, 1992; Greenberg, Watson, Elliot, & Bohart, 2001). Nonetheless, other studies have not confirmed a direct link between therapists' empathy and positive patient outcomes (Bohart, Elliot, Greenberg, & Watson, 2002;

Luborsky et al., 1971; Meltzoff & Kornreich, 1970). The inconsistencies in conceptualization and variation in the measurement of empathy in patient care (see Chaps. 1, 5, and 6) could be among the reasons for inconsistent findings on empathy and patient outcomes reported in some of the aforementioned studies.

A meta-analytic review found that the typical effect size in studies on empathy and psychotherapy outcomes is in the 0.20 s (Bohart et al., 2002). According to the operational definitions of effect sizes (Cohen, 1987; Hojat & Xu, 2004), an effect size of this magnitude is trivial. However, the magnitude of effect size for the relationship between empathy and patient outcomes varies, depending on the conceptualization of empathy (e.g., cognitive or emotional empathy), the instruments for measuring it, the format of the assessment (e.g., self-rated or observer-, peer-, or client-rated), the type of therapy (e.g., group, cognitive, psychoanalytical, behavioral therapy, or eclectic), the therapist's experience, the patient's receptivity, and so on (Bohart et al., 2002).

The aforementioned studies were mostly on the associations between psychotherapists' empathy and patient outcomes. Research is scarce regarding a direct empirical link between physician empathy and the tangible outcomes of medical and surgical treatments (Stewart, 1996). However, some studies have reported on the link between physician empathy and clinical outcomes. For example, it has been reported that internal medicine residents' self-perceived incidents of medical errors were associated with a lower level of their empathy (West et al., 2006). A study (Sultan, Attali, Gilberg, Zenasni, & Hartemann, 2011) found that physicians' accurate understanding of their diabetic patients' beliefs about their illness (as an indicator of empathic understanding) was associated with better self-care among patients (e.g., improved diet, increased blood glucose self-testing).

Staudenmayer and Lefkowitz (1981) found that physicians' empathic concern (determined by peers' ratings on their sensitivity) was related to the length of hospitalization and concerns about medications; highly sensitive physicians were more concerned about the side effects of medications and kept their patients (with asthma and other pulmonary problems) in the hospital for longer periods. MacPherson, Mercer, Scullion, and Thomas (2003) reported that the perceptions of acupuncture patients concerning their care providers' empathy were significantly associated with patients' enablement, which in turn was highly correlated with self-reported patient outcomes.

In a study with 1048 fourth-year medical students, empathic engagement assessed by standardized patients was significantly correlated with patients' level of comfort and feelings of being important (Colliver, Willis, Robbs, Cohen, & Swartz, 1998). In that study, the students whose empathic engagement was assessed as insufficient (judged to be empathic by fewer than three of the seven standardized patients) also received lower ratings concerning their skills in history taking and physical examinations (Colliver et al., 1998).

Levinson (1994) reported that patients' satisfaction and adherence to treatment were directly associated with their physicians' empathic skills, whereas patients' dissatisfaction and malpractice claims were associated with their physicians' lack of those skills. In another study, physicians regarded empathic behavior as the most important quality for being a "good physician" for improving patient outcomes;

however, the physicians themselves listed empathic behavior as the least important factor for being promoted in the hospital setting (Carmel & Glick, 1996).

An experiment conducted in the General Medicine Clinic at Cook County Hospital in Chicago showed that physicians' empathic, as opposed to sympathetic, responses to patients can lead to different measurable influences on their practice behavior and on patient outcomes (Nightingale et al., 1991). The sample in that experiment consisted of 96 residents and fellows whose preference for responding empathically or sympathetically to patients was determined by the following scenario:

> Your next patient enters the office, sits down, and says: "Doctor, my husband/wife died and I feel terrible!" The English language gives you two basic ways to respond to the patient: (A) "I understand how you feel" or words to that effect, or (B) "I feel sorry for you" or words to that effect. Which do you use?

The "A" option was considered to be an empathic response, and the "B" option was considered to be a sympathetic response. The physicians who chose the empathic response (60% of the sample) ordered fewer laboratory tests, performed cardiopulmonary resuscitation for a shorter period of time before declaring their efforts unsuccessful, and showed less preference for intubating a hypothetical patient with end-stage lung disease. The investigators concluded that physicians' empathic or sympathetic responses could lead to significant differences in their style of practice and their use of resources. In another study, it was reported that empathy can reduce the cost of medical care (Yarnold, Greenberg, & Nightingale, 1991).

In a study on the effect of physicians' empathy on patients' satisfaction and compliance with treatment (Kim et al., 2004), a set of questionnaires was administered to 550 outpatients at a university hospital in South Korea. The results indicated that patients' perceptions of physicians' empathy, measured by a modified version of the Barrett-Lennard's Relationship Inventory (Chap. 5), could have a significant influence on patients' satisfaction and compliance. The researchers concluded that enhancement of physicians' empathic communication skills is among the best approaches to improving patient satisfaction and compliance with treatment. In another study, expressions of empathy and support contributed to patients' satisfaction with their physicians (Thompson, Hearn, & Collins, 1992).

Dubnicki (1977) reported that psychotherapists' high scores on Hogan's Empathy Scale (Chap. 5) were predictive of more accurate prognoses. Kendall and Wilcox (1980) found that when therapists formed an empathic relationship with hyperactive and uncontrolled children, the children's behavior improved. Physicians' empathy, determined by positive interactions between pediatricians and the mothers of sick children, improved the mothers' satisfaction with the children's care and reduced their concern about the illness (Wasserman, Inui, Barriatua, Carter, & Lippincott, 1984). Another study found that physicians' empathy, responsiveness, and reliability were significant determinants of patients' satisfaction with their healthcare (Bowers, Swan, & Koehler, 1994).

The majority of studies on the link between clinicians' empathy and patient outcomes relied on the clinicians' self-reported empathy. However, it has been suggested that patients' own perceptions of their healthcare providers' empathy could be a better predictor of clinical outcomes (Free et al., 1985; Kurtz & Grummon,

1972). This was confirmed in a study of 350 patients with the common cold (Rakel et al., 2009) who were treated by six healthcare providers (five family physicians and one nurse practitioner). Patients in this study completed the Consultation and Relational Empathy (CARE) (Mercer, Maxwell, Heaney, & Watt, 2004; Mercer, McConnachie, Maxwell, Heaney, & Watt, 2005, see Chap. 5). After adjustment for patients' gender, race, education, optimism, perceived stress, and hours since first symptom, results showed significant associations between patients' assessment of their healthcare providers' empathy, and clinical outcomes as indicated by shorter duration and reduced severity of cold symptoms along with a positive change in the patients' immune system (Rakel et al., 2009). Authors concluded that "clinician empathy as perceived by patients with the common cold, significantly predicts subsequent duration and severity of illness and is associated with immune system." This was one of the earliest studies on empathy and patient outcomes. In a large-scale meta-analytic review study, Howick and his colleagues reported that greater healthcare providers' empathy or communication of positive messages could have beneficial effects on a range of clinical conditions, including perception of pain (Howick, Moscrop, Mebius, Fanshow, Lewith,…Onakpoya, 2018).

In a study (Yang, Xiao, Wang et al., 2018) using patients with advanced prostate cancer, it was found that urologists' clinical empathy scores (measured by the JSE) were positively associated with patients' self-efficacy and with the natural killer cells' activities, but were negatively associated with patients' anxiety and stigma. Authors concluded that physicians' empathy, through mediating roles of patient anxiety, sigma, and self-efficacy, contributed to improvement of patients' immune cellular function (by natural killer cells' activities).

Physician Empathy and Tangible Patient Outcomes

Most of the abovementioned studies on the association between clinicians' empathy and patient outcomes (with the exception of Yang et al., 2018) are limited for two reasons: (1) empathy of the physician was not measured by a psychometrically sound instrument with face and content validities, developed specifically to measure clinical empathy in the context of patient care; (2) the indicators of patient outcomes were either subjective or self-reported, which could be confounded by judgmental errors.

To the best of our knowledge, there are two published studies in which a significant association was observed between a validated measure of physician empathy (JSE) and tangible patient outcomes extracted from patients' electronic records, independent from patient's subjective judgment.

In the first study (Hojat, Louis, Markham et al., 2011a), electronic records of 891 adult patients with diabetes mellitus who were treated by one of 29 family physicians in the USA were examined, and the results of the most recent tests for hemoglobin A1c and low-density lipoprotein cholesterol (LDL-C) were extracted. Positive clinical outcomes were defined as good control of the disease reflected in A1c test results <7.0% and LDL-C < 100. Findings showed that physicians' scores on the JSE could significantly predict clinical outcomes in the diabetic patients. Patients of physicians with high JSE scores were significantly more likely to have good control of their disease (56% of patients with A1C test results <7.0, and 59% with LDL-C < 100), compared to patients of physicians with low JSE scores (40% with A1c <7.0, and 44% with LDL-C < 100). The association between physicians' scores on the JSE and patient outcomes (results of A1c and LDL-C) remained statistically significant after controlling for physicians' gender and age, as well as for patients' gender, age, and type of health insurance. Summary results are depicted in Figs. 11.1 and 11.2.

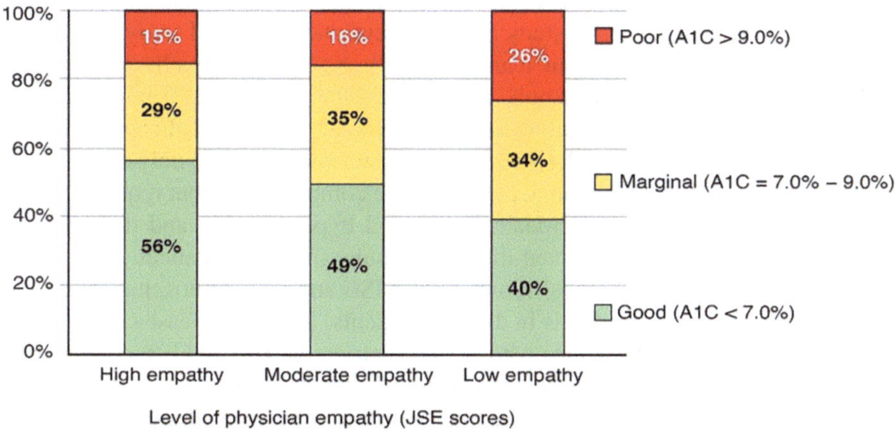

Fig. 11.1 Association between physician empathy and hemoglobin A1C test results for patients with diabetes mellitus (n = 891)

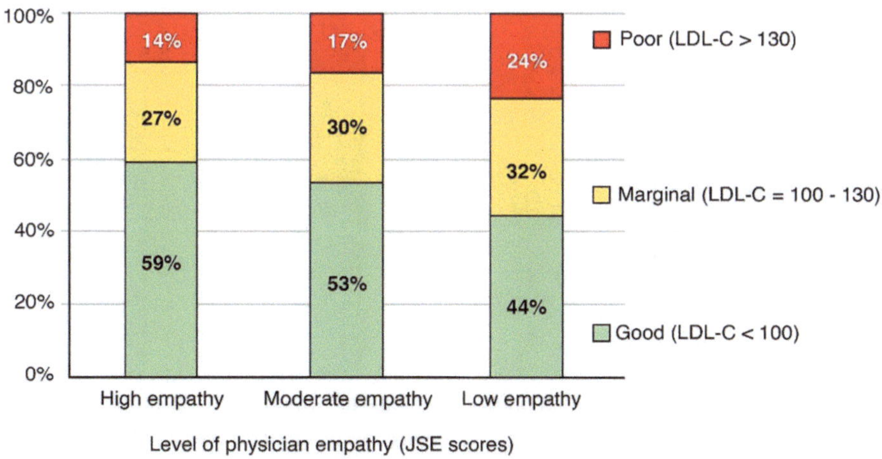

Fig. 11.2 Association between physician empathy and low-density lipoprotein cholesterol (LDL-C) test results for patients with diabetes mellitus (n = 891)

Eight years after publication of our abovementioned study, a group of investigators at the Cleveland Clinic attempted to replicate the study (Chaitoff, Rothberg, Windover, Calabrese, Misra-Herbert & Matrinez, 2019), but failed to find significant associations between physician empathy and patient outcomes. We challenged their findings due to their failure to replicate our study for the following reasons: incompatibility in the study samples of physicians, differences in the case mix of participating patients, analytical dissimilarities, and confounding institutional factors (Hojat, Maio, Markham, Louis & Gonnella, 2019). Markham and Kass (2023) in their review of research on physician empathy and clinical outcomes indicated that the aforementioned Jefferson Study and patient outcomes was cited 1327 times by others (as of 2023) and presented additional reasons for inconsistent findings between the original Jefferson study and the Cleveland replicated study.

In the second study from our team addressing physician empathy and tangible patient outcomes (Del Canale, Louis, Maio, Wang, Rossi, Hojat, & Gonnella, 2012), electronic records of 20,961 adult patients with type 1 or type 2 diabetes mellitus who were treated by one of 242 primary care physicians (in Parma, Italy) were examined, and data were extracted on acute metabolic complications that required hospitalization (e.g., diabetic ketoacidosis, coma, and hyperosmolar) and demographic information. Physicians completed the JSE. Results showed statistically significant associations between physicians' scores on the JSE and rates of hospitalization due to acute metabolic complications in diabetic patients. Rates of disease complication in diabetic patients of physicians who scored high on the JSE (≥112), compared to other physicians with moderate scores (111–197) or low JSE scores (<97), were 4.0, 7.1, and 6.5 per 1000, respectively. Summary results are presented in Fig. 11.3.

The association remained statistically significant after controlling for physicians' gender, age, type of practice (solo or group), geographical location of

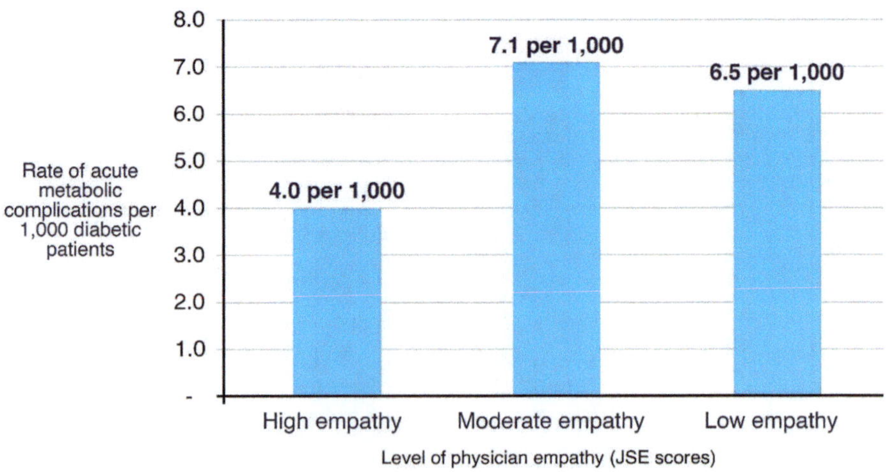

Fig. 11.3 Association between physician empathy (n = 242) and acute metabolic complications in diabetic patients (n = 20,961) in Parma, Italy

practice (plains, hills, mountains), and also patients' gender, age, and duration of time enrolled with the physician. Similarities in findings of the two aforementioned studies on significant associations between physician empathy and patient outcomes are important for the generalization of the findings, given the cultural differences or variation in medical education and healthcare systems in the USA and Italy.

Mechanisms Linking Clinical Empathy and Patient Outcomes

Our conceptualization and definition of clinical empathy implies that empathic engagement in patient care revolves around communication, reciprocity, and mutual understanding, all of which pave the road to interpersonal attunement. Mechanisms involved in connecting clinical empathy and patient outcomes can be described by *psychosocial factors* and *neurobiological responses* that are usually evoked when interpersonal attunement is formed.

At the psychosocial level, interpersonal attunement, resulting from empathic engagement in patient care, lays the foundation for a trusting relationship between the clinician and the patient. Such a trusting relationship will diminish constraints in communication and inhibition in revealing illness narrative without concealment. All these mechanisms lead to achieving a more accurate diagnosis and a greater compliance.

At the neurobiological level, interpersonal attunement in empathic engagement is analogous to a synchronized dance between patient and clinician, which is orchestrated by the tune of neurobiological markers that are described in the "perception-action coupling" model formulated by Preston and deWaal (2002). According to this model, perceptions of another person's cognitive, emotional, and somatosensory states automatically activate representations of those states, unless prohibited (Preston & deWaal, 2002). In addition, the neurobiological stimulation in interpersonal attunement that is formed by empathic engagement can activate hormonal changes (e.g., oxytocin, vasopressin) (Heinrichs & Domes, 2008) that influence the strength of empathic engagement.

Also, a set of neurons, known as the *mirror neuron system*, is discharged (Rizzolatti, Fadiga, Gallase, & Fogassi, 1996; Gallese, 2001) that may play an important role in understanding of experiences of others, which is the key ingredient of empathic engagement in patient care (Hojat, Louis, Maio, & Gonnella, 2013). All of the aforementioned psychosocial and neurobiological activities, and the mirror neuron system, can provide a plausible explanations for the mechanisms involved in linking empathic engagement in patient care and patient outcomes (Hojat, Louis, Maio, & Gonnella, 2013). Figure 11.4 depicts the aforementioned pathways in connecting clinical empathic and healthcare outcomes.

Over a century ago, Theodore Lipps, who brought the concept of empathy ("einfühlung" in the German language) into psychology, proposed that seeing someone else's facial expression triggers the observer to automatically adopt a similar facial expression, known as facial mimicry. These behaviors can be explained by the

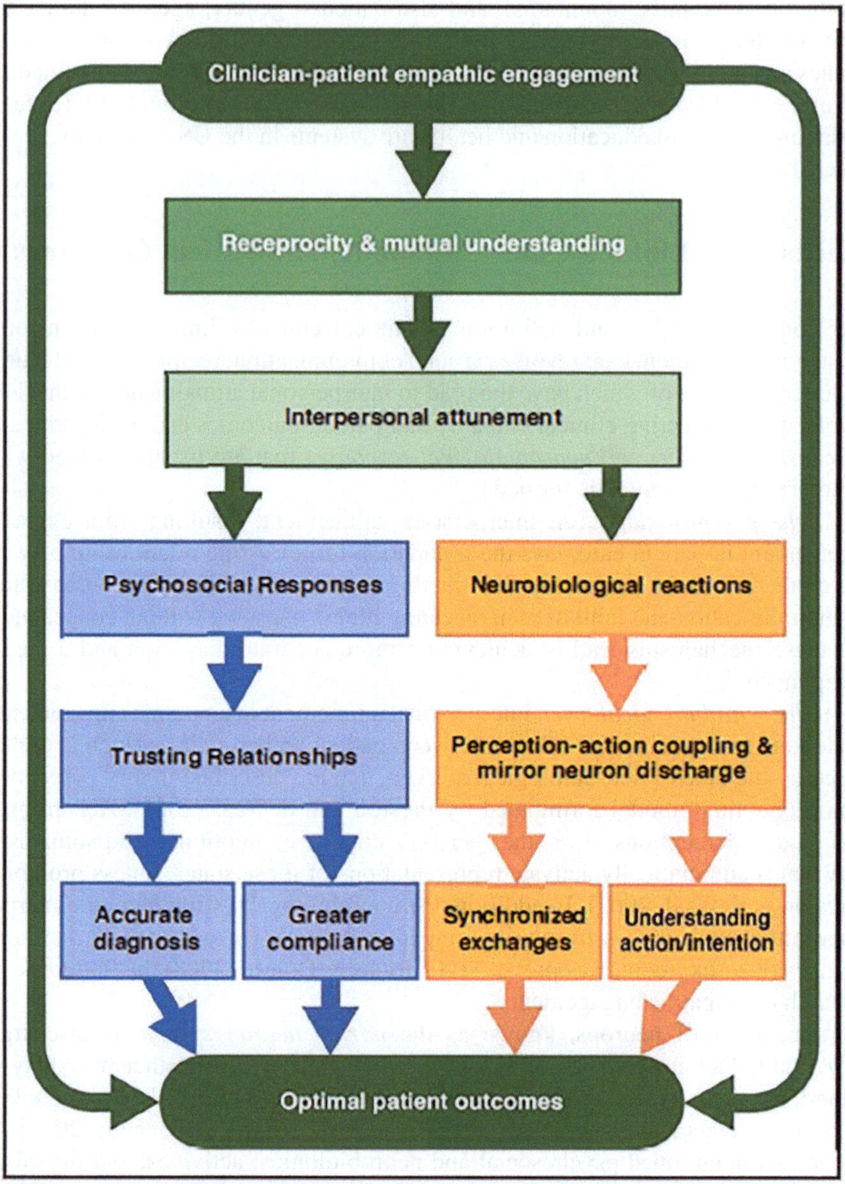

Fig. 11.4 Pathways from clinician-patient empathetic engagement to patient outcomes. Reproduced from Hojat, Maio, Pohl, & Gonnella (2023), ©Authors, Open Access

perception-action model (PAM) formulated by Preston and deWaal (2002). They suggested that perceptions of another person's cognitive, emotional, and somatosensory states automatically activate representations of those states in the observer, unless inhibited. Thus, the PAM can provide physiological explanations for understanding of a patient's pain, suffering, experiences, and concerns, which are among components of empathic engagement in patient care (see Chap. 13). The link between the PAM, the motoneuron system (MNS), and empathy is supported by findings of subconscious mimicry in facial expression, postures, and mannerism; contagious yawning; affect contagion; synchronization in heart rate; mood; and galvanic skin response among interacting individuals, especially among those who are engaged in a goal-directed and meaningful interaction (Hojat, Louis et al., 2013, see also Chap. 13).

In summary, the combined effects of psychosocial and neurobiological mechanisms involved in empathic patient–clinician interactions can help in understanding the mechanisms underlying the beneficial effects of empathic engagement in patient care.

Recapitulation

One can speculate that physicians' positive interpersonal conduct, as an indicator of empathic engagement, is associated with positive patient outcomes, including more accurate diagnoses, greater adherence to treatment regimens, patients' greater satisfaction, and less likelihood of malpractice litigation. Abundant research supports this speculation. Although convincing evidence exists to confirm significant associations between empathic engagement and patient outcomes, empirical research is scarce verifying a direct link between validated measures of clinical empathy in the context of patient care and tangible indicators of patient outcomes. However, two empirical studies of physicians and their diabetic patients in the USA and Italy provided strong evidence in support of positive effects of physician empathy on clinical outcomes in diabetic patients. The question of why a healthcare provider's clinical empathy is associated with patient outcomes was addressed by providing plausible explanations for possible underlying psychosocial and neurobiological underpinnings in empathic engagement in patient care.

Chapter 12
Erosion and Enhancement of Clinical Empathy

The only thing necessary for the triumph of evil is for good men to do nothing.

—(Edmund Burke, cited in Manning, Levine, & Collins, 2007, p. 561).

You couldn't love something you didn't understand.

—(Forrest Carter, 1976, p. 38)

Abstract

- Clinical empathy is viewed as an important element of professionalism in medicine; however, some obstacles to the development and implementation of empathy exist in medical education and practice.
- Health professions education and the healthcare system have become overly reliant on computer-based diagnostic and therapeutic technology that may limit students' and practitioners' vision about the importance of human connection and empathic engagement in patient care.
- It is timely and important to pay serious attention to enhancing and sustaining empathy in health professions education and patient care given the findings that medical students tend to develop a certain cynicism as they progress through their medical education, and clinical empathy tends to erode in medical school and postgraduate medical education.
- Enhancing and sustaining clinical empathy in health profession education and practice of patient care should be considered a mandate that must be acted upon by leaders and educators in health professions academic centers and healthcare institutions.
- Research shows that clinical empathy is an attribute that is amenable to change as a result of targeted educational programs and educational experiences.

M. Hojat, *Clinical Empathy*, https://doi.org/10.1007/978-3-031-87413-0_12

- Some approaches used to enhance clinical empathy in the health professionals-in-training and in-practice are described, including improving interpersonal skills, audio- or video-taping of patient encounters, exposing students to role models, role playing (e.g., aging game), shadowing a patient (patient navigator), hospitalization experiences, improving narrative skills, reflective writing, the Balint method, and studying literature, the arts, and theatrical performances.
- More empirical research is needed to confirm the effectiveness of programs designed to enhance clinical empathy, examine their long-term effects, and develop strategies to sustain enhancement in clinical empathy over time.

Introduction

This chapter begins with a discussion of professionalism in medicine and describes some factors that hamper the development of empathy among students and practitioners in the health professions. It also presents results of findings of empirical research that suggest that empathy tends to erode during medical and some other health professions education. Then, I describe some of the approaches that researchers in health professions education have used to enhance empathy, including 10 specific approaches used more frequently in undergraduate and graduate medical education to improve and sustain empathy among physicians-in-training.

Professionalism in Medicine

Professionalism in medicine is defined as an array of personal qualities beyond the requisite medical knowledge and procedural skills that healthcare professionals must possess to deliver high-quality healthcare to their patients that leads to positive clinical outcomes (Veloski & Hojat, 2006). Medical and health professions educators are encouraged to make every effort to foster professionalism in medicine by offering programs at the undergraduate, graduate, and continuing education levels.

Although no consensus exists regarding the number and nature of personal qualities required for professionalism in medicine, compassionate care and empathy have frequently been mentioned as its key components (Arnold, 2002; Barondess, 2003; Linn, DiMatteo, Cope, & Robbins, 1987). In his book *Humanism and the Physician*, Edmund Pellegrino (1979) described the empathic way of helping patients as an important aspect of the physician's humanistic attributes. Senior residents at Laval and Calgary Universities in Canada listed empathy, respect, and competence as the three most important elements of professionalism in medicine (Brownell & Cote, 2001).

Cultivating humanistic values, including empathy, is among the important goals of education in the healthcare professions. The Medical Schools Objectives Project of the Association of American Medical Colleges (2004) included enrichment of empathy among the educational objectives of medical schools, emphasizing that the schools should strive to produce altruistic physicians who provide compassionate care to patients and demonstrate empathy by conveying their understanding of the patient's perspective. In a position paper, the American Board of Internal Medicine (1983) recommended that humanistic attributes, including empathy, should be instilled in and assessed among residents as an essential part of their medical training. National Board of Osteopathic Medical Examiners (NBOME, 2011) lists exhibition of compassionate treatment, altruism, and empathy among the required competencies in the practice of medicine.

Despite the consensus regarding the healing potential of empathic encounters in patient care, insufficient attention has been given to enhancement of the capacity for empathy in the design of medical education curriculum. Novack (1987) identified this, lamenting that the concept of empathy in patient care seemed to be fading away in modern medical education, but did not seem to be seriously concerned about physicians' losing their healing touch, treating it instead "as if it were a relic of an unscientific past" (Novack, 1987, p. 346).

The lack of attention to clinical empathy in patient care may be partially the result of overreliance on computer-based diagnostic and therapeutic technology and partially the result of changes in the healthcare system with its ripple effect on medical education and the practice of medicine. In the biotechnologically advanced atmosphere of patient care, computer output seems to receive more attention from some practitioners who trust the machines more than their own skills in detecting clinical signs of disease or their patients' narrative accounts of illness.

Although the pathophysiology of disease may be detected by examining computer output and electronic images, an accurate diagnosis of illness is possible by listening to the patient and conducting physical examinations in clinical encounters (Spiro, 1986). The public continued to plead desperately for physicians who were more communicative and empathic in their encounters with patients (Fishbein, 1999). Girgis and Sanson-Fisher (1995) reported that although most physicians were well-equipped to provide high-quality technical services, they were often ill equipped to provide empathic care. Despite the current emphasis on the development of professionalism, enhancement of empathy in the education of healthcare professionals has not yet received systematic and sufficient attention.

Obstacles to Empathy in Patient Care

Some of the factors that impede the development and implementation of empathy in in-training and in-practice health professionals are described in the following sections.

Cynicism

Most medical students embark on a journey to become physicians with idealism and enthusiasm for curing disease and preventing infirmity. Despite the intention of medical school faculty to nurture these qualities, it is ironic that some observed a decline in humanitarianism, enthusiasm, and idealism among students during medical training (Kay, 1990; Maheux & Beland, 1989; Sheehan, Sheehan, White, Leibowitz, & Baldwin, 1990; Silver & Glicken, 1990; Wolf, Balson, Faucett, & Randall, 1989; Zeldow & Daugherty, 1987). This observation has been supported by empirical research showing that students' empathy tends to erode in medical school (Hojat et al., 2004, 2009) and in postgraduate medical education (Bellini, Baime, & Shea, 2002; Bellini & Shea, 2005). More recent research, using the JSE, provided additional evidence in support of the aforementioned findings (see Appendix A). In a national study of osteopathic medical students in the USA (Hojat, Shannon, DeSantis, Speicher et al., 2020), we found a significant decline in the JSE scores in the clinical phase of medical school education, but less pronounced in magnitude than that observed in the US allopathic medical students (Chap. 14).

The effects of medical education on personal qualities have been addressed empirically in a long time ago with some disturbing results (Becker & Geer, 1958; Eron, 1958). One longitudinal study conducted in the 1950s (Eron, 1958) found that medical students became more cynical and less humanitarian as they progressed through medical school, whereas this pattern was not observed among law students! In that study, a typical question used to measure cynicism was, "If you don't look out for yourself, nobody else will," and a typical question for measuring humanism was "When I hear about the suffering of a particular individual or group, I want very much to help."

A similar concern about medical students' progression toward cynicism during medical school was raised in the early 1980s (Silver, 1982). Another study found that as many as three-fourths of medical students became more cynical about academic life and the medical profession as they progressed through medical school (Sheehan et al., 1990). This metamorphosis in the character of medical students was likened to the "battered child syndrome" and was attributed to inappropriate treatment of students by the medical schools (Rosenberg & Silver, 1984; Silver & Glicken, 1990). The terms "dehumanization" (Edwards & Zimet, 1976) and "traumatic deidealization" (Kay, 1990) were also used to describe the cynical transformation that occurred during medical education.

Several additional studies conducted in the 1980s reported other disturbing findings. A study at the University of Texas Health Science Center in San Antonio found that medical students underwent a significant hedonistic change in personality between the freshman and junior years of medical school; they became less inhibited and more self-indulgent (Burnstein et al., 1980). In a longitudinal study conducted at the same medical center, a decline in students' scores on the "need to understand" scale of a personality inventory also raised concern about the negative influence of medical education on students' personal qualities (Whittemore, Burstein, Loucks, & Schoenfeld, 1985). Students in the senior year at the Louisiana

State University School of Medicine reported that the top two changes in attitude during medical school were more cynicism (76%) and more concern about making money (60%) (Wolf et al., 1989).

The alarm bells became even louder in 2002 when a nationwide study found that 61% of residents in American residency training programs believed that they had become more cynical during their medical education (Collier, MaCue, Markus, & Smith, 2002). Cynicism was more prominent among female residents than it was among male residents (63% versus 56%, respectively). In an earlier study, however, residents with children reported less cynicism and more humanistic feelings during their medical education (Sanson-Fisher & Maguire, 1980).

In an atmosphere of declining humanism, the emphasis by some modern medical educators placed on "detached concern" and "affective distance" for the purpose of increasing objectivity in clinical decision making has accelerated the dramatic metamorphosis occurring in medical education and patient care (Coulehan & Williams, 2001; Evans, Stanley, & Burrows, 1993; Farber, Novack, & O'Brien, 1997). Although well intended, the advice of those educators, who encourage "detached concern," in taking care of patients can be misinterpreted, thus adding to the factors contributing to the ultimate depletion of empathy's importance in medical education and practice (Ludmerer, 1999; Starr, 1982). Among other factors found to fuel increased cynicism in medical education are lack of role models (Diseker & Michielutte, 1981; Kramer, Ber, & Moore, 1987) and lack of dedicated educational programs for nourishment of humanistic qualities in patient encounters, which still receive insufficient emphasis in formal medical education curriculum.

Paradigmatic Shift in the Healthcare System

In addition to factors related to physicians and patients, the environment of healthcare delivery exerts a significant influence on physicians' interpersonal behavior and patient outcomes (Gonnella et al., 1993a, 1993b). Developments over time in the organization, financing, and delivery of healthcare, notably in the expansion of managed care, cost containment, and the restriction of physicians' autonomy, have posed challenges that contribute to physicians' discontent with the practice of medicine and a lack of opportunity for empathic engagement in clinical encounters (Burdi & Baker, 1999; Magee & Hojat, 2001).

Anecdotal reports suggest that financial incentives and insurance regulations in the current environment of healthcare have forced a number of physicians to trade off their patients' interest against their will. The golden principle that the patient's best interest must be the primary consideration in patient care has lost its priority in such a market-driven healthcare environment. A survey of physicians found the significant decline in the time physicians spent with patients, their inability to control the length of patients' hospital stays, and their own work schedules exacerbated their dissatisfaction with the existing atmosphere of the healthcare environment (Burdi & Baker, 1999). When Burdi and Baker (1999) compared a sample of physicians surveyed in 1991 with another cohort-matched sample of physicians surveyed in 1996, they found that the number of physicians who said that they would have chosen medicine if they had been college students declined by 10% during the 5-year period. This decline reflected the evolving changes in the healthcare system leading to physician dissatisfaction.

In a survey of 2608 physicians conducted in 2004, 58% of them said that their enthusiasm for medicine had declined in the past few years, and 87% said that their morale had declined because of changes in the healthcare system (Zuger, 2004). The discontent of physicians is an inevitable outcome of the restrictions on their autonomy and use of resources imposed by hospital administrators, the healthcare system, and the health insurance industry (Hojat, Gonnella, Erdmann, Veloski et al., 2000; Kassirer, 1998; Magee & Hojat, 2001). Physicians' discontent with the practice of medicine, especially among those who have been "wounded" by malpractice allegations, matters because it influences the interpersonal quality of care and empathic engagement in clinical encounters. An analysis of how physicians were depicted in the movies showed that their portrayal as positive figures had declined, noting they were often depicted as greedy, egoistic, uncaring, and unethical (Flores, 2002).

The "time" factor is another impediment caused by the growing emphasis on cost containment that has contributed to shortening the duration spent in clinical encounters, thus hindering the formation of empathic relationships. The medical profession, once the most respected of all professions (Thomas, 1985), is now under siege, and physicians are frequently blamed, often mistakenly, for the problems created by nonphysician managers of health insurance organizations. These structural and functional shifts in the healthcare delivery system can hamper the potential benefits of forming empathic clinician–patient relationships. The ripple effect of changes in the American healthcare system has also been shown to have a profound effect on medical students (Hojat, Veloskiet al., 1999) and nurses (Steinbrook, 2002).

Research has shown that physicians' discontent leads to patients' noncompliance with treatment (DiMatteo et al., 1993) and dissatisfaction with their healthcare providers (Hass et al., 2000; Linn, Yager, Cope, & Leake, 1985). Such discontent among physicians can be reflected in pessimism manifested in their communication with patients. Furthermore, research has suggested that pessimism is significantly associated with mortality among physicians as well as their patients (Hollowell & De Ville, 2003).

The paradigmatic shift described earlier has transformed the healthcare delivery system into a profit-driven enterprise with less emphasis on clinician–patient interactions and more emphasis on financial efficiency (Merlyn, 1998). Diminished prestige, loss of autonomy, and deep personal dissatisfaction are among the outcomes of such paradigmatic shifts. Research has shown a widespread "professional malaise" among physicians caught between the desire to provide high-quality care to their patients, on the one hand, and the need to satisfy the insurers and regulators, on the other hand (Zuger, 2004).

According to psychoanalytic theories, this type of approach-avoidance psychic conflict (e.g., a desire to help patients and avoid conflicts with insurers at the same time) can lead to frustration and neurotic-type distress that threatens physicians' physical, mental, and social well-being. Poor clinical management and substandard medical care resulting from a system that restricts physicians' autonomy in dealing with patients inevitably lead to hostile reactions by the public, often directed toward physicians, who themselves are victims of the system's crippling effects.

Added to this paradigmatic shift in the healthcare delivery system is the dramatic rise in the number of malpractice suits. The inevitable result has been greater discontent with medicine among practitioners and even greater dissatisfaction with healthcare services among patients (Mello et al., 2004). In an atmosphere in which the physician–patient relationship resembles an encounter between consumer and retailer, little room obviously is left for compassion and empathy.

The primary concern among powerful players in the healthcare system—notably, nonphysicians employed by government agencies, hospital administrators, and the health insurance industry—is cost containment. The new arrangements created by this shift of emphasis have intruded in the clinical autonomy of physicians, led to the inability of physicians to preserve their altruistic image, and eroded the public's trust and support (Schlesinger, 2002). In a hostile atmosphere where physician–patient encounters are based on fear of allegations of malpractice, rather than on trust, the physician–patient relationship is likely to be shaken at best and violated or broken at worst (Thom, Hall, & Pawlson, 2004). As a result of all the changes occurring in the healthcare system, the adverse effects on the physician–patient relationship threaten the outcomes of care (Simpson et al., 1991). Needless to say, an empathic relationship is highly unlikely to form in an atmosphere in which physicians view each patient as a potential adversary for malpractice litigation (Mello et al., 2004), while patients view their physicians as uncaring and greedy individuals who cannot be trusted.

In 2002, the American Board of Internal Medicine, the American College of Physicians, the American Society for Internal Medicine, and the European Federation of Internal Medicine jointly published a report titled *Medical Professionalism in the New Millennium: A Physician Charter* (Sox, 2002). The report not only confirmed the existence of the problems described here but also underscored their severity by concluding that the "changes in the healthcare delivery systems in countries throughout the industrial world threaten the values of professionalism" (p. 234). These trends in medicine, with their ripple effect on medical education, have resulted in brief consultations, the goal of which is to identify one physical problem as the "chief complaint" (Shorter, 1986), thus shifting the attention from the patient as a "whole person" to a disease as a "case." One hopes that the recent attention to professionalism in medical education and practice will bring empathic engagement between physician and patient to the forefront of healthcare once again.

Overreliance on Biotechnology, Computerized Diagnostics, and Therapeutic Procedures

The new millennium offers either the best or the worst clinical care, depending on whether one views the "glass" as half-full or half-empty. The glass is half-full, given the fact the biotechnological developments can certainly help to prevent many diseases worldwide at a rapid pace, to make more accurate diagnoses much earlier than before, and to treat patients more aggressively. The unprecedented rapid development of vaccine and treatment for COVID-19 pandemic is a recent example of biotechnological contribution to health care. The glass is half-empty because computerized medicine, telemedicine health care, and artificial intelligence technology are gradually replacing "the laying on of hands," trivializing the importance of face-to-face encounters between clinician and patient, and reducing opportunities to form empathic engagement as a result. Even telephone calls to family physicians (who made home visits in the good old days) nowadays are often answered by automatic messages instructing desperate patients to call back during office hours or go to the nearest hospital emergency room for help. Obviously, these trends are not conducive to empathic engagement in patient care.

During visits to a physician's office, patients are often required to undergo a series of laboratory tests, unnecessarily in some cases (Divinagarcia, Harkin, Bonk, & Schluger, 1998; Sandler, 1980), and wait until the physician receives the results and makes a diagnosis, overlooking the clinical signs and symptoms that have been used successfully by physicians for hundreds of years. In this era of overreliance on computerized diagnostic and therapeutic technology, many physicians tend to view the results of laboratory tests and computerized diagnostic procedures as the holy script—despite the well-known errors associated with the sensitivity and specificity of tests—rather than paying more attention to the patients' clinical signs and illness narrative. Thus, patients are treated as objects for technical services (Coulehan & Williams, 2001) rather than as subjects for human care. This style of dealing with patients defies Peabody's stated purpose of patient care: "The treatment of a disease may be entirely impersonal; the care of a patient must be completely personal" (Peabody, 1984, p. 814). In a survey of patients who either changed their physicians or were thinking of changing their physicians, the following comment made by a patient continues to deserve serious attention in medical education: "Students should be taught to use technology as a backup and not as the primary factor of the examination of the patient" (Cousins, 1985, p. 1423).

The shift from the patient's trust in the physician's healing touch to the physician's trust in computerized diagnostic and therapeutic procedures has led to strain in the physician–patient relationship and the public's perception that physicians have become too "detached" to be concerned about their patients (Mangione et al., 2002). As a result, the medical profession has received the criticism that physicians are losing their human touch (Johnston, 1992). Indeed, a number of studies have supported this view by confirming that medical students, residents, and practicing physicians have become more cynical and less compassionate during medical training and practice (Feudtner, Christakis, & Christakis, 1994; Hojat et al., 2004; Kay, 1990; Lu, 1995; Maheux & Beland, 1989; Self, Schrader, Baldwin, & Wolinsky, 1993; Sheehan et al., 1990; Silver & Glicken, 1990; Wolf et al., 1989; Zeldow & Daugherty, 1987). This trend seems to be still ongoing, given the findings of erosion in clinical empathy reported in this chapter and in Appendix A. The uncharted terrain in the healthcare environment, such as telemedicine, virtual patient care, and artificial intelligence technology in health professions education and patient care, call for urgently needed research to explore their effects and challenges and provide convincing empirical evidence and plausible explanations for the development, or demise, of empathic engagement in patient care (see Chap. 15).

The abovementioned issues are only some of the challenges facing medical and health professions education and practice today. However, despite all the bad news, the good news is that it is possible to enhance empathy through dedicated educational programs and through demonstrations of its beneficial effects on patient outcomes.

The Amenability of Clinical Empathy to Change

A number of studies have shown that during the course of medical and health professions education, a students' capacity for empathy can undergo positive, negative, or no change. Although the inconsistent research findings are troublesome and may reflect issues involving conceptualization, measurement, and methodology, the fact that most of the recent studies have noted a change in empathy indicates that this attribute is amenable to change, either positive as a result of implementing targeted interventions (Hojat, Axelrod, Spandorfer, & Mangione, 2013; Van Winkle, Bjork et al., 2012; Van Winkle, Fjortoft, & Hojat, 2012) or negative as a result of negative educational experiences, encounters with dissatisfied patients, and a lack of positive role models (Hojat et al., 2009).

The State-Versus-Trait Debate

The idea of enhancing empathy during education for the health professions depends heavily on the belief that the capacity for empathy is amenable to change. Thus, it is important to address this issue at the outset, otherwise, discussion of educational programs designed to enhance empathy would be pointless if empathy proved to be a stable personality trait that cannot be easily changed.

Psychologists have long been concerned about the possibility of changing people's motivations, attitudes, values, personality, and behavior. It is generally believed that some human attributes are more resistant to change than others. In the behavioral and social sciences, personal qualities, such as excitability, that are highly stable and difficult to change, are often called *traits*, whereas relatively unstable personality attributes that are easy to change, such as moods, are called *states* (Cole, Martin, & Steiger, 2005). The findings of longitudinal research concerning the stability of the so-called traits are inconsistent. For example, some findings suggest that traits can change over time (Roberts & DelVecchio, 2000), and other findings indicate that traits continue to show stability over a period of 15 years (Caspi & Silva, 1995).

The notion that empathy has an evolutionary root (Chap. 3) suggests that under ordinary circumstances, normal individuals are naturally programmed to demonstrate empathy. The extent to which the potential for empathy can be actualized or enhanced in a particular person depends on the interaction of several factors, including the person's constitutional makeup, early life experiences, motivation, and a facilitating environment as well as exposure to specific educational programs. Therefore, empathy, in my view, is neither a highly stable personality trait nor a state that can be changed without effort. In a sense, empathy resembles the notion of attachment, in that it is rooted in evolutionary, genetic, developmental, experiential, situational, and educational ground, and its deficit can be improved by therapeutic or interventional approaches.

Changes in Clinical Empathy During Health Professions Education

Positive Change

Some studies that offered a targeted educational program reported an improvement in empathy. For example, residents who participated in a comprehensive interpersonal skills training course demonstrated greater use of empathy when dealing with patients (e.g., they asked more open-ended questions and provided emotion-related responses) (Kause, Robbins, Heidrich, Abrassi, & Anderson, 1980).

A study of Israeli medical students found that a clerkship in psychiatry improved their scores on Mehrabian and Epstein's Emotional Empathy Scale (Chap. 5) and that the students retained the effect of the program for at least 6 months (Elizur & Rosenheim, 1982). In another study, the investigators noticed that medical students and physicians who participated in an interpersonal skills workshop demonstrated improved empathic engagement, as determined by their increasing use of supportive behaviors, such as listening, responding empathically, and calming patients (Kramer, Ber, & Moore, 1989).

At the University of Missouri School of Medicine in Kansas City, empathy training offered to students in the early years of medical school resulted in increased scores on Carkhuff's Empathic Understanding in Interpersonal Processes Scale (Feighny, Arnold, Monaco, Munro, & Earl, 1998). However, the students' scores on Davis's Interpersonal Reactivity Index (IRI, see Chap. 5) did not increase, probably because of its lower sensitivity in the clinical context. Over the years, training in communication skills provided in various formats (lectures, workshops, and audio- or videotapes) has proven to be useful in improving empathy-related skills (Evans et al., 1993; Fine & Therrien, 1977; Kramer et al., 1989; Sanson-Fisher & Poole, 1978; Winefield & Chur-Hansen, 2000).

Stepien and Baernstien (2006) reviewed articles on empathy education programs in medical schools and found that many of the articles reported an improvement of empathy. However, these authors suggested that research on enhancement of empathy in medical education poses challenges because of the lack of consensus about the conceptualization and definition of empathy; the lack of adequate research designs and control groups; and variation among the instruments used to measure empathy. These limitations may not apply to more recent studies that used a validated measure of empathy (JSE), which relies on an operational definition of empathy in the context of patient care, as described in Chaps. 1 and 6 (e.g., Brazeau, Schroeder, Rovi, & Boyd, 2011; Chen, LaLopa, & Dang, 2008; Hojat, Axelrod et al., 2013; Van Winkle, Fjortoft et al., 2012). More recent studies, using the JSE, have often reported improvements in clinical empathy as a result of health professions students participation in special programs developed for enhancing empathic understanding of patients pain, suffering and concerns (see Appendix A).

Negative Change

Another group of studies showed a decline in empathy among medical students and residents during the course of their medical education in the absence of a targeted educational program. For example, after a period of clinical experience, medical students at the Bowman Gray School of Medicine in North Carolina showed a slight decrease in scores on Hogan's Empathy Scale (Diseker & Michielutte, 1981). Another study reported that a sample of medical students developed a hedonistic personality pattern during medical school that contributed to the decline in empathy (Whittemore et al., 1985).

In a study of changes in empathy, humanism, and professionalism during medical education at a major academic center, Marcus (1999) analyzed approximately 400 dreams reported by healthy medical students and house staff and traced the development of empathy and humanistic attitudes in different years of medical education. Marcus reported that some of the factors that became noticeable among students in the third year of medical school, as inferred from dream analyses, were identification with cold and uncaring role models; increasing reliance on the technological aspects of treatment, rather than on the humanistic side of patient care; and development of a sense of elitism or of belonging to a privileged group.

At the University of Pennsylvania Hospital, Bellini et al. (2002) administered the IRI (see Chap. 5) to first-year residents in internal medicine and reported a decline in the residents' scores on the Perspective Taking and Empathic Concern subscales of the IRI. Conversely, the residents' scores increased on the IRI Personal Distress subscale—a result that was not conducive to empathic patient care. A follow-up study 3 years later showed that the decline in scores on the Empathic Concern scale remained throughout the 3 years of the residency program (Bellini & Shea, 2005).

Similar patterns of decline in empathy were found in most of the other studies in which the JSE was used. For example, in our longitudinal study of 456 medical students at Jefferson, we found an erosion in empathy in the third year of medical school (Hojat et al., 2009). In an earlier longitudinal study of 125 third-year medical students, we also noticed a statistically significant decline in JSE scores from the beginning to the end of the third academic year (Hojat et al., 2004). In a study of residents in internal medicine in three different years of residency at Thomas Jefferson University Hospital, we noticed a progressive decline in JSE scores as the residents progressed from one level of training to the next (Mangione et al., 2002). Although systematic, the observed decline did not reach the conventional level of statistical significance ($p < 0.05$) in this study. Sherman and Cramer (2005) also observed a significant decline in dentistry students' scores on the JSE as the students progressed through dental school.

A number of other researchers have also noticed a statistically significant decline in the JSE scores as medical and other health profession students' progressed through their education in different cultures (see Appendix A). The unfortunate transformation of health professions students to less empathic beings as they progress through health professions education resembles the notion of the "Lucifer effect" described by Zimbardo (2007) about why good people turn bad as a result of environmental conditions, as he observed in his well-known Stanford Prison Experiment (see Chap. 8). (Lucifer was a mythological angel who fell from grace to become Satan.)

One review article claimed that findings on erosion of empathy among medical and other health profession students have been exaggerated (Colliver, Conlee, Verhulst, & Dorsey, 2010a, 2010b). However, such criticism has not been left unchallenged (Newton, 2010; Hojat, Gonnella, & Veloski, 2010; Sherman & Cramer, 2010). Empirical research findings from a number of studies that have confirmed a decline in empathy during health professions education are deeply troubling and should not be viewed as a trivial matter. To restore respect to the medical profession, the most humanistic profession in existence, the factors that contribute to the decline of empathy and other humanistic values must be investigated seriously. A medical education system that produces physicians who are unable to apply the science of medicine in conjunction with the art of healing represents, in my view, "unfinished business." The physician who has learned the science of medicine but has no sense of the art of healing, is, in the words of Saadi (the twelfth-century Persian poet), like one "who ploughs, but sows no seed."

No Change

There is yet a third group of studies showing no change in empathy during medical education. For example, a course in behavioral science offered to medical students did not change the students' orientation toward viewing the patient as a person (Markham, 1979).

Zeldow and Daugherty (1987) observed no significant changes in medical students' empathy measured with the Empathic Concern and Perspective Taking subscales of the IRI. A study in which the IRI was administered to nursing students during their third year of nursing education found no change in their empathy during the 9-month training period (Becker & Sands, 1988). There are also a number of studies with different health professions students in various cultures who reported no significant changes in the JSE scores as a result of implementation of their educational programs aimed at improving empathy (see Appendix A).

In general, the majority of findings reported in the previous sections indicate that empathy is amenable to either positive or negative changes during professional education. Even the negative findings can be viewed optimistically, because if empathy can decline in the absence of appropriate educational programs, it has the potential to increase if appropriate educational remedies are implemented. The possibility of teaching empathy (Spiro, 1992) and other human virtues (Shelton, 1999) during medical and other health professions education has already been discussed. However, do we all agree that educators in the health professions must assume responsibility for improving students' personal qualities, including clinical empathy, in addition to imparting knowledge to them and developing their clinical and procedural skills?

Although this question may generate some debate concerning the applications of behavioral modification with students and practitioners in the health professions, my own answer is an affirmative one because of my belief that medicine (and all other health professions for that matter) is a public service endeavor and therefore must produce professionals who are fully equipped to better serve the public (Hojat, Erdmann, & Gonnella, 2014). Consequently, in addition to opportunities to acquire up-to-date knowledge and develop fine clinical and procedural skills, medical and all other health professions educational programs should provide students with opportunities to develop personal qualities that lead to optimal patient outcomes (Knight, 1981; Shelton, 1999). That, I believe, must be considered as a mandate, not a luxury, not only in health professions education, but also in all other educational programs in any public service disciplines.

As the research findings just described attest, assuming that students in the health professions will automatically develop empathic understanding and other humanistic qualities during their professional education obviously is unrealistic (Hornblow, Kidson, & Ironside, 1988). Therefore, because not everyone develops the capacity for empathy by default, enhancement of empathy among health professions students and practitioners requires targeted educational programs, appropriate experiences, and exposure to humanistic role models.

Approaches to the Enhancement of Clinical Empathy

Many approaches have been used to enhance empathy, most of them by social psychologists and some by medical and nursing educators. Among the many approaches to improving empathy are parental training (Gladding, 1978; Therrien, 1979), skill-development workshops (Black & Phillips, 1982; Hatcher et al., 1994; Kremer & Dietzen, 1991; Pecukonis, 1990), perspective-taking exercises (Coke, Batson, & McDavis, 1978), role taking and role playing (Kalisch, 1971; Moser, 1984), communication or interpersonal skill training (Kause et al., 1980; Yedidia et al., 2003), films and videos (Gladstein & Feldstein, 1983; Simmons, Robie, Kendrick, Schumacher, & Roberge, 1992; Werner & Schneider, 1974; Hojat, Axelrod, Spandorfer et al., 2013), role modeling (Dalton, Sunblad, & Hylbert, 1976; Gulanick & Schmeck, 1977; Shapiro, 2002), or a combination of these and other approaches (Beddoe & Murphy, 2004; Benbassat & Baumal, 2004; Erera, 1997; Kipper & Ben-Ely, 1979).

Although didactic teaching methods are effective for improving beginners' empathic communication skills (Gladstein et al., 1987), more advanced techniques, such as role playing, simulation, and audiovisual methods, are useful for advanced training in empathy. The following sections briefly describe some of the approaches used to enhance empathy in the fields of social and counseling psychology and then discuss some of the methods used among students and practitioners in the health-care professions.

Social and Counseling Psychology

In early laboratory experiments, social psychologists used the classical conditioning paradigm to demonstrate that empathic responses could be elicited. For example, two studies indicated that watching others who appeared to be receiving electric shocks followed by a warning signal could cause observers to form empathic reactions to the warning signal (Berger, 1962; DiLollo & Berger, 1965). The observers terminated the electric shocks more quickly when they believed that they were able to help (Weiss, Boyer, Lombardo, & Stich, 1973). These studies suggest that the empathic response can be elicited by classical and operant conditioning.

An empathy enhancement program for parents who wished to improve their parent–child communication, called Parent Effectiveness Training, was implemented using lectures, tape recordings, role playing, and role modeling (Therrien, 1979). The results showed that parents who participated in the program were able to function at a higher level of empathy, as measured by the Accurate Empathy Scale of Truax and Carkhuff's Relationship Questionnaire. The improvement was maintained over a period of 4 months.

In a series of studies on the use of imagination, Stotland and colleagues demonstrated that when an observer was instructed to "stand in another person's shoes" by simply imagining the pain experienced by a person whose hand was caught in a machine generating painful heat, the observer exhibited a more intense empathic response than did other observers who passively watched the distressed person's actions and appearance (Stotland, 1969; Stotland, Mathews, Sherman, Hansson, & Richardson, 1978). This finding suggests that a cognitive process of perspective taking or imagining the other person's experience (i.e., standing in the other person's shoes) can elicit empathic responses reflected in the role taker's behavior, heartbeat, and skin conductance.

Imagination has also been used as a method of inducing an empathic response. Two kinds of imagination have been used. One kind was imagining another person in a specific situation (e.g., a person whose parents have been killed in an automobile accident). This imagines what the other person might feel and experience (third-person experience). The other kind was imagining oneself experiencing another person's concerns, feelings, and experiences as vividly as possible (first-person experience). Empathic behavior determined by physiological responses or self-reports can be generated by such imaginings.

Since prejudice against specific groups can lead to psychological distance, some psychologists have attempted to reduce prejudice and improve prosocial behavior by enhancing empathy. If an important ingredient of empathy is the ability to understand other people's concern, pain, and suffering, such an understanding can reduce prejudice and bridge the gap between people. Efforts to understand others will diminish hatred toward them, and helping behavior presumably would follow when empathic understanding is formed (Batson, 1991; Batson & Coke, 1981; Davis, 1994).

One approach to understanding others is to read about them—their values, culture, concern, pain, and suffering. Most programs designed to increase cultural sensitivity focus on the simple principle that understanding different cultures reduces prejudice and increases the sense of common identity. In one study, when people were asked to read stories about a particular group of sufferers, such as patients with AIDS, homeless people, or prisoners on death row, they developed more positive attitudes toward these groups as their awareness improved (Batson, Polycarpou et al., 1997).

Those who read vignettes about racial discrimination and were instructed to empathize with the victims (by standing in the other person's shoes) improved their attitudes toward the victims (Stephan & Finlay, 1999). When college students participated in a "dialogue group" to discuss diversity, race, and ethnic issues, the researchers observed both short- and long-term improvements in the students' empathic understanding of minority groups (Gruin, Peng, Lopez, & Nagda, 1999; Lopez, Gurin, & Nagda, 1998). Such dialogues concerning people's similarities and differences can create a sense of a common identity that reduces prejudice and increases helping behavior. Research has also demonstrated that people who participate in multicultural educational programs, read relevant materials, watch videos, and engage in conversation with people from other racial, ethnic, and cultural groups increase their insight and their empathic understanding of the views held by those groups (Banks, 1997).

Bridgman (1981) suggested that prosocial behavior could be measured by cognitive developmental processes through role taking. In a study based on this suggestion, children from different groups who took the role of a person from another group in specially designed educational programs worked cooperatively together and improved their empathic understanding of each other. These findings have implications for education in the health professions with regard to not only improving practitioners' understanding of patients and other staff members from diverse sociocultural backgrounds and experiences but also promoting collaboration and teamwork. Our studies have shown that when medical students and nurses work together, the medical students' understanding of the importance of nursing services to patient care increases and their attitudes about collaborative relationships improve significantly (Hojat et al., 1997; Hojat & Herman, 1985).

Several studies (Krebs (1975) and Stotland and colleagues (Stotland, 1969; Stotland et al., 1978) indicated that taking another person's perspective can lead to increased intensity of the motivation to help and, consequently, to an empathic response. Batson and colleagues reported that empathic behavior could be developed in a two-stage model of training (Batson, Coke, & Pych, 1983; Coke et al., 1978). In Stage 1, adopting the perspective of another person, such as a patient, increased empathic concern. The motivation to help was elicited in Stage 2 as a result of adopting another person's perspective.

Crabb, Moracco, and Bender (1983) developed a training program for lay helpers (church volunteers) based on the micro counseling interviewing technique (Ivey, 1971) and the skilled-helper training method (Egan, 1975), and trained a large group of church volunteers. After administering Carkhuff's Empathic Understanding in Interpersonal Processes Scale to the participants, the authors reported that a large-group format for teaching the skills of empathy can be effective (Crabb et al., 1983).

In another study, undergraduates were taught active listening skills (e.g., identifying expressions of emotion and communicating this understanding verbally) either through training tapes (the self-directed method) or through highly intensive programs presented by teachers (Kremer & Dietzen, 1991). Although both approaches improved the students' empathy skills, the investigators concluded that empathy skills could be taught effectively in a large-group format without intensive programs and with direct contact with a teacher as a necessary component.

Another important finding was that an observer's empathic responses could be demonstrated more vividly when the person observed was involved in a distressing, not pleasant, situation (Stotland et al., 1978). In other words, human beings tend to empathize with people who need help to reduce their pain and suffering, rather than empathize (rejoice) with people who want to share their joy and ecstasy. This finding is relevant to clinician–patient encounters, where there is always a patient in pain and in need of help and a clinician in a position to offer help. Such is the condition in which an empathic relationship is waiting to form.

The Health Professions

Since the 1970s, a number of researchers have argued that empathy is far too important to be taught only to health professionals (Ivey, 1971, 1974). Egan (1975) and Therrien (1979) recommended that everyone should receive empathy training to improve human relationships in general and to face crises of life more effectively. Others have suggested that the capacity for empathy can serve as a foundation for building interpersonal relationships that have a buffering effect against stress and can be an essential step in conflict resolution (Kremer & Dietzen, 1991), regardless of professions.

Researchers in the health professions have attempted to enhance empathy by offering educational programs. Most of the programs address the broader goal of improving students' interpersonal skills and understanding which implicitly means enhancement of the capacity for empathy. It is assumed that the capacity for empathy is an essential prerequisite to demonstrate empathic behavior (Book, 1991). The following studies provide examples of training programs designed to enhance empathy among students and practitioners in the health professions.

In a study at the University of Haifa, social work students participated in an empathy training program developed and implemented for service professionals (Erera, 1997). Designed to enhance participants' sensitivity, the program consisted of four activities: (a) recording students' interviews with clients; (b) reviewing the interviews for the purpose of developing hypotheses or speculating about statements clients made during the interviews; (c) developing hypotheses about the students' statements; and (d) verifying the hypotheses or speculations by analyzing possible reasons for the statements students made during exchanges with clients. For example, "What did the client try to convey by using a specific statement?" or "What did the student infer from the client's statement?" A statistically significant improvement in scores on Mehrabian and Epstein's Emotional Empathy Scale (Chap. 5) was observed among the students who participated in the program.

Sensitivity to nonverbal cues is an important skill in establishing an empathic clinician–patient relationship. When a group of mental health professionals was exposed to a 90-min program designed to increase their ability to interpret nonverbal cues, the results demonstrated that such skills could be learned (DiMatteo, 1979; Rosenthal, Hall, DiMatteo, Rogers, & Archer, 1979). The brief presentation included information about the importance of nonverbal communication in clinical settings, demonstrations of how one can understand nonverbal expressions of affect by noting changes in tone of voice, and practice in judging emotions by observing facial expressions, bodily movements, and postures. The participants had no difficulty learning the apparent meaning of certain nonverbal cues.

In a study designed to improve empathy among nursing students, the students underwent didactic training that involved role playing and exposure to a role model (Kalisch, 1971). Although the investigator noticed an increase in the students' self-reported empathy on Barrett-Lennard's Relationship Inventory, no increase occurred in patients' ratings of the nurses' empathy.

LaMonica, Carew, Winder, Haase, and Blanchard (1976) developed an empathy training program for hospital nursing staff based on Carkhuff's human relationship model (1969). During the brief program, nurses learned to interpret patients' nonverbal behaviors and expressions of anger, engaged in empathic role playing, and practiced responding empathically. Despite a significant increase in the nurses' empathy scores, the authors reported that the majority of participants needed more training.

Layton (1979) attempted to enhance nursing students' empathy by conducting an experiment based on Bandura's observational social learning theory (Bandura,

1977). The students observed interviews with simulated patients that consisted of three components: (a) a modeling component demonstrating the interviewers' empathy (positive modeling) or lack of empathy (negative modeling); (b) a labeling component in which segments of the modeling component were played back, followed by a narrative explaining the presence or absence of empathy depicted on the videotapes; and (c) a rehearsing component, during which the videotapes were stopped briefly after each verbal and emotional expression shown by the patient. During each pause, the students were asked to construct their own responses to the patient's expressions. When the experiment ended, Layton found that the junior-year students' scores on Carkhuff's Empathic Understanding in Interpersonal Processes Scale (Chap. 5) had improved, whereas the scores of the senior students had not. Layton speculated that one explanation for the disparate results was that the modeling approach may have been more effective for less advanced students.

As a result of extensive work in nursing education and research in the 1960s and 1970s, Orlando (1961, 1972) developed a model of therapeutic encounters proposing that when nurses interacted with patients, they should validate their perceptions to ensure that they had an accurate understanding of the patients' experiences. More than two decades later, Olson and Hanchett (1997) adopted Orlando's model as a suitable method of studying empathy and patient outcomes and hypothesized that if nurses understood their patients' needs accurately and shared that understanding with patients, who in turn confirmed its accuracy, patient outcomes would improve. Accordingly, Olson and Hanchett initiated a study involving 70 staff nurses and 70 patients to test the hypothesis that nurses' empathy would reduce patients' distress and overlap with the patients' perceptions of the nurses' empathy, as measured by the Empathic Understanding subscale of Barrett-Lennard's Relationship Inventory. At the end of the study, the authors reported a moderate but statistically significant relationship between the nurses' self-reported empathy and the patients' perceptions of the nurse's empathy; i.e., the hypothesis was confirmed.

In another study, Beddoe and Murphy (2004) exposed nursing students to an 8-week "mindfulness-based stress reduction" program to explore the program's effects on stress and empathy. At the end of the 8 weeks, the authors reported favorable changes in the students' scores on the Personal Distress and Fantasy subscales of the IRI.

Ten Approaches to Enhance Clinical Empathy in Health Professions Education and Practice

In this section, I have selected 10 approaches that are more specific to medical (and all other health professions) education and practice (Hojat, 2009). Consistent with our definition of empathy, the common goal of all of these approaches is to improve the understanding of students and practitioners in the health professions with regard to patients' concern, pain, suffering, and experiences.

Improving Interpersonal Skills

Interpersonal skill development is considered an essential prerequisite to demonstrate empathic behavior (Book, 1991). Researchers in the health professions have attempted to enhance empathy by designing educational programs to improve students' interpersonal skills that implicitly imply enhancement of the capacity for empathy (Evans et al., 1993; Kramer et al., 1989; Poole & Sanson-Fisher, 1980). Suchman, Markakis, Beckman, and Frankel (1997) developed an interpersonal model of empathic communication in the medical interview. Emphasis in this method is placed on the development of three basic communication skills: "recognition" of patient's negative emotions, concerns, and inner experiences; "exploration" of these emotions, concerns, and experiences; and "acknowledging" them to generate a feeling in the patient of being understood. These three skills correspond, respectively, to the keywords of "cognition," "understanding," and "communicating" in our definition of empathy in the context of patient care. The goal of this training is to form an empathic engagement in the caregiver–care–receiver relationship through the caregiver recognizing an "empathic opportunity" when the care receiver directly or implicitly expresses emotions or concerns. The caregiver responds empathetically by explicitly expressing understanding of the care receiver's concerns and communicating to the care receiver that those concerns are understood.

In responding to the empathic opportunity, many untrained physicians may disregard the patient's concerns, thus missing or terminating an opportunity rather than taking advantage of it. The training focuses on capturing the empathic opportunities that provide the caregiver with "windows of opportunities" (Branch & Malik, 1993) while avoiding pitfalls in missing or terminating them. A caregiver can form and maintain the empathic communication dynamics by continuing the conversation about the patient's concerns. This can be done by simply nodding the head to reflect understanding and using simple statements such as "I understand your concern; let's work on it together." In addition to verbal cues, sensitivity to nonverbal cues is an important skill in establishing an empathic clinician–patient relationship. Nonverbal communication in clinical settings can be taught by understanding nonverbal expressions of affect. Such nonverbal expressions include changes in tone of voice, eye contact, gaze and aversion of gaze, silence, laughter, teary eyes, facial expressions, hand and body movements, trembling, touch, physical distance, leaning forward or backward, sighs, or other signs of distress or discomfort. These are important nonverbal cues in clinical encounters (Mehrabian, 1972; Wolfgang, 1979). Psychological effects of nonverbal cues—such as folded arms being more likely to indicate defensiveness, coldness, rejection, or inaccessibility, or moderately open arms being more likely to convey acceptance and warmth—can also be taught in interpersonal skill training programs (DiMatteo, 1979).

Also, teaching clinicians to try to mirror patients' postures, gestures, respiration rates, speech tempo and pitch, and language pattern can contribute to forming an empathic engagement (Matthews, Suchman, & Branch, 1993). Winefield and Chur-Hansen (2000) reported that 81% of medical students who participated in two brief sessions on effective communication with patients felt more prepared to engage in empathic interviews. Yedidia et al. (2003) reported that practicing communication skills and engaging medical students in self-reflection on their performances improved students' overall communication competence as well as their skills in building relationships in patient care. A 5-day communication skills workshop offered to medical students and medical residents in Spain significantly increased scores of participants' empathy (measured by the JSE) compared to a non-participant control group (Fernandez-Olano, Montoya-Fernandez, & Salinas-Sanchez, 2008).

In a randomized clinical trial conducted at the Johns Hopkins University School of Hygiene and Public Health, 69 physicians were assigned to one of the three groups: two experimental groups and one control group (Roter et al., 1995). Physicians in the experimental groups received 8 h of training designed to increase their communication skills and reduce their patients' emotional distress. The patients in one experimental group were actual patients and those in the other group were simulated patients. During the training, the physicians asked patients about their concerns and expectations, reassured them, and acknowledged their psychosocial struggles. The results showed that the empathic skills of the physicians who participated in either training course compared to the control group improved significantly without increasing the time spent with individual patients.

Audio- or Video-Taping of Encounters with Patients

A review and analysis of audio- or video-taping of patient encounters with physicians, nurses, and hospital and office administrators to identify positive and negative interviewing factors demonstrates a valuable learning experience for enhancing empathic engagement. Using the interpersonal empathic communication method (Suchman et al., 1997) described above, Pollak et al. (2007) audio-recorded 398 interviews between advanced cancer patients and their oncologists. They found that oncologists responded with empathy to patient concerns only 27% of the time. Physicians either missed or prematurely terminated the conversation about patients' concerns 73% of the time. In a similar study, Morse, Edwardsen, and Gordon (2008) reported that only 10% of physicians responded to empathic opportunities in their communication with lung cancer patients.

Sanson-Fisher and Poole (1978) of the University of Western Australia Medical School exposed 112 medical students to eight audio-taped empathy training sessions and compared them with 23 students without such exposure. After the training, students' scores on the Accurate Empathy scale of Truax and Carkhuff's Relationship Questionnaire increased significantly compared with the scores of a control group of students who did not participate in the program. Audio-taped conversations between patients and physicians can help identify empathic opportunities and physicians' positive responses, as well as demonstrate missed opportunities, or cases in which the concern-related part of the conversation was terminated. This can have valuable educational benefits for enhancing empathy.

By analyzing videotapes of interviews of 87 first-year medical students with simulated patients at Michigan State University School of Medicine, Werner and Schneider (1974) used a variation of a technique called "Interpersonal Process Recall" to enhance medical students' interviewing skills and awareness of patients' affective messages. The students were videotaped as they interacted with simulated patients with various problems. The videotapes were then played back so the students could view interactions with patients and receive critical analyses from instructors and other students about their interactions with the patient. After each tape-recorded interview, the students joined in a group with their faculty instructors to discuss and analyze different sections of the interview. The videotape could be paused, forwarded, and rewound during the analysis. Werner and Schneider (1974) concluded that analysis of the videotape replay made students increasingly aware of their behavior in communicating with patients and improved students' ability to empathize with patients. They also concluded that the videotape had its greatest impact on students who had the least developed communication skills.

Exposure to Role Models

Some investigators have suggested that faculty in undergraduate and graduate medical education can serve as role models or mentors to improve students' capacity for empathy (Campus-Outcalt, Senf, Watkins, & Bastacky, 1995; Ficklin, Browne, Powell, & Carter, 1988; Skeff & Mutha, 1998; Wright, 1996). Shapiro (2002) interviewed primary care physicians to discern how empathy can be enhanced in medical students and residents. Role modeling was endorsed by almost all research participants as the most effective approach to teaching empathy. Quill (1987) reported that the practice behavior of the ambulatory preceptors, viewed as role models, exerted a broad influence on the residents. A study of medical students in South Africa (Mclean, 2004) found that as the students progressed through medical school, they selected more faculty members as role models. However, the role models they selected most often were their own parents, and notably their mothers who were described as caring, sympathetic, and self-sacrificing mentors. These findings are consistent with the notion I describe in Chap. 4 that mothers are key figures in the development of a child's capacity for empathy.

Despite the fact that exposure to role models is important in the enhancement of empathy, the results of a mailed survey of medical students at four different medical schools in Canada (Maheux, Beaudoin, Berkson, Des Marchais, & Jean, 2000) raised a question about students' exposure to appropriate role models, since 25% of the second-year students and 40% of the seniors said that they did not agree that their medical school faculty behaved as humanistic physicians and teachers. In a study of decline in empathy in medical school, students in response to a question about factors that had negatively influenced their views on patient–physician relationships had indicated that inappropriate role models (faculty and attending physicians) was one of the major factors (Hojat et al., 2009).

Role Playing (Aging Game)

In the 1970s, Hoffman and Reif (1978) introduced a role-playing game to simulate problems perceived by elderly people. McVey, Davis, and Cohen (1989) adapted the technique and developed the "aging game" to increase medical students' understanding of elderly people's sensory deficits and functional dependency. The game generally consists of three stages. In the first stage, students are instructed to imagine that they are old (e.g., 70–99 years old) and use earplugs to simulate hearing loss and goggles covered with vaseline to simulate sight problem.

The second stage begins with a simulation that represents independent living in one area, then proceeds to semi-dependent living in another area, and finally to the third area that simulates dependent living where the students are confined to wheelchairs. In each area, they are confronted with facilitators who play the role of administrators, physicians, or nurses. As they progress through different game levels, the behaviors of the facilitators become more disrespectful.

Stage 3 is a group discussion of the participants' experiences during the previous stages of the game. Results of the original aging game experiment with 112 medical students at Duke University Medical School showed that the medical students gained an increased understanding and sensitivity to the physical and psychosocial problems of the elderly (McVey et al., 1989). It is suggested that role playing results in the development of awareness and increased understanding of elderly patients (Hoffman, Brand, Beatty, & Hamill, 1985; Menks, 1983). Because understanding is the key ingredient in the definition of empathy, it is expected that improvement in understanding leads to enhancement of empathy. Such a link has been reported among medical and dental students by Holtzman, Beck, and Coggin (1978) and Holtzman, Beck, and Ettinger (1981), and among nurses (Marte, 1988).

Pacala, Boult, Bland, and O'Brien (1995) presented a three-hour workshop using a modified version of the aging game with 39 medical students in an ambulatory medicine rotation at the University of Minnesota Medical School. They were then compared with 16 nonparticipating students. Students were asked to assume the identity of elderly persons and used earplugs to simulate hearing loss, heavy athletic stockings to simulate pedal edema, and un-popped popcorn in their shoes to simulate the discomfort of arthritis pain. Scores of a two-item empathy scale (developed by the study authors: "I believe I can truly empathize with older patients" and "I believe I understand what it feels like to have problems associated with aging") increased significantly among participants after completing the workshop.

Varkey, Chutka, and Lesnick (2006) used a variation of the aging game (e.g., students wore heavy rubber gloves to simulate decreased manual dexterity and goggles with films over the lenses to simulate cataracts) with all 84 medical students in two first-year classes. They reported a statistically significant increase in empathy. After 10 years of offering the aging game workshop at the University of Minnesota Medical School, Pacala Boult, and Hepburn (2006) concluded that despite the burden of required personnel and resources to run the aging game workshops, students benefited greatly from their role-playing experiences by developing a long-lasting awareness and understanding of key issues in elderly patients and geriatric medicine.

In a study with students at Purdue University School of Pharmacy (Chen et al., 2008), students were assigned to simulate the life of an underserved patient with multiple chronic medical conditions who had an economic burden (e.g., homeless), cultural differences (e.g., Hispanic), or a communication barrier (illiterate or hearing-impaired). Participation in this experiment increased students' empathy scores. An examination of remarks by students showed that they grew to become more sensitive to patients whose conditions they simulated and developed an understanding of the challenges faced by the patients after "walking in a patient's shoes" (Chen et al., 2008). In another study, medical and pharmacy students participated in a workshop that included a theatrical play performed by their classmates who were coached to enact problems and concerns of elderly patients (a variation of the "aging game"). Statistically significant improvement in the JSE scores was observed among students (Van Winkle, Fjortoft et al., 2012). I will describe this study in more detail in the "Theatrical Performances" section of this chapter.

Shadowing a Patient (Patient Navigator)

The patient navigation program was originally developed at the Harlem Cancer Education and Demonstration Project to help medically underserved cancer patients (Freeman, Muth, & Kerner, 1995). It has been reported that a trained patient navigator, who shadows the patients offering help, contributed to increased satisfaction and decreased anxiety among patients (Ferrante, Chen, & Kim, 2007).

Using the patient navigator paradigm, researchers at the University of Arkansas for Medical Sciences conducted a project in which first-year medical students "shadowed" a patient (with the patient's permission) during visits to a surgical oncologist and observed the patient throughout treatment (Henry-Tillman, Deloney, Savidge, Graham, & Klimberg, 2002). Participants reported that they learned to see patients as people, not as numbers or diseases and 70% said that they experienced feelings of empathy while participating in the program.

In another study, 12 first-year emergency medicine residents at Thomas Jefferson University Hospital were randomly divided into experimental and control groups (Forstater, Chauhan, Allen, Hojat, & Lopez, 2011). Each resident in the experimental group shadowed one patient in the emergency department in the first month of residency training. The control group did not participate in shadowing and followed a routine training schedule. The JSE was completed by all residents 2 and 9 months after the shadowing experiment. No substantial difference was observed on the JSE scores between the two groups 2 months after the experiment (effect size = 0.02); however, a larger decline in empathy scores was noticed in the control group compared to the experimental group (effect size = 0.58), suggesting that the erosion of empathy may be prevented to some extent by shadowing experiences.

Hospitalization Experiences

Sharing common experiences can influence empathic understanding of the patient. The tendency of health professionals to empathize with those with whom they share common experiences has been described as the "wounded healer effect" (Jackson, 2001) (see Chap. 8). Clinicians who have experienced pain have a better understanding of their patients' pain (Gustafson, 1986). Therefore, painful hospitalization experiences can increase their understanding of the hospitalized patient.

At the University of California-Los Angeles Medical School, healthy second-year medical students who had completed their training in the basic sciences and had no previous history of hospitalization participated in a program designed to examine whether the experience of being hospitalized would increase empathy for hospitalized patients (Wilkes, Milgrom, & Hoffman, 2002). The students were admitted to the hospital under an assumed name. Investigators reported that the pseudo-hospitalization experience was useful because it enhanced students' understanding of patients' problems. Interestingly, the students acting as "new patients" gave the nursing staff more favorable patient encounter ratings than they gave to physicians (Wilkes et al., 2002). Because of the effect of hospitalization on a physician's understanding of patients, Ingelfinger (1980) suggested that actual hospitalization experiences could be used as a criterion for admission to medical schools!

On their first day in the Emergency Medicine Department at the University of Florida Health Sciences Center, 25 residents participated in a study in which they were instructed to register as patients (the admission staff and nurses were not aware of the experiment) (Seaberg, Godwin, & Perry, 1999, 2000). Although the study was brief and ended when the emergency room physician entered the examination room, the results suggested that the experience enhanced residents' empathy, as indicated by their reports that the experiment improved their attitude toward patients in the emergency room.

The Study of Literature and the Arts

In his book, *A History of Medicine*, Castiglioni (1941) quoted Hippocrates as saying, "Where there is a love for man, there is also a love for the arts." The statement indicates that there is a bridge connecting the human heart and the arts. Numerous authors have proposed that in addition to reading the medical literature, medical students and physicians should read literature unrelated to medicine because it would expose them to a rich source of knowledge and insights about the emotions, pain, suffering, and perspectives of human beings and would improve their capacity for forming empathic connections (Acuna, 2000; Charon et al., 1995; Herman, 2000; Jones, 1987; Kumagai, 2008; McLellan & Husdon Jones, 1996; Montgomery Hunter, Charon, & Coulehan, 1995; Peschel, 1980; Szalita, 1976) (for an annotated bibliography of works in medical and nonmedical literature, see Montgomery Hunter et al., 1995). In support of the impact of physicians' familiarity with literature and the arts on patient outcomes, Mandell and Spiro (1987, p. 458) suggested that "the humanities will not improve the technical care of our patients, but they may help to civilize that care."

Borrowing from Jungian concepts, Knapp (1984) suggested that by studying classical literature, the reader can develop insight into the "collective unconscious" of the human mind and better understand the archetypal images in myths, legends, literature, and the arts. The simulated worlds presented by famous novels, short stories, poems, plays, paintings, sculptures, music, and films enable us to learn how emotions are expressed in human relationships (Oatley, 2004). Thus, the study of literature and the arts can provide students and practitioners in the health professions with values and experiences in areas of concern in clinical practice, such as aging, death, disability, and dying (Montgomery Hunter et al., 1995). The study of literature and the arts can also aid the development of otherwise hard-to-teach clinical competencies, such as accurate observation, interpretation, imagination, ethical issues, and moral reflection (Montgomery Hunter et al., 1995).

In addition, studying literature and reading poetry not only facilitate clinicians' understanding of other people's feelings and expressions of their inner world but also can be used as an ancillary tool through which both clinician and patient can find different meanings in and ways of expressing emotion, pain, and suffering (Lerner, 1978, 2001). Furthermore, literature and the arts provide clinicians with the ability to use metaphor in encounters with patients that can help them to enhance mutual clinician–patient understanding (Blanton, 1960; Lerner, 2001).

Charon et al. (1995) indicated that in addition to increasing one's understanding of human suffering and ability to use metaphor, studying literature and the arts can help health professionals "contextualize" and "particularize" the ethical issues in patient care. Other authors have indicated that health professionals can gain new insights into the moral and ethical issues posed by their profession through the lens of literature, poetry, and the arts (Calman, Downie, Duthie, & Sweeney, 1988; Charon et al., 1995; Coles, 1989; Flagler, 1997; Marshall & O'Keefe, 1994; Radley, 1992), and recognize that the discoveries of others can lead to the development of self (Kumagai, 2008). The quandaries and decision-making processes of characters in literary narratives are useful for teaching ethical guidelines to students and practitioners in the health professions (Coles, 1989). The thoughts, feelings, sensations, and intuitions influenced by immersing oneself in literature can serve as a powerful impetus toward understanding the human mind (Schneiderman, 2002).

Reading literature can result in higher mental processes leading to greater imagination and better interpretive skills that reinforce empathic understanding (Calman et al., 1988; Charon et al., 1995; Clouser, 1990; Downie, 1991; Radley, 1992; Starcevic & Piontek, 1997; Younger, 1990). Literature can enrich students' moral education, increase their tolerance for ambiguity, and give them a rich grounding for empathic understanding of their patients. Lancaster, Hart, and Gardner (2002) offered a 1-month course in which medical students read works, such as Tolstoy's *The Death of Ivan Ilych*, which improved their narrative skills. When the course ended, the students assigned their highest rating to the enhancement of empathy as a result of their participation in the course. Shapiro, Morrison, and Boker (2004) noticed a significant improvement in first-year medical students' empathy and attitudes toward humanities after participating in a short course in reading and discussion of poetry, skits, and short stories.

Although it is assumed that engagement with literature can deepen medical students' understanding of illness experiences, increase their capacity for self-reflection, and enhance their capacity for empathy, resistance among medical students to a course on literary inquiry has been observed (Wear & Aultman, 2005). Denying the relevance to medicine of studying literature, discounting the value of literary inquiry to patient care, and distancing the arts from science are among the reasons for medical students' resistance to studying literature and improving their narrative skills (Wear & Aultman, 2005). Students' motivation can be improved by convincing them of the link between literary inquiry and medicine. Despite the importance of humanities in enhancing empathy, only a third of all the medical schools in the USA had incorporated literature into their curriculum as of the mid-1990s (Charon et al., 1995; Jones, 1997; Montgomery Hunter et al., 1995). Other medical schools should be encouraged to follow their lead. The development of professionalism in medicine, according to Wear and Nixon (2002), requires an imaginative immersion into others' stories that can be attained by studying literature and the arts.

In a multi-institutional study involving five medical schools in the USA, students who reported more involvement with or exposure to humanities and the arts (e.g., visual arts, singing, playing musical instruments, listening to music, dancing, writing for pleasure, attending theater, museums/galleries) obtained significantly higher scores on the JSE (Mangione, Chakraborti, Staltri et al., 2018). In another study with students from 11 Portuguese medical schools (Fornetti & Barbosa, 2024), it was found that medical students who were more involved in artistic activities (e.g., music, photography, dance, painting, poetry, theater, etc.) scored higher than other classmates on the total score and subtest scores (e.g., Empathic Concern, and Fantasy) of the IRI (see Chap. 5).

Improving Narrative Skills and Reflective Writing

It is said that human beings are storytelling animals (Hurwitz, 2000), that the universe is made of stories (Feldman & Kornfield, 1991), and that physicians are immersed in patients' stories (Steiner, 2005). Humans are described by Dawes (1999, p. 29) as "the primates whose cognitive capacity shuts down in the absence of a story." It is suggested that the human brain evolved to process stories better than any other forms of input (Newman, 2003). Narrative, defined by Smith (1981, p. 228) as "someone telling someone else that something happened," is the royal road to a patient's world.

It is physicians' attentive listening to their patients' narratives of illness (narrative skills), rather than "clinical interrogation," (Kleinman, 1995) that opens a window of opportunity to empathic engagement. In clinician–patient encounters, listening to the patient's stories of illness with the third ear while taking the history of the patient's current illness is described as a "narrative communication" that, when skillfully performed, not only has diagnostic value but therapeutic benefit as well (Adler, 1997). The narrative account of the patient's illness is the beginning of the healing process as well as a pathway to a correct diagnosis (Adler & Hammett, 1973). Patients often carefully monitor the clinician's attentiveness to their illness narrative, detect signs of the clinician's empathic receptiveness, and feel better when the clinician appears to be in tune with the narrative themes (Brody, 1997). In his article "Power of Stories over Statistics," Newman (2003) suggests that narrative skills enable physicians to make empathic connections with their patients.

Clinicians are often witnesses to their patients' pain and suffering: they listen to the patients' stories, and they prepare short narratives of the patients' experiences after taking their history and interviewing them. The clinicians' task, according to Kleinman (1988, p. 50), is "to witness a life story, to validate its interpretation, and to affirm its value." Because the feelings and experiences of others are captured in patients' narratives, their narratives can convey how they view their illness (Bruner, 1990). Evidence suggests that participating in programs on reflective writing and improving narrative skills can improve clinicians' empathic understanding (DasGupta & Charon, 2004; Lancaster et al., 2002; Shapiro & Hunt, 2003). The understanding of patients will improve by adopting their perspectives through their stories and by narrative skills allowing healthcare providers to reflect on the nature of patients' concerns and experiences. According to Kumagai (2008), narratives of illness provide an insight into subjective experiences of others, which fosters perspective-taking ability and identification with patients. According to Steiner (2005), clinical stories can be used to inform, share, inspire, educate, and persuade, with implications not only in forming empathic engagement but also in health research (to find a common theme) and in health policy (to formulate compassionate policies).

Clinicians' narrative skills gained by engaging with stories in literature is pivotal when thinking about case histories in ethics (Charon & Montello, 2002). Charon (2001b) has written extensively about narrative medicine and physicians' narrative competence in recognizing and interpreting the predicaments of their patients. She believes that a bridge exists between narrative skills and the capacity for empathy (Charon, 1993) and that the effective practice of medicine requires narrative competence that includes the ability to understand, absorb, interpret, and act based on the stories and plights of patients (Charon, 2000, 2001a).

Narrative competence in medicine can be acquired by reading, writing, studying the arts, and recognizing that all human beings are vulnerable to illness and death (Charon, 1993). According to DasGupta and Charon (2004), the ability to elicit, interpret, and translate patients' narrative accounts of their illness is the key to empathic communication. Reflective writing and narrative competence offer opportunities for empathic and nourishing medical care (Charon, 2001a). In a study involving 11 second-year medical students, 9 reported that reflective writing (e.g., writing about a personal illness or another person's illness) could enhance their understanding of patients and improve their ability to care for patients (DasGupta & Charon, 2004).

Narrative competence is beneficial not only for the clinicians who write the patients' stories of illness to make accurate diagnoses and select appropriate treatments but for the patients as well. For example, patients with mild or moderately severe asthma or rheumatoid arthritis who wrote about their stressful experiences achieved a significantly better clinical outcome (Smyth, Stone, Hurewitz, & Kaell, 1999). Branch, Pels, and Hafler (1998) suggested that small-group discussions about medical students' narrative reports of critical incidents during encounters with patients could enhance the students' understanding of the clinician–patient relationship.

In another study, 40 staff physicians at the Cleveland Clinic were assigned into one experimental and two control groups (Misra-Hebert et al., 2012). Those in the experimental group participated in a six-session program on narrative medicine and engaged in guided reflective writing. Physicians in one control group received the assigned course reading materials (which were given to the experimental group) but did not participate in the course sessions (control group 1), and those in the second control group neither received the reading materials nor participated in the course sessions. Quantitative analysis showed improvements in the experimental group compared to the two control groups (using the JSE). Qualitative analysis of physicians' reflective writings in the intervention group showed compassionate solidarity and empathic concern and more exploration of negative rather than positive emotions.

Theatrical Performances

Dramatic performances—by real or simulated patients, professional actors portraying patients, or health professions students playing a role—have been used to enhance empathy. For example, Shapiro and Hunt (2003) presented medical students at the University of California-Irvine College experiences with AIDS through narrative and song. Another patient, a survivor of ovarian cancer, described her experiences on hearing the diagnosis, undergoing treatment, and coping with the psychological effects of the ordeal and the spiritual journey on which she embarked while dealing with the illness. After the theatrical presentations, the students reported that watching the theatrical performances increased their empathic understanding of patients with AIDS or ovarian cancer.

In another study with 370 medical and pharmacy students at Chicago College of Osteopathic Medicine and at Chicago College of Pharmacy of Midwestern University (Van Winkle, Fjortoft et al., 2012), students participated in a workshop which included a 10-minute theatrical play performed by their classmates who were coached to enact problems and concerns of elderly patients (a variation of the "aging game"). Subsequent to watching the play, students discussed in small groups their perceptions and feelings about issues of elderly people depicted in the play. Statistically significant increases in the JSE pretest–posttest mean scores were found in both groups of medical and pharmacy students. However, follow-up assessments showed that the improvement in empathy scores did not sustain for a longer time after the workshop.

The performing arts have also been used to increase medical students' understanding of patients' grief (Stokes, 1980) and of death and dying (Holleman, 2000). Dramatic and tragic theatrical performances can generate insights into the observer that arise from climactic intellectual, emotional, or spiritual enlightenment (Golden, 1992). Empathy can arise from the cathartic effects of other peoples' tragedies. In his theory of catharsis, Aristotle explained that observing the hero's tragic experiences can generate a calming effect (a catharsis) that serves to separate the observer from the hero's suffering while understanding the hero's pain. A healthy society needs the performing arts, and students and practitioners in the healthcare professions need them for the same reason—because they learn about the experiences of others and can experience catharsis by being drawn into their patients' tragic stories while remaining separate from patients (Trautmann Banks, 2002). In other words, empathy can arise from the cathartic effects of these stories.

Another explanation for the beneficial effects of the performing arts on empathy is the involvement of the human mirror neuron system. As I described in Chap. 13, when a person observes another person performing an act, the mirror neuron system is activated in the observer's brain and contributes to empathic understanding of the observed person. It is also well known, particularly from studies involving hypnosis and imagery, that imagination can produce real physiological effects (Wester & Smith, 1984). These neurological and physiological activities may explain how watching theatrical or cinematic performances can induce neurophysiological effects leading to a greater empathic understanding.

There is a notion of teaching health professions students performing arts to cultivate empathic skills. It is assumed that developing skills to act and think like another human being (e.g., doctors, patients) can improve understanding of those whose acts and thoughts are simulated. The idea seems to be similar to Gestalt-Therapy technique introduced by Frederick Perls (1969/1992). The basic principle in this therapeutic technique is to teach therapists and clients phenomenological awareness (being in the here and now) by placing oneself in another person's shoes, but simultaneously retaining one's own sense of identity. Acting nonjudgmentally as if one is another person, without losing the "as if" condition (Rogers, 1959, 1975), is the guiding acting role to experience another person's feelings and concerns. Based on premises from theater and performing arts education, a technique, called "Facilitated Simulation Education and Evaluation," has been introduced to improve interpersonal communication skills and enhance empathic understanding in physicians-in-training (Eisenberg, Rosenthal, & Schlussel, 2015).

Balint Method

The Balint training program was developed by Michael Balint at the Tavistock Institute in London for general practitioners. Balint designed a program to counteract a problem that Houston (1938) had described nearly two decades earlier. The training is based on the notion that medical trainees often spend their entire training in the laboratory and the hospital ward where they do not have sufficient opportunity to develop skills in interpersonal aspects of patient care. To compensate for deficits in interpersonal communication and awareness of psychosocial aspects of illness, Balint suggested that they meet in small groups of 10 to discuss cases they felt were difficult, particularly in relation to the physician–patient relationship (Balint, 1957). The program provides opportunities to enhance understanding of patients' experiences and concerns.

Activities in the original Balint method included 1–2 h of unstructured, open, and supportive small-group meetings every 1–3 weeks, for 1–3 years. The primary focus in these meetings was on behavioral, cognitive, and emotional issues related to communication between patients, physicians, and other personnel. The discussions (often coordinated by a psychoanalyst or psychologist) focused on the patient as a person rather than his or her disease as a case and on difficulties experienced in patient–resident encounters. In addition to patient–physician communication, participants were also encouraged to discuss issues related to interprofessional collaboration and hospital administration.

The Balint method, and particularly shorter variations of it, has received attention in some residency programs in the USA, particularly in family medicine (Brock & Salinsky, 1993; Cataldo, Peeden, Geesey, & Dickerson, 2005). In a study of family medicine residents in the USA, no significant difference on the scores of the JSE was observed between those who participated in a Balint training program and those who did not (Cataldo et al., 2005).

Other Approaches to Enhance Clinical Empathy in Health Professions Students and Practitioners

There are other innovative approaches used to sustain and enhance empathy among health professions students and practitioners. For example, in an experimental study of 248 second-year medical students at Jefferson (Hojat, Axelrod et al., 2013), students were divided into experimental and control groups and participated in a two-phase study. In phase 1, students in the experimental group watched and discussed video clips of patient encounters (selected from commercial movies) meant to enhance empathic understanding; those in the control group watched a documentary film. Ten weeks later in phase 2 of the study, students who were in the experimental group were divided into two groups.

One group attended a lecture on the importance of empathy in patient care, and the other plus those in the control group watched a movie about racism. The JSE was administered pre-post in phase 1 and posttest in phase 2. Results showed a statistically significant increase in the JSE mean scores for the experimental group in phase 1. No significant change in the JSE scores was found in the control group. In phase 2 of the study, the JSE mean score improvement was sustained in the group who attended the lecture on importance of empathy in patient care, but not in the experimental group who watched a movie about racism in this phase of the study. Also, no significant change of empathy was observed in the control group in the second phase of the study. It was concluded that enhancement of empathy in medical students can be sustained by additional educational reinforcements.

In another study, 57 residents from 16 family medicine programs (Magee & Hojat, 2010) were offered the opportunity in the second year of their training to choose one of their indigent pregnant patients, in the second trimester of pregnancy, to receive the free gift of a glider rocking chair. Shortly after the baby was born, 10 of the residents agreed to make a prearranged home visit to the mother of the newborn to assist in assembling the chair while talking with the mother in a friendly manner about child care and well-being. Compared to the residents who did not make such a home visit, the simple home visit experience contributed to an impressive increase in posttest JSE scores among those residents who made such a home visit.

In a study conducted at the University of Missouri-Kansas City School of Medicine, medical students participated in a three-stage multidimensional training program on empathy (Feighny et al., 1998). In Stage 1, the students developed a clinical presentation of an illness, such as diabetes, from a patient's perspective (cognitive empathy). In Stage 2, the students tried to experience the situation as if they were patients (emotional empathy). In Stage 3, the students were provided with corrective feedback about their communication skills (behavioral empathy). The investigators noted that the students' scores improved significantly on Carkhuff's Empathic Understanding in Interpersonal Processes Scale but did not change significantly on the IRI. The investigators attributed the discrepancy to the IRI's lack of sensitivity in the context of patient care. In her doctoral dissertation at Iowa University, Stebbins (2005) reported that exposure to interactive interpersonal communication enhanced empathy among second-year osteopathic medical students.

Platt and Keller (1994) developed a program to enhance empathic communication among physicians facing difficult encounters with patients who expressed strong negative emotions (e.g., anger, fear, sadness) and were unwilling to assume responsibility for their own health. During the program, the participants attempted to increase their awareness of a patient's emotional clues by trying to understand the emotion, naming the emotion for the patient to ensure that they had identified the emotion correctly, acknowledging and justifying the patient's emotion, and affirming the patient's behavior and offering help. The authors concluded that empathic communication is a teachable and learnable skill.

In summary, the major premise of all of the aforementioned approaches is the improvement of understanding, which is the key ingredient in the definition of empathy. Therefore, at a conceptual level, it makes sense to assume that all of these approaches can lead to the cultivation of empathy. However, in their review of the literature on effects of educating for empathy in medicine, Stepien and Baernstien (2006) concluded that most studies that attempted to provide empirical evidence in support of improving empathy suffer from inappropriate design, methodological limitations, uncertainty about conceptualization and measurement of empathy, and small nonrepresentative samples. More convincing empirical evidence is needed to confirm the short- and long-term effects of these programs on health professions education and practice.

Effectiveness of the Programs

Although some studies cited in this chapter indicate that empathy can be enhanced, some clues suggest that the improvement cannot be sustained without practice or reinforcement (Engler et al., 1981; Hojat, Axelrod et al., 2013). Thus, the popular saying "Use it or lose it" may be applicable to empathy that has been enhanced as a result of an educational program. Furthermore, it is also important to bear in mind that when assessing any educational program designed to enhance empathy, it is desirable to examine not only the short-term but also, more importantly, the long-term effects of the program. Although some studies have indicated that educational training programs designed to enhance empathy may have a relatively long-term effect (Kramer et al., 1989; Poole & Sanson-Fisher, 1980), the long-lasting effects of empathy training programs await more empirical scrutiny.

At a conceptual level, it makes sense to believe that targeted educational programs can cultivate empathy. However, Skelton, Macleod, and Thomas (2000) were not satisfied with empirical evidence to verify the truth of this assumption. With regard to this challenge, McManus (1995) suggested that investigators who attempt to conduct empirical assessments of the humanities' contribution to medical outcomes must "bite the bullet" of definition and measurement. However, recent research subsequent to the development of the JSE (Chap. 7) can relieve us, to some extent, of the need to bite that bullet (see Appendix A).

Recapitulation

Although the emphasis on professionalism in medicine places a high value on enhancement of clinical empathy in patient care, most students in the existing medical education system in the USA do not routinely acquire the skills needed to demonstrate clinical empathy and assess its development as students progress through medical school. However, research shows that empathy can be effectively enhanced by targeted educational programs. Counteracting the trends in medical education and practice that are not conducive to enhancing clinical empathy in patient care requires a mandate for the development and implementation of educational programs at all levels of training (undergraduate, graduate, and continuing education) in all health professions academic centers and hospitals. Only then will the public be better served and all health professionals regain the utmost respect they rightly deserve.

Chapter 13
In Search of Neurological Underpinnings of Clinical Empathy

Empathy is a biological concept par excellence.

—(Leslie Brothers, 1989, p. 17)

Neurons that fire together wire together.

—(attributed to Carla Shatz, cited in Doidge, 2007, p. 63)

Neurons that fire apart wire apart/neurons out of sync fail to link.

—(cited in Doidge, 2007, p. 64)

Abstract

- During its long evolution history, the human brain has evolved to understand other person's state of mind, feelings, perspectives, and intentions. Such an understanding has survival value and facilitates empathic relationships.
- Evidence suggests a neurophysiobehavioral substructure exists in human beings that serves as a precursor and facilitator for understanding others, evident by a newborn's reactive crying, inborn capacity for mimicry and imitation, physiological synchronicity in interpersonal interactions, perception–action coupling, propensity to understand other's state of mind reflected in the theory of mind, and findings of a new line of research on the mirror neuron system.
- Empirical findings from brain imaging studies, brain lesion research, empathy deficiency in neurological disorders (e.g., autism, Asperger's syndrome, and alexithymia), and pain research suggest that certain brain areas can be implicated in forming or failing to form empathic connection.
- A search for neurological underpinnings of empathy is highly desirable for better understanding of neurological factors that contribute to the development or arrest of the capacity for empathy. Outcomes of such research will have important educational as well as medical implications.

M. Hojat, *Clinical Empathy*, https://doi.org/10.1007/978-3-031-87413-0_13

- From brain imaging research, it can be speculated that certain cortical areas of the brain (e.g., regions for cognitive processing in the medial prefrontal cortex, dorsolateral, and mirror neuron region in the premotor areas) could be implicated in cognitive empathic responses.
- Findings also suggest that the regions for emotional processing, i.e., the orbitofrontal cortex and older structures of the brain, such as the limbic system, and specifically areas known as the pain matrix (e.g., amygdala, insula, and anterior cingulate cortex), could be implicated in emotional empathic reactions. However, these speculations await further experimental verification.

Introduction

Along with the emergence of a new discipline of social cognitive neuroscience and advances in neuroimaging technology, there has been growing research on the neurological underpinnings of empathy. Social cognitive neuroscience is an interdisciplinary branch of science that combines the technology from neuroscience with theories and views from behavioral, social, cognitive, political, and economics sciences to explore the neural bases of perceptions, understanding one's self and others, and social interactions (Copland & Goldie, 2014; Lieberman, 2007).

Advancements in brain imaging technology have provided a unique opportunity to examine neural activities associated with cognitive and affective states. Locating the areas of the brain that are implicated in empathic engagement will have important educational and medical implications for enhancing clinical empathy in health professions students and practitioners and for diagnosis and treatment of empathy deficit disorders. Views from the ideomotor principle postulated by William James (1890), neuron cell assembly advanced by Donald Hebb (1946), perception–action coupling proposed by Preston and deWaal (2002), and the discovery of the mirror neuron system (MNS) (Iacoboni et al., 1999; Rizzolatti, Fadiga, Gallese, & Fogassi, 1996) suggest that neurological activities are involved in empathic engagement. The following factors provide evidence in support of the existence of neurological roots of empathy: universal human capacity for expression and understanding of emotions; mimicry and imitation starting at an early age; synchronization in body postures in interpersonal interactions (see Chap. 3) and in physiological functions (e.g., heartbeat and galvanic skin response); as well as findings on neurological activities in social interactions in general, and in pain research in particular. This chapter examines the theoretical bases and empirical evidence in the search for neurological underpinnings of empathy.

Neuroanatomy

The human brain, according to Keysers (2011), is "wired to be empathic." (p. 216). According to Brothers (1989, p. 11), empathy as a social behavior is a concept that "appears to have a great potential utility in bringing together neural and psychological data." To achieve a better understanding of empathy, we must expand our knowledge about the cellular mechanisms involved in interpersonal relationships. In an article on a new intellectual framework for psychiatry, Eric Kandel (1998) proposed a basic principle that all mental, cognitive, and emotional processes, without exception, derive from neurological operations of the brain. He further suggested that this principle applies to both individual and social behaviors. Thus, as an attribute that is manifested in interaction with others, empathy falls well within the scope of the brain's neurological operations.

The human brain is a complex command-and-control center for cognition and emotions. Although the three divisions of the brain (brainstem, limbic system, and cerebral cortex) are structurally and evolutionarily distinct, they are closely interconnected through a complex neurological network. The brainstem (reptilian brain), phylogenetically the oldest section of the brain, controls the physiology of survival (e.g., heartbeat and breathing). The next oldest section, the limbic system, wraps around the brainstem and functions as the primary center for emotion and social behavior (MacLean, 1990). The limbic brain has an abundance of opiate receptors that not only can reduce physical pain but also can diminish the excruciating psychological and social pains arising from a broken interpersonal relationship (Lewis, Amini, & Lannon, 2000).

Included in the limbic system are a number of interconnected substructures, such as the amygdala, insula, hippocampus, hypothalamus, and cingulate gyrus. Among the substructures of the limbic system, the role of the amygdala is important in understanding the neurology of social behavior because of its contribution to detect social signals. The amygdala is an almond-shaped structure consisting of a highly interconnected cluster of neurons situated deep in the medial temporal lobes. It is implicated in producing emotional reactions, expressions of emotion, and responses to social signals (Milner, Squire, & Kanel, 1998). The amygdala is a gateway to a person's view of the social environment (Nauta & Feirtag, 1986) and plays a crucial role in the fight-or-flight response (Siegel, 1999).

The newest component of the brain, the cerebral cortex, which is largest in humans, has a great deal to do with complex cognitive behavior, abstract thinking, reasoning, language, and other high-level activities of the human brain. One striking change that occurred in the course of the brain's evolution is the tremendous increase in the complexity and size of the cerebral cortex in vertebrates in general and in human beings in particular (Nolte, 1993). The newest layers of the cerebral cortex, the neocortex, stem from complex social living (Keverne, Nevison, & Martel, 1997). These layers allow engagement in voluntary social behavior based on cognitive understanding (akin to clinical empathy as conceptualized in Chaps. 1, 3, and 6).

Cognition is more likely to be linked to cortical activities, whereas emotion is more likely to be associated with subcortical activities and the limbic system (Nathanson, 1996). Most cognition occurs in the thalamic–neocortical axis (the thinking brain), whereas primary emotions are largely registered within the hypothalamic–limbic axis (the feeling brain) (Moore, 1996). Thus, one can speculate that the limbic system is more likely to be implicated in emotional empathy (synonymous to sympathy, see Chaps. 1 and 3), whereas the neocortex is more likely to be implicated in cognitive empathy (differences between cognitive and emotional empathy are described in Chaps. 1 and 3, and their implications for patient care are discussed in Chap. 6). Consistent with this speculation, in a functional magnetic resonance imaging (fMRI)-based quantitative meta-analytic study, Fan, Duncan, de Greck, and Northoff (2011) reported that cognitive and emotional empathy can be distinguished by the different regional activation of the brain. They identified the dorsal anterior midcingulate cortex to be recruited more frequently in the cognitive empathy, and the right anterior insula in the emotional empathy. Similar results were reported by Eres, Decety, Louis, and Molenberghs (2015), who found that higher scores on cognitive empathy were associated with greater gray matter density in the midcingulate cortex and adjacent dorsomedial prefrontal cortex, and higher scores on emotional empathy were associated with greater gray matter density in the insula cortex.

A long evolutionary path that resulted in the development of the capacity for bonding and interpersonal relationships must have left durable footprints in the human central nervous system. It is now beyond dispute that our cognition and emotions (empathy and sympathy, respectively) are inextricably woven into the structure and function of the human brain (Damasio, 2003). Behavioral scholars and social cognitive neuroscientists benefiting from advanced brain imaging technology are able to view social and interpersonal behaviors from a neurological perspective (Bennett, 2001).

Using advanced biomedical technology and brain imaging technology, a new and interesting line of research is shedding light on the issue of neurology of empathy. New technologies, such as positron emission tomography (PET) and, in particular, fMRI, allow noninvasive exploration of the human brain at a high level of resolution that helps investigators understand not only the structural aspects but also the functional activities of the brain that are associated with empathic engagement. However, given the current research findings, we are still far from confidently knowing the neurological roots of empathy. Despite all of the biotechnological advances at the present time, we have only a hint of what the neurological underpinnings of empathy might be.

Theoretical Foundations

The following four theoretical perspectives provide foundations for exploring the neurological underpinnings of empathy.

William James Ideomotor Principle

In his book "Principles of Psychology" William James postulated the ideomotor principle, proposing that mental representation of a movement can lead to the actual movement to some degree. In other words, merely observing or even thinking of an action increases the likelihood of performing the act (James, 1890). The ideomotor principle, according to Iacoboni (2009a) can also account for imitation and mimicry which pave the road to empathic understanding (see Chap. 3). Research findings suggest that those who are good at imitation are better in recognizing emotions in others, which is a pillar of empathic understanding (Iacoboni, 2009a). There is a strong tendency in humans for imitation, i.e., facial or postural mimicry, to align themselves with others in social interactions (Lieberman, 2007). Thus, a link can be expected between the ideomotor principle, imitation and mimicry, and empathic understanding.

Neuron Cell Assembly Theory

Donald Hebb (1946) postulated that "any two cells or systems of cells that are repeatedly active at the same time will tend to become 'associated,' so that activity in one facilitates activity in the other." (p. 70). The Hebb's neuron cell assembly theory indeed can be summarized in the quotation cited in the epigraph of this chapter: "Neurons that fire together wire together" (attributed to Carla Shatz, cited in Doidge, 2007). The notion of firing together-wiring together can also provide neurological explanations for not only the perception–action model (PAM, introduced previously in Chap. 11 and described in the following section), but also for habit formation, observational learning, and the influences of sociocultural and educational experiences on the development of the capacity for empathy.

Perception–Action Model

The PAM, formulated by Preston and deWaal (2002) to describe the ultimate and proximate causes of empathy, specifies that perceptions of another person's cognitive, emotional, and somatosensory states automatically activate representations of those states in the observer, unless inhibited. The integrated PAM is recognized as a function with precursors such as mimicry and imitation (Goubert et al., 2005), which help to illustrate mechanisms involved in empathic engagement. Mimicry and imitation (see Chap. 3) are indeed recognized as facilitators of empathic understanding (Iacoboni, 2009a).

Empirical research suggests that perception–action coupling could sometimes function in a peculiar way. For example, in an experiment on perception and activation of motor behavior, research participants performed a scrambled-sentence language task. One group was exposed to words that typically could be associated with elderly people and retirement (e.g., old, gray, bingo, Florida, forgetful, and retired). The other group was exposed to neutral words (e.g., thirsty, private, and clean). At the end of the experiment, the researchers recorded the time to walk back from the experimental room to the elevator to leave the building. It was noticed that those who were exposed to the words associated with older age walked slower than the other group (Bargh, Chen, & Burrows, 1996). These findings support the PAM, suggesting that words that evoke perceptions that are associated with older age can significantly influence the corresponding motor function of the perceivers, showing that empathic understanding can be reflected in actual behavior.

Consistent with the PAM, Craig and Weiss (1971) suggested that perception of others in pain (e.g., observing a patient in pain) can activate cognitive, emotional, and somatosensory representations of the pain, which in turn has a significant effect on the observer's understanding of the patient's pain and suffering. Over a century ago, Theodore Lipps stated that "when I observe a circus performer walking on a tight rope, I feel I am inside him" (cited in Carr, Iacoboni, Dubeau, Mazziotta, & Lenzi, 2003, p. 5502). This statement is a vivid example of linking the PAM to empathic understanding of others through cognitive, affective, and somatosensory activation. The theory that observation can lead to action is further explained by the MNS, which will be discussed in the following section.

The Mirror Neuron System

The ideomotor principle, the neuron cell assembly theory, and the PAM laid the foundation for the discovery of the Mirror Neuron System (MNS). Indeed, one of my colleagues, Dr. Nuno Sousa, Professor of Neuroscience at Minho University in Portugal, believes that MNS is the underlying substrate of the PAM (personal communication, e-mail dated 8/27/2015). In one of the early studies on the MNS, Di Pellegrino, Fadiga, Fogassi, Gallese, and Rizzolutti (1992) noticed that a set of neurons in primates' brains was activated when primates performed a goal-oriented act (e.g., reaching for an object) and also the same set of neurons was activated when another primate observed the act without performing it.

Subsequent to the observation of Di Pellegrino et al. (1992), neuroscientist Giacomo Rizzolatti and colleagues at the University of Parma, Italy, were the leading investigators who systematically studied and discovered the MNS in macaque monkeys (Gallese, Fadiga, Fogassi, & Rizzolatti, 1996; Rizzolatti et al., 1996). They discovered that a specific set of neurons in the ventral premotor cortex of the monkey's brains (known as the F5 area) discharged when the monkey observed another monkey performing hand actions, such as grasping, tearing, holding, or manipulating an object. The same set of neurons (dubbed as "mirror neurons") discharged when the monkey actually performed the hand action (Gallese et al., 1996; Rizzolatti et al., 1996).

Accordingly, Gallese, Keysers, and Rizzolatti (2004, p. 396) concluded that "the observation of an action leads to the activation of parts of the *same* cortical neural network that is implicated during its execution" (emphasis added). This brain mechanism serves as a bridge to the understanding of another's action, and is considered as the neural basis of social cognition (Gallese et al., 2004).

Other studies led by Marco Iacoboni at the University of California at Los Angeles and other neuroscientists demonstrated the existence of a similar system of mirror neurons in humans (Buccino et al., 2001; Gallese, 2003; Hari et al., 1998; Iacoboni et al., 1999; Iacoboni, 2009b). The results of these studies led to the assumption that a region of the human brain, analogous to the F5 area of a monkey's brain, is activated when we observe actions performed by others *as if* we were performing the actions ourselves. The discovery of the mirror neurons indeed provided the link between social cognition and neuroscience (Gallese et al., 1996; Keysers & Perrett, 2004; Rizzolatti et al., 1996). Research findings on the MNS presented the first convincing neurological evidence to show neurological activities for perception–action coupling (Jackson & Decety, 2004; Rizzolatti & Craighero, 2004).

Brain imaging studies in humans have shown that the mirror neurons matching the hand action fire in the following sectors of the cortical network: Broca's region, premotor cortex, and posterior parietal cortex (Buccino et al., 2001; Gallese, 2003). Considering the homology between the F5 area of a monkey's brain and Broca's region in the inferior frontal lobe (involved in speech control) of the human brain (Hari et al., 1998; Kohler et al., 2002), one can find similarities in the mirror neuron matching system in monkeys and humans.

Two key studies improved our understanding of the generalized function of the MNS. In the first key study, Umilta et al. (2001) carried out an experiment to examine if mirror neurons are involved in understanding "intention" or the "goal" of an action. This was the first experimental study to explore if the mental representation of an action with intended purpose can trigger the neuron system representing that action and its purpose. In other words, can the intended goal (final part) of the action be inferred when it is hidden from view? In one part of the experiment, the monkey was shown a fully visible action (grasping an object) ("full vision" condition). In the other part of the experiment, the same action was presented to the monkey, but the final grasping of the object was blocked by a screen, thus hidden from being directly observed ("hidden" condition).

The results showed that the majority of the mirror neurons fired in the full vision also responded in the hidden condition, suggesting that mirror neurons were involved in action recognition and could correctly infer the intention of the action (in the hidden condition). Similar results were obtained with human subjects, suggesting that the MNS is not only involved in action recognition but also in understanding the intention of others (Iacoboni, 2009b; Iacoboni et al., 2005). These findings generally indicate that the MNS has a mediating role not only in the understanding of others' actions, but also in predicting the goals, intention, and consequences of such actions, which are important ingredients of empathic understanding. If monkeys have the capacity to predict the intention of an action, then humans are certainly bestowed with a capacity to understand others' states of mind (mind reading) (see Chap. 4, for a relevant discussion of the theory of mind).

Another relevant finding with regard to the MNS is that the observed acts must be goal-directed to better recruit mirror neurons, suggesting that random acts or acts performed by robots are less likely to activate the MNS (Tai, Scherfler, Brooks, Sawamoto, & Castiello, 2004). Goal-directed, non-repetitive robot acts, however, can activate the MNS (Gazzola, Rizzolatti, Wicker, & Keysers, 2007). Also, it has been shown that the MNS processes biological (or realistic) and nonbiological (or unrealistic) movements differently. For example, Castiello, Lusher, Mari, Edwards, and Humphreys (2002) reported that the brain reacts differently to a grasping action performed by a human compared to a robotic hand. Similarly to humans, a monkey's brain encodes the grasping actions performed by a person differently from grasping by a tool or a mechanical device (Castiello, 2003).

The second key study on generalization of the MNS function was conducted by Kohler et al. (2002) in which they found that the MNS in monkeys could recognize actions even from their sound (e.g., ripping a piece of paper and cracking a nut) without seeing the action. The MNS response to the auditory stimulus prompted Rizzolatti and Arbibi (1998) to speculate that the mirror neurons have an evolutionary link to language acquisition. This speculation seems reasonable given that the core area of MNS (F5) in monkey's brains corresponds anatomically to the Broca's area in the human brain, which is the language processing center.

Therefore, the MNS was found to be the key neurophysiological indicator in gestural communication (Kohler et al., 2002), which is another key ingredient of empathic understanding. Further studies showed that not only motor actions and auditory stimulus but also more abstract intentions embedded in the contexts, such as drinking a cup of tea in the context of a tea party, cleaning a cup after the party (Iacoboni et al., 2005), or observation of emotional states (Carr et al., 2003), can also recruit the same areas which contain the MNS. It has also been demonstrated that components of the MNS (including the inferior frontal cortex) are involved in the imitation and expressions of emotions (Carr et al., 2003).

Neurological Roots

Brain studies provide plausible explanations as to why we flinch, wince, cringe, or recoil when observing others in pain and almost "feel" the pain of others (Valeriani et al., 2008). It has been demonstrated that affective brain regions (anterior cingulate cortex and anterior insula) are activated by observing a loved one receiving a painful electric shock (Singer et al., 2004). It is interesting to note that research participants with higher scores on measures of cognitive and emotional empathy (e.g., Interpersonal Reactivity Index and Balanced Emotional Empathy Scale) showed stronger activations in pain-related areas when observing their partners being subjected to painful stimuli (Singer et al., 2004).

Wicker et al. (2003) discovered that observing another person's expression of emotions such as disgust (produced by unpleasant odors) could activate the neural representation of the emotion, as well. By using fMRI, Wicker and colleagues concluded that anatomical and functional data provided evidence that the insula was the common neural basis of seeing and feeling disgust, which is a pathway to emotional empathy. Heins, Engelmann, Vollberg, and Tobler (2016) found that receiving help from an out-group member elicits a signal in the anterior insular cortex, which can contribute to a subsequent increase in empathy for the out-group members.

According to Carr et al. (2003), the insula is a plausible candidate for relaying information about action representation to the area of the limbic system that processes emotional content. Lesions in this circuit can lead to impaired understanding of other people's emotions, thus blocking the pathway to emotional empathy. Therefore, it makes intuitive sense that the observer and the observed person experience similar sensations and emotions that can lead to a common understanding (Goubert et al., 2005), which is the foundation of empathic engagement. Watching a spider crawling on another person's face can make the observer shiver as if the spider were crawling on his or her own face. Keysers et al. (2004) attributed this "tactile empathy" to brain activities in the secondary somatosensory cortex. Gallese (2003, p. 176) proposed that "sensations and emotions by others can also be 'empathized,' and therefore *implicitly* understood through a mirror matching mechanism."

The notion that perception of a behavior in another person can activate one's own representation of that behavior is not new (Decety & Jackson, 2004); however, providing objective neurological evidence linking empathy to brain activities is new with broad implications. The MNS plays an important role in understanding the experiences of others; thus, it opens a gateway to understanding neurological pathways to empathy.

A number of studies suggest that understanding the mental state of others (see Chap. 4), which is the backbone of empathic engagement (Chap. 4, theory of mind), appears to be localized to areas of the frontal cortex (Platek, Keenan, Gallup, & Mohamed, 2004), especially the right frontal lobe (Stuss, 2001). Aspects of cognitive empathy, such as perspective taking and role taking skills, are linked to functions of the frontal lobe, whereas aspects of emotional empathy have been hypothesized to be associated with the orbitofrontal areas (Eslinger, 1998). The prefrontal cortex is particularly vital to empathic engagement, and the dorsolateral region of the frontal cortex is linked to people's ability to understand other people's experiences (more relevant to cognitive empathy), and that the orbitofrontal region of the brain could be related to people's emotional responsiveness and sensitivity to the emotional states of others (more relevant to emotional empathy) (Eslinger, 1998).

The dorsolateral prefrontal cortex is known for its role in decision-making and context evaluation (Rahm, 2006). It has been suggested that prefrontal damage may result in impaired perspective-taking ability. The medial prefrontal cortex plays a critical role in reading others' intentions (Shallice, 2001). Several authors have demonstrated that theory of mind is associated with a cerebral pattern of activity involving the medial prefrontal cortex. It has been reported that lesions in prefrontal cortex, particularly in orbitoprefrontal area, can lead to "acquired sociopathy" (Shamay-Tsoory, Tomer, Goldsher, Berger, & Aharon-Peretz, 2004).

Both the prefrontal and orbitofrontal cortex are involved in integrating cognitive operations in interpersonal relationships and decision-making (de Quervain et al., 2004). Research indicates that dorsolateral lesions are associated with a deficit in empathy as well as impaired cognitive flexibility, whereas patients with orbitofrontal cortex lesions are more impaired in emotional empathy than in cognitive flexibility (Decety & Jackson, 2004). The orbitofrontal cortex has been implicated in the regulation of emotion that contributes to emotional empathic engagement (Cahill, 2005). Singer and Frith (2005) reported that seeing pictures of unknown people getting hurt (e.g., a hand trapped in a car door, or someone's hand being pierced by a needle) elicited brain activities in the affective brain section (anterior cingulate cortex). In their discussion of the "painful side of empathy," these authors suggested that neural activities are elicited even when people think about the pain of others.

In a pain study, using fMRI, Jackson, Meltzoff, and Decety (2005) found that observation of pain in others was associated with significant bilateral changes in activities in the anterior cingulate cortex, the anterior insula, and the cerebellum, which prompted them to conclude that their findings help to understand the neurological mechanisms that are implicated in empathy for pain. Carr et al. (2003) used fMRI to confirm that to form empathic relationships, people need to evoke the representation of actions in the brain associated with the conditions they observe in others. In other words, it is necessary to place oneself in another person's shoes to form empathic understanding. In a review article: "The Functional Architecture of Human Empathy," Decety and Jackson (2004, p. 80) concluded that "part of the neural network mediating pain experiences is shared when empathizing with pain in others." In summing up the findings on neurological underpinnings of empathy, Decety (2015) concluded that circuits connecting the brainstem, amygdala, basal ganglia, anterior cingulate cortex, insula, and orbitofrontal cortex are involved in some forms of empathic responses.

The Role of the Right Hemisphere

A number of studies suggest that the right hemisphere is more involved in empathy than the left hemisphere (Rankin et al., 2006; Ruby & Decety, 2004; Shamay-Tsoory, Tomer, Berger, & Aharon-Peretz, 2003). Interpersonal signals, such as facial expressions of emotion, are recognized best in the right cerebral hemisphere, and, most mechanisms associated with regulating emotions are activated in the right hemisphere as well (Perry et al., 2001). Also, it has been reported that the ability to recognize emotions from facial expressions is impaired in patients whose right hemisphere has been damaged (Kolb & Taylor, 1981). Recognition of facial expressions and empathic understanding were impaired in patients with atrophy of the right temporal lobe (Perry et al., 2001). Greater empathy deficit has been observed in those with anterior temporal lobe atrophy in the right compared to the left hemisphere (Perry et al., 2001). Expression and perception of nonverbal communication appears to be mediated by the right hemisphere, whereas verbal communication is mediated predominantly by the left hemisphere (Siegel, 1999). It is generally believed that the posterior region of the right hemisphere plays a special role in perceptions of emotion and recognition of emotional clues (Buck & Ginsburg, 1997a, 1997b).

In an interesting experiment in search of the comforting substrate of the right brain, Horton (1995) hypothesized that the comforting substrate is located in the right hemisphere of the brain. The hypothesis was based on the notion that the calming effectiveness of holding the baby on the left side of the chest against the beating heart is an indication of the baby's specific need to be comforted. In this experiment, Horton (1995) gave the option to 60 research participants to choose between two identical red balls (one on the left and one on the right). Results showed that only 20% of the right-handed subjects chose the left ball. Participants were also given the choice between two identical white teddy bears which were described as grieving because they lost their mothers, upset, scared, and in need of being soothed. In this experimental condition, the majority of the participants chose the left bear. Also, two-thirds of the participants who were mothers in this study chose the left bear. Results support the view that the comforting attitude has its origin in the right brain (by choosing the left bear) suggesting the possibility that right brain lateralization of the comforting substrate is more pronounced, especially in mothers.

It is also interesting to note that a great majority of mothers, regardless of whether they are right- or left-handed (approximately 90% of people are right-handed), carry their infants against the left side of their chest (Salk, 1960). It may be argued that an evolutionary factor prompted mothers to place their infants to the left of their chest closer to their hearts, or to have their dominant right hand free to defend the child against predators. However, from a neurological perspective, placing a child on the left activates the left visual field which can lead to more direct communication to the right hemisphere of the brain (Sieratzki & Woll, 1996). Some believe that this suggests that the right brain may have a more significant role than the left brain in human attachment and interpersonal relationships (Sieratzki & Woll, 1996; Swain, Lorberlaum, Kose, & Strathearn, 2007).

Lesion research showed that while damage to the right hemisphere resulted in greater impairment in cognitive empathy than damage to the left hemisphere, damage to the right prefrontal cortex did not have a significant impairment in emotional empathy (Shamay-Tsoory et al., 2004). Rankin et al. (2006) reported a large scale lesion study of investigating the neural basis of empathy. Their findings suggest that the right anterior temporal and medial frontal regions are neurological roots to empathic behavior. Further support was provided by Tranel, Bechara, and Denburg (2002), who found that the right compared to left ventromedial prefrontal cortex is more directly involved in social behavior and decision-making.

Dementia patients with right-sided brain damage were also more likely than patients with left brain damage to show deficits in empathy and other aspects of interpersonal behavior (Rankin et al., 2006). It has been reported that damage to the right hemisphere is frequently associated with impairment in social interactions

(Edwards-Lee & Saul, 1999) and with impaired judgment of facial expressions (Adolphs, Damasio, Tranel, Cooper, & Damasio, 2000). Also, according to Decety and Chaminade (2003), right parietal cortices are involved with the capacity for understanding other's emotions. Rankin et al. (2006) found that empathy scores (measured by the IRI, see Chap. 5) correlated significantly with the volume of the gray matter in the right brain areas. The aforementioned studies generally indicate that the role of the right brain hemisphere seems to be more important in manifesting empathy.

Neurological Impairment and Empathy: Lesion Studies

The inability to recognize one's own emotions and the emotions of others can impair capacity to form empathic relationships. This is often observed in patients with certain developmental, neurological, and psychiatric disorders. If, as research suggests, empathy is a function of cellular activities in the brain, it would be reasonable to assume that certain neurological damage in the brain could impair capacity for empathy. This assumption has been supported by studies of patients with brain lesions or certain neurological problems. The well-known case of Phineas Gage is a classic example of impaired social skills associated with lesions of the frontal lobe (Benton, 1991; Damasio, Grabowski, Frank, Galaburda, & Damasio, 1994; Hamilton, 1984). Gage was the foreman of a railroad construction company. In 1848, as a result of an accidental explosion, an iron bar was propelled completely through his skull and landed some 25–30 yards behind him (Macmillan, 2000). Although he recovered physically and survived for $11^1/_2$ years after the injury, he never regained his capacity for forming empathic relationships. The following neurological conditions have been linked to impairment in the capacity for empathy.

Autism

Of all the developmental disorders, autism is among the best clinical examples for studying the neurological basis of empathy. Poor social skills are among the core features of autistic individuals, and the central pathology of autism is an impaired capacity for empathy (Brothers, 1989). A defect in social interaction is a primary criterion for the diagnosis of autism (Frances, First, & Pincus, 1995). It has been observed that autistic children never respond to their mother's smile, indicating that they do not exhibit a capacity to respond empathically to others (Decety & Jackson, 2004). Autistic infants are born with some deficit in forming attachment and social interactions (Tucker, Luu, & Derryberry, 2005).

Empirical and clinical evidence suggests that, compared to the general population, autistic individuals obtain lower scores on tests measuring the ability to understand facial expressions displayed in photographs of people with happy, sad, or fearful faces and display a seriously impaired capacity for empathy (Baron-Cohen, 2003). Autistic children show a profound cognitive impairment to understand the perspectives and intentions of other people, which is a cognitive impairment (Tucker et al., 2005). In a study by Dziobek et al. (2008) using the Multifaceted Empathy Test (MET), it was noticed that adults with Asperger's syndrome (a condition within the autism spectrum disorders, but typically with a milder phenotype), compared to a healthy control group, also displayed impaired empathy, but more pronounced in cognitive empathy rather than emotional empathy. The MET includes a set of pictures depicting individuals in emotionally charged situations (e.g., being threatened). For the assessment of cognitive empathy, participants are asked to infer the mental status on the individual(s) shown in the pictures. For the assessment of emotional empathy, participants are asked to identify and rate their emotional reaction to the event shown in the picture.

Alexithymia

Alexithymia is a condition that impairs patients' perception of other people's affective status. Sufferers usually have difficulty recognizing and labeling emotions and feelings, which are associated with impairment in capacity for empathy (Mann, Wise, Trinidad, & Kohanski, 1994). Guttman and LaPorte (2002) reported that patients with alexithymia scored low on empathy measured by the Interpersonal Reactivity Index (Chap. 5). Also, a significant association has been reported between alexithymia and autism (Hill, Berthoz, & Frith, 2004). Most etiological models of alexithymia have proposed a dysfunction of the right hemisphere to account for the characteristic pattern observed in patients with alexithymia (Jessimer & Markham, 1997).

Although no specific brain lesion has been identified as the cause of alexithymia, case studies of patients with alexithymia should be of interest to empathy researchers to examine underlying mechanisms involved in a lack of capacity to recognize emotions which is a main feature of alexithymia.

Other Empathy Deficit Disorders

It has been reported that many pervasive developmental, personality, and neurological disorders such as elective mutism, Tourette's syndrome, anorexia nervosa, schizophrenia, psychopathy, post-traumatic brain injury, and stroke are associated with deficits in empathy (Charman et al., 1997; Mullins-Nelson, Salekin, & Leistico, 2006; Rankin et al., 2006). In a study by Grattan and Eslinger (1989), significant empathic change (measured by Hogan's Empathy Scale, see Chap. 5) was associated with brain injury, which resulted in acquired disabilities featured by cognitive inflexibility.

Eslinger (1998) reported that more than half of the neurologically damaged patients scored more than two standard deviations below the mean on a measure of empathy. In a study involving patients with neurological damage caused by head injuries, ischemic hemispheric strokes, encephalitis, or multiple sclerosis, Eslinger et al. (1996) found that both cognitive and emotional empathy were impaired by the neurological damage. Brothers (1989) hypothesized that the impairment of empathy observed in certain neurological conditions, such as autism or in certain lesions of the cortex in the right cerebral hemisphere, suggests that empathy has neurophysiological roots.

Evidence presented by Anderson, Bechara, Damasio, Tranel, and Damasio (1999) suggests that individuals with early-onset prefrontal lesions (before 16 months of age) resemble patients with comparable adult-onset lesions in a number of ways. Those individuals failed to acquire complex social knowledge during the regular development period. Unlike adult-onset patients, however, early-onset patients could not retrieve complex social knowledge at the factual level, and may never have acquired such knowledge (Anderson et al., 1999).

It has been reported that acquired cerebral damage, such as focal damage to the prefrontal cortex in adulthood and damage to the frontal lobe in early childhood, can disturb social behavior, including the capacity for empathy (Eslinger, 1998). Research showed that empathic understanding was impaired subsequent to focal lesions of the prefrontal cortex (Decety & Jackson, 2004; Eslinger, 1998). Some research findings concerning the neuroanatomical basis of social behavior indicated that after damage to the frontal lobe, patients became profoundly inept in their social behavior in general (Grattan & Eslinger, 1989) and in their capacity for empathy in particular (Eslinger, 1998).

In a study of character changes in patients with multiple sclerosis, a decline in empathy (measured by the Hogan Empathy Scale) was observed that was attributed to a neurogenic frontal lobe syndrome (Benedict, Priore, Miller, Munschauser, & Jacobs, 2001). In another study, it was reported that affective agnosia in patients with lesions in the right temporoparietal area rendered patients unable to understand emotions conveyed by vocal quality (Heilman, Scholes, & Watson, 1975). Another condition, aprosodic-agestural syndrome (an inability to express felt emotions through voice intonation), caused by lesions in the right hemisphere, makes patients unable to express themselves through gestures (Ross & Mesulam, 1979). Yet another group of patients includes those with lesions in the left hemisphere that impair the ability for symbolic communication and make patients unable to pantomime.

Empathy deficit is often a feature of psychopathic personality. Although a psychopath may have the skill to understand another person's perspective and have the ability to manipulate others, they often lack concern for the welfare of others and can inflict pain and suffering with no apparent remorse (Tucker et al., 2005); thus, all psychopaths have empathy deficit disorder.

Developmental history of many patients who are psychopaths shows clear evidence of abuse and neglect in their childhood and a lack of quality attachment with a primary caregiver. However, it is reported that in addition to the aforementioned factors, lesions in prefrontal cortex and particularly in the orbitoprefrontal area can also lead to "acquired psychopathy" (Shamay-Tsoory et al., 2004; Tucker et al., 2005) with severe empathic deficiency. Rankin, Kramer, and Miller (2005) found that patients with semantic dementia showed low levels of both cognitive and emotional empathy, whereas patients with frontotemporal dementia showed deficits only in cognitive empathy, as measured by the Interpersonal Reactivity Index. In a study by Shamay-Tsoory et al. (2004), impairment in cognitive empathy (measured by the Interpersonal Reactivity Index) and emotional empathy (measured by Mehrabian and Epstein's Emotional Empathy Scale) was assessed in patients with brain lesions. It was found that patients with prefrontal lesions (especially those with lesions involving orbitoprefrontal and medial regions) were significantly impaired in both cognitive and affective empathy. In particular, patients with lesions in the prefrontal cortex had significantly low empathy scores. Damage to the right hemisphere resulted in greater impairment in cognitive empathy, whereas damage to the right prefrontal cortex did not exert significant impairment in affective empathy (Shamay-Tsoory et al., 2004).

Gillberg (1992, 1996) grouped conditions that could lead to empathy deficiency in a category labeled "disorders of empathy." Gillberg (1996) assumed that humans have an "empathy quotient" that, like the intelligence quotient (IQ), has a normal distribution in the general population (a bell-shaped curve with a mean of 100 and a standard deviation of 15). Accordingly, Gillberg (1996) suggested that, similar to the classification of intellectual abilities (IQ), autism could be arbitrarily classified as an empathic deficiency equivalent to a quotient below 50 (people with an IQ below 50 are classified as either moderately, severely, or profoundly impaired), and Asperger's syndrome (a milder form of autism) would be equivalent to a quotient in the range of 50–70 (people with an IQ between 50 and 70 are classified as mildly impaired).

Empathy for Pain

Before describing the neurological underpinning of empathy, it is important to notice that research findings indicate that patient's higher ratings of physician empathic engagement in rendering care were associated with less pain experiences in patients with chronic pain (Licciardone, Tran, Ngo, Toledo, 2024). Neurological basis of empathic engagement has been explored in a number of pain studies. Understanding the pain and suffering of patients is the backbone of empathic relationships in patient care. Neuroimaging studies have generally shown that in mentally healthy people, observing others in pain activates similar brain areas that are implicated in the person in pain (Jackson, Brunet, Meltzoff, & Decety, 2006). Various painful personal experiences, ranging from being pin-pricked to feeling an aching phantom limb or suffering from social loss, are represented in a complex neural network referred to as the "pain matrix " which is a fluid system jointly activated by pain, composed of several interacting networks including anterior cingulate cortex, anterior insula, as well as frontal and parietal areas (Melzack, 1990).

Pain is an interesting model for incorporating the previously described notions of the ideomotor principle, neuron cell assembly, perception–action coupling, and MNS. A shared representation of others' pain is suggested by the findings that neuron cells in the human cingulate cortex fire when pain is inflicted and when a person observes another person in pain. Empathy for pain can also be a function of the situations, attitudes, and personal relationships. For example, Englis, Vaughan, and Lanzetta (1982) reported that empathy for pain was elicited when the observer had a cooperative (as opposed to competitive) relationship with the person in pain. In a study by Singer et al. (2006), male and female participants engaged in an economic game with two confederates who were professional actors; one confederate played fairly, but the other confederate played unfairly. Brain activities of the participants were recorded when the confederates received painful stimulus to the hand. Both male and female participants showed brain activities in the pain-related brain areas (frontoinsular and anterior cingulate cortices) toward fair players. However, pain-related brain activation was less pronounced for male participants when observing the unfair player receiving pain. These findings suggest that empathic response to pain in men is a function of their attitudes toward social behavior of others in pain. Hein and Singer (2008) reported that the amplitude of perception of other's pain is modulated by the intensity of emotion, characteristics of the suffering person, gender, and perceived fairness.

In a pain study, a series of pictures of hands and feet in painful situations and another series of pictures of hands and feet in non-painful situations were shown to research participants (Jackson et al., 2005). The fMRI images showed activation of several brain regions in the observers that are known to play a significant role in pain processing (e.g., anterior cingulate cortex, anterior insula, and the cerebellum). Brain regions associated with feeling an emotion can also be influenced by seeing the facial expression of that emotion, a phenomenon described as emotional contagion or sympathy (Singer et al., 2004).

Several neuroimaging studies have demonstrated commonalities in pain matrix activation when subjects experience pain themselves and when they observe others in pain (Morrison, Lloyd, di Pellegrino, & Roberts, 2004). Common areas include thalamus, anterior cingulate cortex, anterior insula, and prefrontal cortex. This is especially true when the person in pain is a significant figure, like a family member, friend, or partner (Holden, 2004). For example, mothers listened to recorded infant cries and white noise control sounds. The fMRI results indicated that the mothers showed significantly greater anterior cingulate cortex activity upon hearing the baby cries compared to white noise. This finding demonstrates the plasticity or reactivity of the pain matrix to internal psychological factors.

In an fMRI study, it was observed that when subjects received pain or were signaled that loved ones were experiencing pain, the bilateral anterior insula, rostral anterior cingulate cortex, brainstem, and cerebellum were activated. It was also noted that activation intensity in brain areas, when observing others in pain, was correlated with individual empathy scores (Singer et al., 2004).

Evidence also suggests that empathic engagement is more contingent upon the frontocortical brain areas, which have been implicated in mentalization and the theory of mind (Nummenmaa et al., 2008; Wellman, 1991). The medial prefrontal cortex has also been implicated in the theory of mind (Gallagher & Frith, 2003), suggesting that this area of the brain may constitute a partial system for empathy (Nummenmaa et al., 2008). The medial prefrontal cortex appears to play a role in the ruminative focus on pain and apprehension about pain's implications.

Research showed sympathetic involvement with a person in pain increased activity in the anterior insula and thalamus, which are involved in processing negative or unpleasant emotions (Nummenmaa et al., 2008). It is also interesting to note that pain-related areas in the anterior cingulate cortex have extensive output connections to premotor areas, a brain region observed to contain much of the MNS in macaque monkeys (Morrison et al., 2004). Some of the same neural activities in the experience of physical pain are also involved in the experience of social pain (e.g., separation, rejection, social exclusion, and losing a significant person) (Eisenberger, Leiberman, & Williams, 2003). Thus, the expression of being *hurt* by experiencing loneliness, rejection, and separation is not metaphoric only, but real in nature and operates by sharing common neuroanatomical underpinnings with physical pain. Studies have demonstrated that sadness, social exclusion, and physical pain activate similar limbic regions (e.g., anterior cingulate cortex and anterior insula) (Loggia, Mogil, & Bushnell, 2008). It should also be mentioned that in addition to the somatosensory, cognitive, and emotional factors, other variables such as genetics, gender, and culture contribute to the perception of pain and to the physicians' approach in the treatment of pain (Grossman & Wood, 1993; Safdar et al., 2009; Weisman & Teitlebaum, 1985).

Avenanti, Bueti, Galati, and Aglioti (2005) showed that empathy for pain increased the blood oxygen level dependent (BOLD) signal in the anterior insula and anterior cingulate cortices, which are part of the affective division of the pain matrix. Neural activity in the affective pain network was also reported in fMRI studies where subjects observed pictures or movies in which potentially painful stimuli were delivered to hands or other human body parts (Jackson et al., 2005; Morrison et al., 2004; Singer et al., 2004).

Approaches to Study the Neurobiophysiology of Pain

Three approaches have often been used in social cognitive neuroscience research in studying perception of pain: (1) studying pain parameters when the person is experiencing pain (self-pain); (2) recording biological, physiological, and psychological changes and neurological activities when observing another person in pain and imagining oneself actually experiencing the other person's pain (self-perspective or first-person representation); (3) recording biological, physiological, and psychological changes and neurological activities when observing another person in pain, but imagining how that person would experience pain (other-perspective or third-person representation).

Understanding perception of self-pain versus self-perspective of other's pain versus other-perspective of pain requires a distinction between self and others when merging with self, and when separating other's pain from one's own. These different perspectives on pain involve different forms of perceptions, which lead to different consequences (Batson, Early, & Salvarini, 1997). For example, research in social psychology (Batson et al., 2003; Underwood & Moore, 1982) has documented this distinction by showing that self-perspective is likely to induce personal distress (akin to emotional empathy), whereas other-perspective is likely to evoke perspective taking (akin to cognitive empathy).

In the conceptualization of empathy, researchers have often failed to make a distinction between the self- and other-oriented perspective taking (Coplan, 2014). The two types of perspective taking are not only conceptually different, but also recruit different neurological mechanisms. For example, other-oriented perspective taking requires greater mental flexibility and emotional regulation, whereas self-oriented perspective taking is likely to lead to egocentric affective response and emotional exhaustion (Coplan, 2014; Jackson, Brunt, et al., 2006), which is akin to sympathetic reaction. For a true empathic engagement, it is essential to make a clear distinction between self- and other-oriented perspective taking.

One of the earlier experiments on perception of pain in others was conducted by Stotland (1969) in which three groups of participants viewed a subject whose hand was strapped in a heat generating machine. One group was instructed just to watch the event non-judgmentally (neutral observation). The second group was instructed to imagine their own hand strapped in the machine (self-perspective). The third group was told to imagine how the person whose hand was strapped was feeling (other-perspective). It was found that imagining the pain of others could generate cognitive and emotional empathic connections, and produce similar tangible physiological responses which corresponded to perception of pain as predicted by PAM (e.g., palm sweating and galvanic skin response). Data from functional brain imaging studies show that imagining pain in one's self and others, in the absence of any painful stimulus, activates critical brain areas involved in pain perception (Ochsner et al., 2008).

It has been consistently reported that observing someone in pain activates neurons in the observer similar to those that are firing in the person experiencing pain (Botvinick et al., 2005; Jackson et al., 2005). Findings in pain research have generally showed that both the self-perspective and the other-perspective were associated with activation in the neural network involved in pain processing, including the parietal operculum, anterior medial cingulate, and the anterior insula (Derbyshire, 2000; Lamm et al., 2007). However, the self-perspective yielded higher pain ratings and involved the pain matrix more extensively in the secondary somatosensory cortex, the posterior part of the anterior cingulated cortex, and the middle insula (Derbyshire, 2000).

In one study, participants received painful stimuli in some trials, and in other trials participants observed a signal that their partner, who was present in the same room, would receive the same stimuli (Singer et al., 2004). The anterior medial cingulated cortex, the anterior insula, and the cerebellum were activated during both conditions. Similar results were reported by Morrison et al. (2004), who applied a moderately painful pinprick stimulus to the fingertips of their participants and in a second condition showed them a video clip showing another person undergoing similar stimulation. Both conditions resulted in common activities in pain-related areas of the cingulated cortex.

In another study, participants were shown photos depicting right hands and feet in painful or neutral situations, and were asked to imagine the level of pain that these situations would generate (Jackson et al., 2005). Significant activation was detected in regions involved in the pain matrix network, notably in the anterior cingulated cortex and the anterior insula. Yet in another study (Lamm et al., 2007), participants were requested to watch the videos adopting two different perspectives, that is, either imagining how they themselves would feel if they were in the place of the other (imagine self), or imagining how the other feels (imagine other). Results supported the view that response to the pain of others can be a function of cognitive and motivational factors. In other words, observing others in pain can either evoke empathic response and altruistic motivation, or personal distress and egoistic motivation to reduce one's own distress, depending upon the capacity for self–other differentiation and cognitive appraisal (Lamm et al., 2007). For example, perception of pain via the self-perspective approach is likely to evoke an egoistic motivation to reduce personal distress associated with the activated brain that controls emotional pain response, whereas the other-perspective approach is likely to instigate an altruistic motivation to help (Batson, 1991; Dovidio, 1991; Goubert et al., 2005). Altruistic motivation is more aligned with our characterization of cognitively defined empathy, which allows planning, whereas egoistic motivation fits better with our description of emotionally defined sympathy (or emotional empathy), which is more likely to be spontaneous (see Chap. 1).

Research Challenges

It is important to notice that in neurological research of empathy, with the exception of a very few studies (Dziobek et al., 2008; Nummenmaa et al., 2008; Shamay-Tsoory et al., 2004), no clear distinction has been made between cognitive and emotional empathy (Morelli, Rameson, & Lieberman, 2014) and their differential motivational factors and especially their different consequences in the context of patient care (see Chap. 6). No wonder that the results of most studies on the neurological underpinnings of empathy are inconsistent because of conceptual ambiguity (associated with conceptualization and definition) and methodological shortcomings (associated with measurement of the concepts and research design). Thus, research outcomes cannot be specifically attributed to only one of the two forms of cognitive or emotional empathy (or empathy and sympathy, respectively).

It is difficult to dissociate cognitive and emotional empathy within the traditional pain paradigm because they are somewhat correlated (Jackson et al., 2005), but if we fail to make such a distinction we can never find the correct answer in our search for neurological underpinnings of empathy (as opposed to sympathy). The challenge ahead is to propose agreeable conceptualizations and definitions of cognitive and emotional empathy and their corresponding measurements; and then develop new research paradigms to evoke cognitive empathic responses for one and emotional empathic reactions for the other (e.g., using event-related brain imaging). Finally, we can be in a better position to examine similarities and differences in brain activation in response to scenarios that evoke cognitive or emotional empathy. Based on the characterization of the two concepts (see Chaps. 1, 3, and 6), and based on some of the neurological findings reported in this chapter, distinct brain activations can be expected in cognitive empathic responses (e.g., most likely in the premotor and prefrontal cortex) and in emotional empathic reactions (e.g., most likely in the amygdala, insular, and cingulate cortex).

Furthermore, brain lesion research may also shed light on the detrimental effects on cognitive and emotional empathy of damage to cortical or limbic structures, respectively. Admittedly, this is a very simplistic view of a complex behavioral-social concept (such as empathy), which is certainly more complicated, and convoluted by many biophysioneurological, personal, social, cultural, and educational factors and their interactions. It is a real challenge to tease out the psychological effects of emotion from cognition, and empathy from sympathy in our search for neurological underpinnings of empathy. We can hope for the best meaningful outcomes because even the sky is no limit in the realm of scientific inquiry.

Recapitulation

Human beings are evolved to understand and to be understood for survival. Theoretical views on ideomotor principle, neuron cell assembly, perception–action coupling, and MNS, as well as empirical findings in social cognitive neuroscience, support the notion that neurological activities are involved in the process of understanding others and being understood by others. Brain imaging, brain lesion studies, and research findings on brain activities involved in perception of pain provide tangible evidence in support of neurological underpinnings of empathy. Research findings, however, are not consistent, probably due to conceptual ambiguity (e.g., a lack of distinction between cognitive and emotional empathy, or empathy and sympathy, respectively) and methodological shortcomings (e.g., measurement and research design issues). Future explorations on neurological underpinnings of empathy should clarify the conceptual ambiguity, and measurement issues, as well as development of appropriate research paradigms to address neurological underpinnings of empathy. Without such conceptual and methodological rigor, we may never find a satisfactory answer in our search for neurological roots of empathy.

Chapter 14
The Project in Osteopathic Medical Education and Empathy (POMEE): A Landmark Nationwide Study of Clinical Empathy in United States Medical Students

To be understood is a basic human need
that can be fulfilled when an empathic connection is formed.

—(Hojat, 2016, p. 77)

Abstract

- This chapter briefly describes the "*Project in Osteopathic Medical Education and Empathy*" *(POMEE)*, a groundbreaking nationwide study of clinical empathy and medical education research on the largest scale ever undertaken. POMEE was designed to address correlates, group differences, enhancement and erosion of clinical empathy, and pertinent personal qualities associated with clinical empathy in osteopathic medical students in the United States.
- The unique features of POMEE include: participation of large nationwide samples, representative of corresponding populations of US osteopathic medical students in all years of medical school education; use of a content-specific and context-relevant psychometrically sound instrument (JSE S-Version) for measuring clinical empathy; and statistical control to mitigate the effect of social desirability response bias, implemented for the first time in a national study of medical education. These unique features add to our confidence about internal and external validity, utility, reproducibility, and generalizability of POMEE findings.
- POMEE was designed as a two-phased project. Phase I was a cross-sectional (2-year) study, and Phase II was a longitudinal (5-year) project. Goals of both phases of POMEE are described in this chapter. A web-based study survey was administered to students who voluntarily participated in the project.
- Highlights of findings of POMEE showed significant differences in clinical empathy by gender, race/ethnicity, academic background, and career interest;

M. Hojat, *Clinical Empathy*, https://doi.org/10.1007/978-3-031-87413-0_14

and significant associations with pertinent personal qualities such as attitudes toward interprofessional collaboration, orientation toward lifelong learning, and burnout experiences.
- A significant decline in clinical empathy was found in the clinical phase of medical education that was less pronounced among osteopathic compared to allopathic medical students.
- National norm tables for clinical empathy scores were developed for osteopathic medical students at different years of medical school education from matriculation to graduation.
- A new instrument that we developed in POMEE-Phase II for measuring attitudes toward osteopathic medicine is described, and its psychometrics are reported in this chapter.
- Measurement properties, psychometrics, and national norm tables were presented for the first time in osteopathic medical school matriculants for pertinent personal quality measures that yielded significant associations with clinical empathy, such as attitudes toward interprofessional collaboration, orientation toward physician lifelong learning, and burnout experiences.
- POMEE-Phase II was not completed as planned due to premature termination of funding and some of its major goals remain unfulfilled.

Introduction

Based on my 40 plus years of involvement in medical education research, I consider the *Project in Osteopathic Medical Education and Empathy* (POMEE) a landmark and unique nationwide medical education research study, because of its special features that I will describe in this chapter. I served as the principal investigator of this landmark project, which aimed to study the development of clinical empathy during medical school education, its correlates, group differences, and outcomes.

This chapter describes a brief history of the project, and some of its special features. It reports highlights of selected published and unpublished findings and their implications for medical education. It also describes the major goals of the project that were successfully achieved, and those that, due to unforeseeable events, remain unfulfilled!

How the Project Was Initiated

I believe it was sometime in 2016 that I received a telephone call in my office from a soft-spoken man who introduced himself as Len Calabrese, calling from the Cleveland Clinic. After greetings, he expressed admiration for my published research on clinical empathy and mentioned his interest in research on the topic of empathy in osteopathic medical education. He also indicated his plan to travel to the

City of Brotherly Love to meet me at Jefferson in my office to chat about his ideas of large-scale research on the topic, and the possibility of a collaborative project.

I found the conversation cordial, and his amiable words and friendly tone of his voice favorably inclined me to meet him in-person. However, not knowing him well, I endeavored to learn more about the caller's academic background, research interest, and professional position. Thus, I responded that I would check my calendar to find a few dates that could work for both of us to meet in the near future to discuss the possibility of a collaborative research project.

To learn more about Len Calabrese, I navigated a few search engines, including Google, and found that Leonard Calabrese, DO, was a distinguished professor of medicine at the Cleveland Clinic Lerner College of Medicine of Case Western University; Chairman of Osteopathic Research and Education; R.J. Fasenmyer Chair of Clinical Immunology; and Vice Chair of Department of Rheumatic and Immunology Diseases at the Cleveland Clinic, with an impressive record of publications and presentations.

I called Dr. Calabrese to tell him that I was impressed by his record of scholarly work, patient care, and research; thus, instead of him coming to Jefferson to see me, I would be happy to go to the Cleveland Clinic to meet him and his team and present some of my clinical empathy research findings, and also discuss the possibility of collaborative research. That meeting at the Cleveland Clinic went well, and I found that Dr. Calabrese had an ambitious research idea in mind to undertake a large-scale study of clinical empathy in osteopathic medical education. Particularly, I found him genuinely concerned about training empathic physicians.

To pursue the idea of a large-scale study of clinical empathy in osteopathic medical students, assess willingness of deans of osteopathic medical colleges, and seek funding sources for the project, Dr. Calabrese developed a plan for a national meeting. He scheduled a national conference in Scottsdale, Arizona (November 17, 2016), and invited deans of colleges of osteopathic medicine, a few key figures from the American Association of Colleges of Osteopathic Medicine (AACOM) and the American Osteopathic Association (AOA), and a few researchers interested in clinical empathy (including Helen Riess, M.D., and Richard Frankel, Ph.D.). The meeting at the beginning did not go as well as we expected, mainly because most of the participating deans estimated very low response rates by medical students in web-based surveys (in the range of 20%).

In a break during the meeting, I found Dr. Calabrese in a kind of disappointed mood. After a couple of toasts, I tried to cheer him up and discussed my idea of how to proceed before giving up the idea of a nationwide project. I suggested that we propose a two-phased project, using Phase I as a pilot study for Phase II to get an idea about the willingness of the US colleges of osteopathic medicine to participate in the project and willingness of osteopathic medical students to complete web-based study surveys. In the proposal, we specified that pursuing Phase II of the project would be conditional upon the success of Phase I. We both agreed that obtaining a participation rate of more than 50% of all US colleges of osteopathic medicine and a response rate of at least 50% of medical students from participating colleges would give us a green light to pursue Phase II.

This approach could provide insights surrounding the issue of participation and response rates raised by deans of osteopathic medical colleges at the Scottsdale conference. This suggestion made Dr. Calabrese less worried about the deans' concerns on response rates. We had another toast! Dr. Calabrese patted me gently on my shoulder in response to my suggestion and said: "Let's pursue it!" It was also Dr. Calabrese who suggested the title for the study: "*Project in Osteopathic Medical Education and Empathy,*" and its abbreviation: "POMEE."

I could never have imagined that a short conversation between Dr. Calabrese and me that day at a meeting break in Scottsdale could lead to a groundbreaking project in medical education research on clinical empathy. We decided to prepare a draft of the POMEE proposal for funding purposes. And...this was how POMEE was initiated!

A short time after the Scottsdale conference, Dr. Calabrese invited me to travel to the headquarters of the AACOM for a meeting with its leadership (including Dr. Shannon, then the president and CEO of the AACOM) to present the idea of a nationwide project on medical education and clinical empathy and discuss the research plan and how to proceed. It was also decided to gather key medical education leaders from the AACOM to visit our Center for Research in Medical Education and Healthcare at Jefferson and discuss a collaborative project.

In that meeting, it was suggested that I develop an initial proposal for Phase I of the project and its goals, research design, sampling design, study survey, data collection procedures, statistical analyses, implications of the findings for medical education, and a plan for dissemination of results for publication or presentations. The proposal was promptly funded by the AACOM with a shared contribution from the AOA, in collaboration with the Cleveland Clinic and the Sidney Kimmel Medical College of Thomas Jefferson University. Therefore, POMEE did not go through regular steps of initially responding to a request for proposal (RFP) to secure funding. It was indeed an invited project by the funding organizations through the efforts of Dr. Calabrese.

Development of a Two-Phased Project

In consultation with Dr. Calabrese, we planned for the two-phased project in which Phase I would be a 2-year *cross-sectional study* of clinical empathy in US osteopathic medical students in all 4 years of medical schools. Phase I would lay the foundation for Phase II (a 5-year *longitudinal study*), to ensure that representative samples of osteopathic medical colleges would be willing to participate, and that a reasonably large number of students, representing the populations of osteopathic medical students in different years of medical school education, would be willing to complete a web-based and relatively long study survey.

Special Features of POMEE

POMEE uniquely benefits from the following special features:

1. Research participants included large nationwide samples of osteopathic medical students in all 4 years of medical school education, resembling the national population of osteopathic medical students in the US, based on their age, gender, and race/ethnicity (Hojat, Shannon, DeSantis, Speicher et al., 2019).
2. To measure clinical empathy, it used a well-established psychologically sound instrument, the *Jefferson Scale of Empathy* (JSE), tailored specifically for medical students (JSE S-Version, see Chap. 7, also Appendix A). The JSE S-Version at the present time is the only content-specific and context-relevant instrument for measuring clinical empathy in medical students, with strong evidence in support of its validity and reliability (Chap. 7). Also, as part of POMEE (Hojat, DeSantis, Shannon et al., 2018), we provided further evidence in support of the measurement properties and psychometrics of the JSE-S version in osteopathic medical students, which will be briefly described in this chapter.
3. Statistical control to mitigate the effect of the social desirability response bias from respondents' attempts to provide "good impression" responses, by using the "Infrequency" scale from the *Zuckerman–Kuhlman Personality Questionnaire* (ZKPQ) (Zuckerman, 2002; Hojat, Zuckerman, Gonnella, Mangione et al., 2005).
4. Another advantage and feature of POMEE was that it provided a unique opportunity to examine consistencies (or inconsistencies) in findings from its different nationwide samples (e.g., in different years of medical school education) which could provide evidence for the generalization of the findings and enable comparing POMEE findings with other published studies on clinical empathy in allopathic medical students.

Specifically, the aforementioned features increase our confidence about the internal validity (true relationships amongst study variables) and external validity (generalization of findings) of clinical empathy in medical students, thus providing more definitive answers to clinical empathy issues that are of interest to medical education researchers.

A brief description of POMEE was posted on the following link on the AACOM website: https://www.aacom.org/programs-events/programs-initiatives/project-in-osteopathic-medical-education-and-empathy.

The Major Goals of POMEE-Phase I

This phase of the project was a *cross-sectional* study, designed to address the following issues:

1. Provide further evidence in support of measurement properties and psychometrics of the JSE S-Version in osteopathic medical students.

2. Collect descriptive statistics of the JSE S-Version scores in osteopathic medical students and examine group differences on the JSE scores by gender, year in medical school, specialty interest, race/ethnicity, and academic background.
3. Compare findings from osteopathic students with previous findings from allopathic medical students to examine similarities and differences in pattern of changes of clinical empathy scores (decline or increase) in different years of medical school education.
4. Develop national norm tables for scores of the JSE S-Version.

The Major Goals of POMEE-Phase II

POMEE-Phase II was a *longitudinal study*, designed to achieve the following objectives:

1. Examine changes (increase or decline) in clinical empathy, emotional empathy, and selected personal quality measures (e.g., attitudes toward osteopathic medicine, attitudes toward interprofessional collaboration, orientation toward physician lifelong learning, and burnout experiences) as the study cohort progress through medical school.
2. Explore reasons for positive and negative changes in clinical empathy, reported by the study cohort in their medical school education.
3. Examine the magnitude of associations between clinical and emotional empathy with personal quality measures such as attitudes toward osteopathic medicine, attitudes toward interprofessional collaboration, orientation toward physician lifelong learning, and burnout experiences as the study cohort progresses through medical school education from matriculation to graduation.
4. Investigate contributions of selected variables on changes in clinical empathy, such as: school's specific admissions policies, old versus new schools, geographical location, specific medical education curriculum, special programs in communication skills, etc.
5. Assess the effects of targeted educational programs for enhancing clinical empathy.

The Study Survey for POMEE-Phase I

A web-based study survey was specifically developed for Phase I, and an expanded version of the survey was developed for Phase II of the project. The study survey in Phase I consisted of questions about students' gender, age, race and ethnicity, academic background, and career interest, plus the following two instruments:

1. The *Jefferson Scale of Empathy Medical Student Version* (JSE S-Version) for measuring clinical empathy (a 20-item instrument described in detail in Chap. 7).

2. *The Infrequency Scale* (10 items) from the Zuckerman–Kuhlman Personality Questionnaire (ZKPQ) (Zuckerman, 2002) was used to mitigate the effect of social desirability response bias, by identifying respondents who attempt to give socially desirable responses that are unlikely to be true (e.g., "I never met a person I didn't like"), indicating questionable validity for that respondent's record.

Expansion of the Study Survey in POMEE-Phase II

In addition to the *JSE S-Version*, and the *Infrequency Scale* of the ZKPQ, we included the following five instruments to the study survey of POMEE-Phase II:

1. *Attitudes Toward Osteopathic Medicine Scale* (ATOMS): We developed a new 13-item survey to measure respondents' attitudes toward the tenets and philosophy of osteopathic medicine that included the following three components, based on the results of factor analysis: "Perceptions of Osteopathic Medicine," "Osteopathic Diagnosis and Treatment," and "Holistic Care." Measurement properties and psychometrics of the ATOMS were reported, using a nationwide sample of first-year students, as part of POMEE-Phase II (Hojat, DeSantis, Cain et al., 2021). This instrument will be described later in this chapter.
2. *Emotional Empathy*: We selected two subscales, "Empathic Concern" and "Personal Distress" from the *Interpersonal Reactivity Index* (IRI) (Davis, 1983, 1994) for measuring emotional empathy (used by permission). These subscales measure emotional empathy according to the author of the IRI (Davis, 1983, p. 114), and particularly "Empathic Concern" assesses feeling of sympathy and concern for others (See Chap. 5 for a brief description of the IRI).
3. *Jefferson Scale of Attitudes Toward Interprofessional Collaboration* (JeffSATIC): This 20-item instrument that we developed at Jefferson measures attitudes or orientation toward interprofessional collaboration and teamwork in health professions students and practitioners. Strong support for its measurement properties and psychometrics has been reported in a multi-institutional and multi-national study of health professions students (Hojat, Ward, Spandorfer et al., 2015).
4. *Jefferson Scale of Physician Lifelong Learning* (JeffSPLL): This is a 14-item instrument we developed at Jefferson for measuring orientation toward lifelong learning in medical students and physicians. Evidence in support of its psychometrics has been reported in medical students (Wetzel, Mazmanian, Hojat et al., 2010) and physicians (Hojat, Nasca, Gonnella, Frisby et al., 2003; Hojat, Veloski, & Gonnella, 2009, 2010, 2012).
5. *Shirom–Melamed Burnout Measure* (SMBM): This is a 14-item instrument (used by permission) to measure burnout experiences (Shirom & Melamed, 2006; Melamed, Sharom, Toker et al., 2006; Gerber, Colledge, Mucke et al., 2018).

Data Collection

In both POMEE phases, medical students in participating osteopathic medical colleges were informed by their college's assigned research coordinators, leadership, and local newsletters/publications about the importance of the nationwide project (POMEE). Students were encouraged to voluntarily participate in the project, and were reminded that they would receive the link to the study survey via their student email address. They were also assured that personal data would be treated with strict confidentiality. No additional personal identity information was solicited from respondents in the study surveys, with the exception of a voluntary option for respondents to enter their email address to receive feedback on their JSE scores, and for the purpose of merging data (by email address) from the study cohort in different years of medical school in Phase II-POMEE.

Study Participants in POMEE-Phase I

Overall, 16,760 completed surveys were received in the 2017–2018 academic year, comprising new matriculants ($n = 6009$), and students at the end of the first-year ($n = 3616$), second-year ($n = 2764$), third-year ($n = 2413$), and fourth-year ($n = 1958$) of medical school education in 41 of 48 US campuses of colleges of osteopathic medicine (the number of observations in different statistical analyses varies due to availability of data in the corresponding analyses).

Study Cohort in POMEE-Phase II

The study cohort in POMEE-Phase II included 5696 first-year matriculants from 46 campuses of US colleges of osteopathic medicine in the 2019–2020 academic year, who voluntarily participated in the project. And according to the longitudinal study design, this cohort was to be followed-up during their medical school education and possibly after medical school.

Published Studies from POMEE-Phase I

Selected findings from POMEE-Phase I were reported in four articles published prior to the ending date of the project, which are described below.

Measurement Properties and Psychometrics of the JSE S-Version

The *first* publication reported measurement properties and psychometrics of the JSE S-Version in osteopathic medical students (Hojat, DeSantis, Shannon, Mortensen et al., 2018). Because the study samples of almost all other studies on psychometrics of the JSE S-Version included students from allopathic medical schools, it was necessary to provide evidence supporting measurement properties and psychometrics of the JSE S-Version in osteopathic medical students. POMEE provided a unique opportunity, and the results were very encouraging.

Participants of this study included 6009 first-year students who voluntarily completed the study survey at the beginning of medical school (2017–2018 academic year). The web-based study survey was administered to all first-year matriculants of participating campuses of US colleges of osteopathic medicine.

Descriptive Statistics

Descriptive statistics and Cronbach's coefficient alpha for men and women and for the total sample are reported in Table 14.1. The JSE mean score for the total study cohort was 116.54 ($SD = 10.85$). The mean score for men was 114.40 ($SD = 11.34$); for women it was 118.78 ($SD = 9.78$). The gender difference was statistically significant ($p < 0.01$). Results remained unchanged by using analysis of covariance, controlling for the social desirability response bias (scores of the Infrequency Scale of the ZKPQ, as a covariate). The magnitudes of Cronbach's coefficient alpha were 0.82, 0.83, and 0.81 for the total sample, men, and women, respectively.

Table 14.1 Descriptive statistics of the JSE S-Version scores in a nationwide sample of 6009 first-year students at the beginning of the 2017–2018 academic year from 41 campuses of US colleges of osteopathic medicine

Statistics	Men ($n = 3175$)	Women ($n = 2795$)	Total ($n = 5970$)[a]
Mean	114.40	118.78	116.54
Median	115	120	117
Mode	116	119	119
Standard deviation	11.34	9.78	10.85
Possible range	20–140	20–140	20–140
Actual range	26–140	69–140	26–140
Skewness	−0.54	−0.61	−0.60
Kurtosis	1.29	0.58	1.15
Cronbach's coefficient Alpha	0.83	0.81	0.82

Reproduced from Hojat, DeSantis, Shannon et al. (2018). ©Authors, Open Access

[a]Thirty-nine respondents who did not specify their gender or reported other gender categories were excluded from statistical analysis

Although the obtained mean scores for the first-year matriculants in osteopathic medical schools, shown in Table 14.1, were slightly higher than those for their counterparts in a large sample of one allopathic medical school (Hojat & Gonnella, 2015, also see Chap. 7), the pattern of other findings reported in Table 14.1 is close to those reported in allopathic medical students (reported in Chap. 7).

Item-Total Score Correlations and Effect Sizes of Item Discrimination Indices

Pearson correlation coefficients were calculated to examine correlations between each item score and the total score of the JSE. For that purpose, we calculated the corrected item-total score correlations (by excluding the corresponding item from the total JSE score). Corrected item-total score correlations ranged from a low of 0.20 to a high of 0.61 (median = 0.46). The item with the highest item-total score correlation was: "Physicians' understanding of the emotional status of their patients, as well as that of their patients' families is one important component of physician-patient relationship" ($r = 0.61$), and the item with lowest item-total score correlation was: "Physicians should not allow themselves to be influenced by strong personal bonds between their patients and their patients family members" ($r = 0.20$). All correlations were positive and statistically significant ($p < 0.01$). Summary results are reported in Table 14.2. The pattern of findings is similar to that reported for the first-year students in an allopathic medical school (Hojat & Gonnella, 2015).

To address the discrimination power of each item, we calculated the item discrimination index. For that purpose, we divided the sample into two groups of approximately top-third high scorers on the JSE (score > 122, $n = 2096$) and bottom-third low scorers (JSE score < 112, $n = 2028$). For each item, we calculated the difference of its mean scores between the top- and bottom-third scoring groups, then divided the mean difference for each item by the pooled standard deviation of the item scores to calculate the item discrimination effect size index (similar to the Cohen's *d*, [Cohen, 1987]).

Effect size estimates of the item discrimination indices are reported in Table 14.2. The item discrimination effect size indices ranged from a low of 0.67 to a high of 1.42 (median = 1.14). According to operational definitions on the magnitude of effect size estimates (*d*), suggested by Cohen (1987), all of the item discrimination effect size estimates reported in Table 14.2 are considered substantial and practically important. As expected, the item-total score correlations and the effect size estimates of the item discrimination indices were highly correlated ($r = 0.97$, $p < 0.01$). The pattern of findings is similar to that reported in a large sample of first-year students in an allopathic medical school (Hojat & Gonnella, 2015).

Table 14.2 Corrected item-total score correlations[a] and effect size estimates of item discrimination indices[b] for the Jefferson Scale of Empathy in a national sample of 6009 first-year students at the beginning of the 2017–2018 academic year from 41 campuses of US colleges of osteopathic medicine

Abbreviated JSE items[c]	Corrected item-total score correlation	Effect size of discrimination index
Understanding emotions in patient–clinician relationship (16)	0.61	1.42
Empathy as a therapeutic factor (20)	0.60	1.37
Attention to patients' personal experiences (8)	0.54	1.30
Nonverbal cues and body language in understanding patients (13)	0.53	1.29
Patient–physician emotional ties in medical treatment (11)	0.53	1.24
Place of emotion in medical treatment (14)	0.53	1.14
Understanding is therapeutic to patient (10)	0.51	1.27
Standing in patients' shoes (9)	0.51	1.27
Life events in understanding physical complaints (12)	0.49	1.33
Attention to patients' emotions (7)	0.47	1.13
Empathy and clinical success (15)	0.45	1.18
Understanding makes patients feel better (2)	0.43	1.02
Thinking like patients for better care (17)	0.41	1.14
Understanding body language in communication (4)	0.38	0.98
Understanding patients' feelings influences treatment (1)	0.38	1.03
Taking patients' perspectives (6)	0.26	0.81
Viewing patients' perspectives (3)	0.26	0.78
Enjoy literature and arts (19)	0.25	0.77
Sense of humor and clinical outcomes (5)	0.21	0.67
Physician influenced by patients' personal bonds (18)	0.20	0.67
Mean (Median)	0.43 (0.46)	1.09 (1.14)

Reproduced from Hojat, DeSantis, Shannon et al. (2018). ©Authors, Open Access

[a]Correlations between scores on each item and the JSE total score by excluding the corresponding item from the total score. All correlations are statistically significant ($p < 0.01$)

[b]In calculation of the effect size estimate (Cohen's *d*) of the discrimination index, the item mean score of the JSE high scorers (top 33%, $n = 2096$) was subtracted from JSE low scorers (bottom 33%, $n = 2028$), divided by the pooled standard deviation of the corresponding item

[c]Numbers in parentheses correspond to the item numbers in the JSE

Underlying Factors of the JSE S-Version

To examine underlying factors (components) of the JSE S-Version in the study sample, we randomly divided the sample into two groups. Data for the first group ($n = 3004$) were used for exploratory factor analysis to determine underlying components of the JSE, and data for the second group ($n = 3005$) were used for confirmatory factor analysis to confirm the latent variable structure of the JSE. Before performing factor analyses, we compared the two groups and found no significant differences in gender, age, ethnicity/race, and their scores on the JSE and the Infrequency Scale of the ZKPQ. For detailed description of procedures and results of exploratory and confirmatory factor analyses, see Hojat, DeSantis, Shannon et al. (2018).

Exploratory and Confirmatory Factor Analysis of the JSE S-Version

The three-factor model ("Perspective Taking," "Compassionate Care," and "Walking in Patient's Shoes") which emerged in most other factor analytic studies of the JSE with allopathic medical and other health professions students (see Chap. 7) also emerged in the exploratory factor analysis of POMEE data (see Table 14.3). More detailed findings from exploratory factor analysis are depicted in Fig. 14.1.

Table 14.3 Rotated factor pattern[a] for the JSE S-Version using a national sample of 6009 first-year students at the beginning of the 2017–2018 academic year from 41 campuses of US colleges of osteopathic medicine

	Factors[b]		
Abbreviated JSE items[c]	Factor 1	Factor 2	Factor 3
Standing in patients' shoes (9)	**0.66**	−0.03	0.00
Understanding is therapeutic to patient (10)	**0.62**	0.01	0.01
Understanding emotions in patient–clinician relationship (16)	**0.61**	0.16	0.00
Thinking like patients for better care (17)	**0.60**	−0.08	−0.03
Nonverbal cues and body language in understanding patients (13)	**0.57**	0.10	0.00
Empathy as a therapeutic factor (20)	**0.54**	0.20	0.00
Understanding makes patients feel better (2)	**0.53**	0.01	−0.01
Understanding body language in communication (4)	**0.48**	−0.04	0.07
Empathy and clinical success (15)	**0.44**	0.10	0.00
Sense of humor and clinical outcomes (5)	**0.35**	−0.09	−0.01
Attention to patients' personal experiences (8)	0.03	**0.65**	−0.02
Patient–physician emotional ties in medical treatment (11)	0.03	**0.64**	−0.01
Place of emotion in medical treatment (14)	0.03	**0.62**	0.00
Understanding patients' feelings influences treatment (1)	−0.09	**0.59**	−0.08
Life events in understanding physical complaints (12)	0.05	**0.54**	0.06
Attention to patients' emotions (7)	0.03	**0.52**	0.07

(continued)

Table 14.3 (continued)

Abbreviated JSE items[c]	Factors[b] Factor 1	Factor 2	Factor 3
Enjoy literature and arts (19)	−0.02	0.28	0.05
Physician influenced by patients' personal bonds (18)	−0.01	0.21	0.05
Taking patients' perspectives (6)	−0.03	0.05	**0.77**
Viewing patients' perspectives (3)	0.03	−0.01	**0.72**
Eigenvalues	5.52	1.66	1.39

Reproduced from Hojat, DeSantis, Shannon et al. (2018). ©Authors, Open Access
[a]Principal component factor analysis with oblique rotation used for half of the sample (n = 3004). Confirmatory factor analysis was performed in the other half of the sample (n = 3005)
[b]Items are listed by descending order of magnitude of factor coefficients with each factor. Factor coefficients ≥0.35 are shown in **bold**. Items were scored using a seven-point Likert-type scale. Half of the items are reversed scored
[c]Numbers in parentheses refer to the item number in the JSE

In addition, confirmatory factor analysis supported the three-factor model in this national sample of osteopathic medical students (Hojat, DeSantis, Shannon et al., 2018). Findings were consistent with those of most other factor analytic results in allopathic medical students (Hojat & Gonnella, 2015, see Chap. 7). However, in a large-scale exploratory and confirmatory factor analytic study in multiple allopathic medical schools in the US (Stansfield et al., 2016), the three-factor model was suggested as an acceptable fit for preclinical years, but in that study, a four-factor model emerged as a better fit for clinical years in allopathic medical students.

Similarities in factor patterns of the JSE S-Version in different samples, medical education systems, and in different countries (see Chap. 7 and Appendix A) indicate that the underlying components of the JSE are relatively stable, regardless of cultural variation and differences in medical education systems (Hojat, DeSantis, Shannon et al., 2018).

Findings from this nationwide study generally provide evidence supporting stability of the results of measurement properties and psychometrics of the JSE in both osteopathic and allopathic medical students, described as the first goal of POMEE-Phase I. The additional psychometric support of the JSE S-Version from POMEE adds to the confidence of its users in the construct and criterion-related validities, and internal consistency reliability in measuring clinical empathy.

Clinical Empathy as Related to Gender, Age, Race/Ethnicity, Academic Background, and Career Interest

The *second* publication of data collected in POMEE-Phase I included 10,751 students (49% women) from 41 campuses of US osteopathic medical schools in different years of medical school (3616 first-year; 2764 second-year; 2413 third-year, and 1958 fourth-year students) who completed the web-based study survey at the end of the 2017–2018 academic year (Hojat, DeSantis, Shannon et al., 2020). Selected highlights of the findings are reported in the following sections.

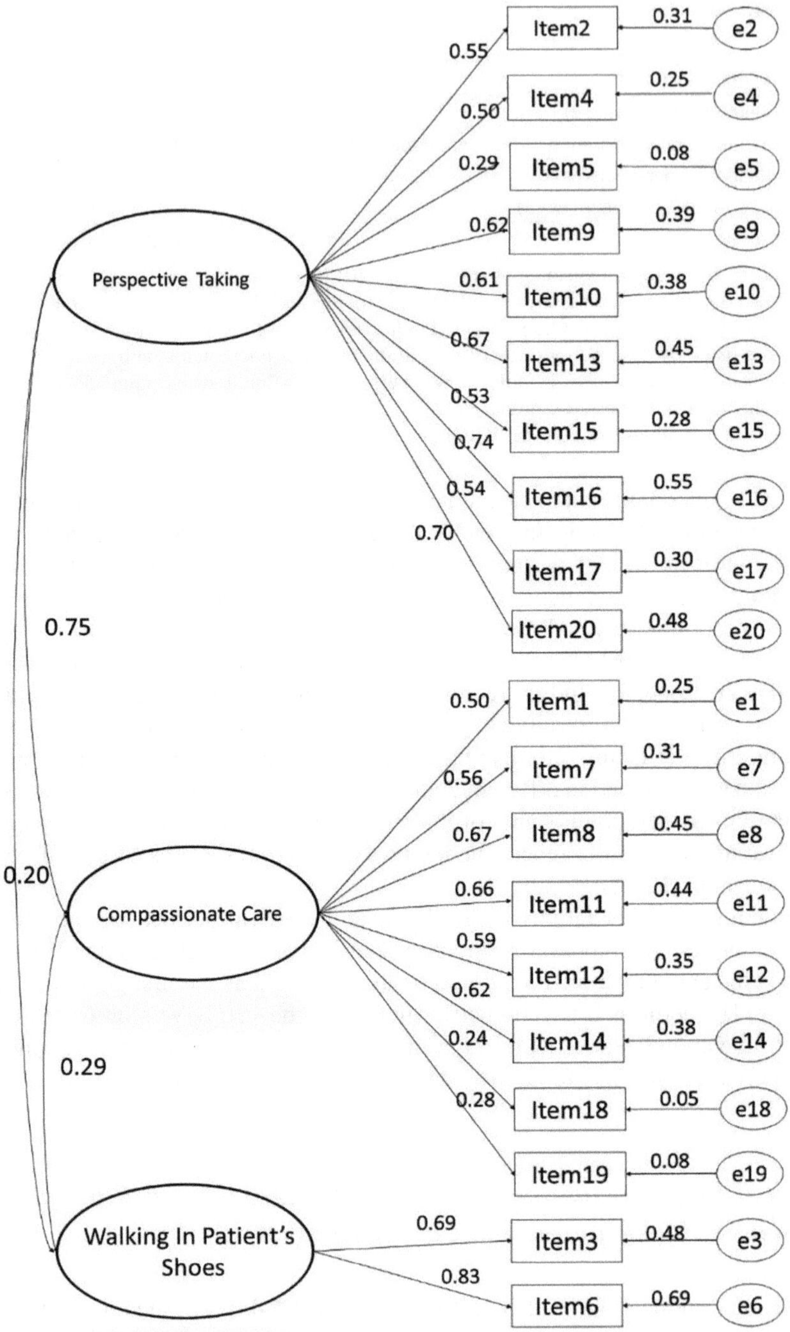

Fig. 14.1 Three-factor model of the JSE S-Version (latent variable structure) in a national sample of 6009 first-year students at the beginning of 2017–2018 academic year from 41 campuses of US colleges of osteopathic medicine. Reproduced from Hojat, DeSantis, Shannon et al. (2018). ©Authors, Open Access

Clinical Empathy and Gender

Composition of gender by year of medical school education in this study is reported in Table 14.4. Means and standard deviations of the JSE for students in each year of medical school and for the total sample are also reported in the table. We used analysis of covariance to control for the effect of social desirability response bias, by using scores of the Infrequency Scale of the ZKPQ as a covariate.

As shown in Table 14.4, and in Fig. 14.2, the mean scores of the JSE for women were consistently higher than those for men, in each of the different years of medical school and in the total sample; differences were statistically significant and practically important based on the magnitudes of the effect size estimates (Cohen's *d*). The finding of higher clinical empathy scores in women in this nationwide study is consistent with most studies reported by others in samples of physicians-in-training and in-practice (see Chaps. 7 and 10). More detailed descriptions of findings and comparisons with previous studies are reported in the original article (Hojat, DeSantis, Shannon et al., 2020). The gender difference in empathy has often been attributed to social learning and cultural factors; however, evidence regarding gender-specific inclination and behavior observed in infants and toddlers suggest that women's empathic inclination could have hard-wired roots, in addition to social learning and cultural factors (Hojat, DeSantis, Shannon et al., 2020) (also see Chap. 10).

Table 14.4 Means[a] and standard deviations of scores on the JSE S-Version for men and women[b] in national samples from 41 campuses of US colleges of osteopathic medicine

	Sample 1[b]		Sample 2[b]		Sample 3[b]		Sample 4[b]		Total	
Gender	*N* (%)	*M (SD)*	*N* (%)	*M (SD)*	*N* (%)	*M (SD)*	*N* (%)	*M (SD)*	*N* (%)	*M (SD)*
Men	1839 (51)	112.43 (13.14)	1348 (49)	112.34 (12.63)	1198 (50)	111.12 (13.58)	966 (50)	110.74 (14.04)	5351 (50)	111.82 (13.30)
Women	1738 (48)	118.03 (10.60)	1383 (50)	117.19 (10.60)	1180 (49)	116.09 (11.06)	970 (50)	115.79 (11.07)	5271 (49)	116.96 (10.82)
Other[c]	39 (1)		33 (1)		35 (1)		22 (1)		129 (1)	
Adjusted *F*-ratio	$F_{(1,3574)} =$ 192.65**		$F_{(1,2728)} =$ 116.19**		$F_{(1,2375)} =$ 96.32**		$F_{(1,1933)} =$ 76.87**		$F_{(1,10619)} =$ 472.68**	

$^{**}p < 0.01$

[a]Mean scores were adjusted by using analysis of covariance to control for the effect of "good impression" response bias. Scores of the Infrequency Scale of the Zuckerman–Kuhlman Personality Questionnaire served as covariate

[b]Samples 1–4 included students in the first, second, third, and fourth years of medical school, respectively, who completed the study survey at the end of the 2017–2018 academic year

[c]Respondents who did not report their gender were excluded from the statistical analysis of this table

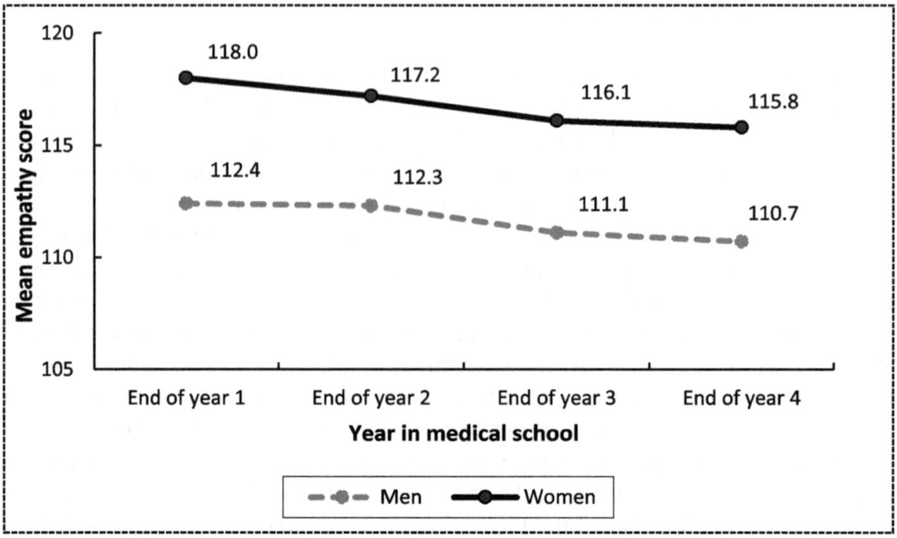

Fig. 14.2 Comparison of JSE S-Version scores for men and women in national samples of students in 41 campuses of US colleges of osteopathic medicine. Mean empathy scores were adjusted to control for "good impression" response bias effects by using ANCOVA. Scores for the Infrequency Scale of the Zuckerman–Kuhlman Personality Questionnaire served as covariate. Results of ANCOVA indicated higher mean empathy scores for women compared to men. Year 1: Adjusted $F_{(1,3574)} = 192.7$, $p < 0.01$. Year 2: Adjusted $F_{(1,2728)} = 116.2$, $p < .01$. Year 3: Adjusted $F_{(1,2375)} = 96.3$, $p < 0.01$. Year 4: Adjusted $F_{(1,1933)} = 76.9$, $p < 0.01$. Reproduced from Hojat, Shannon, DeSantis et al. (2020). ©Authors, Open Access

Clinical Empathy and Age

Empirical research on clinical empathy and age is scarce. In the nationwide sample in POMEE, we did not find a significant association between JSE scores and respondents' age (Hojat, DeSantis, Shannon et al., 2020). Negligible associations between clinical empathy and age in physicians-in-training could be an artifact of the "restriction of range" phenomenon in students' age distribution, which does not allow the corresponding correlations to capture the true relationship (Hojat, DeSantis, Shannon et al., 2020).

Clinical Empathy and Race/Ethnicity

Frequency distributions by race/ethnicity and summary results of statistical analyses of the JSE scores by race/ethnicity are reported in Table 14.5.

As shown in the table, the majority of respondents identified themselves as White/Caucasian (65%, $n = 7022$), followed by Asian (21%, $n = 2304$), Hispanic/Latino/Spanish (5%, $n = 485$), and Black/African-American (3%, $n = 324$). About 1% ($n = 129$) identified themselves as American Indian/Alaskan, or Hawaiian/Pacific Islander. Means and standard deviations and summary results of statistical

Table 14.5 Means[a] and standard deviations of scores on the JSE S-Version by race/ethnicity[b] in national samples from 41 campuses of US colleges of osteopathic medicine

Race/ethnicity category	Sample 1[c] N (%)	Sample 1[c] M (SD)	Sample 2[c] N (%)	Sample 2[c] M (SD)	Sample 3[c] N (%)	Sample 3[c] M (SD)	Sample 4[c] N (%)	Sample 4[c] M (SD)	Total N (%)	Total M (SD)
White/Caucasian	2283 (63)	115.34 (12.08)	1805 (65)	114.76 (11.95)	1609 (67)	113.66 (12.31)	1325 (68)	113.38 (12.82)	7022 (65)	114.44 (12.27)
Black/African American	107 (3)	117.08 (11.50)	83 (3)	118.66 (12.26)	78 (3)	117.63 (11.39)	56 (3)	115.19 (13.42)	324 (3)	117.28 (12.01)
Hispanic/Latino/Spanish	207 (6)	116.56 (11.74)	114 (4)	115.87 (10.29)	100 (4)	113.84 (13.63)	64 (3)	116.17 (11.92)	485 (5)	115.77 (11.88)
Asian	842 (23)	114.32 (12.88)	607 (22)	114.47 (11.82)	470 (19)	112.69 (13.74)	385 (20)	112.07 (12.74)	2304 (21)	113.66 (12.80)
Other[d]	177 (5)		155 (6)		156 (6)		128 (6)		616 (6)	
Adjusted *F*-ratio	$F_{(3,3434)}$ = 3.25*		$F_{(3,2604)}$ = 3.40*		$F_{(3,2252)}$ = 3.57*		$F_{(3,1825)}$ = 2.72*		$F_{(3,10130)}$ = 10.78**	

Reproduced from Hojat, DeSantis, Shannon et al. (2020). ©Authors, Open Access

$*p < 0.05$, $** p < 0.01$

[a]Mean scores were adjusted by using analysis of covariance to control for the effect of "good impression" response bias. Scores of the Infrequency Scale of the Zuckerman–Kuhlman Personality Questionnaire served as covariate

[b]Respondents who did not report their ethnicity or who were included in the "other" category were excluded from statistical analysis

[c]Samples 1–4 included students in the first, second, third, and fourth years of medical school, respectively, who completed the study survey at the end of the 2017–2018 academic year

[d]Includes students who did not report their race/ethnicity and those who identified as American Indian/Alaskan or Hawaiian/Pacific Islander

For Sample 1: Asian < all ethnic groups; for Sample 2: Black/African American > Asian, Black/African American > White/Caucasian; for Sample 3: Black/African American > all ethnic groups; for Sample 4: Hispanic/Latino/Spanish > Asian. In the total sample (samples 1–4 combined), all pairwise comparisons were statistically significant with the exception of Hispanic/Latino/Spanish compared to Black/African American which showed no statistical difference in adjusted mean scores

analyses on the JSE scores for students in each of the race/ethnicity groups by year of medical school education are reported in Table 14.5. Analysis of covariance was used, and scores on the Infrequency Scale of the ZKPQ served as a covariate to mitigate the social desirability response bias.

Results reported in Table 14.5 show the highest JSE mean score for the total participants was obtained by Black/African-American students, and the lowest by Asian students. A similar pattern of differences was also observed among students in each year of medical school education, with the exception of year 4 in which the Hispanic/Latino/Spanish students obtained a significantly higher JSE mean score, closely followed by Black/African-American students.

The higher JSE scores in the underrepresented Black/African-American and Hispanic/Latino/Spanish minority groups may be explained by the notion of the "wounded healer effect" (Laskowski & Pellicore, 2002), which describes that those who have experienced suffering can better understand the pain and suffering of others by sharing common experiences. This effect suggests that those who have experienced discrimination and social injustice could be more sensitive to the suffering of others and develop a more empathic understanding of the concerns of others who are in need of help.

Empirical research is scarce on differences in clinical empathy by race/ethnicity in physicians-in-training and in-practice. One reason, we speculate, is that often sufficient numbers of observations in underrepresented minority samples are unavailable in single institutions to undertake credible research with meaningful statistical analyses. Therefore, to our knowledge, this large nationwide project is the first clinical empathy study in which a sufficient number of observations in different racial/ethnic groups were available for meaningful statistical comparisons. More detailed analyses and comparisons with other research findings are reported in Hojat, DeSantis, Shannon et al. (2020).

Clinical Empathy and Academic Background

POMEE examined clinical empathy and participants' academic backgrounds, i.e. their undergraduate majors. However, for international readers with different medical school education systems (e.g., European system of medical school education), a brief explanation is needed about the academic background of medical students. In the United States (and Canada), a college degree (B.S. or B.A.) is a prerequisite for applicants to medical school, with rare exceptions for special programs in some medical schools. Medical school education in the USA, under normal circumstances, is a 4-year program. To determine the academic background of participants, we grouped them into the following broad categories: "Biological Sciences," "Chemical/Physical Sciences," "Social/Behavioral Sciences," "Arts and Humanities," and "Other" disciplines. Frequency distribution of participants' academic background (undergraduate majors) is reported in Table 14.6.

As shown in the table, the majority of participants majored in Biological Sciences (60%, 6423), and the fewest majored in Arts and Humanities (4%, $n = 401$). Means and standard deviations of the JSE scores by academic background in different years of medical school, and summary statistical analyses are reported in Table 14.6.

The highest JSE mean scores for the total participants were obtained by students with undergraduate majors in "Social/Behavioral Sciences," and "Arts and Humanities"; the lowest JSE mean score was obtained by students with undergraduate majors in "Chemical/Physical Sciences." A similar pattern of findings was observed for students in different years of medical school. Although the differences were statistically significant for students in years 1 and 2, and for the total sample, they were practically unimportant, as indicated by the magnitudes of effect size estimates ($d < 0.20$). The differences in the JSE mean scores by academic background were not statistically significant for students in years 3 and 4 of medical school (see Table 14.6).

Table 14.6 Means[a] and standard deviations of scores on the JSE S-Version by undergraduate major[b] in national samples from 41 campuses of US colleges of osteopathic medicine

	Sample 1[c]		Sample 2[c]		Sample 3[c]		Sample 4[c]		Total	
Undergraduate major	*N* (%)	*M (SD)*	*N* (%)	*M (SD)*	*N* (%)	*M (SD)*	*N* (%)	*M (SD)*	*N* (%)	*M (SD)*
Biological Sciences	2177 (60)	115.04 (12.52)	1617 (58)	114.40 (12.02)	1488 (62)	113.43 (13.18)	1141 (58)	113.13 (12.68)	6423 (60)	114.17 (12.60)
Chemical/ Physical Sciences	545 (15)	114.02 (12.98)	466 (17)	113.47 (12.86)	345 (14)	112.48 (13.47)	312 (16)	112.43 (14.41)	1668 (16)	113.23 (13.34)
Social/ Behavioral Sciences	246 (7)	116.29 (12.00)	213 (8)	116.56 (12.39)	163 (7)	114.59 (12.13)	153 (8)	115.17 (12.59)	775 (7)	115.80 (12.25)
Arts & Humanities	117 (3)	117.10 (11.62)	101 (4)	116.68 (11.27)	109 (5)	114.25 (12.57)	74 (4)	113.31 (13.63)	401 (4)	115.53 (12.24)
Other[d]	531 (15)		367 (13)		308 (12)		278 (14)		1484 (14)	
Adjusted *F*-ratio	$F_{(3,3080)}$ = 3.09*		$F_{(3,2392)}$ = 4.29**		$F_{(3,2100)}$ = 1.20		$F_{(3,1675)}$ = 1.57		$F_{(3,9262)}$ = 8.95**	

Reproduced from Hojat, DeSantis, Shannon et al. (2020). ©Authors, Open Access

$*p < 0.05$, $** p < 0.01$

[a]Mean scores were adjusted by using analysis of covariance to control for the effect of "good impression" response bias. Scores of the Infrequency Scale of the Zuckerman–Kuhlman Personality Questionnaire served as covariate

[b]Respondents who did not report their undergraduate major or who reported majors in the "other" category were excluded from statistical analysis

[c]Samples 1–4 included students in the first, second, third, and fourth years of medical school, respectively, who completed the study survey at the end of the 2017–2018 academic year

[d]Includes those who did not report their undergraduate major, and those who reported the following majors: Double Major in Science/Non-Science, General Studies, Honors Program, Interdisciplinary, Pre-Med, Other, and No Major

For Sample 1: Arts & Humanities > Chemical/Physical Sciences, Social/Behavioral Sciences > Chemical/Physical Sciences; for Sample 2: Arts & Humanities > Chemical/Physical Sciences, Social/Behavioral Sciences > Biological Sciences, Social/Behavioral Sciences > Chemical/Physical Sciences. No statistically significant differences were observed in Samples 3 and 4. In the total sample (samples 1–4 combined), each pairwise comparison was statistically significant, with the exception of Arts & Humanities compared to Social/Behavioral Sciences which showed no statistical difference in adjusted mean scores

Empirical research on clinical empathy and students' academic background is scarce. To our knowledge, this is the first large-scale study to examine associations between clinical empathy and academic background in medical students. Interestingly, in the POMEE, we found that differences in clinical empathy among students with different academic backgrounds were significant only in the preclinical phase of medical school education (years 1 and 2), but the differences became non-significant as students progressed to the clinical phase of medical school education (years 3 and 4). These findings suggest that the effects of academic background on clinical empathy prior to medical school could last only during early years of medical school education but fade away in the last 2 years of medical school education. Further research is needed to confirm this finding.

Clinical Empathy and Career Interest

To obtain students' career interests, in the study survey we presented a list of 23 specialties most frequently pursued by graduates of osteopathic medical schools. We classified the specialties into the following broad categories: "People-Oriented" (including Family Medicine, General Internal Medicine, Obstetrics and Gynecology, and Pediatrics); "Technology/Procedure-Oriented" (including Anesthesiology, Dermatology, General Surgery, Neurology, Ophthalmology, Orthopedics, Otolaryngology and Facial Plastic Surgery, Pathology, Plastic Surgery, and Radiology); and "Other" specialties. We retained "Psychiatry" in its own category because in previous research, psychiatrists obtained the highest scores on the JSE (Hojat, Gonnella, Nasca, Mangione, Vergare, & Magee et al., 2002), and we were interested to ascertain if it was also the case with osteopathic medical students. Grouping specialties into broad categories of "People-Oriented" and "Technology/Procedure-Oriented" has previously been used in medical education research (Hojat, Gonnella, Nasca, Mangione et al., 2002; Lieu, Schroeder, & Altman, 1989).

Frequency distributions of students interested in each specialty category; means and standard deviations of the JSE scores; and summary results of statistical analyses for the total study sample and for students in each year of medical school are reported in Table 14.7.

As shown in the table, the most frequently chosen specialty category was "People-Oriented" (45%, $n = 4867$ of the total participating sample). The proportion expressing an interest in pursuing a "People-Oriented" specialty (mostly a primary care specialty) was higher for students in later years of medical school education, compared to those in an earlier year (35% in the first, and 63% in the last year of medical school).

The mean scores of the JSE (adjusted for social desirability response bias) reported in Table 14.7 show that students who obtained the highest mean scores were interested in pursuing "Psychiatry" and "People-Oriented" specialties, and their JSE scores were significantly different from those who were interested in pursuing "Technology/Procedure-Oriented" specialties. The differences were also practically important, indicated by the magnitude of the effect size estimates; and the pattern of findings was similar for students in different years of medical school (for more detailed analyses, see Hojat, DeSantis, Shannon et al., 2020). Findings in this large-scale nationwide study confirmed previous findings for samples of allopathic medical students (Hojat et al., 2002) and practicing physicians (Hojat, Gonnella, Nasca, Mangione, Vergare et al., 2002) (also, see Chap. 9).

Findings of associations between clinical empathy and gender, race/ethnicity, academic background, and specialty interest have important implications for identifying medical students who may need additional help to enhance and sustain their empathic orientation toward patient care (Hojat, DeSantis, Shannon et al., 2020). Given the limited resources for offering remedial targeted educational programs to enhance clinical empathy, it is important to identify students who have less propensity for empathic engagement and may need more help than others to benefit from such goal-directed educational remedies. Also, the findings have implications for

Table 14.7 Means[a] and standard deviations of scores on the JSE S-Version by specialty plan[b] in national samples from 41 campuses of US colleges of osteopathic medicine

	Sample 1[c]		Sample 2[c]		Sample 3[c]		Sample 4[c]		Total	
Specialty	*N* (%)	*M* (*SD*)	*N* (%)	*M* (*SD*)	*N* (%)	*M* (*SD*)	*N* (%)	*M* (*SD*)	*N* (%)	*M* (*SD*)
People-oriented[d]	1257 (35)	116.73 (11.65)	1102 (40)	116.41 (10.89)	1277 (53)	114.56 (12.45)	1231 (63)	114.17 (12.29)	4867 (45)	115.43 (11.92)
Technology/procedure-oriented[e]	705 (19)	112.28 (13.35)	427 (15)	111.95 (13.66)	495 (20)	110.13 (14.41)	273 (14)	110.53 (15.40)	1900 (18)	111.41 (14.03)
Psychiatry	72 (2)	117.58 (12.81)	88 (3)	117.27 (13.54)	134 (6)	116.64 (12.10)	102 (5)	116.21 (11.11)	396 (4)	116.93 (12.28)
Other specialties[f]	740 (20)		501 (18)		441 (18)		342 (17)		2024 (19)	
Undecided	842 (23)		646 (23)		66 (3)		10 (<1)		1564 (15)	
Adjusted *F*-ratio	$F_{(2,2030)}$ = 31.00**		$F_{(2,1613)}$ = 23.03**		$F_{(2,1902)}$ = 25.36**		$F_{(2,1602)}$ = 11.29**		$F_{(2,7159)}$ = 78.88**	

Reproduced from Hojat, DeSantis, Shannon et al. (2020). ©Authors, Open Access
** $p < 0.01$
[a]Mean scores were adjusted by using analysis of covariance to control for the effect of "good impression" response bias. Scores of the Infrequency Scale of the Zuckerman–Kuhlman Personality Questionnaire served as covariate
[b]Respondents who did not report their specialty plan, those who were undecided, or those who reported specialties in the "other" category were excluded from statistical analysis
[c]Samples 1–4 included students in the first, second, third, and fourth years of medical school, respectively, who completed the study survey at the end of the 2017–2018 academic year
[d]People-oriented specialties included: Family Medicine, Internal Medicine, Obstetrics/Gynecology, and Pediatrics
[e]Technology/procedure-oriented specialties included: Anesthesiology, Dermatology, Neurological Surgery, Ophthalmology, Orthopedic Surgery, Otolaryngology/Facial Plastic Surgery, Pathology, Plastic Surgery, Radiology, and Surgery
[f]Includes those who did not report their specialty plan, those who selected "Other" specialty, or those who selected specialties that were chosen by <20 students

career counseling and guiding students in choosing specialties more aligned with their clinical empathic orientation (Hojat, DeSantis, Shannon et al., 2020).

Erosion of Clinical Empathy in Medical School

A *third* publication from the POMEE-Phase I database examined the decline of clinical empathy in a cross-sectional study by year of medical school education (Hojat et al., 2020). Participants in this study included 10,751 students enrolled in 41 campuses of US osteopathic medical colleges (3616 first-year; 2764 second-year; 2413 third-year; and 1958 fourth-year), who completed the JSE at the end of the 2017–2018 academic year. Comparisons on scores of the JSE among students in different years of medical school, using analysis of covariance (controlling for the

Table 14.8 Cross-sectional comparison of scores of the JSE S-Version for students in different years of medical school in national samples from 41 campuses of US colleges of osteopathic medicine

Medical school year[a]	*N*	Adjusted mean[a]	Standard deviation
By year in medical school[b]			
End of year 1	3616	115.04	12.46
End of year 2	2764	114.68	12.13
End of year 3	2413	113.38	13.03
End of year 4	1958	113.04	13.21
By clinical phase in medical school[c]			
Years 1 & 2 (Preclinical)	6380	114.88	12.32
Years 3 & 4 (Clinical)	4371	113.22	13.11

Reproduced from Hojat, Shannon, DeSantis et al. (2020). ©Authors, Open Access
[a]Mean scores are adjusted to control for the effect of the "good impression" response bias. Scores on the Infrequency Scale of the Zuckerman–Kuhlman Personality Questionnaire served as covariate
[b]Adjusted $F_{(3,10746)} = 15.79$, $p < 0.01$. Post-hoc mean comparison test indicated that (Year 1 = Year 2) > (Year 3 = Year 4), $p < 0.01$
[c]Adjusted $F_{(1,10748)} = 45.31$, $p < 0.01$, $d = 0.13$

effect of social desirability response bias, by using scores on the Infrequency Scale of the ZKPQ as a covariate), showed a statistically significant decline in scores of the JSE from the preclinical years (1 and 2) to the clinical years (3 and 4). We reported adjusted JSE mean scores and standard deviations for students in each year of medical school; in preclinical and clinical phases of medical school education; and summary results of statistical analyses in this cross-sectional study (Table 14.8).

Decline of clinical empathy in each year by gender is depicted in Fig. 14.2. As shown, the trend of decline in the JSE scores in different years of medical school is similar in men and women (for more detailed data, see Hojat, Shannon, DeSantis et al., 2020). Also, a similar pattern of decline in clinical empathy scores was observed for students who were interested in pursuing "People-Oriented" and "Technology/Procedure-Oriented" specialties (see Fig. 14.3).

Comparisons of Decline in Clinical Empathy in Osteopathic and in Allopathic Medical Students

Findings from POMEE data, compared to those collected from allopathic medical schools in the US, showed some similarities in the pattern of decline; however, it was also noticed that the decline of the JSE scores was less pronounced in osteopathic medical students than that reported for allopathic medical students (for more detailed analyses, see Hojat, Shannon, DeSantis et al., 2020).

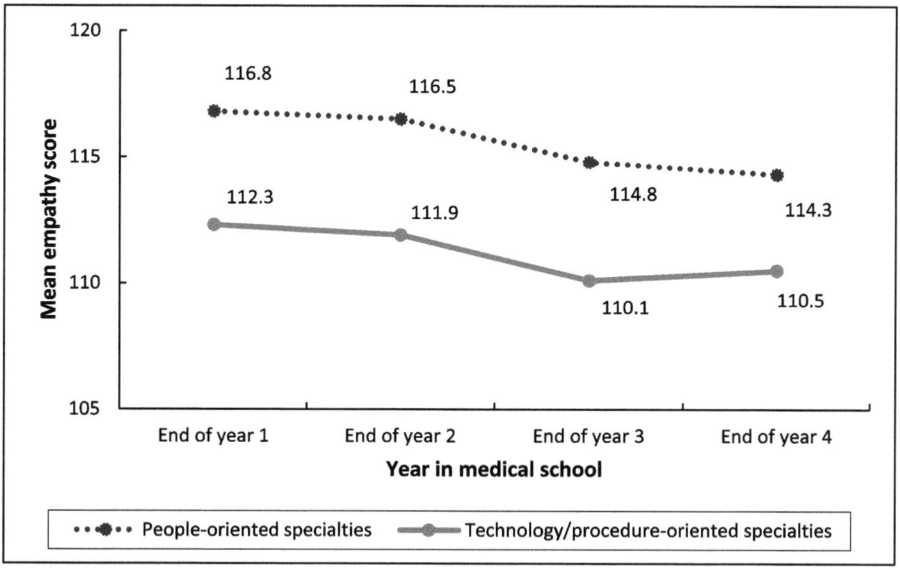

Fig. 14.3 Comparison of JSE S-Version scores for students by career interest in national samples of students in 41 campuses of US colleges of osteopathic medicine. Mean empathy scores were adjusted to control for "good impression" response bias effects by using ANCOVA. Scores of the Infrequency Scale of the Zuckerman–Kuhlman Personality Questionnaire served as covariate. Results of ANCOVA indicated higher mean empathy scores for students pursuing people-oriented (e.g., family medicine, psychiatry, pediatrics, etc.) compared to technology/procedure-oriented (e.g., pathology, radiology, surgery, etc.) specialties. Year 1: Adjusted $F_{(1,2031)} = 61.7$, $p < 0.01$. Year 2: Adjusted $F_{(1,1614)} = 45.6$, $p < 0.01$. Year 3: Adjusted $F_{(1,1903)} = 47.5$, $p < 0.01$. Year 4: Adjusted $F_{(1,1603)} = 20.1$, $p < 0.01$. Reproduced from Hojat, Shannon, DeSantis et al. (2020). ©Authors, Open Access

National Norm Tables of the JSE Scores for Osteopathic Medical Students

The *fourth* publication from data collected in POMEE-Phase I presented national norms of the JSE scores for osteopathic medical students in the US at different levels of medical school education, from matriculation to graduation. Norms for the assessments of clinical empathy, based on performance of large and representative samples from well-defined target populations, can be used to place individual or group performance against the corresponding national normative population. POMEE provided this unique opportunity for the first time to establish national norm tables on a valid and reliable instrument (JSE S-Version), specifically developed for administration to medical students for measuring an important personality attribute that could predict clinical competence in medical school (Hojat, Gonnella, Mangione, Nasca, Veloski et al., 2002) and patient outcomes (Hojat, Louis, Maxwell, Markham et al., 2010; Del Canale et al., 2012).

Participants in this national norm study included five samples from 41 US osteopathic medical college campuses comprising a total of 16,149 students who completed the study survey at matriculation and at the end of the first-year (samples 1 and 2, respectively); and at the end of the second-, third-, and fourth-year of medical school (samples 3, 4, and 5, respectively) in the 2017–2018 academic year. Data confirmed that the study samples were similar to their respective national populations regarding age, gender, and race/ethnicity (for more detailed information, see Hojat, Shannon, DeSantis, Speicher et al., 2019).

To minimize confounding effects of social desirability response bias in the national norm tables, we excluded those students (2–3%) who scored higher than 3 on the Infrequency Scale of the ZKPQ, recommended by the author of the test as the cutoff for questionable validity of a respondent's record due to attempts to give socially desirable responses (Zuckerman, 2002, p. 383). Also, because we found notable gender differences in the JSE scores in POMEE samples and in some other studies (see Chaps. 7 and 10), we reported norm data for men and women separately in all of the norm tables.

In addition, because we found no substantial differences on the JSE score in preclinical years (years 1 and 2 of medical school education), we combined data for these 2 years to generate a norm table for students in the preclinical component of medical school ($n = 6115$; Table 14.9). Similarly, we combined data for students in years 3 and 4 of medical school ($n = 4216$; Table 14.10) to generate a norm table for students in the clinical component of medical school education (Hojat, Shannon, DeSantis, Speicher et al., 2019). A separate norm table was also developed for matriculants to osteopathic medical school, prior to their exposure to formal medical school curriculum; it may be used for admission purposes if JSE is considered as a complementary measure for admission decisions ($n = 5818$; Table 14.11) (for more detailed information, see Hojat, DeSantis, Shannon et al., 2018; Hojat, Shannon, DeSantis et al., 2019).

Using Norm Tables

These norm tables can be used to find the corresponding national rank of an individual student's raw score on the JSE S-Version. If the student's gender is known, the gender-specific percentile rank can be used from the corresponding norm table. However, if a student's gender is not known, then the percentile rank reported in the norm tables for men and women combined can be used as an estimate. For example, if a score of 125 is obtained by a third-year male medical student, first we must find the raw score interval on the corresponding norm table for third-year medical students (e.g., reported interval score of 125–126 in Table 14.10). Then, the corresponding percentile rank should be found by looking across the 125–126 score interval for men (in Table 14.10); this reads 88, meaning that a score of 125 on the JSE S-Version for a third-year male osteopathic medical student places him in the 88th percentile of all male students in the population of third-year male students in

Table 14.9 National norms for the JSE S-Version for first- and second-year osteopathic medical students (preclinical years) in national samples from 41 campuses of US colleges of osteopathic medicine[a]

JSE	Men ($n = 3042$)			Women ($n = 3073$)			Combined ($n = 6115$)		
Raw score	*f*	*cf*	Percentile rank	*f*	*cf*	Percentile rank	*f*	*cf*	Percentile rank
≤80	58	58	2	10	10	<1	68	68	1
81–82	19	77	2	2	12	<1	21	89	1
83–84	18	95	3	9	21	1	27	116	2
85–86	19	114	3	5	26	1	24	140	2
87–88	22	136	4	6	32	1	28	168	3
89–90	36	172	5	15	47	1	51	219	3
91–92	35	207	6	13	60	2	48	267	4
93–94	46	253	8	19	79	2	65	332	5
95–96	62	315	9	18	97	3	80	412	6
97–98	77	392	12	40	137	4	117	529	8
99–100	82	474	14	39	176	5	121	650	10
101–102	100	574	17	65	241	7	165	815	12
103–104	152	726	21	93	334	9	245	1060	15
105–106	163	889	27	99	433	12	262	1322	19
107–108	163	1052	32	126	559	16	289	1611	24
109–110	182	1234	38	138	697	20	320	1931	29
111–112	189	1423	44	173	870	25	362	2293	35
113–114	201	1624	50	185	1055	31	386	2679	41
115–116	195	1819	57	201	1256	38	396	3075	47
117–118	205	2024	63	219	1475	44	424	3499	54
119–120	181	2205	70	230	1705	52	411	3910	61
121–122	167	2372	75	257	1962	60	424	4334	67
123–124	152	2524	80	239	2201	68	391	4725	74
125–126	136	2660	85	204	2405	75	340	5065	80
127–128	103	2763	89	190	2595	81	293	5358	85
129–130	87	2850	92	175	2770	87	262	5620	90
131–132	81	2931	95	149	2919	93	230	5850	94
133–134	51	2982	97	82	3001	96	133	5983	97
135–136	28	3010	98	43	3044	98	71	6054	98
137–138	22	3032	99	19	3063	99	41	6095	99
139–140	10	3042	>99	10	3073	>99	20	6115	>99

Reproduced from Hojat, Shannon, DeSantis et al. (2019). ©Authors, Open Access
cf cumulative frequency, *f* frequency
[a]Excluded were respondents who did not specify their gender as "male" or "female" (1%) and those with scores >3 on the Infrequency Scale of the Zuckerman–Kuhlman Personality Questionnaire (for identifying respondents who attempted to make a good impression)

Table 14.10 National norms for the JSE S-Version for third- and fourth-year osteopathic medical students (clinical years) in national samples from 41 campuses of US colleges of osteopathic medicine[a]

JSE	Men (n = 2099)			Women (n = 2117)			Combined (n = 4216)		
Raw score	*f*	*cf*	Percentile rank	*f*	*cf*	Percentile rank	*f*	*cf*	Percentile rank
≤80	64	64	3	14	14	1	78	78	2
81–82	15	79	3	5	19	1	20	98	2
83–84	13	92	4	7	26	1	20	118	3
85–86	21	113	5	4	30	1	25	143	3
87–88	19	132	6	5	35	2	24	167	4
89–90	27	159	7	9	44	2	36	203	4
91–92	39	198	9	13	57	2	52	255	5
93–94	28	226	10	13	70	3	41	296	7
95–96	39	265	12	21	91	4	60	356	8
97–98	51	316	14	36	127	5	87	443	9
99–100	74	390	17	37	164	7	111	554	12
101–102	90	480	21	56	220	9	146	700	15
103–104	77	557	25	62	282	12	139	839	18
105–106	118	675	29	67	349	15	185	1024	22
107–108	124	799	35	117	466	19	241	1265	27
109–110	137	936	41	97	563	24	234	1499	33
111–112	126	1062	48	130	693	30	256	1755	39
113–114	108	1170	53	156	849	36	264	2019	45
115–116	145	1315	59	166	1015	44	311	2330	52
117–118	134	1449	66	162	1177	52	296	2626	59
119–120	141	1590	72	147	1324	59	288	2914	66
121–122	120	1710	79	154	1478	66	274	3188	72
123–124	96	1806	84	130	1608	73	226	3414	78
125–126	78	1884	88	136	1744	79	214	3628	84
127–128	65	1949	91	126	1870	85	191	3819	88
129–130	53	2002	94	97	1967	91	150	3969	92
131–132	39	2041	96	60	2027	94	99	4068	95
133–134	31	2072	98	47	2074	97	78	4146	97
135–136	4	2076	99	30	2104	99	34	4180	99
137–138	14	2090	99	9	2113	>99	23	4203	99
139–140	9	2099	>99	4	2117	>99	13	4216	>99

Reproduced from Hojat, DeSantis, Shannon et al. (2019). ©Authors, Open Access
f frequency, *cf* cumulative frequency
[a]Excluded were respondents who did not specify their gender as "male" or "female" (<1%), and those with scores >3 on the Infrequency Scale of the Zuckerman–Kuhlman Personality Questionnaire (for identifying respondents who attempted to make "good impression")

Table 14.11 National norms for the JSE S-Version for first-year matriculants in a national sample from 41 campuses of US colleges of osteopathic medicine at the beginning of medical school[a]

JSE	Men (n = 3071)			Women (n = 2747)			Combined (n = 5818)		
Raw score	*f*	*cf*	Percentile rank	*f*	*cf*	Percentile rank	*f*	*cf*	Percentile rank
≤80	19	19	<1	5	5	<1	24	24	<1
81–82	12	31	1	2	7	<1	14	38	1
83–84	7	38	1	1	8	<1	8	46	1
85–86	8	46	1	3	11	<1	11	57	1
87–88	8	54	2	5	16	<1	13	70	1
89–90	24	78	2	5	21	1	29	99	1
91–92	26	104	3	5	26	1	31	130	2
93–94	34	138	4	8	34	1	42	172	3
95–96	31	169	5	21	55	2	52	224	3
97–98	70	239	7	30	85	3	100	324	5
99–100	79	318	9	35	120	4	114	438	7
101–102	102	420	12	34	154	5	136	574	9
103–104	125	545	16	70	224	7	195	769	12
105–106	139	684	20	78	302	10	217	986	15
107–108	183	867	25	110	412	13	293	1279	19
109–110	199	1066	31	115	527	17	314	1593	25
111–112	211	1277	38	153	680	22	364	1957	31
113–114	218	1495	45	147	827	27	365	2322	37
115–116	221	1716	52	204	1031	34	425	2747	44
117–118	203	1919	59	207	1238	41	410	3157	51
119–120	208	2127	66	237	1475	49	445	3602	58
121–122	198	2325	72	211	1686	58	409	4011	65
123–124	175	2500	79	212	1898	65	387	4398	72
125–126	144	2644	84	203	2101	73	347	4745	79
127–128	119	2763	88	206	2307	80	325	5070	84
129–130	89	2852	91	161	2468	87	250	5320	89
131–132	92	2944	94	117	2585	92	209	5529	93
133–134	59	3003	97	82	2667	96	141	5670	96
135–136	37	3040	98	48	2715	98	85	5755	98
137–138	16	3056	99	28	2743	99	44	5799	99
139–140	15	3071	>99	4	2747	>99	19	5818	>99

Reproduced from Hojat, DeSantis, Shannon et al. (2018). ©Authors, Open Access
f frequency, *cf* cumulative frequency
[a]Excluded were respondents who did not specify their gender as "male" or "female" (<1%) and those with scores >3 on the Infrequency Scale of the Zuckerman–Kuhlman Personality Questionnaire (for identifying respondents who attempted to make a good impression)

a US osteopathic medical school. In other words, 88% of male students scored below 125 on the JSE S-Version in this particular norm group.

To my knowledge, this was the first nationwide study in medical education research in the US in which national norms were developed for a validated instrument

(JSE S-Version) for the assessment of an individual's score in different levels of medical school education for different genders.

The national norms developed in this study have important implications for assessing osteopathic medical students' individual and group scores against national norms. Percentile ranks in norm tables corresponding to students' raw scores can provide supplementary information for admissions to medical school or postgraduate medical education programs.

Looking forward, national norms could also serve as a tie-breaker in admissions decision-making for applicants with similar academic qualifications (Hojat, 2014). Moreover, the national norm tables could help to identify the degree of students' need for remedial education to enhance their clinical empathy. In addition, national norm tables could potentially be used to assess the outcomes of educational programs, interventions, or remedies implemented in different years of osteopathic medical school training. Thus, not only can these norm tables be used to assess individuals' scores against national norms, but they can also help to evaluate group changes in percentile ranks over time to assess outcomes of targeted educational programs.

Recognition of a POMEE Publication by the AOA with Medical Writing Award

Our POMEE publication on national norms for a clinical empathy measure, published in the *Journal of American Osteopathic Association* (Hojat, Shannon, DeSantis, Speicher, Bragan, & Calabrese, 2019), was recognized by the American Osteopathic Association House of Delegate as the 2020 recipient of the George W. Northup, DO, Medical Writing Award. Results of POMEE reported in this section confirmed that the major goals of Phase I of the project were successfully achieved. In addition, the project enjoyed broad publicity in print and digital media, in addition to several invited interviews about the project, its findings, and implications of findings that were published or posted on several websites. Despite the tremendous success of POMEE-Phase 1 in achieving its major goals, POMEE-Phase II had a different destiny.

Findings from Data Collected in POMEE-Phase II

Because of the limitations of cross-sectional research in investigating changes over time, POMEE-Phase II was designed as a longitudinal study to overcome those limitations and re-examine changes (erosion or enhancement) in clinical empathy as the study cohort progresses through medical school education, and to search for factors/events that are associated (positively or negatively) with erosion/enhancement of clinical empathy. Also, it was intended to explore better approaches to enhance clinical empathy in medical students.

However, the 5-year longitudinal project was abandoned after the first year due to unexpected circumstances that will be described later. Thus, only the following single article was published from data collected in the first year of POMEE-Phase II. A few additional studies on correlates of clinical empathy, that were in the pipeline to be prepared for publication in professional journals in the second year of the POMEE-Phase II, are also briefly reported in this section; these could be of value to future researchers of clinical empathy.

Development of a New Instrument to Measure Attitudes Toward Osteopathic Medicine (ATOMS)

We endeavored to examine relationships between clinical empathy and degree of orientation toward osteopathic medical education and practice, but this required a psychometrically sound instrument to measure attitudes toward osteopathic medicine.

Thus, we undertook a comprehensive review of the literature to find a psychometrically sound instrument to quantify attitudes of osteopathic medical students and practitioners of osteopathic medicine toward principles of osteopathic medicine, osteopathic approaches in diagnosis and treatment, and integrative and holistic care, which are among the tenets of osteopathic medicine (Carey, Motyka, Garret, & Keller, 2003; Noll, Ginsberg, Elahi & Cavalieri, 2016). We could not find any established instrument with sufficient psychometric support to serve that purpose. The rich database of the POMEE national study provided the opportunity to develop such an instrument that could also have important implications for the assessment of osteopathic medical education programs.

The study sample included first-year matriculants (n = 5696) of the 2019–2020 academic year from participating osteopathic medical colleges. This national sample for the POMEE-Phase II longitudinal study was defined as the "study cohort" who, according to the research protocol, were to be followed up during their course of medical school education, possibly through postgraduate medical education, and even in their practice of medicine, if such long-term research interest continues.

For the use in POMEE-Phase II, and for possible use by other osteopathic medical education researchers, we developed a 13-item instrument: *Attitudes Toward Osteopathic Medicine Scale* (ATOMS). Items are answered on a seven-point Likert scale (1 = Strongly Disagree, 7 = Strongly Agree, see Fig. 14.4). Details about the development of the ATOMS were described in the original publication (Hojat, DeSantis, Cain, Speicher et al., 2021). This chapter briefly describes highlights of measurement properties and psychometrics of ATOMS.

Instructions: Please indicate the extent of your agreement or disagreement with each of the following statements by checking the appropriate circle, using the following 7-point scale (a higher number indicates more agreement)

1-------2-------3-------4-------5-------6-------7

Strongly Disagree ***Strongly Agree***

	①②③④⑤⑥⑦
1. The osteopathic philosophy of holistic care greatly influenced my decision to attend an osteopathic school.	○
2. Patients whose physicians are knowledgeable of multiple medical systems and complementary and alternative practices, in addition to conventional medicine, do better than patients whose physicians are only familiar with conventional medicine.	○
3. Therapeutic touch has been discredited as a healing modality.	○
4. Physicians with a balanced lifestyle (i.e. Attending to their own health, social, family and spiritual needs, as well as interests beyond medicine) generate improved patient outcome.	○
5. Osteopathic Manipulation often makes patients "feel" better temporarily, but does not lead to objective improvement in long-term outcomes for patients.	○
6. A strong relationship between patient and physician is an extremely valuable therapeutic intervention that leads to improved outcomes.	○
7. Instilling hope in patients is a physician's duty.	○
8. Osteopathic manipulative therapy is a valuable method for resolving a wide variety of musculoskeletal problems (beyond back pain).	○
9. Information about the relative effectiveness of treatments that is obtained by research methods other than randomized controlled trials has little value to physicians.	○
10. Physicians who strive to understand themselves provide better care than those who do not.	○
11. Psychosocial factors are as important as biomedical factor in health and illness.	○
12. Medical problems need specific medical and surgical interventions, thus, holistic approaches to medical problems cannot be as beneficial as targeted biomedical treatment.	○
13. Touch and tactile approaches may not serve a significant purpose in patient care.	○

Fig. 14.4 Attitudes Toward Osteopathic Medicine Scale (ATOMS). Reproduced from Hojat, DeSantis, Cain, Speicher, Bragan, Shannon, & Calabrese (2021). ©2021 Authors. Open Access

Psychometrics of the Attitudes Toward Osteopathic Medicine Scale (ATOMS)

The mean and standard deviation of ATOMS scores for the total study sample (n = 5669, excluding those with incomplete ATOMS surveys) were 73.9 and 9.5, respectively. The possible score range was 13–91, and actual range was 29–91. Cronbach's reliability coefficient was 0.83, which is in the acceptable range of educational and psychological tests (see Hojat, DeSantis, Cain et al., 2021 for more descriptive data).

Item-Total Score Correlations

The corrected item-total score correlations of the 13-item ATOMS were calculated based on the correlation between each item score and the total ATOMS score, excluding the corresponding item from the total score. These were all statistically significant ($p < 0.01$) and moderately high, ranging from a low of 0.29 for this item: "Therapeutic touch has been discredited as a healing modality" (a reverse-scored item) to a high of 0.61 for this item: "Osteopathic manipulative therapy is a valuable method for resolving a wide variety of musculoskeletal problems." The median item-total score correlation was 0.49 (see Table 14.12 for more detailed data).

Table 14.12 Rotated factor loadings[a], corrected item-total score correlations[b], and effect sizes of item discrimination indices[c] for the Attitudes Toward Osteopathic Medicine Scale (ATOMS) in a national sample of first-year matriculants of 46 campuses of US colleges of osteopathic medicine ($n = 5696$)

Item	Factor 1	Factor 2	Factor 3	Corrected item-total score correlation	Item discrimination index effect size
Physicians who strive to understand themselves provide better care than those who do not. (10)	**0.75**	0.00	−0.02	0.51	1.40
Physicians with a balanced lifestyle (i.e., Attending to their own health, social, family, and spiritual needs, as well as interests beyond medicine) generate improved patient satisfaction. (4)	**0.68**	−0.02	0.04	0.49	1.25
A strong relationship between patient and physician is an extremely valuable therapeutic intervention that leads to improved outcomes. (6)	**0.65**	0.08	0.02	0.54	1.44
Psychosocial factors are as important as biomedical factor in health and illness. (11)	**0.54**	0.09	0.04	0.47	1.25
Instilling hope in patients is a physician's duty. (7)	**0.42**	−0.11	0.13	0.31	1.02
Medical problems need specific medical and surgical interventions; thus, holistic approaches to medical problems cannot be as beneficial as targeted biomedical treatment. (12)	0.05	**0.67**	−0.05	0.48	1.56

(continued)

Table 14.12 (continued)

Item	Factor 1	Factor 2	Factor 3	Corrected item-total score correlation	Item discrimination index effect size
Touch and tactile approaches may not serve a significant purpose in patient care. (13)	0.08	**0.62**	0.03	0.54	1.55
Osteopathic manipulation often makes patients "feel" better temporarily, but does not lead to objective improvement in long-term outcomes for patients. (5)	−0.12	**0.52**	0.32	0.54	1.67
Information about the relative effectiveness of treatments that is obtained by research methods other than randomized controlled trials has little value to physicians. (9)	−0.02	**0.48**	−0.03	0.32	1.15
Therapeutic touch has been discredited as a healing modality. (3)	−0.01	**0.46**	−0.05	0.29	1.09
Osteopathic manipulative therapy is a valuable method for resolving a wide variety of musculoskeletal problems (beyond back pain). (8)	0.07	0.06	**0.71**	0.61	1.72
The osteopathic philosophy of holistic care greatly influenced my decision to attend an osteopathic school. (1)	0.05	0.00	**0.66**	0.51	1.42
Patients whose physicians are knowledgeable of multiple medical systems and complementary and alternative practices, in addition to conventional medicine, do better than patients whose physicians are only familiar with conventional medicine. (2)	0.18	−0.06	**0.54**	0.49	1.45
Eigenvalue	4.41	1.59	1.04		

Reproduced from Hojat, DeSantis, Cain et al. (2021). ©Authors, Open Access

[a]Based on the content of items with high factor loadings, Factor 1 was entitled "Perspectives on Osteopathic Medicine," Factor 2: "Osteopathic Diagnosis and Treatment," and Factor 3: "Holistic-Integrative Care." Items are sorted by descending order of factor loadings within each factor. Factor coefficients ≥0.42 are shown in **bold**. Number in parentheses refers to the appearance of the items in the ATOMS instrument

[b]Correlations between scores on each item and the ATOMS total score by excluding the corresponding item from the total score; all were statistically significant ($p < 0.01$)

[c]Effect size estimate (Cohen's *d* statistic) of the discrimination index was calculated by subtracting the item mean score of the ATOMS high scorers (top 33%) from the item mean score of the ATOMS low scorers (bottom 33%), divided by the pooled standard deviation of the corresponding item

Effect Sizes of Item Discrimination Indices

The effect sizes of item discrimination indices were calculated by subtracting the item mean score for the top 33% ATOMS scorers from the mean score of the same item obtained by the bottom 33% ATOMS scorers, divided by the pooled standard deviation of the corresponding item. These effect sizes are analogous to the Cohen's *d* statistics (Cohen, 1987). All of the effect sizes were substantially large (>1.01), indicating that the difference in mean item scores between high and low ATOMS scorers was both statistically significant in the favor of high scorers, and practically important, as evidenced by large effect sizes (see Table 14.12).

Exploratory Factor Analysis

We examined the underlying construct of the 13-item ATOMS by conducting exploratory factor analysis, principal components with oblique (promax) rotation to allow correlations among the factors. Summary results of exploratory factor analysis are reported in Table 14.12. Three factors emerged, each with an eigenvalue greater than one (Kaiser Criterion). The eigenvalues before rotation were 4.41, 1.59, and 1.04, and accounted for 34%, 12%, and 8% of the total variance, respectively. The scree test showed that the plot of eigenvalues leveled off after the third extracted factor, supporting retention of the three factors. The Kaiser–Meyer–Olkin measure of sampling adequacy (MSA) showed an overall index of 0.88, indicating that data were adequate for factor analysis. The Bartlett's test for sphericity indicated that the intercorrelation matrix was factorable ($\chi^2_{(42)} = 463.82$, $p < 0.01$).

The first factor was entitled "Perspectives on Osteopathic Medicine" (rotated factor loadings ≥0.42 among its five items). A typical item representing this factor is: "A strong relationship between patient and physician is an extremely valuable therapeutic intervention that leads to improved outcomes." The second factor, "Osteopathic Diagnosis and Treatment" included five items with factor loadings ≥0.46. A typical item representing this factor is: "Touch and tactile approaches may not serve a significant purpose in patient care" (a reverse-scored item). The third factor, "Holistic-Integrative Care" included three items with factor loadings ≥0.54. A typical item representing this factor is: "The osteopathic philosophy of holistic care greatly influenced my decision to attend an osteopathic school." The Cronbach's coefficient alphas for the three extracted factors were 0.77, 0.71, and 0.73, respectively (see Hojat, DeSantis, Cain et al., 2021 for more detailed discussion).

Group Differences in ATOMS Scores

Scores of the ATOMS were compared for research participants by gender, race/ethnicity, academic background, and career interest.

Gender

The ATOMS mean score for men was 71.5 (*SD* = 10.0) and for women was 76.1 (*SD* = 8.3). The gender difference in favor of women was statistically significant ($p < 0.01$). The gender difference was also practically important as indicated by the effect size of 0.51 (see Table 14.13).

Race/Ethnicity

The highest mean score on ATOMS was obtained by Black/African-American students ($M = 77.3$, $SD = 9.2$), and the lowest by Asian students ($M = 72.9$, $SD = 9.5$). The mean scores of the White and Hispanic/Latino/Spanish origin groups were in

Table 14.13 Mean scores on the Attitudes Toward Osteopathic Medicine Scale (ATOMS) by gender, race/ethnicity, academic background, and career interest in a national sample of first-year matriculants of 46 campuses of US colleges of osteopathic medicine

	N	Mean	SD	*F*-ratio	*p*
Gender[a]					
Men	2653	71.5	10.0	$F_{(1,5615)} = 362.31$	<.01
Women	2964	76.1	8.3		
Race/Ethnicity[b]					
White/Caucasian	3386	73.9	9.4	$F_{(3,5099)} = 15.80$	<.01
Asian	1315	72.9	9.5		
Hispanic/Latino/Spanish origin	235	75.8	8.4		
Black/African American	167	77.3	9.2		
Academic Background[c]					
Biological Sciences	2833	74.1	9.3	$F_{(3,3939)} = 13.04$	<.01
Chemical/Physical Sciences	755	71.8	9.7		
Social/Behavioral Sciences	264	74.5	9.7		
Arts and Humanities	91	74.3	9.9		
Career Interest[d]					
People-oriented	2347	75.2	9.0	$F_{(2,5110)} = 40.21$	<.01
Technology/Procedure-oriented	1542	72.5	9.9		
Other	1224	73.2	9.6		

Reproduced from Hojat et al. (2021). ©Authors, Open Access
[a]Women > Men, effect size = 0.51
[b]Black/African American > Hispanic/Latino/Spanish origin > White/Caucasian and Asian, effect size between the highest and lowest mean scores = 0.47
[c]Chemical/Physical Sciences < all others, effect size between the highest and lowest mean scores = 0.28
[d]People-oriented > Other > Technology/Procedure-oriented, effect size between the highest and lowest mean scores = 0.28

between the other two groups. The differences in favor of the Black/African-American group versus Asian, White, and Hispanic/Latino/Spanish origin groups were statistically significant ($p < 0.01$). Also, the Hispanic/Latino/Spanish origin group obtained mean scores which were significantly higher than those obtained by White and Asian groups. The racial/ethnic differences were practically important (effect size between the highest and lowest scoring groups = 0.47) (see Table 14.13).

Academic Background

Respondents were asked to report their undergraduate major by choosing from a list of 56 undergraduate majors (sorted alphabetically). For statistical analysis, we grouped the undergraduate majors into the following four broad categories: "Biological Sciences," "Chemical/Physical Sciences," "Social/Behavioral Sciences," and "Arts and Humanities." We compared respondents with different undergraduate majors on their ATOMS scores.

The majority reported their undergraduate degree in "Biological Sciences" ($n = 2833$), followed by those who majored in "Chemical/Physical Sciences ($n = 755$), "Social/Behavioral Sciences" ($n = 264$), and "Arts and Humanities" ($n = 91$). The lowest ATOMS mean score was obtained for those who majored in "Chemical/Physical Sciences" ($M = 71.8$, $SD = 9.7$), which was significantly lower than the scores in the other three academic background groups ($p < .01$) (see Table 14.13).

Career Interest

Respondents were asked to choose from a list of 33 specialties (most frequently pursued by graduates of colleges of osteopathic medicine) that they planned to pursue after graduation from medical school. We divided the specialties into three broad categories: "People-Oriented" (e.g., family medicine, internal medicine, obstetrics and gynecology, and pediatrics); "Technology/Procedure-Oriented" (e.g., anesthesiology, dermatology, ophthalmology, orthopedic surgery, radiology, and surgery); and "Other" (including specialties chosen by fewer than 20 matriculants). This classification of specialties has been used in other studies with allopathic (Hojat, Gonnella, Nasca, Mangione, Veloski et al., 2002) and osteopathic medical students (Hojat, Shannon, DeSantis, Speicher et al., 2020).

Summary results of statistical analyses (reported in Table 14.13) showed that the highest ATOMS mean score was obtained by those who were interested in pursuing "People-Oriented" specialties ($M = 75.2$, $SD = 9.0$), and the lowest by those who planned to pursue "Technology-/Procedure-Oriented" specialties ($M = 72.5$, $SD = 9.9$) (see Table 14.13).

Associations Between ATOMS Scores and Personal Quality Measures

Bivariate correlations between the JSE and ATOMS scores, and the following personal quality measures are reported in Table 14.14: Emotional Empathy (measured by sum of the scores of two subscales-Empathic Concern and Personal Distress) from the *Interpersonal Reactivity Index* (IRI) (Davis 1983, 1994); the *Jefferson Scale of Attitudes Toward Interprofessional Collaboration* (JeffSATIC) (Hojat, Ward, Spandorfer, Arenson et al., 2015); The *Jefferson Scale of Attitudes Toward Physician Lifelong Learning* (JeffSPLL) (Hojat, Veloski, & Gonnella, 2009; Wetzel, Mazmanian, Hojat et al., 2010); and the *Shirom–Melamed Burnout Measure* (SMBM) (Shirom & Melamed, 2006; Melamed, Shirom et al., 2006). Summary results of statistical findings are reported in Table 14.14.

We also used multiple regression analysis to examine the unique contribution of each of the personal quality measures in predicting scores on the ATOMS. Table 14.14 shows bivariate correlations and results of multiple regression analyses such as standardized regression coefficients (β), unstandardized regression coefficients, standard errors, *t*-values, and statistical significance for unique contributions of the regressors in predicting ATOMS scores.

As shown in the table, all obtained bivariate correlations were statistically significant ($p < 0.01$), ranging from highs of 0.60 for interprofessional collaboration

Table 14.14 Summary results of multiple regression analysis[a] in a national sample of first-year matriculants of 46 campuses of US colleges of osteopathic medicine ($n = 5660$)

Regressors	Bivariate correlation[b]	Standardized regression coefficient (β)[c]	Unstandardized regression coefficient[d]	Standard error	*t*-Value
JSE	0.58**	0.30	0.25	0.01	23.00**
IRI	0.17**	0.08	0.13	0.02	7.50**
JeffSATIC	0.60**	0.33	0.25	0.01	25.08**
JeffSPLL	0.36**	0.13	0.22	0.02	11.73**
SMBM	−0.29**	−0.12	−1.27	0.11	−11.57**
Intercept	–	0	3.62	1.33	2.73*

Reproduced from Hojat, DeSantis, Cain et al. (2021). ©Authors, Open Access

JSE Jefferson Scale of Empathy, *IRI* Interpersonal Reactivity Index, *JeffSATIC* Jefferson Scale of Attitudes Toward Interprofessional Collaboration, *JeffSPLL* Jefferson Scale of Physician Lifelong Learning, *SMBM* Shirom–Melamed Burnout Measure

$^{**}p < 0.01$, $^{*}p < 0.05$, adjusted multiple $R = 0.68$, $p < 0.01$

[a]Scores on the Attitudes Toward Osteopathic Medicine Scale (ATOMS) as the dependent variable, and personal quality measures as regressors

[b]Bivariate correlation between the ATOMS scores and other personality measures shown in the table

[c]Standardized regression coefficients (β) are calculated from score distributions converted to a standard distribution for all regressors with a mean of zero and standard deviation of 1 for comparability purposes

[d]Unstandardized regression coefficients are calculated from raw score distributions

and 0.58 for clinical empathy, to a low of 0.17 for emotional empathy. The correlation between scores of the ATOMS and burnout measure was statistically significant and negative ($r = -0.29$, $p < 0.01$).

The largest unique and positive contributors to predicting ATOMS scores in the multivariate regression model included measures of interprofessional collaboration ($\beta = 0.33$) and clinical empathy ($\beta = 0.30$); the least contributors included orientation toward lifelong learning ($\beta = 0.13$) and emotional empathy ($\beta = 0.08$). Burnout showed a statistically significant negative contribution, meaning that lower scores on the ATOMS can lead to higher burnout experiences in osteopathic medical students. The adjusted multiple correlation was $R = 0.68$, meaning that 46% ($R^2 = 0.68^2 = 46\%$) of the variation in the ATOMS scores could be accounted for by the five regressors (Table 14.14). The results of statistical analyses reported in Table 14.14 provide support for the criterion-related validity of the ATOMS, given the direction and magnitude of empathy scores and other predictors consistent with expectation.

The bivariate correlations reported in Table 14.14 show that scores of the JSE-S-Version have statistically significant correlations with all other personal quality variables. The highest correlations were found between ATOMS scores and those of the JeffSATIC ($r = 0.60$) and JSE ($r = 0.58$); the lowest correlations were observed between ATOMS scores and the JeffSPLL ($r = 0.36$) and emotional empathy ($r = 0.17$). Also, a negative correlation was found between ATOMS scores and burnout experiences ($r = -0.29$). All of the correlations are in the expected direction. The aforementioned findings provide support for measurement properties and psychometrics of the ATOMS in a nationwide sample of osteopathic medical students.

National Norm Table for ATOMS Scores

The national sample in this study provided a unique opportunity to develop national norms for the ATOMS scores to determine the percentile rank of any new matriculant to osteopathic medical schools. Because of gender difference on ATOMS scores observed in this study, we calculated percentile ranks for the norm table for men and women separately (Table 14.15). For example, if the ATOMS score of a male matriculant is 80, first find the score interval that includes a score of 80 (79–80 score interval in Table 14.15), then find the corresponding national percentile rank displayed in the row for that score interval in the table. The corresponding national percentile rank in the table for a male matriculant with an ATOMS score of 80 is 78%, meaning that a score of 80 places a male matriculant in the 78th percentile rank of all first-year male matriculants. However, a female matriculant with an ATOMS score of 80 would be at the 61st percentile rank among female matriculants. If the gender is unknown, then the percentile rank on the norm table for men and women combined can be used as an estimate.

Table 14.15 National norm table for the Attitudes Toward Osteopathic Medicine Scale (ATOMS) in a national sample of first-year matriculants of 46 campuses of US colleges of osteopathic medicine

ATOMS	Men (n = 2653)			Women (n = 2964)			Combined (n = 5617)		
Raw score	*f*	*cf*	%tile Rank	*f*	*cf*	%tile Rank	*f*	*cf*	%tile Rank
≤46	17	17	<1%	1	1	<1%	18	18	<1%
47–48	14	31	1%	1	2	<1%	15	33	<1%
49–50	25	56	2%	5	7	<1%	30	63	1%
51–52	52	108	3%	25	32	1%	77	140	2%
53–54	46	154	5%	10	42	1%	56	196	3%
55–56	65	219	7%	18	60	2%	83	279	4%
57–58	75	294	10%	25	85	2%	100	379	6%
59–60	99	393	13%	42	127	4%	141	520	8%
61–62	109	502	17%	74	201	6%	183	703	11%
63–64	119	621	21%	84	285	8%	203	906	14%
65–66	157	778	26%	97	382	11%	254	1160	18%
67–68	183	961	33%	135	517	15%	318	1478	23%
69–70	186	1147	40%	172	689	20%	358	1836	29%
71–72	230	1377	48%	248	937	27%	478	2314	37%
73–74	220	1597	56%	256	1193	36%	476	2790	45%
75–76	212	1809	64%	259	1452	45%	471	3261	54%
77–78	181	1990	72%	238	1690	53%	419	3680	62%
79–80	146	2136	78%	249	1939	61%	395	4075	69%
81–82	148	2284	83%	251	2190	70%	399	4474	76%
83–84	89	2373	88%	279	2469	79%	368	4842	83%
85–86	111	2484	92%	217	2686	87%	328	5170	89%
87–88	94	2578	95%	151	2837	93%	245	5415	94%
≥ 89	75	2653	99%	127	2964	98%	202	5617	98%

Respondents who did not specify their sex as "male" or "female" (<1%) were excluded in this table
f frequency, *cf* cumulative frequency
Reproduced from Hojat et al. (2021). ©Authors, Open Access

Psychometrics of Personal Quality Measures Used in POMEE-Phase II and Their Associations with Clinical Empathy

The POMEE provided a unique opportunity to examine, for the first time, associations between students' scores in clinical empathy and personal quality measures on a national level. Evidence is also provided in support of the measurement properties and psychometrics of the following personal quality measures: *JeffSATIC, JeffSPLL, and SMBM* in national samples of osteopathic medical students.

Attitudes Toward Interprofessional Collaboration and Teamwork

The *Jefferson Scale of Attitudes Toward Interprofessional Collaboration* (JeffSATIC) is a 20-item instrument for measuring attitudes or orientation toward teamwork and interprofessional collaboration in health professions students and practitioners. Each item is answered on a seven-point Likert scale. Evidence supporting measurement properties and psychometrics of this instrument has been reported in allopathic medical students and other health professions students (Hojat, Ward, Spandorfer, Arenson et al., 2015).

The study sample was the cohort of POMEE-Phase II, excluding students with incomplete JSE and JeffSATIC surveys and those with surveys of questionable validity (determined by score > 3 on the Infrequency Scale of the ZKPQ). The final sample for statistical analyses included 5675 students; 2656 self-identified as male (47%); 2967 (52%) as female; and 52 (<1%) declined to report their gender.

Descriptive Statistics

The mean and standard deviation of JeffSATIC scores for the study sample were 121.9 and 12.6, respectively. The possible score range was 20–140 and actual range was 35–140. Cronbach's reliability coefficient was 0.90, which is in the acceptable range for educational and psychological tests. These findings are comparable to those reported in health professions students in the US (Hojat, Ward, Spandorfer, Arenson et al., 2015).

Item-Total Score Correlations

The corrected item-total score correlations of the 20-item JeffSATIC were calculated based on the correlation between each item score and the total score, excluding the corresponding item from the total score. All of these correlations were statistically significant ($p < 0.01$) and moderately high. They ranged from a low of 0.34 for this item: "Health professionals working together cannot be equally accountable for the care/service they provide," (a reverse-scored item) to a high of 0.68 for this item: "Health professionals should be made aware that their colleagues in other health-related disciplines can contribute to the quality of care." The median correlation was 0.53. Summary results are reported in Table 14.16.

Table 14.16 Corrected item-total score correlations[a] and effect sizes of item discrimination indices[b] for the Jefferson Scale of Attitudes Toward Interprofessional Collaboration (JeffSATIC) in a national sample of first-year matriculants of 46 campuses of US colleges of osteopathic medicine ($n = 5675$)

Item	Corrected item-total score correlation	Item discrimination index effect size
Health professionals should be viewed as collaborators rather than superiors or subordinates.	0.47	1.25
All health professionals should have responsibility for monitoring the effects of interventions on their patients/clients.	0.54	1.47
Teamwork in healthcare cannot be an outcome of interdisciplinary education.	0.45	1.32
Academic institutions should develop interdisciplinary educational programs to enhance collaborative practice.	0.57	1.62
Health professionals should not question decisions made by colleagues even if they feel that it might have detrimental effects on the patient/client.	0.47	0.96
All health professionals can contribute to decisions regarding the well-being of patients/clients.	0.55	1.58
Collaborative practice always works best when health professionals develop working relationships to achieve agreed upon goals.	0.60	1.55
Interdisciplinary education and interprofessional collaboration are not linked to one another.	0.58	1.60
The primary function of other health professionals is to follow, without question, orders by the physicians who are treating the patients/clients.	0.51	1.28
Interprofessional collaboration which includes mutual respect and communication improves the work environment.	0.63	1.25
All health professionals should contribute to decisions regarding improving care of their patients/clients.	0.57	1.71
Job satisfaction has nothing to do with interprofessional collaborative practices.	0.48	1.27
Health professionals should be made aware that their colleagues in other health-related disciplines can contribute to the quality of care.	0.68	1.95
Health professionals should be involved in making policy decisions concerning their work.	0.48	1.26
Because of role differentiation, there are not many overlapping areas of responsibility among health professionals in providing care to their patients/clients.	0.46	1.33
To promote the best interest of the patient/client, health professionals should use their own judgment rather than consulting their colleagues in other health-related disciplines.	0.50	1.39
Medical errors will be minimized when collaboration exists among health professionals.	0.54	1.41

(continued)

Table 14.16 (continued)

Item	Corrected item-total score correlation	Item discrimination index effect size
All health professionals have their own special expertise to render quality care to their patients/clients.	0.39	1.09
Health professionals working together cannot be equally accountable for the care/service they provide.	0.34	1.15
During their education, all health profession students should have experience working in teams with other health profession students in order to understand their respective role.	0.60	1.44
Mean (Median)	0.52 (0.53)	

[a]Correlations between scores on each item and the JeffSATIC total score by excluding the corresponding item from the total score; all were statistically significant ($p < 0.01$)
[b]Effect size estimate (Cohen's *d* statistic) of the discrimination index was calculated by subtracting the item mean score of the JeffSATIC high scorers (top 33%, scores > 127, $n = 1946$) from the item mean score of the JeffSATIC low scorers (bottom 33%, scores < 119, $n = 1969$), divided by the pooled standard deviation of the corresponding item

Effect Sizes of Item Discrimination Indices

The effect sizes of item discrimination indices were calculated by subtracting the item mean score for the top 33% JeffSATIC scorers from the mean score of the same item obtained by the bottom 33% JeffSATIC scorers, divided by the pooled standard deviation of the corresponding item. These effect sizes are analogous to the Cohen's *d* statistic (Cohen, 1987). All of the effect sizes were substantially large (>0.95) indicating that the differences in mean item scores between high and low JeffSATIC scorers were both statistically significant in the favor of high scorers, and practically important, as evidenced by large effect sizes (see Table 14.16).

Exploratory Factor Analysis

We explored the underlying components of the JeffSATIC by using an exploratory factor analysis ($n = 5675$). We used principal components factor analysis with oblique rotation (promax) to allow correlations among the extracted variables.

The scree test was used to determine the number of factors to retain, which showed that the plot of eigenvalues levels off after the third factor was extracted. Thus, we limited the number of retained factors to three. The Kaiser–Meyer–Olkin measure of sampling adequacy (MSA) was used, which showed an overall index of 0.95, indicating that data were adequate for factor analysis. Also, the Bartlett's test for sphericity indicated that the intercorrelation matrix was factorable ($x^2_{(133)} = 1897.18$, $p < 0.01$).

The eigenvalues for the three retained factors before rotation were 6.93, 1.53, and 1.02, accounting for 35%, 8%, and 5% of the total variance, respectively. The first factor, "Working Relationships," included nine items with factor coefficients equal to or greater than 0.43. The second factor, "Accountability," included eight items with factor coefficients equal to or greater than 0.34. These factors emerged in samples of a multi-institutional study of health professions students in the US and Australia (Hojat, Ward, Spandorfer, Arenson et al., 2015). The third factor was a residual factor that included three items with factor coefficients equal to or greater than 0.38 that address authority, monitoring, and interdisciplinary education. The Cronbach's coefficient alphas for the three factors were 0.85, 0.78, and 0.68, respectively. Summary results of factor analysis are reported in Table 14.17.

Group Differences in JeffSATIC Scores

Scores of the JeffSATIC were compared for research participants by gender, race/ethnicity, academic background, and career interest. Summary statistical results are reported in Table 14.18.

Gender

The JeffSATIC mean score for men was 119.52 (SD = 13.28) and for women was 124.18 (SD = 11.25). The gender difference in favor of women was statistically significant ($p < 0.01$). The gender difference was not negligible as indicated by the effect size of 0.38 (see Table 14.18). Significant gender differences in JeffSATIC scores in favor of women were observed in samples of a multi-institutional study of health professions students in the US and Australia (Hojat, Ward, Spandorfer, Arenson et al., 2015).

Race/Ethnicity

The highest mean score on JeffSATIC was obtained by Black/African-American students (M = 124.32, SD = 12.87) and the lowest by Asian students (M = 121.34, SD = 12.84). The mean scores of the White and Hispanic/Latino/Spanish origin groups were in between the other two groups. The differences in favor of the Black/African-American group versus Asian and White groups were statistically significant ($p < .05$). The effect size of the difference between the highest and lowest scoring groups was low: 0.23 (see Table 14.18).

Table 14.17 Rotated factor loadings[a] for the Jefferson Scale of Attitudes Toward Interprofessional Collaboration (JeffSATIC) in a national sample of first-year matriculants of 46 campuses of US of colleges of osteopathic medicine ($n = 5675$)

Item	Factor 1	Factor 2	Factor 3
Health professionals should be made aware that their colleagues in other health-related disciplines can contribute to the quality of care. (13)	**0.63**	0.10	0.10
Health professionals should be involved in making policy decisions concerning their work. (14)	**0.60**	0.06	−0.12
Interprofessional collaboration which includes mutual respect and communication improves the work environment. (10)	**0.59**	0.17	−0.01
Collaborative practice always works best when health professionals develop working relationships to achieve agreed upon goals. (7)	**0.55**	0.04	0.15
All health professionals have their own special expertise to render quality care to their patients/clients. (18)	**0.53**	−0.07	−0.02
All health professionals should contribute to decisions regarding improving care of their patients/clients. (11)	**0.51**	−0.06	0.26
Medical errors will be minimized when collaboration exists among health professionals. (17)	**0.49**	0.06	0.09
All health professionals can contribute to decisions regarding the well-being of patients/clients. (6)	**0.49**	−0.02	0.22
During their education, all health profession students should have experience working in teams with other health profession students in order to understand their respective role. (20)	**0.43**	0.13	0.18
Health professionals should not question decisions made by colleagues even if they feel that it might have detrimental effects on the patient/client. (5)	0.15	**0.59**	−0.18
Interdisciplinary education and interprofessional collaboration are not linked to one another. (8)	−0.02	**0.58**	0.18
Because of role differentiation, there are not many overlapping areas of responsibility among health professionals in providing care to their patients/clients. (15)	−0.05	**0.56**	0.07
The primary function of other health professionals is to follow, without question, orders by the physicians who are treating the patients/clients. (9)	0.03	**0.55**	0.05
To promote the best interest of the patient/client, health professionals should use their own judgment rather than consulting their colleagues in other health-related disciplines. (16)	0.09	**0.55**	−0.03
Teamwork in healthcare cannot be an outcome of interdisciplinary education. (3)	−0.02	**0.51**	0.07
Job satisfaction has nothing to do with interprofessional collaborative practices. (12)	0.13	**0.46**	−0.01
Health professionals working together cannot be equally accountable for the care/service they provide. (19)	−0.11	**0.34**	0.22
Health professionals should be viewed as collaborators rather than superiors or subordinates. (1)	0.07	0.00	**0.60**
All health professionals should have responsibility for monitoring the effects of interventions on their patients/clients. (2)	0.23	−0.01	**0.50**

(continued)

Table 14.17 (continued)

Item	Factor 1	Factor 2	Factor 3
Academic institutions should develop interdisciplinary educational programs to enhance collaborative practice. (4)	0.18	0.19	**0.38**
Eigenvalue	6.93	1.53	1.02

[a]Factor 1 was entitled "Working Relationships," Factor 2: "Accountability," and Factor 3 was a residual factor. Items are sorted by descending order of factor loadings within each factor. Numbers in parentheses refer to the appearance of the items in the JeffSATIC instrument
Factor coefficients ≥0.34 are shown in **bold**

Table 14.18 Means and standard deviations of the Jefferson Scale of Attitudes Toward Interprofessional Collaboration (JeffSATIC) by gender, race/ethnicity, academic background, and career interest in a national sample of first-year matriculants of 46 campuses of US colleges of osteopathic medicine

	N	Mean	SD
Gender[a]			
Men	2656	119.52	13.28
Women	2967	124.18	11.25
Race/ethnicity[b]			
White/Caucasian	3390	122.03	12.28
Asian	1316	121.34	12.84
Hispanic/Latino/Spanish origin	234	122.84	12.23
Black/African American	167	124.32	12.87
Academic background[c]			
Biological Sciences	2830	121.55	12.56
Chemical/Physical Sciences	756	121.25	12.66
Social/Behavioral Sciences	266	122.69	12.77
Arts and Humanities	91	121.04	13.28
Career interest[d]			
People-oriented	2347	123.04	12.02
Technology/procedure-oriented	1544	120.04	13.27
Other	1226	122.15	12.08

[a]Women > Men, effect size = 0.38
[b]Black/African American > White/Caucasian and Asian, effect size = 0.23
[c]No differences
[d]People-oriented > Other > Technology-oriented, effect size = 0.24

Academic Background

We grouped the students' undergraduate majors into the following four broad categories: "Biological Sciences," "Chemical/Physical Sciences," "Social/Behavioral Sciences," and "Arts and Humanities." We compared respondents with different undergraduate majors on the JeffSATIC scores. No significant differences were observed in the JeffSATIC scores among students with different academic backgrounds (see Table 14.18).

Career Interest

Respondents were asked about the specialty they were planning to pursue after graduation from medical school. As described previously, we divided the reported specialties into three broad categories: "People-Oriented" (e.g., family medicine, internal medicine, obstetrics and gynecology, and pediatrics); "Technology-/Procedure-Oriented" (e.g., anesthesiology, dermatology, ophthalmology, orthopedic surgery, radiology, and surgery); and "Other" (including specialties chosen by fewer than 20 matriculants). This classification of specialties has been used in other studies with allopathic (Hojat, Gonnella, Nasca, Mangione, Veloski et al., 2002) and osteopathic medical students (Hojat, Shannon, DeSantis, Speicher et al., 2020). Summary results of statistical analyses, reported in Table 14.18, showed that the highest JeffSATIC mean score was obtained by those who were interested in pursuing "People-Oriented" specialties ($M = 123.04$, $SD = 12.02$) and the lowest by those who planned to pursue "Technology-/Procedure-Oriented" specialties ($M = 120.04$, $SD = 13.27$). The difference was statistically significant ($p < 0.01$) and the effect size estimate between mean scores of those interested in "People-Oriented" versus "Technology-/Procedure-Oriented" specialties was 0.24.

The JeffSATIC Scores, Clinical Empathy, Attitudes Toward Osteopathic Medicine, and Personal Quality Measures

Correlations between scores of the JeffSATIC and scores of clinical empathy and other personal quality measures are reported in Table 14.19.

Reported in the table are bivariate correlations between JeffSATIC scores, JSE scores, and the following personal quality measures: emotional empathy (measured by sum of the scores of two subscales, Empathic Concern and Personal Distress) from the Interpersonal Reactivity Index (IRI) (Davis 1983, 1994; see Chap. 5); JeffSPLL (Hojat, Veloski, & Gonnella, 2009; Wetzel, Mazmanian, Hojat et al., 2010); and the SMBM (Shirom & Melamed 2006; Melamed, Shirom et al., 2006).

We used multiple regression analysis to examine the unique contribution of each of the personal quality measures in predicting scores on the JeffSATIC. Table 14.19 shows Pearson bivariate correlations and results of multiple regression analyses, such as standardized regression coefficients (β), unstandardized regression coefficients, standard errors, *t*-values, and statistical significance for unique contributions of the regressors in predicting JeffSATIC scores.

As shown in Table 14.19, all obtained bivariate correlations were statistically significant ($p < 0.01$), ranging from a high of 0.64 for clinical empathy to a low of 0.15 for emotional empathy. The correlation between scores on the JeffSATIC and the burnout measure was statistically significant and negative ($r = -0.24$, $p < 0.01$).

The largest unique and positive contributors to predicting JeffSATIC scores in the multivariate regression model were scores on the JSE ($\beta = 0.42$) and ATOMS (β

Table 14.19 Summary results of multiple regression analysis[a] in a national sample of first-year matriculants of 46 campuses of US colleges of osteopathic medicine ($n = 5653$)

Regressors	Bivariate correlation[b]	Standardized regression coefficient[c]	Unstandardized regression coefficient[d]	Standard error	t-Value
JSE	0.64**	0.42	0.47	0.01	35.74**
IRI	0.15**	0.01	0.03	0.02	1.35
ATOMS	0.60**	0.31	0.40	0.02	25.08**
JeffSPLL	0.35**	0.11	0.26	0.02	10.96**
SMBM	−0.24**	−0.03	−0.41	0.14	−2.91**
Intercept	–	0	24.80	1.66	14.95**

Excludes students with incomplete responses, and those who scored > 3 on the Infrequency Scale of the ZKPQ to mitigate the effect of social desirability response bias

JSE Jefferson Scale of Empathy, *IRI* Interpersonal Reactivity Index, *ATOMS* Attitudes Toward Osteopathic Medicine Scale, *JeffSPLL* Jefferson Scale of Physician Lifelong Learning, *SMBM* Shirom–Melamed Burnout Measure

**$p < 0.01$, adjusted multiple $R = 0.71$, $p < 0.01$

[a]Scores on the Jefferson Scale of Attitudes Toward Interprofessional Collaboration (JeffSATIC) as the dependent variable, and personality measures as regressors

[b]Bivariate correlation between the JeffSATIC scores and other personality measures shown in the table

[c]Standardized regression coefficients (β) are calculated from score distributions converted to a standard distribution for all regressors with a mean of zero and standard deviation of 1 for comparability purposes

[d]Unstandardized regression coefficients are calculated from raw score distributions

= 0.31), and the least contributors were emotional empathy (β = 0.01) and JeffSPLL (β = 0.11). The Burnout measure showed a statistically significant negative contribution, meaning that lower scores on the JeffSATIC predict higher burnout experiences in osteopathic medical students. The adjusted multiple correlation was $R = 0.71$, meaning that 50% ($R^2 = 0.71^2 = 50\%$) of the variation in the JeffSATIC scores could be accounted for by the five regressors (Table 14.19).

In the multiple regression analysis, with the exception of emotional empathy, all other regressors (listed in Table 14.19) contributed significantly and uniquely to the prediction of the JeffSATIC scores. Summary results of statistical analyses reported in Table 14.19 provide support for the criterion-related validity of the JeffSATIC in a nationwide sample of osteopathic medical students. The magnitude and direction of associations are mostly consistent with our expectations.

National Norm Table for JeffSATIC Scores

The national sample in POMEE provided an opportunity to develop national norms for JeffSATIC scores to determine the percentile ranks of new matriculants to osteopathic medical schools. Because of the observed gender differences on JeffSATIC in this study, we calculated percentile ranks for the norm table for men and women separately (Table 14.20). For example, if the JeffSATIC score of a male matriculant is 128, first locate the score interval that includes a score of 128 (e.g., 127–128 score interval in Table 14.20), then find the corresponding national percentile rank displayed in the row for that score interval in the table. The

Table 14.20 National norm table for the Jefferson Scale of Attitudes Toward Interprofessional Collaboration (JeffSATIC) in a national sample of first-year matriculants of 46 campuses of US colleges of osteopathic medicine ($n = 5623$)

	Men only ($n = 2656$)			Women only ($n = 2967$)			Men & women combined		
JeffSATIC score	*f*	*cf*	%tile rank	*f*	*cf*	%tile rank	*f*	*cf*	%tile rank
≤80	35	35	1%	15	15	0%	50	50	0%
81–82	11	46	2%	1	16	1%	12	62	1%
83–84	14	60	2%	7	23	1%	21	83	1%
85–86	12	72	2%	0	23	1%	12	95	2%
87–88	15	87	3%	4	27	1%	19	114	2%
89–90	8	95	3%	6	33	1%	14	128	2%
91–92	16	111	4%	8	41	1%	24	152	2%
93–94	22	133	5%	12	53	2%	34	186	3%
95–96	21	154	5%	9	62	2%	30	216	4%
97–98	38	192	7%	13	75	2%	51	267	4%
99–100	50	242	8%	22	97	3%	72	339	5%
101–102	44	286	10%	26	123	4%	70	409	7%
103–104	66	352	12%	38	161	5%	104	513	8%
105–106	56	408	14%	51	212	6%	107	620	10%
107–108	83	491	17%	57	269	8%	140	760	12%
109–110	87	578	20%	72	341	10%	159	919	15%
111–112	99	677	24%	97	438	13%	196	1115	18%
113–114	128	805	28%	102	540	16%	230	1345	22%
115–116	158	963	33%	119	659	20%	277	1622	26%
117–118	168	1131	39%	128	787	24%	296	1918	31%
119–120	156	1287	46%	169	956	29%	325	2243	37%
121–122	157	1444	51%	195	1151	36%	352	2595	43%
123–124	156	1600	57%	175	1326	42%	331	2926	49%
125–126	150	1750	63%	230	1556	49%	380	3306	55%
127–128	175	1925	69%	205	1761	56%	380	3686	62%
129–130	143	2068	75%	188	1949	63%	331	4017	68%
131–132	149	2217	81%	220	2169	69%	369	4386	75%
133–134	123	2340	86%	260	2429	77%	383	4769	81%
135–136	108	2448	90%	191	2620	85%	299	5068	87%
137–138	98	2546	94%	180	2800	91%	278	5346	93%
139–140	110	2656	98%	167	2967	97%	277	5623	98%

Excluded were students with incomplete JSE and JeffSATIC, those who scored > 3 on the Infrequency Scale of the ZKPQ, and those who did not report their gender
f frequency, *cf* cumulative frequency

corresponding national percentile rank in the table for a male matriculant with a JeffSATIC score of 128 is 69%, meaning that a score of 128 places a male matriculant in the 69th percentile rank of all first-year male matriculants. However, a female matriculant with a JeffSATIC score of 128 would be placed at the 56th percentile rank of female matriculants. If the gender is unknown, then the percentile rank on the norm table for men and women combined can be used as an estimate.

Orientation Toward Lifelong Learning

The 14-item *Jefferson Scale of Physician Lifelong Learning* (JeffSPLL) was used to measure attitudes or orientation toward lifelong learning in medical students and physicians. Evidence supporting measurement properties and psychometrics of this instrument has been reported in medical (Hojat, Nasca, Gonnella, Frisby et al., 2003; Hojat, Veloski, & Gonnella, 2009, 2010, 2012; Wetzel et al., 2010) and other health professions students and practitioners. It has also been translated into several languages (e.g., Arabic, Chinese, Hebrew, Korean, Portuguese, and Spanish).

The usable sample included the cohort of POMEE-Phase II. Students with incomplete surveys (on the JSE and JeffSPLL) or with records of questionable validity (determined by their score of >3 on the Infrequency Scale of the ZKPQ) were excluded. Therefore, the final sample for statistical analysis in this study included 5669 students (2654 men; 2963 women; and 52 students who declined to specify their gender).

Descriptive Statistics

The mean and standard deviation of the JeffSPLL scores for the study sample were 45.4 and 5.4, respectively. The possible score range was 14–56, and the actual score range was 19–56. The Cronbach's reliability coefficient alpha was 0.83, which is in the accepted range of educational and psychological tests. These figures are comparable to those reported for allopathic medical students in the US (Witzel, Mazmanian, Hojat et al., 2010).

Item-Total Score Correlations

The corrected item-total score correlations of the 14 items of JeffSPLL and item discrimination indices are reported in Table 14.21. The corrected correlations are calculated based on the correlation between each item score and the total score of the JeffSPLL, excluding the corresponding item from the total score. All corrected item-total score correlations were statistically significant ($p < 0.01$) and moderately

Table 14.21 Corrected item-total score correlations[a] and effect sizes of item discrimination indices[b] for the Jefferson Scale of Physician Lifelong Learning (JeffSPLL) in a national sample of first-year matriculants of 46 campuses of US colleges of osteopathic medicine ($n = 5669$)

Item	Corrected item-total score correlation	Item discrimination index effect size
Searching for the answer to a question is, in and by itself rewarding. (1)	0.40	1.18
Lifelong learning is a professional responsibility of all physicians. (2)	0.33	0.71
I enjoy reading articles in which issues of medicine are discussed. (3)	0.54	1.64
I routinely attend meetings of student study groups. (4)	0.39	1.21
I read medical literature in journals, websites, or textbooks at least once every week. (5)	0.51	1.61
I routinely search computer databases to find out about new developments in medicine. (6)	0.54	1.58
I believe that I would fall behind if I stopped learning about new developments in medicine. (7)	0.42	1.23
One of the important goals of medical school is to develop students' lifelong learning skills. (8)	0.37	0.94
Rapid changes in medical science require constant updating of knowledge and development of new professional skills. (9)	0.41	1.07
I always make time for learning on my own, even when I have a busy class schedule and other obligations. (10)	0.48	1.56
I recognize my need to constantly acquire new professional knowledge. (11)	0.51	1.49
I routinely attend optional sessions, such as grand rounds, guest lectures, or clinics where I can volunteer to improve my knowledge and clinical skills. (12)	0.50	1.53
I take every opportunity to gain new knowledge/skills that are important to medicine. (13)	0.61	1.96
My preferred approach in finding an answer to a question is to consult a credible resource such as a text, computer database, or colleague. (14)	0.41	1.22
Mean (Median)	0.46 (0.45)	

Numbers in parentheses refer to the appearance of the items in the JeffSPLL instrument

[a]Correlations between scores on each item and the JeffSPLL total score by excluding the corresponding item from the total score, all were statistically significant ($p < 0.01$)

[b]Effect size estimate (Cohen's *d* statistic) of the discrimination index was calculated by subtracting the item mean score of the JeffSPLL high scorers (top 33%) from the item mean score of the JeffSPLL low scorers (bottom 33%), divided by the pooled standard deviation of the corresponding item

high, ranging from a low of 0.33 for this item: "Life-long learning is a professional responsibility of all physicians" to a high of 0.61 for the item: "I take every opportunity to gain new knowledge/skills that are important to medicine." The median for corrected item-total score correlation was 0.45.

Effect Sizes of Item Discrimination Indices

The effect sizes of item discrimination indices were calculated by subtracting the item mean score for the top 33% JeffSPLL scorers from the mean score of the same item obtained by the bottom 33% JeffSPLL scorers, divided by the pooled standard deviation of the corresponding item. These effect sizes are analogous to the Cohen's *d* statistics (Cohen, 1987). All of the effect sizes were substantially large (>0.70), indicating that the difference in mean item scores between high and low JeffSPLL scorers were both statistically significant in the favor of high scorers, and practically important, evident from large effect sizes (see Table 14.21).

Exploratory Factor Analysis

We explored the underlying components of the JeffSPLL in a nationwide sample of matriculants of osteopathic medical schools by using an exploratory factor analysis ($n = 5669$). We used principal components factor analysis with oblique rotation (promax) to allow correlations among the extracted variables (see Table 14.22).

The scree test was used to determine the number of factors to retain, which showed that the plot of eigenvalues levels off after the second factor is extracted. Thus, we limited the number of retained factors to two. The Kaiser–Meyer–Olkin measure of sampling adequacy (MSA) was used, which showed an overall index of 0.87, indicating the data were adequate for factor analysis. Also, the Bartlett's test for sphericity indicated that the intercorrelation matrix was factorable ($x^2_{(64)} = 2016.88$, $p < 0.01$). The eigenvalues for the two retained factors before rotation were 4.47, and 1.87, accounting for 32% and 13% of the total variance, respectively.

The first factor, "Attention to Learning Opportunities," included seven items with factor coefficients equal to or greater than 0.38. The second factor, "Learning Beliefs and Motivation," included seven items with factor coefficients equal to or greater than 0.32. These factors were similar to those that emerged in samples of allopathic medical students and physicians (Hojat, Veloski, Gonnella, 2009, 2010, 2012; Wetzel et al., 2010). The Cronbach's coefficient alphas for these two factors were 0.79 and 0.77, respectively (Table 14.22).

Table 14.22 Rotated factor loadings[a] for the Jefferson Scale of Physician Lifelong Learning (JeffSPLL) in a national sample of first-year matriculants of 46 campuses of US colleges of osteopathic medicine ($n = 5669$)

Item	Factor 1	Factor 2
I routinely search computer databases to find out about new developments in medicine. (6)	**0.75**	−0.10
I read medical literature in journals, websites, or textbooks at least once every week. (5)	**0.72**	−0.09
I routinely attend optional sessions, such as grand rounds, guest lectures, or clinics where I can volunteer to improve my knowledge and clinical skills. (12)	**0.59**	0.03
I take every opportunity to gain new knowledge/skills that are important to medicine. (13)	**0.59**	0.18
I routinely attend meetings of student study groups. (4)	**0.48**	−0.01
I always make time for learning on my own, even when I have a busy class schedule and other obligations. (10)	**0.45**	0.16
I enjoy reading articles in which issues of medicine are discussed. (3)	**0.38**	0.32
Rapid changes in medical science require constant updating of knowledge and development of new professional skills. (9)	−0.07	**0.73**
One of the important goals of medical school is to develop students' lifelong learning skills. (8)	−0.08	**0.68**
Lifelong learning is a professional responsibility of all physicians. (2)	−0.11	**0.66**
I recognize my need to constantly acquire new professional knowledge. (11)	0.18	**0.55**
My preferred approach in finding an answer to a question is to consult a credible resource such as a text, computer database, or colleague. (14)	0.13	**0.47**
I believe that I would fall behind if I stopped learning about new developments in medicine. (7)	0.22	**0.36**
Searching for the answer to a question is, in and by itself rewarding. (1)	0.23	**0.32**
Eigenvalue	4.47	1.87

[a]Factor 1 was entitled "Attention to Learning Opportunities," and Factor 2: "Learning Beliefs and Motivation." Items are sorted by descending order of factor loadings within each factor. Numbers in parentheses refer to the appearance of the items in the JeffSPLL instrument
Factor coefficients ≥0.32 are shown in **bold**

Group Differences in JeffSPLL Scores

Scores of the JeffSPLL were compared for research participants by gender, race/ethnicity, academic background, and career interest. Summary statistical results are reported in Table 14.23.

Gender

The JeffSPLL mean score for men was 45.23 ($SD = 5.6$), and for women was 45.55 ($SD = 5.3$). Although gender difference in favor of women was statistically significant ($p < 0.05$), it was practically negligible (Cohen's effect size of $d = 0.06$).

Table 14.23 Jefferson Scale of Physician Lifelong Learning by gender, race/ethnicity, academic background, and career interest in a national sample of first-year matriculants of 46 campuses of US colleges of osteopathic medicine ($n = 5669$)

	N	*Mean*	*SD*	*F*-ratio	*p*
Gender[a]					
Men	2654	45.23	5.6	$F_{(1,5615)} = 4.90$	<.05
Women	2963	45.55	5.3		
Race/ethnicity[b]					
White/Caucasian	3387	45.45	5.3	$F_{(3,5098)} = 8.39$	<.01
Asian	1314	44.83	5.7		
Hispanic/Latino/Spanish origin	235	46.53	4.9		
Black/African American	166	45.60	5.4		
Academic background[c]					
Biological Sciences	2831	45.24	5.3	$F_{(3,3936)} = 0.71$	0.54
Chemical/Physical Sciences	755	45.01	5.5		
Social/Behavioral Sciences	263	45.29	5.9		
Arts and Humanities	91	45.77	5.7		
Career interest[d]					
People-oriented	2344	45.22	5.3	$F_{(2,5108)} = 4.16$	<.05
Technology-oriented	1544	45.69	5.5		
Other	1223	45.62	5.6		

[a]Women > Men, effect size = 0.06
[b]Hispanic/Latino/Spanish origin > all others, effect size = 0.31
[c]No statistically significant differences
[d]People-oriented < all others, effect size = 0.09

Race/Ethnicity

The highest mean score on the JeffSPLL was obtained by the Hispanic/Latino/Spanish origin group ($M = 46.53$, $SD = 4.9$); that was significantly higher than other groups, but practically unimportant due to the low magnitude of the effect size estimate ($d = 0.31$).

Academic Background

As described previously, we grouped the students' undergraduate majors into the following four broad categories: "Biological Sciences," "Chemical/Physical Sciences," "Social/Behavioral Sciences," and "Arts and Humanities." We compared respondents with different undergraduate majors on their JeffSPLL scores. No significant differences were observed among students with different academic backgrounds (see Table 14.23).

Career Interest

Respondents were asked about the specialty they were planning to pursue after graduation from medical school. As described previously, we divided the reported specialties into three broad categories: "People-Oriented" (e.g., family medicine, internal medicine, obstetrics and gynecology, and pediatrics); "Technology-/ Procedure-Oriented" (e.g., anesthesiology, dermatology, ophthalmology, orthopedic surgery, radiology, and surgery); and "Other" (including specialties chosen by fewer than 20 matriculants).

Summary results of statistical analyses are reported in Table 14.23. Mean scores were very close among the three comparison groups; there were statistically significant differences that were practically negligible (effect size estimate = 0.09).

The JeffSPLL Scores, Clinical Empathy, Attitudes Toward Osteopathic Medicine, and Personal Quality Measures

Reported in Table 14.24 are Pearson bivariate correlations between scores on the JeffSPLL, clinical empathy (JSE), and the selected personal quality measures. Multiple regression analysis was used to examine the unique contribution of each of the regressors reported in the table in predicting scores on the JeffSPLL. Summary results of statistical analyses are presented in Table 14.24.

As shown, with the exception of emotional empathy (combined scores on the Empathic Concern and Personal Distress of the IRI subscales), all other obtained bivariate correlations were modest in magnitude and statistically significant ($p < 0.01$), with highs of 0.36 (for the ATOMS) and 0.35 (for the JeffSATIC) to a low of 0.01 (for the emotional empathy). The correlation between scores of the JeffSPLL and burnout measure was statistically significant and negative ($r = -0.29$, $p < 0.01$). The largest unique and positive contributions to predicting JeffSPLL scores in the multivariate regression model were scores on the ATOMS ($\beta = 0.19$) and JeffSATIC ($\beta = 0.18$).

The burnout measure showed a statistically significant and negative contribution ($\beta = -0.18$), meaning that lower scores on the JeffSPLL predicted higher burnout experiences in osteopathic medical students. The adjusted multiple correlation was $R = 0.44$, meaning that 19% ($R^2 = 0.44^2 = 19\%$) of the variation in the JeffSPLL scores could be accounted for by the five regressors (Table 14.24). In the multiple regression analysis, except for emotional empathy, all other regressors listed in Table 14.24 contributed significantly and uniquely to the prediction of the JeffSPLL scores. The results of statistical analyses reported in Table 14.24 generally provide support for the criterion-related validity of the JeffSPLL in a nationwide sample of osteopathic medical students. The magnitude and direction of associations are mostly consistent with our expectations.

Table 14.24 Summary results of multiple regression analysis[a] in a national sample of first-year matriculants of 46 campuses of US colleges of osteopathic medicine in predicting JeffSPLL scores[a] ($n = 5653$)

Regressors	Bivariate correlation[b]	Standardized regression coefficient[c]	Unstandardized regression coefficient[d]	Standard error	*t*-Value
JSE	0.28**	0.02	0.01	0.01	1.25
IRI	0.01	−0.03	−0.03	0.01	−2.44*
JeffSATIC	0.35**	0.18	0.08	0.01	10.96**
ATOMS	0.36**	0.19	0.11	0.01	11.73**
SMBM	−0.29**	−0.18	−1.09	0.08	−14.12**
Intercept	–	0	30.25	0.84	35.89**

Excluded were students with incomplete surveys of the six measures, or those who scored > 3 on the Infrequency Scale of the ZKPQ

JSE Jefferson Scale of Empathy, *IRI* Interpersonal Reactivity Index, *JeffSATIC* Jefferson Scale of Attitudes Toward Interprofessional Collaboration, *ATOMS* Attitudes Toward Osteopathic Medicine Scale, *SMBM* Shirom–Melamed Burnout Measure

**$p < 0.01$, *$p < 0.05$, adjusted multiple $R = 0.44$, $p < 0.01$

[a]Scores on the Jefferson Scale of Physician Lifelong Learning (JeffSPLL) as the dependent variable, and personality measures as regressors

[b]Bivariate correlations between the JeffSPLL scores and other personality measures shown in the table

[c]Standardized regression coefficients (β) are calculated from score distributions converted to a standard distribution for all regressors with a mean of zero and standard deviation of 1 for comparability purposes

[d]Unstandardized regression coefficients are calculated from raw score distributions

National Norm Table for JeffSPLL Scores

Because we observed no practically important gender difference on the JeffSPLL scores, we did not prepare the norm table separately by gender. Table 14.25 presents national percentile ranks of the JeffSPLL scores for the total study sample, regardless of gender for first-year matriculants of US colleges of osteopathic medicine.

The norm table should be used like other norm tables for other personal quality measures presented in this chapter. For example, if the JeffSPLL score of a matriculant (regardless of gender) is 51, first find the score interval that includes a score of 51 (e.g., 51–52 score interval in Table 14.25), then find the corresponding national percentile rank displayed in the row for that score interval in the table. The corresponding national percentile rank in Table 14.25 for the 51–52 interval is 86%, meaning that a score of 51 places the matriculant in the 86th percentile rank of all first-year matriculants.

Table 14.25 National norm table for the Jefferson Scale of Physician Lifelong Learning (JeffSPLL) in a national sample of first-year matriculants of 46 campuses of US colleges of osteopathic medicine ($n = 5669$)

JeffSPLL	*f*	*cf*	%tile rank
≤30	25	25	<1%
31–32	39	64	1%
33–34	80	144	2%
35–36	151	295	4%
37–38	279	574	8%
39–40	488	1062	14%
41–42	645	1707	24%
43–44	755	2462	37%
45–46	756	3218	50%
47–48	759	3977	63%
49–50	655	4632	76%
51–52	466	5098	86%
53–54	319	5417	93%
55–56	252	5669	98%

Excluded were students with incomplete surveys (JSE and JeffSPLL), or students who scored > 3 on the Infrequency Scale
f frequency, *cf* cumulative frequency

Burnout Measure

We used the 14-item *Shirom–Melamed Burnout Measure* (SMBM) instrument to quantify burnout experiences in medical students (Shirom & Melamed, 2006; Melamed, Shirom et al., 2006). The items were answered on a seven-point Likert scale, and the final score, according to the suggestion by its authors, is the average of the item scores. The POMEE provided this unique opportunity, for the first time, to examine measurement properties and psychometrics of this instrument in a nationwide sample of matriculants to osteopathic medical colleges.

The study sample for statistical analyses of this measure was POMEE-Phase II cohort, including 5672 students (2653 men; 2967 women; and 52 who did not identify their gender) and completed a web-based survey at the beginning of the first year of medical school (academic year 2019–2020). Respondents with incomplete surveys, or with records of questionable validity (determined by their score of greater than 3 on the Infrequency Scale of the ZKPQ) were excluded from the study sample.

Descriptive Statistics

The mean and standard deviation of the SMBM scores for the total study sample were 2.70 and 0.90, respectively. The possible score range was 1–7; the actual score range was also 1–7. The Cronbach's reliability coefficient alpha was 0.93, which is in the higher range of educational and psychological tests.

Item-Total Score Correlations

The corrected item-total score correlations of the 14 items of the SMBM and item discrimination indices are reported in Table 14.26. The corrected correlations are calculated based on the correlation between each item score and the total score of the SMBM (excluding the corresponding item from the total score). All corrected item-total score correlations were statistically significant ($p < 0.01$), and relatively high, ranging from a low of 0.51 for this item: "I feel I am not capable of investing emotionally in coworkers and customers," to a high of 0.78 for this item: "I feel I'm not thinking clearly." The median correlation was 0.70.

Effect Sizes of Item Discrimination Indices

The effect sizes of item discrimination indices were calculated by subtracting the item mean score for the top 33% SMBM scorers from the mean score of the same item obtained by the bottom 33% SMBM scorers, divided by the pooled standard deviation of the corresponding item. These effect sizes are analogous to the Cohen's *d* statistics (Cohen, 1987). All of the effect sizes were substantially large (>1.29), indicating that the differences in mean item scores between high and low SMBM scorers were both statistically significant, and practically important, evident from large effect sizes (see Table 14.26).

Exploratory Factor Analysis

We explored the underlying components of the SMBM by using an exploratory factor analysis ($n = 5672$). We used principal components factor analysis with oblique rotation (promax) to allow correlations among the extracted variables.

The scree test was used to determine the number of factors to retain, which showed that the plot of eigenvalues levels off after the third factor was extracted. Therefore, we limited the number of retained factors to three. The Kaiser–Meyer–Olkin MSA was used, which showed an overall index of 0.93, indicating the data

Table 14.26 Corrected item-total score correlations[a] and effect sizes of item discrimination indices[b] for the Shirom–Melamed Burnout Measure (SMBM) in a national sample of first-year matriculants of 46 campuses of US colleges of osteopathic medicine ($n = 5672$)

Item	Corrected item-total score correlation	Item discrimination index effect size
I feel tired. (1)	0.57	1.58
I have no energy for going to work in the morning. (2)	0.63	1.90
I feel physically drained. (3)	0.70	2.20
I feel fed up. (4)	0.70	2.15
I feel like my "batteries" are "dead." (5)	0.75	2.59
I feel burned out. (6)	0.72	2.27
My thinking process is slow. (7)	0.71	2.30
I have difficulty concentrating. (8)	0.70	2.25
I feel I'm not thinking clearly. (9)	0.78	2.62
I feel I'm not focused in my thinking. (10)	0.76	2.60
I have difficulty thinking about complex things. (11)	0.70	2.20
I feel I am unable to be sensitive to the needs of coworkers and customers. (12)	0.52	1.37
I feel I am not capable of investing emotionally in coworkers and customers. (13)	0.51	1.39
I feel I am not capable of being sympathetic to coworkers and customers. (14)	0.52	1.30
Mean (Median)	0.66 (0.70)	

Numbers in parentheses refer to the appearance of the items in the SMBM instrument

[a]Correlations between scores on each item and the SMBM total score (calculated as the sum of scores on each item) by excluding the corresponding item from the total score; all were statistically significant ($p < 0.01$)

[b]Effect size estimate (Cohen's d statistic) of the discrimination index was calculated by subtracting the item mean score of the SMBM high scorers (top 33%, scores > 3.01, $n = 1953$) from the item mean score of the SMBM low scorers (bottom 33%, scores < 2.22, $n = 1946$), divided by the pooled standard deviation of the corresponding item

were adequate for factor analysis. Also, the Bartlett's test for sphericity indicated that the intercorrelation matrix was factorable ($x^2_{(52)} = 2069.22$, $p < 0.01$). The eigenvalues for the three retained factors before rotation were 7.27, 1.91, and 1.28, accounting for 52%, 14%, and 9% of the total variance, respectively.

The first factor, "Exhaustion," included six items with factor coefficients equal to or greater than 0.64. A typical item under this factor is, "I feel like my 'batteries are dead.'" The second factor, "Concentration Issues," included five items with factor coefficients equal to or greater than 0.70. A typical item under this factor is, "I feel I'm not focused in my thinking." The third factor, "Interpersonal Issues," included three items with factor coefficients equal to or greater than 0.82. A typical item under this factor is, "I feel I am unable to be sensitive to the needs of coworkers and customers." The Cronbach's coefficient alphas for the three factors were 0.90, 0.92, and 0.91, respectively. Summary results of factor analysis are reported in Table 14.27.

Table 14.27 Rotated factor loadings[a] for the burnout measure in a national sample of first-year matriculants of 46 campuses of US colleges of osteopathic medicine ($n = 5672$)

Item	Factor 1	Factor 2	Factor 3
I feel like my "batteries" are "dead." (5)	**0.86**	0.01	0.04
I feel physically drained. (3)	**0.85**	0.02	−0.05
I feel burned out. (6)	**0.69**	0.09	0.10
I feel tired. (1)	**0.67**	0.11	−0.13
I have no energy for going to work in the morning. (2)	**0.66**	0.09	−0.01
I feel fed up. (4)	**0.64**	0.05	0.17
I feel I'm not focused in my thinking. (10)	0.02	**0.90**	−0.01
I feel I'm not thinking clearly. (9)	0.07	**0.84**	0.03
I have difficulty concentrating. (8)	0.10	**0.79**	−0.07
I have difficulty thinking about complex things. (11)	0.03	**0.71**	0.13
My thinking process is slow. (7)	0.13	**0.70**	0.02
I feel I am not capable of being sympathetic to coworkers and customers. (14)	−0.01	−0.01	**0.92**
I feel I am not capable of investing emotionally in coworkers and customers. (13)	−0.01	0.02	**0.89**
I feel I am unable to be sensitive to the needs of coworkers and customers. (12)	0.02	0.03	**0.82**
Eigenvalue	7.27	1.91	1.28

Numbers in parentheses refer to the order of appearance of the items in the SMBM instrument
[a]Items are sorted by descending order of factor loadings within each factor. Factor coefficients ≥0.64 are shown in **bold**. Factor 1 was entitled "Exhaustion," Factor 2: "Concentration Issues," and Factor 3: "Interpersonal Issues"

Group Differences in SMBM Scores

Research participants were compared on their SMBM scores by gender, race/ethnicity, academic background, and career interest. Summary statistical results are reported in Table 14.28.

Gender

No statistically significant gender difference was observed between men ($n = 2653$) and women ($n = 2967$) on scores of the SMBM.

Race/Ethnicity

Comparing the SMBM scores by race/ethnicity, the lowest mean score on SMBM was obtained by students in the Black/African-American group ($M = 2.57$, $SD = 0.86$), and the highest mean score was in the Asian group ($M = 2.81$, $SD = 0.94$). The differences among racial/ethnic groups were statistically significant ($p < 0.01$) with a moderate effect size estimate ($d = 0.26$) (Table 14.28).

Table 14.28 Means and standard deviations of the Shirom–Melamed Burnout Measure (SMBM) by gender, race/ethnicity, academic background, and career interest in a national sample of first-year matriculants of 46 campuses of US colleges of osteopathic medicine ($n = 5672$)

	N	*Mean*	SD	*F*-ratio	*p*
Gender[a]					
Men	2653	2.70	0.90	$F_{(1,5618)} = 0.18$	0.67
Women	2967	2.69	0.91		
Race/ethnicity[b]					
White/Caucasian	3387	2.66	0.88	$F_{(3,5101)} = 10.32$	<.01
Asian	1316	2.81	0.94		
Hispanic/Latino/Spanish origin	236	2.61	0.89		
Black/African American	166	2.57	0.86		
Academic background[c]					
Biological Sciences	2834	2.67	0.88	$F_{(3,3940)} = 3.30$	<.05
Chemical/Physical Sciences	755	2.77	0.96		
Social/Behavioral Sciences	264	2.72	0.92		
Arts and Humanities	91	2.82	0.91		
Career interest[d]					
People-oriented	2349	2.72	0.90	$F_{(2,5110)} = 0.99$	0.37
Technology-oriented	1543	2.67	0.91		
Other	1221	2.70	0.89		

[a]No significant differences
[b]Asian > all others, effect size = 0.26
[c]No differences were observed in the post-hoc means comparisons (Duncan's multiple range test)
[d] No significant differences

Academic Background

We compared students with undergraduate majors in the following four broad categories: "Biological Sciences," "Chemical/Physical Sciences," "Social/Behavioral Sciences," and "Arts and Humanities" on their SMBM scores. The highest mean score was found for students with an academic background in Arts and Humanities ($M = 2.82$, $SD = 0.91$), and the lowest mean score was observed for students with an academic background in Biological Sciences ($M = 2.67$, $SD = 0.88$). Although the differences among the four groups with different academic backgrounds were statistically significant ($p < 0.05$), the post-hoc pairwise mean comparison test did not show any significant pairwise differences on their SMBM scores (see Table 14.28).

Career Interest

We divided specialties of interest to medical students into three broad categories: "People-Oriented" (e.g., family medicine, internal medicine, obstetrics and gynecology, and pediatrics); "Technology-/Procedure-Oriented" (e.g., anesthesiology, dermatology, ophthalmology, orthopedic surgery, radiology, and surgery); and "Other" (including specialties chosen by fewer than 20 matriculants). Summary results of statistical analyses on SMBM scores are reported in Table 14.28. No statistically significant difference was found in the SMBM scores among students with different specialty interests.

Burnout Measure, Clinical Empathy, Attitudes Toward Osteopathic Medicine, and Personal Quality Measures

Bivariate correlations between scores on the SMBM and clinical empathy (JSE), emotional empathy and other personal quality measures; and results of multiple regression analysis to examine the unique contribution of each of those measures in predicting SMBM scores are reported in Table 14.29.

As shown in the table, bivariate correlations between SMBM and clinical empathy scores were negative and statistically significant. It is also interesting to note that, with the exception of emotional empathy, all other variables used in the statistical analysis in Table 14.29 contributed negatively to predicting SMBM scores,

Table 14.29 Summary results of multiple regression analysis[a] in a national sample of first-year matriculants of 46 campuses of US colleges of osteopathic medicine ($n = 5653$)

Regressors	Bivariate correlation[b]	Standardized regression coefficient[c]	Unstandardized regression coefficient[d]	Standard error	t-Value
JSE	−0.21**	−0.05	−0.00	0.00	−3.09**
IRI	0.14**	0.19	0.03	0.00	15.32**
JeffSATIC	−0.24**	−0.05	−0.00	0.00	−2.91**
JeffSPLL	−0.29**	−0.19	−0.03	0.00	−14.12**
ATOMS	−0.29**	−0.19	−0.02	0.00	−11.57**
Intercept	–	0	5.50	0.14	39.17**

Excluded were students with incomplete surveys on any of the six measures, or those who scored > 3 on the Infrequency Scale of the ZKPQ

JSE Jefferson Scale of Empathy, *IRI* (scores of Empathic Concern and Personal Distress subscales of the Interpersonal Reactivity Index), *JeffSATIC* Jefferson Scale of Attitudes Toward Interprofessional Collaboration, *JeffSPLL* Jefferson Scale of Physician Lifelong Learning, *ATOMS* Attitudes Toward Osteopathic Medicine Scale

**$p < 0.01$, adjusted multiple $R = 0.40$, $p < 0.01$

[a]Scores on the Shirom–Melamed Burnout Measure (SMBM) as the dependent variable, and personality measures as regressors

[b]Bivariate correlations between the SMBM scores and other personality measures shown in the table

[c]Standardized regression coefficients (β) are calculated from score distributions converted to a standard distribution for all regressors with a mean of zero and standard deviation of 1 for comparability purposes

[d]Unstandardized regression coefficients are calculated from raw score distributions

meaning that higher scores on those regressors (the exception is the measure of emotional empathy) predicted lower burnout experiences.

The negative association observed between scores on clinical empathy (JSE) and burnout experiences, in contrast to the positive relationship between emotional empathy (IRI, synonymous to sympathy) and burnout experiences is interesting and deserves further attention that will be briefly addressed later in the analysis of the underlying construct of empathy and personal quality measures.

National Norm Table for the SMBM Scores

Because we found no significant gender difference on the SMBM scores, we did not prepare the norm table for this instrument separately by gender. Table 14.30 presents national norm percentile ranks for the total study sample, regardless of gender, in first-year matriculants of US colleges of osteopathic medicine.

The norm table for the SMBM should be used like other norm tables described in this chapter. For example, if the SMBM score of a matriculant is 3.9, first find the score interval that includes a score of 3.9 (e.g., 3.6–4.0 score interval in Table 14.30), then find the corresponding national percentile rank displayed in the row for that score interval in the table. The corresponding national percentile rank in Table 14.30 for the 3.6–4.0 score interval is 87%, meaning that a score of 3.9 on the SMBM places the matriculant in the 87th percentile rank of all first-year matriculants in US colleges of osteopathic medicine.

Table 14.30 National norm table for the Shimon–Melamed Burnout Measure (SMBM) in a national sample of first-year matriculants of 46 campuses of US colleges of osteopathic medicine ($n = 5672$)

SMBM score	*f*	*cf*	% tile rank
1	75	75	1%
1.1–1.5	467	542	5%
1.6–2.0	857	1399	17%
2.1–2.5	1194	2593	35%
2.6–3.0	1126	3719	56%
3.1–3.5	889	4608	73%
3.6–4.0	672	5280	87%
4.1–4.5	264	5544	95%
4.6–5.0	76	5620	98%
≥5.1	52	5672	99%

Excluded were students with incomplete surveys, or students who scored > 3 on the Infrequency Scale of the ZKPQ (indicating questionable validity of responses)
f frequency, *cf* cumulative frequency

Associations Among Scores of Clinical Empathy, Emotional Empathy, Attitudes Toward Osteopathic Medicine, and Personal Quality Measures in a Global Statistical Model

Intercorrelation Matrix

We calculated bivariate Pearson correlation coefficients among clinical empathy (JSE scores), emotional empathy (combined scores on Empathic Concern and Personal Distress subscales of the IRI), attitudes toward osteopathic medicine (scores on the ATOMS), and the three personal quality measures: attitudes toward interprofessional collaboration and teamwork (scores on the JeffSATIC), orientation toward lifelong learning (scores on the JeffSPLL), and self-reported burnout experiences (scores on the SMBM) (intercorrelation matrix is presented in Table 14.31).

As shown in the table, JSE scores (clinical empathy) yielded the highest positive and statistically significant correlations with the JeffSATIC scores ($r = 0.64$) and ATOMS ($r = 0.58$). Conversely, clinical empathy yielded an inverse correlation with SMBM ($r = -0.21$). Also, burnout experiences (SMBM scores) showed negative correlations with scores of JeffSATIC ($r = -0.24$) and JeffSPLL ($r = -0.29$). All were statistically significant ($p < 0.01$).

Data reported in Table 14.31 show a positive correlation between clinical and emotional empathy that is statistically significant but low in magnitude ($r = 0.21$). However, while associations between clinical empathy and burnout were negative

Table 14.31 Intercorrelation matrix of the clinical empathy scores and other study variables in a national sample of first-year matriculants of 46 campuses of US colleges of osteopathic medicine

	JSE	IRI	JeffSATIC	JeffSPLL	SMBM	ATOMS
JSE	1.00					
IRI	0.21**	1.00				
JeffSATIC	0.64**	0.15**	1.00			
JeffSPLL	0.28**	0.01	0.35**	1.00		
SMBM	−0.21**	0.14**	−0.24**	−0.29**	1.00	
ATOMS	0.58**	0.17**	0.60**	0.36**	−0.29**	1.00

In this intercorrelation matrix, JSE scores (clinical empathy) yielded the highest positive correlations with the JeffSATIC scores (Attitudes Toward Interprofessional Collaboration) ($r = 0.64$), and ATOMS (Attitudes Toward Osteopathic Medicine Scale) ($r = 0.58$). Conversely, the burnout measure (SMBM) yielded inverse correlations with scores on clinical empathy (JSE) ($r = -0.21$), JeffSATIC (Interprofessional Collaboration) ($r = -0.24$), and JeffSPLL (Orientation Toward Lifelong Learning) ($r = -0.29$)

JSE Jefferson Scale of Empathy (a measure of clinical empathy), *IRI* (scores of Empathic Concern and Personal Distress subscales of the Interpersonal Reactivity Index, a measure of emotional empathy), *JeffSATIC* Jefferson Scale of Attitudes Toward Interprofessional Collaboration, *JeffSPLL* Jefferson Scale of Physician Lifelong Learning, *SMBM* Shirom–Melamed Burnout Measure, *ATOMS* Attitudes Toward Osteopathic Medicine Scale

** $p < 0.01$

(meaning that higher scores on clinical empathy are associated with less burnout experiences), the correlation between emotional empathy and burnout was positive (meaning that higher scores on emotional empathy are associated with greater burnout experiences).

Underlying Construct of Clinical Empathy, Emotional Empathy, Attitudes Toward Osteopathic Medicine, and Personal Quality Measures

We explored the underlying construct of the six instruments used in POMEE-Phase II, by using an exploratory factor analysis ($n = 5653$). We used principal components factor analysis with varimax rotation to extract independent factors.

The scree test was used to determine the number of factors to retain, which showed that the plot of eigenvalues leveled off after the second factor was extracted. The Kaiser–Meyer–Olkin MSA was used, which showed an overall index of 0.77, indicating that data were adequate for factor analysis. Also, the Bartlett's test for sphericity indicated that the intercorrelation matrix was factorable ($x^2_{(4)} = 72.75$, $p < 0.01$).

The eigenvalues for the two retained factors before rotation were 2.63 and 1.19, accounting for 44% and 20% of the total variance, respectively. The first factor, entitled "Positive Attributes," included four scales (JSE, JeffSATIC, ATOMS, and JeffSPLL) with factor coefficients equal to or greater than 0.40. The second factor, including scores on emotional empathy and burnout, entitled "Negative Attributes," had the largest factor coefficient of 0.60 using the SMBM. The emotional empathy scores had rotated factor coefficients of 0.25 (on factor 1) and 0.36 (on factors 2). Summary results of factor analyses are reported in Table 14.32.

Notably, emotional empathy (synonymous to sympathy, see Chaps. 1 and 6) emerged as an independent factor from clinical empathy (JSE scores, or cognitive empathy). This explains the findings of a positive relationship between burnout and measures of emotional empathy found in some studies (Hojat, Maio, Pohl, Gonnella, 2023; Williams, 1989).

A few researchers, using empathy measuring instruments other than the JSE, reported a positive association between scores of empathy and burnout experiences (Williams, 1989), meaning that higher empathy leads to more burnout experiences which is counterintuitive (Hojat, Spandorfer, Louis, & Gonnella, 2011). However, those finding are in line with an idea that empathic engagement in patient care can lead to "compassion fatigue," a "secondary traumatic stress disorder" and burnout, an unverified assumption that was advanced by Figley (1995), who claimed, that "those who have enormous capacity for feeling and empathy tend to be more at risk of compassion stress" (Figley, 1995, p. 1). In his book "Against Empathy," Bloom (2016) without acknowledging the consequential differences between cognitive and emotional empathy (see Chaps. 1 and 6) claimed that "empathy is a negative in

Table 14.32 Rotated factor loadings[a] of clinical empathy and measures of personal quality in a national sample of first-year matriculants of 46 campuses of US colleges of osteopathic medicine (*n* = 5653)

Scale	Factor 1	Factor 2
JSE	**0.79**	0.03
JeffSATIC	**0.79**	0.07
ATOMS	**0.76**	−0.13
JeffSPLL	**0.40**	−0.30
SMBM	−0.27	**0.60**
IRI (Empathic Concern & Personal Distress)	0.25	**0.34**
Eigenvalues	2.63	1.19

Excluded were students with incomplete surveys on any of the six measures, or those who scored > 3 on the Infrequency Scale of the ZKPQ (indicating questionable validity of responses)
JSE Jefferson Scale of Empathy (a measure of clinical empathy), *IRI* (scores of Empathic Concern and Personal Distress subscales of the Interpersonal Reactivity Index, a measure of emotional empathy), *JeffSATIC* Jefferson Scale of Attitudes Toward Interprofessional Collaboration, *JeffSPLL* Jefferson Scale of Physician Lifelong Learning; SMBM: Shirom–Melamed Burnout Measure, *ATOMS* Attitudes Toward Osteopathic Medicine Scale
[a]Factor coefficients ≥0.34 are shown in **bold.** Factor 1 was entitled "Positive Attributes" and Factor 2 was entitled "Negative Attributes"

human affairs. It's sugary soda, tempting and delicious and bad for us" (Bloom, 2016, p. 13). However, a 2022 study, consistent with our abovementioned findings, reported that cognitive empathy, as opposed to emotional empathy, significantly predicted a lower degree of burnout and stronger mental resilience in medical students (Wu et al., 2022).

Our correlational and factor analytic findings from POMEE provide empirical support for the notion that it is not clinical empathy (conceptualized as a "cognitive" in Chaps. 1 and 6) that leads to burnout. However, it is "emotional" empathy (conceptualized in Chaps. 1 and 6 as an "affective" or "emotional" attribute, synonymous to sympathy) that, in excess, could lead to exhaustion and burnout (Hojat, Maio, Pohl, & Gonnella, 2023). This misunderstanding of a positive association between empathy and burnout, in the context of patient care, is the result of using a measure of emotional rather than cognitive empathy; and making a misleading remark that empathy is detrimental to health care education and patient care. The controversial reports on empathy and burnout call for further research to examine the associations of clinical and emotional empathy measures with other personal qualities (including burnout) that are germane to patient care, and more importantly to tangible clinical outcomes.

The Fate of POMEE-Phase II

On March 23, 2020, I was unpleasantly surprised to receive an email message from then senior vice president for medical education and research at the AACOM, informing me about termination of funding for the POMEE-Phase II, because, as indicated in the message, one of the funding organizations did not continue its share of financial support of the project.

Subsequent to the termination of the project, Dr. Calabrese, who significantly contributed to the initiation of POMEE, expressed his disappointment with the termination decision and wrote: "What you have accomplished is formidable and probably the most robust academic collaborative effort in osteopathic medical history. I owe you greatly." After termination of the funding, I suggested to the leadership of the AACOM not to abandon this landmark project, recommended to continue collecting data, and advised them to, at least, accomplish the first three objectives of POMEE-Phase II. Five years after termination of funding (March 25, 2025), I received a message from the AACOM, inviting me to invigorate the POMEE and to wrap it up, using data collected after termination of funding. It is an ongoing project at the present time.

Recapitulation

POMEE was a groundbreaking endeavor in medical education research with important implications for selection of applicants to medical schools and also for averting erosion in clinical empathy and enhancing empathic understanding of physicians-in-training. Findings from POMEE-Phase I showed significant differences in clinical empathy scores by gender, race/ethnicity, and academic background. Also, a significant difference in clinical empathy was found in favor of those interested in "People-Oriented" specialties as opposed to their counterparts interested in "Technology-/Procedure-Oriented" specialties. A decline in clinical empathy was observed during the clinical phase of medical school, as opposed to the preclinical phase. Although the pattern of decline in empathy was similar to that observed in allopathic medical students, the decline was less pronounced in osteopathic medical students. National norm tables for clinical empathy scores, developed for osteopathic medical students at different levels of medical school education, could have implications for admissions decisions and for program assessment purposes.

POMEE-Phase II was not completed as planned because of the interruption in funding.

Chapter 15
Parting Thoughts: A Systemic Paradigm of Clinical Empathy, Implications, and Future Research Directions

Everything in the system is dependent on the previous state of the system.

—(Robert Lilienfeld, 1978, p. 14)

By becoming more and more aware of our roles in patient–doctor relationship—i.e., of our side-effects as drugs—our therapeutic efficiency will grow apace.

—(Michael Balint, 1957, p. 688)

Abstract

- Clinical empathy in health professions education and patient care is viewed from a broader and more comprehensive perspective of systems theory.
- Using a systemic paradigm of empathy in patient care, this chapter discusses the contributions of major subsets of the system (e.g., clinician-related, nonclinician-related, social learning, and education) and their related elements to clinical encounters that lead to functional or dysfunctional system outcomes.
- An agenda for future research is outlined which includes: (1) exploration of additional components of empathy in the context of health professions education and patient care; (2) the investigation of additional variables that are beneficial or detrimental to empathy in patient care; (3) consideration of empathy as a criterion for admissions, selection, and employment; (4) the study of empathy as a predictor of career choice, and academic and professional success; (5) the development and evaluation of approaches to enhance and sustain empathy in health professions education and patient care; (6) development of approaches to maximize empathy and regulate sympathy; (7) the development of national norm tables and cutoff scores to identify JSE high and marginal scorers; (8) consideration of patients' and peers' perspectives in outcomes of clinical empathy; (9) further explorations of neurological underpinnings of empathy; and

M. Hojat, *Clinical Empathy*, https://doi.org/10.1007/978-3-031-87413-0_15

(10) challenges in undertaking empirical research and providing plausible explanations for empathic engagement without in-person patient–clinician encounter through telemedicine, virtual care, digital healthcare, and artificial intelligence technologies.

- It is suggested that the implementation of remedies for enhancing and sustaining empathy is a mandate that must be acted upon, not only by academic medical centers but by all other educational institutions.

Introduction

Empathy is an attribute that is distributed unevenly in the population. Human beings are not created equal with regard to their capacity for empathy. It is a gift bestowed in abundance on some and in only meager amounts on others. It is an endowment that can grow like a huge tree if the conditions are right. In this book, we embarked on a journey to find out why people differ with respect to their capacity to form empathic connections, how capacity for empathy is developed, how empathy can be quantified in the context of health professions education and patient care, and what are the correlates and clinical outcomes of empathy.

Now that we have come so far and are approaching the final destination of our journey, I would like to reflect on what I have said so far. We embarked on this journey without even knowing the terrain we hoped to discover. Faced with the confusion reflected in research on the conceptualization and measurement of empathy, we attempted to achieve a better vision by resolving the confusion. We visited empathy's historical roots, developmental trajectories, psychosocial correlates, and other related factors in our search of the terrain. In traveling these paths, we learned about the antecedents, development, measurement, and consequences of clinical empathy in health professions education and patient care. Many other terrains remain to be explored, however.

On the basis of the premise that research findings are vulnerable to serious challenge when the definition of the phenomenon under study is unclear, I offered a definition of empathy in the context of patient care (Chap. 6). Although I do not expect my conceptual characterization of clinical empathy to remain unchallenged, let us hope that it can help, to some extent, to resolve the long-standing and unsettled debate regarding the conceptualization and definition of clinical empathy that has always haunted empathy researchers.

The concept of empathy as having both cognitive and emotional components, adopted uncritically from social psychology by educators in the health professions, fits poorly with the clinical reality in clinician–patient encounters (Morse et al., 1992). The golden principle of patient care, "Above all, do not harm" (*primum non nocere*), rules out intense emotional engagement between clinician and patient that may jeopardize the outcomes of patient care. In studying empathy in social psychology in the context of prosocial behavior, emotions can often facilitate, rather than jeopardize, the positive outcomes. However, as I described in Chaps. 1 and 6, in medical and surgical treatment, emotions must be curbed to maintain objectivity. No wonder that regulation of emotions in patient care was strongly recommended by Sir William Osler (1932), who advised, "In the physician or surgeon no quality takes rank with imperturbability [which] means coolness and presence of mind under all circumstances and the physician who has the misfortune to be without it loses rapidly the confidence of his patient." (pp. 3–4). Thus, to achieve optimal patient outcomes, empathy in the context of patient care should be guided primarily by cognition rather than emotion.

Without a distinction between cognition and emotion, we will be wrestling forever with the challenge of how to separate the two in the context of patient care. With that in mind, we also need to recognize that clinicians cannot remain completely emotionless when dealing with their patients. As part of human nature, emotions always play a role in any kind of human relationship. The challenging issue that remains to be explored is the extent to which emotions would be beneficial in clinical situations and to determine the point from which emotions become detrimental to patient outcomes (see Chaps. 1 and 6).

To avoid more confusion on conceptualization of empathy and sympathy in the context of patient care, I have used alternative words that are commonly used in empathy literature, namely cognitive empathy (sometimes also recognized as "clinical empathy" in the context of patient care), and emotional (or affective) empathy (synonymous to sympathy). In the definition of empathy in the context of patient care, I placed the emphasis on "understanding" patient's pain, suffering, experiences, and concerns. In the definition of emotional empathy (akin to sympathy), I placed the emphasis on "feeling" of patient's pain and suffering. This distinction, described in detail in Chaps. 1, 3, and 6, can help to reduce the ambiguity associated with the terms and their respective consequences in patient care, as well as in the search for their neurological underpinnings (Chap. 13).

A complex concept, such as clinical empathy, cannot be the subject of scientific inquiries in the absence of an instrument that produces quantifiable results. An instrument intended to measure clinical empathy in patient care cannot pass the litmus test of face and content validity unless its contents are not only consistent with its definition, but also relevant to the context of patient care. In addition, psychometric evidence must provide convincing support for the validity and reliability of the instrument. Over time, the *Jefferson Scale of Empathy* (JSE), the instrument described in Chap. 7, has helped us resolve the measurement issues that have caused the uncertainty and have impeded empirical scrutiny of clinical empathy in medical and other health professions education and patient care research.

Complex human attributes are not isolated entities; they always function in relation to other factors. As we learned in previous chapters, empathy is a multifaceted attribute deeply rooted in human evolution; it has genetic traces and a long history of development from conception to grave. Furthermore, as was discussed earlier (Chap. 4), environmental, cultural, experiential, and educational factors contribute independently and interactively to the makeup of the attribute called empathy. More importantly, empathic engagement, or the lack of it, in the context of patient care can lead to virtually opposite clinical outcomes (Chap. 11).

Despite its deep evolutionary roots and genetic component, the capacity for empathy is amenable to change, positively or negatively, to some extent when the conditions are right or wrong. Therefore, as I discussed in Chap. 12, targeted educational programs, appropriate experiences, and environmental facilitators can enhance the capacity for empathy in health professionals-in-training and in-practice; and detrimental factors can erode it. Frequent reinforcements are also needed to sustain the enhanced orientation toward empathic engagement in patient care (Hojat, Axelrod, Spandorfer & Mangione, 2013).

Viewed from a broader perspective, a complex concept, such as empathy in patient care, requires a comprehensive model to depict its important elements, their interactions, and their outcomes. For that purpose, we can turn to systems theory to present a heuristic paradigm of empathy in the context of patient care.

A Systemic Paradigm of Clinical Empathy in Patient Care

The developmental trajectories and outcomes of a complex concept, such as empathy in patient care, can be viewed from the vista of systems theory. According to Pollak (1976), a systemic approach is the professional way of dealing with complexity. A system is defined as a set of interrelated subsets, each with an array of elements, no subset of which is unrelated to any other subset, and each element within a subset is related directly or indirectly to every other element in the system (Ackoff & Emery, 1981). A system will be functional only when all its subsets and all the elements within and between subsets function properly; otherwise, the system will be dysfunctional. A functional system has a purpose. The systemic purpose of empathy in patient care is to enhance mutual understanding between clinician and patient so that a trusting relationship develops between them (see Chap. 11), and the goal of positive and optimal patient outcomes can be achieved.

Gordon Allport (1960) suggested that human personality must be treated as an open system that should be viewed with an open mind. Active systems are often considered to be open systems because they are dynamic and therefore capable of responding and adapting to changes in the environment (Siegel, 1999). The combined functions of the elements within each subset of the system and the interrelationships among subsets prompt the system to generate a totality, a *gestalt*, in which the whole is greater than the sum of its parts. To achieve a better understanding of the antecedents, development, and outcomes of empathy in patient care, it seems desirable to view the concept of empathy in patient care, its subsets, and the elements within each subset as an open system.

A complete understanding of any system requires an understanding of the subsets within the system and the nature of their interacting elements. For example, as Bateson (1971) indicated, if the family is viewed as a complex system, then an effective intervention in the context of family therapy requires a complete understanding of all subsets and elements of the subsets, including the roles, responsibilities, interactions, and functions of all family members within the family structure.

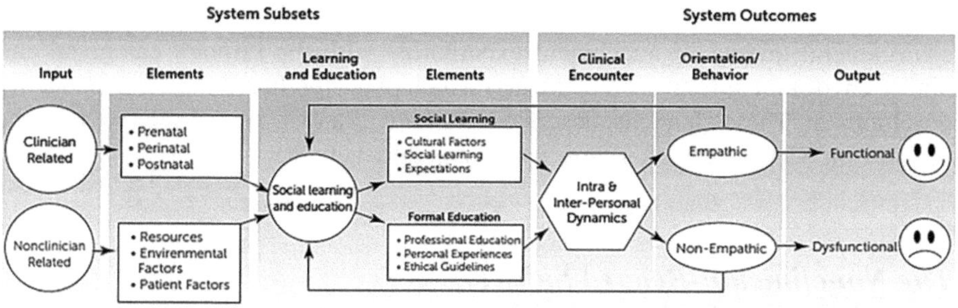

Fig. 15.1 A systemic paradigm of empathy in the context of health professions education and patient care

Similarly, in the context of patient care, as described in Chaps. 4 and 8, the act of seeking help brings to the surface a need for connectedness that generates the energy to set the system of clinical empathic engagement in motion. A clinician–patient encounter represents an open system in need of equilibrium brought about by the energy discharged in interpersonal connection. Achieving positive patient outcomes would indicate that the system is functional (i.e., a state of equilibrium), whereas negative patient outcomes would indicate that the system is dysfunctional (i.e., a state of disequilibrium). Empathic engagement in the clinician–patient relationship is the first step in maintaining systemic equilibrium. Figure 15.1 depicts a systemic paradigm of clinical empathy in the context of patient care. It illustrates the major subsets of the system and the major elements within each subset that ultimately determine the functional or dysfunctional outcome of the system.

Major Subsets of the System

Let us elaborate briefly on the paradigm depicted in Fig. 15.1. Assuming that empathy in patient care resembles an open and purposeful system (i.e., a system that is amenable to change for the purpose of positive patient outcomes), the system would be set in motion by two interacting subsets: a clinician-related subset and a nonclinician-related subset (depicted on the left side of the figure as the entry to the model). Social learning and education are other subsets in the system.

The Clinician-Related Subset

This subset consists mainly of elements related to the clinician's personal qualities, which are offshoots of evolutionary, genetic, and constitutional factors (prenatal elements); events during childbirth (perinatal elements) that can contribute to later physical, mental, and social development; and such factors as the early rearing environment, quality of attachment experiences with the primary caregiver, and family environment (postnatal elements) which play significant roles in personality development. These elements, described in Chaps. 3 and 4, are considered to be the bedrock on which a person's capacity for empathy is built.

The Nonclinician-Related Subset

According to Kurt Lewin (1936), manifestations of behavior are a function of personal qualities, environmental demands, and situational factors. In a paradigm of physicians' performance, Gonnella, Hojat, Erdmann, and Veloski (1993b) proposed that in addition to clinician's knowledge, clinical-procedural skills, and personal qualities, other factors contribute to patient outcomes that are not related to the clinician and often are not under the clinician's control. Hence, the term "nonclinician-related subset." The elements of this subset have often been ignored in evaluations of outcomes of health professions education, appraisal of clinicians' performance, and the assessments of patient outcomes. These elements include the availability of (a) *human resources*, such as technical and professional assistance, and teamwork; (b) *technical resources*, such as diagnostic and treatment facilities, surgical equipment, and availability of laboratory tests; (c) *environmental facilitators* such as physical facilities and facilitating rules and regulations formulated by healthcare institutions, health insurance agencies, and governmental authorities; and (d) patient factors, such as patients' personality, cultural values, attitudes, and lifestyle; willingness to seek timely help; the severity of the disease; and adherence to preventive guidelines and treatment regimens.

The Social Learning and Educational Subsets

The social learning subset consists mainly of elements related to cultural and social norms and values (e.g., ascribed social roles and modes of social behavior) and expectations (e.g., belief in a supernatural power, in the healthcare system, in healthcare providers, and in optimistic or pessimistic expectation of outcomes).

The education subset consists of an array of elements related to formal education and training experiences, such as professional education (e.g., undergraduate, graduate, and continuing education), personal educational experiences (e.g., influence of role models, observations, and clinical experiences, factors in the so-called hidden curriculum, Hafferty, 1998), and professional ethical codes of conduct (e.g., ethical guidelines of professional organizations, such as the American Medical Association and the American Psychological Association). Targeted educational programs and educational experiences designed to enhance the capacity for empathy (see Chap. 12) also are among the elements of this subset.

The Clinical Encounter

Armed or disarmed with the elements of the aforementioned subsets, a clinician encounters a patient who is in a state of disequilibrium and is reaching out to someone for help. The system of empathic engagement begins to form. The intrapersonal and interpersonal dynamics described in Chap. 8 are triggered into operation during exchanges between the clinician and the patient. To form a functional system, the clinician should be armed with the skills needed to understand the patient's concerns and be motivated (an intrapersonal factor) to communicate this understanding to the patient (an interpersonal factor) with a genuine intention to help. As depicted in Fig. 15.1, all elements of clinician-related, nonclinician-related, social learning, and education subsets come together in clinical encounters that can lead to either empathic or nonempathic clinician–patient engagements that, in turn, ultimately determine patient outcomes that will be positive in a functional system or negative in a dysfunctional system.

Outcomes

The interaction between intrapersonal and interpersonal dynamics described in Chap. 8 brings about cognitive processes that can lead to an orientation or a behavior. When the orientation or behavior is empathic, the likelihood of a positive patient outcome will increase. In this case, the system will achieve its purpose, and we can conclude that the system is functional. However, if the intrapersonal and interpersonal dynamics resting on the clinician-related, nonclinician-related, social learning, and formal educational subsets lead to a nonempathic orientation or behavior, the likelihood of a positive patient outcome will be drastically reduced. In this case, the system will fail to achieve its purpose, and we can conclude that the system is dysfunctional.

However, I must emphasize that because other unpredicted elements may intervene, the pathway to empathic engagement between clinician and patient is more complicated than the model depicted in Fig. 15.1. Nonetheless, I hope that the systemic view of empathy just described can serve as a heuristic model illustrating the major components that set the system in motion and show the complexity of empathy in the context of patient care.

An Agenda for Future Research

Training humane clinicians has been a concern of education in the health professions. Because of general societal changes that are taking place, particularly in the industrialized world, there is a trend, directly or indirectly, toward weakening of the importance of the social support systems (see Chap. 2). Also, due to the changes that are transpiring in the healthcare system and leading toward detached care (see Chap. 12), research on factors that contribute to the understanding and enhancement of empathy in patient care is now more important and timely than ever before.

Research on empathy in patient care deserves serious attention, not only because of its importance in training humane clinicians, but also because of its implications for the selection and education of clinicians-in-training and in-practice. Empirical research on empathy in patient care is still evolving; therefore, much more research is needed to enhance our understanding of empathy in patient care. The questions addressed below present only a few of the areas that need to be addressed in the future research on clinical empathy.

What Additional Constructs Are Involved in Clinical Empathy?

According to the findings obtained in our factor analytic studies (Hojat, Gonnella, Nasca, Mangione et al., 2002; Hojat & LaNoue, 2014; Hojat, DeSantis, Shannon, Mortensen et al., 2018) and by others (see Appendix A), empathy in patient care is a multidimensional concept involving at least three factors: "perspective taking," "compassionate care," and "standing in the patient's shoes." Similar factors emerged in a factor analytic study in which the JSE was administered to dental students (Sherman & Cramer, 2005), and in another study with a large sample of medical students in Mexico (Alcorta-Garza, Gonzalez-Guerrero, Tavitas-Herrera, Rodrigues-Lara, & Hojat, 2005) as well as studies by others in the USA and abroad (see Appendix A). These findings added to our confidence concerning the stability of the factors underlying empathy in different groups of health professionals and in different countries. However, we need more evidence to support the factor structure of empathy in groups of students and practitioners in the various health professions (e.g., nursing, dietetics, psychology, and social work).

It is important to bear in mind that the factors extracted in factor analytic studies obviously are a function of the contents and number of the items that are included in the clinical empathy measuring instruments. Therefore, the three underlying factors of empathy identified by the JSE reflect the contents and intercorrelations of the 20 items included in the instrument. Adding a sufficient number of items to address other factors, such as sociability, trust, and ethics, could result in a scale with a different underlying factor structure. More important, whether the current factor structure of the JSE saturates the scale to the point where additional factors cannot account for more than a negligible amount of the variance or whether additional factors would contribute significantly to the scale's incremental validity (i.e., increase its criterion-related and predictive validity) needs to be carefully addressed in future research.

What Additional Variables Are Associated with Clinical Empathy?

As described in Chap. 9, research has shown that empathy is linked to a number of demographic and psychosocial variables, indicators of clinical competence, and career interests. Evidence also suggests that empathic engagement in patient care is associated with physicians' diagnostic accuracy and patients' adherence to treatment, increased satisfaction with their healthcare providers, a reduced tendency to file malpractice claims, and more importantly to patient outcomes (Chap. 11). Also, as was described in Chaps. 4 and 8 and depicted in Fig. 15.1, family environment, early attachment relationships, human and material resources, and environmental, social, and cultural factors contribute to the development and manifestation of clinical empathy in patient care situations (Chap. 4).

It is important to study empirically—and, ideally, with prospective longitudinal research designs—the relative contribution of early experiences; the quality of early and late attachment relationships; and social, cultural, educational, and other factors that can significantly predict empathy scores. This line of research would have important implications for the development of programs to retain and enhance the capacity for clinical empathy.

Clinical empathy also was found to predict ratings of clinical competence among medical students and physicians (Chap. 9). However, further research is needed to address other indicators of academic and professional performance that are significantly associated with clinical empathy scores and patient outcomes. It is desirable to use prospective longitudinal studies to examine the relationship between empathy scores and different measures of academic and professional success or failure (e.g., academic dropout and dismissal; cheating and unethical behavior; disciplinary action against healthcare providers) at different levels of health professions education.

Furthermore, the findings on gender differences in empathy scores (Chap. 10) call for more empirical research to discern whether the differences are more likely to be related to "intrinsic" gender characteristics or to "extrinsic" sex-role socialization and their interactions. Such research is needed because determining the proportion of the variance in clinical empathy scores that is accounted for by intrinsic or extrinsic factors in the analyses of gender differences is an important issue. The answer would potentially have different implications in relation to the selection and education of caring health professionals.

Further investigations also are needed on the unique contribution of empathy to accurate diagnoses, improved compliance, better patient satisfaction, reduced malpractice claims (Chap. 11), and other tangible clinical outcomes regarding control of chronic diseases, such as essential hypertension, diabetes mellitus, and treatment of other chronic and acute illnesses. These outcomes are important to be studied, not only because of their impact on mortality and morbidity, but also because of the economic impact on the patients, their families, and society at large. Two other areas that need to be empirically investigated are the extent of the short- and long-term impact of clinical empathy enhancement programs for health professions students and practitioners, and empathic engagement in patient care without in-person clinician–patient encounters (e.g., telemedicine and digital healthcare that will be briefly described later).

It is also highly desirable, although complicated, to examine the relative contribution of the following factors to the capacity for clinical empathy: genetic factors; quality of early attachment relationships; early life experiences (e.g., parental divorce, death in the family, maternal employment, and day care experiences); later personal life experiences (e.g., traumatic events, peer relationships, marital relationships, and role models); environmental and social factors (e.g., sociopolitical conditions, cultural norms, and ascribed roles); cultural and cross-cultural factors, particularly among immigrants; formal education; and the interactions among these and other factors. It would also be interesting to explore if documented "unethical" behavior during medical school (Papadakis et al., 2005) is significantly associated with a lower level of capacity for clinical empathy.

Gonnella and colleagues (Gonnella & Hojat, 2001; Gonnella, Hojat, Erdmann, & Veloski, 1993a, 1993b; Hojat, Erdmann, & Gonnella, 2014) proposed that to achieve optimal patient outcomes, a physician must perform three roles: clinician, educator, and resource manager. Thus, determining the extent to which each of these roles is associated more with capacity for clinical empathy is also important. Furthermore, it would be desirable to investigate the relative contribution of different factors of clinical empathy (e.g., perspective taking, compassionate care, and standing in the patient's shoes) to each of the three roles of a physician as well as to academic and professional success.

Should Empathy Be Considered for Admissions/ Selection Purposes?

Almost all North American medical schools place great emphasis on applicants' undergraduate grade-point averages and scores on the Medical College Admission Test (MCAT) for the purpose of screening applicants to medical and other health professions schools. Although grade-point averages and MCAT scores are relatively good predictors of a student's academic performance in the early years of medical school (sometimes described as the preclinical or pre-clerkship phase of medical school education), they have poor predictive validity regarding a student's performance in the later years of medical school (sometimes described as the clinical phase of medical school education) (Glaser, Hojat, Veloski, Blacklow & Goepp, 2004; Hojat et al., 2014; Hojat, Erdmann et al., 2000; Hojat, Veloski, & Zeleznik, 1985). The poor long-term predictive validity of the MCAT is not surprising because the test was developed to predict success in the preclinical component of medical education when attrition is most likely in the US medical schools. In addition, because of the "restriction of the range" issue as a result of attrition in the first 2 years, the predictive validity coefficients cannot capture the true relationships with indicators of clinical competence in later years of medical school.

It is obvious that the most qualified candidates who wish to embark on a journey to become caring physicians are those who in addition to medical knowledge and procedural skills possess personal qualities that can generate trust, which ultimately leads to optimal clinical outcomes. However, there is a lingering doubt among medical education leaders about the role of personal qualities in academic success and clinical outcomes. In an article entitled "Building a better physician," Kaplan, Satterfield, and Kington (2012), suggested that just as an understanding of biology and chemistry needs some basic background, which is often assessed in admission tests to medical schools, we also need to assess candidates' understanding of social and behavioral sciences and also improve such understanding as part of professional development of physicians-in-training. It is interesting to notice that the Association of American Medical Colleges (AAMC) which sponsors the MCAT, only in 2015 recognized the importance of the role of psychosocial factors in health and illness; and included a new section (Psychological, Social, and Biological Foundations of Behavior) to the MCAT (starting in 2015) to assess applicants' understanding of psychosocial factors in health and illness. However, much research is needed to examine predictive validity of this new section of the MCAT in students' clinical skills.

In addition to understanding psychosocial factors in health and illness, it is more important to assess the *possession* of psychosocial qualities pertinent to patient care (Hojat et al., 2014). Research shows that the contribution of such personal qualities, including clinical empathy, to the assessment of medical students' performance is greater in the clinical than preclinical phase of medical education (for a review see Hojat et al., 2014, also see Chap. 7). Some may argue that personal qualities can be easily assessed from admission interviews, letters of recommendation, essays, and personal statements. However, there is inadequate evidence in support of the validity of such conventional approaches; some of their shortcomings are described below.

Admissions Interview

Face-to-face interviews are required as part of the admission process in almost all medical schools and residency programs in the USA and Canada. A great majority of these interviews are unstructured with no uniform questions and no standard assessment procedures. It is believed that interviews provide an opportunity to include the human touch in decision-making and that they help in assessing personal qualities (Albanese, Snow, Skochelak, Huggett, & Farrell, 2003). It is proposed that the admissions interviews provide important information in selecting potential students (Eddins-Folensbee, Harris, Miller-Wasik, & Thompson, 2012; Puryear & Lewis, 1981). However, convincing empirical evidence is not yet available to confirm the validity and reliability of admission interviews (Ferguson, James, & Madeley, 2002; Kanter, 2012). Compounding this issue is the fact that medical students themselves, without any training, sometimes perform interviews with new applicants in order to supplement the staff and faculty resources needed for interviewing a large number of applicants. Interestingly, no significant difference has been observed between faculty and students' interview ratings (Eddins-Folensbee et al., 2012; Elam & Johnson, 1992; Gelmann & Stewart, 1975).

The purpose of interviewing candidates for residency programs is to assess their humanistic qualities, attitudes, motivation, and other personal qualities; however, guidelines for assessing such qualities are often vague or nonexistent. Interviews are often not structured to assess those human qualities, or the interviewers are not specifically trained to detect them (Hojat et al., 2014). Information on humanistic qualities of candidates is often available from evaluations of students' behavior in clinical clerkships. Letters of evaluation that medical school deans write for graduates not only should summarize the students' academic attainment but also should include assessments of graduates' humanistic qualities when dealing with patients.

Reliance on interviews conducted by untrained staff or students can jeopardize the validity of the selection process by giving advantage to those applicants who play a better role in presenting themselves well in interview settings. The unstructured interviews by untrained interviewers with no standard scoring guidelines may predict nothing other than an applicant's skills in role playing (Musson, 2009). No wonder that the predictive validity of admission interviews has been reported to be disappointingly low (Walton, 1987). It is interesting to note that despite all of the aforementioned limitations, a national survey of residency program directors in the USA showed an applicant's interview was considered the most important selection criterion (Wagoner, Suriano & Stoner, 1986). The use of interviews in the undergraduate and graduate selection processes provides a unique opportunity to talk with applicants and may be helpful in observing a candidate's reaction to questions, but uncertainties remain open regarding the validity and practical outcomes of admission interviews (Antonovsky, Anson, & Bernstein, 1979; Green, Peters, & Webster, 1991; Hobfolls & Benor, 1981).

More information about applicants' interpersonal skills and capacity for empathy can be probed during admissions interviews once interviewers are trained to assess these qualities. Also, the issue of whether undergraduate elective courses or majors could predict capacity for empathy needs to be empirically addressed. In addition, the issue of whether training those who interview medical school applicants can lead to the selection of more empathic students needs to be studied.

Letters of Recommendation

Most medical schools in North America require letters of recommendation to be submitted by those who are fairly familiar with the academic performance and personal qualities of the applicants. Letters of evaluation written by medical school deans also play a great role in the selection of candidates for residency. To date, there is no convincing empirical evidence in support of the predictive validity of letters of recommendation in medical schools. In our own empirical study using a multivariate statistical model, we found that the level of recommendation contained in the letters written by undergraduate premedical education advisors did not contribute significantly to the prediction of academic performance in medical school beyond the grades obtained prior to medical school (Zeleznik, Hojat, & Veloski, 1983). Furthermore, it has been reported that letters of recommendation may be biased and flattering with no substantial empirical link to later performance (Walton, 1987). Although one purpose of letters of recommendation is to describe personal qualities of the applicant, our research confirmed that too often these letters fail to add anything about applicant's personality beyond a summary of the student's academic performance (Hojat et al., 2014; Zeleznik et al., 1983). Those who prepare recommendation letters should be advised to include information about applicants' interpersonal skills in the letter.

Personal Statements, Letters of Intent, and Essay

Medical schools in the USA often require applicants to write an essay, letter of intent, or some personal statements about, for example, their interest in medicine, career goals, and future plans. There are very few studies on the predictive value of essays or personal statements. In one study, the content of candidates' personal statements was analyzed, and no evidence was found to support its predictive validity (cited in Ferguson et al., 2002). Typically, letters of intent or essays submitted by applicants are evaluated by untrained readers and are assessed on informal criteria (Musson, 2009). Even more questionable is whether candidates themselves, without any help, write the statements, essays, and letters of intent (Musson, 2009). Because of the aforementioned shortcomings, Haque and Waytz (2012) suggest that one appropriate approach for the assessment of personality of physicians-in-training is to administer psychometrically sound instruments for assessing personal qualities pertinent to patient care, including empathy.

Kupfer, Drew, Curtis, and Rubinstein (1978) reported that, when deciding which applicants should be admitted to medical school, considering personal qualities, including empathy, would be likely to lead to excellence in the practice of medicine. Streit-Forest (1982) recommended that once a significant relationship has been established between personal qualities and indicators of academic and professional success, the personal qualities of applicants to medical school should be included among the criteria for admission. In longitudinal studies of medical students, we have shown that measures of personal qualities (e.g., sociability, satisfactory interpersonal relationships, and self-esteem) and measures of academic aptitude (e.g., grade-point averages and MCAT scores) can equally predict performance measures in the first 2 years of medical school. However, the measures of personal qualities could predict ratings of clinical performance in the third year of medical school more accurately than grade-point averages or MCAT scores (Hojat, Robeson, Damjanov et al., 1993; Hojat, Glaser, & Veloski, 1996; Hojat, Vogel, Zeleznik, & Borenstein, 1988). In other words, incremental validity can be improved significantly by including indicators of interpersonal skills and measures of personal qualities in multiple regression models (Hojat et al., 1988, 1993; Zeleznik et al., 1988).

Our research on empathy (using the JSE) has shown that empathy scores are significantly associated with ratings of clinical competence in medical school (Hojat, Gonnella, Mangione et al., 2002) and with tangible clinical outcomes in the practice of medicine (Del Canale et al., 2012). To my knowledge, no empirical study on grade-point averages prior to medical school or the MCAT is available to show that science attainment could predict patient outcomes and clinical competence. There is, however, one study in which we showed that the assessments of MCAT writing samples (no longer included in the new MCAT exam) could significantly predict a student's clinical competence in medical school (Hojat, Erdmann et al., 2000).

Stern, Frohna, and Gruppen (2005) reported that none of the data on academic performance that are often used for admissions to medical schools could predict medical students' professional behavior. However, in that study, findings showed that medical students' unprofessional behavior observed by faculty, clerkship directors, and fellow students could be predicted by students' failure to complete required course evaluations and to report immunization compliance. In another study by Papadakis et al. (2005), it was found that disciplinary action taken against physicians by state medical boards was strongly associated with unprofessional behavior recorded in medical school. These findings support the notion that indicators of personal qualities can predict professional behavior beyond measures of academic attainment. Essential humanistic qualities, such as empathy, elude the measures of undergraduate academic achievement that are commonly used when selecting applicants for admission to medical schools.

Undergraduate academic institutions do not routinely provide information about medical school applicants' interpersonal skills or other personal qualities relevant to the capacity for empathy. However, an examination of undergraduate elective courses or baccalaureate majors can provide clues about applicants' interests in humanities and literature, which are associated with the capacity for empathy (Chap. 14).

Graduate medical education programs often consider indicators of academic attainment in medical school and scores on medical licensing examinations, such as Steps 1 and 2 of the United States Medical Licensing Examinations (formerly the National Board of Medical Examiners), as important determinants in the selection of residents. A residency candidate's personal qualities are often either overlooked or ignored completely.

Jamison and Johnson (1975) suggested that the public would be better served if volunteers for public services were selected on the basis of their capacity for empathy. Because medicine is a public service profession and the professional behavior of physicians includes compassionate care and empathy, why is empathy not a criterion for selection of medical students and residents, or even for employment of physicians? This question deserves serious research attention (Hojat et al., 2014). If social desirability response bias which is considered as a shortcoming of the self-reported personality tests is an excuse to hesitate using clinical empathy scores for selection purposes, we have used an approach to control or mitigate the possible effect of the social desirability response bias (Hojat, DeSantis, Shannon et al., 2018, 2020; Hojat, Shannon, DeSantis et al., 2019, 2020; Hojat, DeSantis, Cain et al., 2021); or at least we can use the clinical empathy scores as a tie-breaker for those applicants with similar qualifications on other admission measures (Hojat et al., 2014).

If further research provides convincing empirical evidence that incorporating empathy into the criteria for selecting applicants to medical schools and residency programs can lead to the advancement of professionalism in medicine, we should set aside our hesitation and include important pertinent personal qualities, such as empathy, when selecting our future healthcare workforce. One positive result could be that healthcare professionals might regain the respect that has been fading away along with the changes taking place in society in general and in the healthcare system in particular. Meanwhile, we also need to study the long-term implications of using empathy as a criterion for selecting applicants to medical schools and residency programs.

Does Clinical Empathy Predict Career Choice?

Findings on differences in clinical empathy among physicians in various specialties (Chap. 9) and among medical students who planned to pursue different specialties after graduation from medical school (Chap. 14) call for further research. The question of whether health professionals choose specific specialties because of differences in their capacity for clinical empathy prior to their professional education or because of effects of their professional education needs further investigation. The answer to the question will have implications in academic health centers for selection of students and trainees; career counseling; and curriculum development. If capacity for clinical empathy predicts career choice and interest in particular specialties, any attempt to select empathic candidates or to enhance empathy could potentially influence the distribution of physician workforce and other health professionals in the different specialties.

How Can Clinical Empathy Be Enhanced and Sustained During Professional Education?

In the absence of dedicated educational programs, studies have found that clinical empathy among medical students and residents tends to decline as they progress through medical education (Bellini et al., 2002, Bellini & Shea, 2005; Hojat et al., 2009, 2004, also see Appendix A), particularly when students are involved with patient contact, which raises serious concerns. Consequently, prospective research is needed to investigate whether empathy scores erode *systematically* or *randomly* during the course of medical education. It also is important to determine what factors would contribute to the systematic decline or variation in empathy in different individuals at different levels of health professions education. In addition, it is important to determine which factors may be detrimental and which factors may be beneficial to individuals. If the detrimental and beneficial factors do not affect all individuals equally, determining what individual characteristics or experiences account for the variation would be an important research goal.

Finally, more research is needed to identify the most appropriate methods or the best combinations of approaches for enhancing empathy among students and practitioners (e.g., development of interpersonal skills, exposure to hospitalization experiences, role playing, exposure to role models, specifically targeted video or audio materials, workshops on perspective taking, theatrical approaches, study of literature and the arts, improvement of narrative skills, etc.; see Chap. 12). Furthermore, both formative and summative evaluations are needed to confirm that programs developed to enhance empathy have achieved their stated goals and, more importantly, that not only the short-term, but also long-term effects of such programs have been carefully evaluated.

The unfortunate erosion of empathy reported among the health professionals in-training, and in-practice raised an alarming red flag that must not be ignored in future research. What are the underlying reasons for this transformation of some of the enthusiastic students into cold-hearted practitioners? Is it related to the "Lucifer effect" that Zimbardo (2007) coined (see Chap. 8) in which good-hearted people turn bad as a result of environmental conditions, role expectations, arrogance, sense of belonging to a privileged group, etc.? Added to the seriousness of the erosion of empathy issue are the findings of a meta-analytic study involving 72 samples of American college students, including 13,737 participants, that reported American college students' empathy had declined between 1979 and 2009 on the Perspective Taking and Empathic Concern scales of the IRI (Konrath, O'Brien, & Hsing, 2011). The decline was most pronounced after the year 2000. Empirical research is needed to explore reasons for these unfortunate changes. Why is our young generation regressing rather than progressing in their capacity for empathy?

Should We Maximize Empathy and Regulate Sympathy in Patient Care?

Because they have different consequences in patient care, I tried to make a distinction throughout this book between cognitive empathy (or clinical empathy in the context of patient care) and emotional empathy (synonymous to sympathy in the layman's term). Some may argue that the findings on the decline in empathy during health professions education and the practice of patient care could be a result of psychological defense mechanisms to adjust to the emotional drain involved in taking care of seriously ill patients. Well, this argument may be true when it concerns hardening hearts against emotional (not cognitive) empathy. However, I would use a different term: "emotional regulation" (rather than "decline") for such an adjustment in emotional empathy (sympathy). Research indicates that those who are able to regulate their emotions are more likely to form empathic engagement and also act in a heightened moral fashion (Decety & Lamm, 2006; Eisenberg et al., 1994).

In an fMRI study, physicians who practice acupuncture were compared to others while observing animated visual stimuli showing needles being inserted into the mouth region, hands, and feet of patients (Cheng et al., 2007). Experts in acupuncture knew that such procedure could be painful to their patient and had learned in their training to regulate their emotions in order not to be distressed and overwhelmed with emotional exhaustion. Thus, as expected, in these acupuncture experts, brain regions involved in the emotional aspect of pain processing (e.g., anterior insula and anterior cingulated cortex, see Chap. 13) did not show increased activation. Instead brain regions associated with emotional regulation and cognitive control (e.g., the medial and dorsolateral prefrontal cortices) showed activation in the acupuncture-practicing physicians (Cheng et al., 2007). The control participants, compared to expert physicians, showed significantly higher pain intensity, activation of the pain matrix, and unpleasant ratings when watching body parts being pricked by needles as opposed to being touched by a Q-tip. Investigators also observed an enhanced self-other distinction in the expert physicians by activation of the right temporoparietal junction, which is known to play a role in self-other differentiation, metacognition, and the theory on mind (Cheng et al., 2007). These findings support the notion that professional training experiences can improve emotional regulation, which helps to prevent burnout and emotional exhaustion.

A decline in cognitive empathy (or clinical empathy) is never justifiable and can never be beneficial to either clinician or patient. Thus, the agenda for future research should include studying approaches not only to enhance (or maximize) and sustain cognitive empathy, but also regulate (or optimize) emotions (or emotional empathy) in health professions education and patient care.

Should We Respond to a Need for Norm Data and Cutoff Scores?

As the developers of the JSE, we have been frequently asked by potential national and international users about the availability of norm data and cutoff scores for identifying high and low scorers. For the development of national norm tables and determining cutoff scores, large and representative samples from the target populations are needed. By using a large sample of entering medical students ($n = 2637$) who entered Sidney Kimmel Medical College at Thomas Jefferson University, we developed proxy norm tables and tentative cutoff scores for men and women matriculants separately (Hojat & Gonnella, 2015, also see Chap. 7). Obviously, data from one medical school cannot serve that purpose; instead, large-scale longitudinal studies are needed with national representative samples of medical and other health professions students, physicians, and other practicing health professionals to develop national and international norm tables and cutoff scores by gender, specialties, and country to identify low and high JSE scorers for the purpose of assessments of professional development, admission, and employment.

As reported in Chap. 14, we developed, for the first time, national norms for osteopathic medical students in the USA by gender in different years of medical school education (from matriculation to graduation) that can be used for the assessment purposes of the JSE scores against national norms (within a medical school, and between medical schools) (Hojat, Shannon, DeSantis, Speicher et al., 2019). Similar research to develop norm tables (and cutoff scores) would be beneficial for the assessment of clinical empathy for allopathic medical students (Hojat & Gonnella, 2015), all other health professions students, and healthcare practitioners.

Do Patients' Perspectives and Peers' Evaluations Contribute to Clinical Outcomes?

Optimal and suboptimal clinician–patient relationships cannot be comprehensively studied if we fail to understand patients' expectations and perspectives regarding the empathy of their healthcare providers. In Chap. 11, I pointed out that a large majority of medical malpractice claims filed is the result of patients' negative views of the relationship with their healthcare providers. Thus, it is important to study clinical outcomes with respect not only to clinicians' self-reported empathy but also to patients' perceptions of their caregivers' empathy and to peers' evaluations of clinicians' empathy. Indeed, a systematic meta-analytic review study in which survey data from patients' assessments of their caregivers' relational empathy was used (by the CARE instrument, see Chap. 5), Howick and colleagues (Howick, Steinkopt, Ulyte et al., 2017) reported patients' assessments of their healthcare providers' empathy vary with patients' gender, providers' discipline (e.g., physicians versus allied health professionals), and providers' nationality (e.g., U.S., U.K., Austria, and Hong Kong). These findings indicate that exogenous factors can confound patients' perceptions of their healthcare providers' empathy that could contribute to clinical outcomes.

Furthermore, it is important to examine healthcare providers' specific behaviors, such as punctuality, sense of humor, nonverbal behavior, and verbal expressions that patients regard as significant determinants of an empathic engagement. The patients' perspectives are particularly important because one key concept in the definition of empathy was clinicians' ability to communicate their understanding to their patients (Chap. 6). Thus, future research should focus on the relationship among three sets of variables: (a) clinicians' self-reported empathy, (b) patients' expectations and perceptions of clinicians' empathy, and (c) peers' evaluations of clinicians' empathy. To enhance our understanding of factors that determine final outcomes of rendering care, the relative contribution of these variables to patient outcomes must be investigated.

What Are the Neurological Underpinnings of Cognitive and Emotional Empathy?

A better understanding of the neurobiological underpinnings of empathy will lead to improving empathy. Brain imaging experiments to find the roots of empathy are flourishing which may shed light on the issues of enhancing and sustaining empathy, and on prevention and treatment of empathy deficit disorders. The discovery of mirror neurons that are activated in the brain when a person sees another person performing a goal-directed act or hears another person who is in distress (Carr, Iacoboni, Dubeau, Mazziotta, & Lenzi, 2003; Kohler et al., 2002) opens a new window for the examination of the neural mechanisms of empathy in human relationships (Chap. 13). With the technical advancements in functional brain imaging, it is now possible to observe and record the neurophysiological indicators of empathy. These exciting discoveries should prove to be extremely valuable in future research designed to identify the structural (neuroanatomical), functional (neurophysiological), and psychosocial aspects of empathy in the human brain.

In addition, based on the studies cited in Chap. 13, both the limbic system and neocortex areas of the brain have often been implicated in neuroanatomical studies of empathy. However, future research must make a distinction between clinical empathy (described in this book as cognitive empathy) and emotional empathy (synonymous to sympathy) and further examine whether different areas of the brain are activated by empathic or sympathetic responses. As I suggested in Chap. 13, intuitively one can speculate that the neocortex is more likely to be implicated in cognitive empathy and the limbic system is more likely to be implicated in emotional empathy (sympathy), but this speculation needs further empirical verification.

Is it Plausible to Develop Empathic Engagement in the Era of Telemedicine, Virtual Care, and Artificial Intelligence?

We are on the brink of a new era of patient care marked by an increasing use of computerized technology. In addition, the advent of new approaches to patient care such as telemedicine, virtual patient care, digital healthcare, and artificial intelligence technologies can provide services to patients faster but raise questions about their short- and long-term outcomes. Furthermore, the COVID-19 pandemic contributed to the rapid expansion of telemedicine, virtual patient care, and digital healthcare, aimed at preventing spread of a highly contagious disease, leading to the lockdown orders mainly for avoiding in-person contacts.

Such uncharted terrain in the healthcare environment, characterized by minimized human contact (or sometimes by no human contact at all!), calls for urgently needed research to explore its challenges and provide convincing empirical evidence and plausible explanations for the development, or demise, of empathic engagement in patient care.

A recently published study (Ayers, Poliak, Dredze et al., 2023) attempted to address this concern. In that study, responses to the patient questions were given either by physicians or by artificial intelligence chatbot (ChatGPT). Investigators compared responses from real physicians and from ChatGPT by having a small team of licensed health professionals (who were blind to the source of responses: physician or ChatGPT) to review responses to patients' questions and rate them (using a 5-point Likert-scale) for quality of the empathic responses and of the quality of information in the responses. Researchers concluded that the ChatGPT responses were assessed by the licensed health professionals as more empathic than responses from physicians. It was also reported that the quality of information in ChatGPT responses was rated significantly higher than that of responses from physicians. Although findings on the quality of information given by ChatGPT responses may seem reasonable, findings on their superiority in empathic response, compared to human beings' responses, needs plausible explanation. Could such findings be explained by the limitations in study design, lack of methodologic rigor, participation of physicians with marginal empathic understanding, invalid assessments of those who judged the quality of responses given by real physicians or ChatGPT, or other factors? Such unexpected outcomes cannot be considered credible without convincing explanation.

It would be challenging to provide convincing data and plausible explanations for superiority of computer-generated empathic engagement, compared to in-person patient–clinician encounters, given features of clinical empathy that were presented in this book, such as *mutual understanding*; *reciprocal communication*; *interpersonal attunement*; *development of trust*; involvement of *psychological factors*; *neurobiological reactions*; *synchronized exchanges* between patient and clinician and observation of nonverbal behavior (see Fig. 11.4 in Chap. 11, and also Chaps. 1, 2, 4, and 6); and taking into consideration the interaction of clinician and nonclinician elements described in the systemic paradigm of clinical empathy (depicted in Fig. 15.1 in this chapter). Thus, the question of whether it is possible to develop empathic engagement in patient care with no in-person encounters is important and challenging, and needs urgently to be addressed by further empirical research. One can use the analogy of giving a *warm* "long-distance" hug to another human being through a computer program without in-person contact and expecting it to be perceived as a more empathic engagement than a real hug, involving patting the back and eye-to-eye contact! In addition, given the exponential growing of artificial intelligence technology in patient care, other challenging issues to address are who would be legally accountable in the case of misdiagnosis and therapeutic error; and how can the balance in diversity, equity, and inclusiveness be maintained in digital patient care and the artificial intelligence environment?

It is interesting to notice that an instrument has also been developed (Schmidmaier, Rupp, Cvetanova, & Mayer, 2024) to quantify clinical empathy of technology, or artificial intelligence, or computerized patient care, called the *Perceived Empathy of Technology Scale* (PETS)! For example, items such as "The system showed interest in me" (as an indication of "emotional responsiveness" factor), and "I trusted the system" (as a measure of "understanding and trust" factor) answered by the users are included in this instrument. Such instruments for the assessment of empathy need careful examination of their face, content, construct, criterion-related and predictive validity to detect empathic deficiencies in different technologic devices, and create approaches to enhance clinical empathy in patient care rendered by digital technology!

New approaches to health professions education and patient care such as telemedicine, virtual care, and artificial intelligence may contribute negatively to the quality of patient–clinician relationships that need to be carefully examined quantitatively and qualitatively before it is too late.

Recapitulation

We embarked on a journey into the terrain of empathy with the hope of exploring the roads leading to empathy (its antecedents) and the paths spreading from empathy (its outcomes). Like the wings that evolved to allow birds to fly high in search of food or the long necks that evolved to allow giraffes to feed on leaves high on trees that other species could not reach, empathy, we learned, has evolutionary roots that sprouted for the purpose of survival.

Similarly, we learned that empathy—like hearing, vision, taste, and smell—has neurological and biophysiological underpinnings. Empathy, like human love, connects people more closely, reduces interpersonal space, and fulfills the human need for affiliation, support, and understanding. In the context of patient care, empathy is no longer a vague concept because an operational definition offered in this book has clarified its meaning, and it is no longer an abstract entity because it can be quantified with a valid and reliable instrument described in this book.

Empathy can increase altruistic, prosocial, and helping behaviors; reduce aggressive behavior; encourage avoidance of conflict; improve conflict management; and promote understanding (Larson & Yao, 2005). Medicine, once considered by the public as one of the most highly respected professions of all, is losing ground (Thomas, 1985), partly because of the failure of medical education to train empathic doctors and partly due to the failure of some health professionals to preserve their altruistic image (Schlesinger, 2002). At the turn of twentieth century, George Bernard Shaw equated the image of the medical profession to the faith in God by declaring that “We have not lost faith, but we have transferred it from God to the medical profession.” This is no longer the case, given the current image of physicians held by public.

In the past few decades, the public’s trust in medicine has eroded and the image of physicians has transformed from compassionate healers to technicians and interpreters of medical tests, influenced by profound changes in medical education and the healthcare system; an imbalance in teaching the science and the art of medicine; undue financial considerations to contain cost; increasing commercialization of medical care; health insurance policies formulated by nonmedical administrators; the emergence of “defensive” medicine; and the replacement of the human presence caring for patients with computerized diagnostic and therapeutic technology (Schlesinger, 2002). Perhaps medicine can regain some of its well-deserved reputation, and physicians can reclaim their altruistic image by paying greater attention to the role of empathy in the selection, education, practice, and professional development of physicians (Hojat et al., 2014).

In the context of patient care, empathy can eliminate the constraints of the clinician–patient relationship. It can bridge the gap between givers and receivers of help and contribute to the physical, mental, and social well-being of both patient and clinician. Like height, weight, eye color, and type of hair, empathy varies among humans. However, a sense of unity can emerge from diversity among human beings once empathic understanding prevails, once one can view the world from the other person's perspective, once one can stand in another person's shoes.

The following saying has been attributed to Albert Einstein: "A person starts to live when he (sic) can live outside himself." Empathic engagement takes a person outside of himself or herself and allows the person to hear others with the third ear and to view the world of others with the mind's eye. Empathic engagement brings unity from diversity, making all of us akin regardless of gender, age, race, culture, religion, or other differentiating and potentially divisive factors. So, that is why any attempt toward empathic understanding of a fellow human being is a step toward enhancing the physical, mental, and social well-being of all in society. Thus, the lesson to be learned is that actual implementation of remedies for enhancement of empathy—not just declaration of their desirability without action—is a mandate that must be acted upon, not only by teachers and healers of human infirmity, but by all members of the human race for the sake of healing human ills unto eternity.

Appendices

M. Hojat, *Clinical Empathy*, https://doi.org/10.1007/978-3-031-87413-0

Appendix A: Annotated Bibliography on the JSE

Science begins in the nothingness of ignorance, and moves toward truth by gathering more and more information, constructing theories as facts accumulate.

—(Steven Jay Gould, 1981, p. 321)

Since the first publication on psychometrics of the JSE in 2001, an increasing number of empirical, conceptual, and review articles have been published in the USA and abroad in which the JSE was used, reviewed, or reported. The following annotated bibliographical list of such studies includes 326 entries, including 61 coauthored by me with my national/international colleagues or research team (marked by an asterisk*) and the rest by researchers from other academic centers either in the USA or abroad.

I grouped these studies into the following seven categories: psychometrics of the JSE (53 entries); correlates of the JSE scores (80 entries); group comparisons on the JSE scores (25 entries); changes in clinical empathy (32 entries); interventions to enhance clinical empathy (74 entries); tangible clinical outcomes associated with physicians' empathy (3 entries); or a combination of some of the aforementioned categories and other miscellaneous findings (59 entries). Some of these studies also used the *Jefferson Scale of Patient Perceptions of Physician Empathy* (JSPPPE). The entries in each category are listed in alphabetic order by the author name. There are also a number of doctoral dissertations or a few theses which were made available to me by their authors, or through *ProQuest Dissertation & Theses Global* in which the JSE was used as a major instrument (50 entries).

I selected the studies that were written in English (or at least were accompanied by an English abstract) and were accessible to me (either were sent by the study's author or were accessible from journals' websites or publishers without hefty charges). In each bibliographic entry for empirical studies, I included crucial information such as research participants, major instrument(s) used, intervention if any, and a brief highlight of major findings. These studies of course vary with respect to their quality; some can be ranked as excellent and some may be marginal regarding their quality. However, I tried not to be judgmental with regard to the quality in the selection of the articles, particularly when there are no agreed upon inclusion criteria to judge the merit of the studies. This bibliography not only provides a summary of most of the publications on the JSE as of publication date of this book, but also can serve as a source for meta-analytic research on clinical empathy, with an important advantage that a uniquely validated instrument was used in all of these studies—a desirable feature of any meta-analytic research.

Studies on Psychometrics of the JSE

*Alcorta-Garza, A., Gonzalez-Guerrero, J. F., Tavitas-Herrera, S. E., Rodrigues-Lara, F. J., & Hojat, M. (2005). Validación de la escala de empatia medica de Jefferson en estudiantes de medicina Mexicanos [Validity of the Jefferson Scale of Physician Empathy among Mexican Medical Students]. *Salud Mental [Mental Health], 28*, 57–63.

Participants included 1022 first-, third-, and fifth-year medical students (494 women) at the School of Medicine, Autonomous University of Nuevo Leon in Monterrey, Mexico, who completed a Spanish translation of the JSE. Results showed that the JSE mean score for the entire sample was 110.4 (SD = 14.1). Women obtained a significantly higher JSE mean score ($M = 111.9$, SD = 13.9) than men ($M = 109.1$, SD = 14.1). Cronbach's alpha coefficient for this sample was 0.74. No significant correlation was observed between scores on the JSE and respondents' ages. Exploratory factor analysis resulted in the same three factors emerging in most studies in the US samples, namely "Perspective Taking," "Compassionate Care," and "Standing in Patient's Shoes."

Ameh, P. O., Uti, O. G., & Daramola, O. O. (2019). Empathy among dental students in a Nigerian institution. *European Journal of Dental Education: Official Journal of the Association for Dental Education in Europe. 23*(2), 135–142. https://doi.org/10.1111/eje.12412.

This study examined the validity and reliability of the JSE HPS-Version as a tool to measure the empathy levels in undergraduate dental students in Nigeria. Research participants ($n = 212$) completed the JSE HPS-Version. The internal reliability (Cronbach's α-coefficient) was 0.84. "Compassionate Care," "Standing in Patients' Shoes," and "Perspective Taking" emerged in factor analysis of the JSE. There was a significant difference in empathy scores between the second- and the fourth-year students. The mean JSE HPS-Version score was comparable to those reported for dental, medical, and other health professions students and physicians. This study provided evidence for the construct validity and reliability of the JSE-HPS for measuring empathy among Nigerian dental students.

Blanco, J. M., Caballero, F., García, F. J., Lorenzo, F., & Monge, D. (2018). Validation of the Jefferson Scale of Physician Empathy in Spanish medical students who participated in an early clerkship immersion programme. *BMC Medical Education, 18*(1), 209. https://doi.org/10.1186/s12909-018-1309-9.

The purpose of this study was cultural adaptation and validation of the Spanish JSE. Research participants included 506 first-, second-, third-, and fifth-year medical students who completed the JSE. Results indicated that item-total score correlations were all positive and statistically significant (median 0.45, $p < 0.01$). Cronbach's alpha coefficient was 0.82. The test–retest intraclass correlation coefficient was 0.68. Confirmatory factor analysis confirmed the three original factors' structure: "perspective taking," "compassionate care," and "standing in the patient's shoes." Women outscored men. The JSE scores were significantly correlated with scores on the IRI ($r = 0.32$). The results support the validity and reliability of JSE in Spanish medical students.

Díaz-Narváez, V. P., Calzadilla-Núñez, A., Reyes-Reyes, A., Lastre Amell, G., Castellón-Montenegro, H., Andrade Valles, I., Fernández-Aragón, S., Fajardo-Ramos, E., Santander Díaz, K., Torres-Martínez, P., Muñoz Gámbaro, G., Borja González, J., & Arispe-Alburqueque, C. (2023). Empathy, psychometrics, cut-off points in nursing students from Latin America. *International Nursing Review*, *70*(2), 185–193. https://doi.org/10.1111/inr.12783.

The purpose of this multicenter study was to examine psychometrics of the JSE. Participants included 3712 students from 11 Latin American nursing schools. The JSE was administered, and multi-dimensionality of the JSE was confirmed by confirmatory factor analysis. The study provided an opportunity to develop cutoff scores to identify high and low empathy-scoring students. It was concluded that the JSE has adequate measurement properties in samples of nursing students in Latin America.

Díaz Valentín, M. J., Garrido Abejar, M., Fuentes Chacón, R. M., Serrano Parra, M. D., Larrañaga Rubio, M. E., & Yubero Jiménez, S. (2019). Validation to the Spanish of the Jefferson empathy scale health professions students version and its psychometric properties in nursing students. *Nurse Education in Practice, 40*, 102629. https://doi.org/10.1016/j.nepr.2019.102629.

This study aimed to evaluate the psychometric properties of the Spanish version of the JSE HPS-Version and to reexamine its factor structure in a sample of nursing students ($n = 422$). Results showed that the scale has a factorial structure with three dimensions. The prominent factor, "Perspective Taking" included 10 items; the second factor, "Compassionate Care," included 6 items, and the third factor, "Standing in the Patient's Shoes," included 3 items. The results of the confirmatory factor analysis suggested that the Spanish version of the JSE-HPS is a valid and reliable instrument to evaluate the empathic inclination in nursing students.

Díez, N., García Del Barrio, L., Cristina Rodríguez-Díez, M., Martín-Lanas, R., Gea, A., & João Costa, M. (2022). Validation of the Jefferson Scale of Patient Perception of Physician Empathy Spanish (Spain) Version in Primary Care. *Family Medicine*, *54*(8), 621–628. https://doi.org/10.22454/FamMed.2022.169675.

The aim of this study was to translate into Spanish and examine psychometrics of the Jefferson Scale of Patient Perceptions of Physician Empathy (JSPPPE) in primary care setting. Participants included 369 patients treated by 21 primary care physicians in Spain, who completed the Spanish versions of the JSPPPE and the Consultation and Relational Empathy Measure (CARE). Results showed a Cronbach's alpha of 0.87, and all corrected item-total correlations were statistically significant (>0.30). Confirmatory factor analysis corroborated the one-factor structure of the instrument. The scores on the Spanish JSPPPE were significantly correlated with scores on the CARE ($r = 0.65$) and with ratings of overall patient satisfaction ($r = 0.50$). The results provide support for the reliability and validity of the Spanish version of the JSPPPE in primary care setting.

*Di Lillo, M., Cicchetti, A., Lo Scalzo, A., Taroni, F., & Hojat, M. (2009). The Jefferson Scale of Physician Empathy: Preliminary psychometrics and group comparisons in Italian physicians. *Academic Medicine*, *84*, 1198–1202.

Participants included 289 Italian physicians (60 women) from three hospitals in Rome, Italy, who completed an Italian translation of the JSE. Results showed that the corrected item-total score correlations of the JSE were all positive and statistically significant, ranging from 0.34 to 0.69. The JSE mean score for the total sample was 115.1 (SD = 15.5), and the Cronbach's alpha coefficient was 0.85. Exploratory factor analysis resulted in six factors, including Perspective Taking, Compassionate Care, and Standing in Patient's Shoes, plus residual factors. Women obtained a higher JSE mean score (*M* = 117.5, SD = 14.6) than did men (*M* = 114.5, SD = 15.6), but the difference was not statistically significant. Physicians practicing surgical specialties scored lower (*M* = 114.2, SD = 15.5) than their counterparts in medical specialties (*M* = 117.5, SD = 15.0). The difference, however, did not reach an accepted level of statistical significance.

Fashami, F. M., Nili, M., Mottaghi, M., & Farahani, A. V. (2023). Measuring empathy in Iranian pharmacy students using the Jefferson Scale of Empathy-Health Professions Student Version. *American Journal of Pharmaceutical Education, 87*(2), ajpe8687. https://doi.org/10.5688/ajpe8687.

The purpose was to assess validity of the Farsi-translated version of the JSE HPS-Version in Iranian pharmacy students. Participants included 496 Iranian pharmacy students. Confirmatory (CFA) and exploratory factor analysis (EFA) were used to explore the underlying components and construct validity of the JSE-HPS. Three factors emerged in the EFA, and confirmed in CFA: compassionate care, perspective taking, and standing in a patient's shoes. Two items in the JSE-HPS did not show sufficiently large factor coefficients. Empathy scores were significantly higher among female pharmacy students. The findings provided support for the validity of the Farsi version of the JSE-HPS among Iranian pharmacy students.

*Fields, S. K., Mahan, P., Hojat, M., Harris, J., Tillman, P., & Maxwell, K. (2011). Measuring empathy in healthcare profession students using the Jefferson Scale of Physician Empathy: Health Provider-Student Version. *Journal of Interprofessional Care, 25*, 287–293. doi: https://doi.org/10.3109/13561820.2011.566648.

Participants included 265 undergraduate nursing students (233 women) at the College of Health Professions, Armstrong Atlantic State University in Savannah, Georgia, USA, who completed the JSE (HPS-Version). Results showed that corrected item-total score correlations were all positive and statistically significant (with the exception of one item), ranging from 0.09 to 0.62, with a median of 0.42. Overall, the JSE mean score for this sample was 111.5 (SD = 12.2). Cronbach's alpha coefficient was 0.78, test–retest reliability with a 3-month interval between testing was 0.58, and it was 0.69 with a 6-month interval. Women scored significantly higher than men (*M* = 112.5, SD = 11.0 and *M* = 104.1, SD = 17.1, for women and men, respectively). Older students obtained a higher JSE mean score, and no statistically significant associations were found between JSE scores and ethnicity, religiosity, or previous non-nursing degree.

*Fjortoft, N., Van Winkle, L. J., & Hojat, M. (2011). Measuring empathy in pharmacy students. *American Journal of Pharmaceutical Education, 75*(6), Article 109. doi: https://doi.org/10.5688/ajpe756109.

Participants included 187 first-year pharmacy students at Midwestern University, Chicago College of Pharmacy, who completed the JSE HPS-Version. Results showed a mean score of 110.7 (SD = 12.1), and Cronbach's alpha coefficient = 0.84. Women obtained a significantly higher JSE mean score (*M* = 112.8, SD = 11.3) than did men (*M* = 106.3, SD = 13.1). Corrected item-total score correlations ranged from 0.09 to 0.69, with a median of 0.55. In exploratory factor analysis, based on the scree test, two factors were retained: "perspective-taking" and "compassionate care." It was concluded that psychometric support of the JSE HPS-Version in pharmacy students can bolster researchers' confidence in using a validated instrument for empathy research in pharmacy education.

Ghardallou, M., Zedini, C., Sahli, J., Ajmi, T., Khairi, H., & Mtiraoui, A. (2022). Psychometric properties of a French version of the Jefferson Scale of Empathy. *International Journal of Medical Education, 13*, 205–214. https://doi.org/10.5116/ijme.62d2.8497.

This study assessed the reliability and construct validity of a French version of the JSE-S. Research participants included 833 medical students in Tunisia. Results showed an acceptable level of internal consistency, with an overall Cronbach's alpha of 0.78. The findings support the construct validity of the French version of the JSE-S. It was concluded that the JSE S-Version appears to be useful for the assessment of clinical empathy among French-speaking populations.

Giménez-Espert, M. D. C., & Prado-Gascó, V. J. (2020). Empathy in nurses: Spanish adaptation of the JSE (JSE) on nurses. *Contemporary Nurse, 56*(3), 255–265. https://doi.org/10.1080/10376178.2020.1813046.

The purpose of this study was to adapt and explore the psychometric properties of the JSE for nursing students in a sample of 500 Spanish nurses. In factor analysis of the instrument, three factors emerged entitled: "Perspective Taking" (Cronbach's alpha = 0.87), "Compassionate Care" (alpha = 0.78), and "Thinking as the Patient" (alpha = 0.63). The study provided psychometric support for the JSE in Spanish nurses.

Gosselin, E., Paul-Savoie, E., Lavoie, S., & Bourgault, P. (2017). Evaluation of Nurse Empathy Perceived by the Standardized Patient in Simulation: A French Validation of the Jefferson Scale of Patient Perceptions of Physician Empathy. *Journal of Nursing Measurement, 25*(2), 152–161. doi/10.1891/1061-3749.25.2.152.

The aim was to provide psychometric evidence for a French version of the Jefferson Scale of Patient Perceptions of Physician Empathy (JSPPPE). Research participants included 26 intensive care nurses in a standardized clinical simulation. For each nurse, a standardized patient completed the JSPPPE and three observers filled out the French version of the Reynolds Empathy Scale (RES). An expert committee confirmed that the JSPPPE has good content validity. The internal consistency was acceptable. A positive correlation was observed between scores on the JSPPPE and the RES, suggesting a good convergent validity. It was concluded that the French translation of the JSPPPE used by standardized patients is the first reliable and valid instrument available in the French language for measuring patient's perception of nurse's empathy in the intensive care unit.

*Gonnella, J. S., Mangione, S., Magee, M., Nasca, T. J., & Hojat, M. (2005). Empathy scores in medical school and ratings of empathic behavior in residency training 3 years later. *The Journal of Social Psychology, 145*, 663–672.

Participants included 106 physician residents who graduated from Jefferson (now Sidney Kimmel) Medical College (45 women) who had completed the JSE in the third year of medical school, and their empathy was rated by their program directors 3 years later at the completion of the first year of residency training. Results showed that the JSE mean score for this sample was 117.8 (SD=10.9). A statistically significant association was found between students' self-reported empathy in the third year of medical school (JSE scores) and ratings of their empathy given by the directors of residency training programs approximately 3 years later.

Gonullu, P., & Oztuna, D. (2012). A Turkish adaptation of the student version of the Jefferson Scale of Physician Empathy. *Marmara Medical Journal, 25*, 87–92. doi:

https://doi.org/10.5472/MMJ.2012.02272.1. Accessible from: http://www.mmj.dergisi.org/pdf/pdf_MMJ_634.pdf.

A Turkish translation of the JSE was administered to 752 (378 women) first- to fifth-year medical students at the Ankara University School of Medicine in Turkey. Confirmatory factor analysis confirmed the three-factor model found in most studies with the USA and abroad. The item "physicians should not allow themselves to be influenced by strong personal bonds between their patients and their family members" did not fit into the model, which was attributed to the possibility of inaccurate translation. Cronbach's alpha coefficients were 0.83, 0.70, and 0.60 for the three factors of Perspective Taking, Compassionate Care, and Standing in Patient's Shoes, respectively. Women scored higher than men on the Perspective-Taking factor, but men outscored women on the two other factors.

*Hojat, M., DeSantis, J., Shannon, S., Mortensen, L.H., Speicher, M., Bragan, L., LaNoue, M., & Calabrese, L.H. (2018). The Jefferson Scale of Empathy: A nationwide study of measurement properties, underlying components, latent variable structure, and national norm in medical students. *Advances in Health Sciences Education, 23,* 899-920. https://doi.org/10.1007/s10459-018-9839-9.

This study was designed to examine measurement properties, underlying components, and latent variable structure of the JSE-S in a nationwide sample of first-year matriculants at US colleges of osteopathic medicine, and to develop a national norm table for the assessment of JSE-S scores. A web-based survey was administered at the beginning of the academic year which included the JSE, and a scale to detect "good impression" responses. Usable surveys were received from 6009 students enrolled in 41 college campuses (median response rate = 92%). The JSE mean score and standard deviation for the sample were 116.54 and 10.85, respectively. Item-total score correlations were positive and statistically significant ($p < 0.01$), and Cronbach $\alpha = 0.82$. Significant gender differences were observed on the JSE scores in favor of women. Also, significant differences were found on item scores between top and bottom third scorers on the JSE. Three factors of Perspective Taking, Compassionate Care, and Walking in Patient's Shoes emerged in an exploratory factor analysis by using half of the sample. Results of confirmatory factor analysis with another half of the sample confirmed the 3-factor model. Also, a national norm table was developed which is the first to assess medical students' JSE-S scores against national data.

*Hojat, M., Gonnella, J. S., Nasca, T. J., Mangione, S., Veloski, J. J., & Magee, M. (2002). The Jefferson Scale of Physician Empathy: Further psychometric data and differences by gender and specialty at item level. *Academic Medicine* (Suppl.), *77*, s58–s60.

Participants included 704 physicians (26% women) who completed the JSE. Results of statistical analyses at item level showed that the item mean scores ranged from 4.8 to 6.5 (on a 7-point Likert scale). Although respondents used the full range of possible responses (1–7) on all items, response distributions for each item were skewed toward the upper end of the scale. Corrected item-total score correlations were all positive and statistically significant, ranging from 0.30 to 0.60, with a median of 0.40. Statistically significant differences were observed on six out of the 20 items of the JSE in favor of women; however, effect size estimates of gender differences were modest. Also, statistically significant differences were observed on 11 of the 20 items of the JSE between physicians in "people-oriented" specialties ($n = 462$, e.g., family medicine, internal medicine, pediatrics, psychiatry, obstetrics and gynecology, emergency medicine) and "technology-oriented" specialties ($n=242$, e.g., anesthesiology, radiology, pathology, surgery, and surgical specialties) in favor of physicians in "people-oriented" specialties (effect size estimates ranged from 0.17 to 0.41).

*Hojat, M. Gonnella, J. S., Nasca, T. J., Mangione, S., Vergare, M., & Magee, M. (2002). Physician empathy: Definition, components, measurement, and relationship to gender and specialty. *American Journal of Psychiatry, 159*, 1563–1569.

Participants included 704 physicians (179 women) in the Jefferson Health System affiliated with Thomas Jefferson University Hospital, who completed the JSE HP-Version. Results showed an overall JSE mean score of 120 (SD=12, $M=121$, score range=50–140), Cronbach's alpha coefficient of 0.81, and test–retest reliability of 0.65 (within a 3- to 4-month interval between testing, $n=71$ physicians). Women scored slightly higher than men (for women: $M=120.9$, SD=12.2; for men: $M=119.1$, SD=11.8), but the difference did not reach statistical significance. Psychiatrists obtained the highest JSE mean score ($M=127.0$, SD=5.5), followed by physicians in internal medicine ($M=121.7$, SD=10.6); pediatrics ($M=121.5$, SD=12.2); emergency medicine ($M=121.0$, SD=10.7); and family medicine ($M=120.5$, SD=12.6). The lowest JSE mean scores were obtained by physicians in anesthesiology ($M=116.1$, SD=12.0); orthopedic surgery ($M=116.5$, SD=12.9); neurosurgery ($M=117.3$, SD=9.5); and radiology ($M=117.9$, SD=13.1). Controlling for physicians' gender, psychiatrists obtained a JSE mean score that was significantly higher than those obtained by physicians in anesthesiology, orthopedic surgery, neurosurgery, radiology, cardiovascular surgery, obstetrics and gynecology, and general surgery. Exploratory factor analysis of data resulted in three factors of Perspective Taking, Compassionate Care, and Standing in the Patient's Shoes.

*Hojat, M., & LaNoue, M. (2014). Exploration and confirmation of the latent variable structure of the Jefferson Scale of Empathy. *International Journal of Medical Education, 5*, 73–81. doi: https://doi.org/10.5116/ijme.533f.0c41.

Participants included 2612 students (1322 women) who entered Jefferson Medical College between 2002 and 2012 and completed the JSE at the entry to medical school. They were divided into two groups: Matriculants between 2002 and 2007 ($n=1380$) and between 2008 and 2012 ($n=1232$). Data for 2002–2007 matriculants were subjected to exploratory factor analysis (principal component factor extraction with oblique rotation), and data for 2008–2012 matriculants were used for confirmatory factor analysis (structural equation modeling and root mean square error for approximation). The exploratory factor analysis resulted in three factors of "perspective-taking," "compassionate care," and "walking in patient's shoes," replicating the three-factor model reported in most of the previous studies. The confirmatory factor analysis showed that the three-factor model was an acceptable fit that confirmed the latent variable structure which emerged in the exploratory factor analysis. Corrected item-total scores correlations for the total sample were all positive and statistically significant, ranging from 0.13 to 0.61 with a median of 0.44. Cronbach's alpha coefficient for the total sample was 0.80, ranging from 0.75 to 0.84 for matriculants of different years.

*Hojat, M., Mangione, S., Nasca, T. J., Cohen, M J. M., Gonnella, J. S., Erdmann, J. B., Veloski, J. J., & Magee, M. (2001). The Jefferson Scale of Physician Empathy: development and preliminary psychometric data. *Educational and Psychological Measurement, 61*, 349–365.

This is the first publication on psychometrics of the original version of the Jefferson Scale of Physician Empathy (JSPE). Participants included three groups: 55 physicians, 41 residents, and 193 medical students. Based on an extensive review of the relevant literature, a preliminary version of the JSPE (90 items) was developed and sent to 100 physicians in 1999 to examine face and content validities (55 responded). Based on feedback received, 45 items were retained after modifications for clarity suggested by the respondents. The modified version plus three scales of the Interpersonal Reactivity Index (IRI) (Perspective Taking, Empathic Concern, and Fantasy), two scales of the NEO PI-R (Warmth and Dutifulness), Faith-in-People (misanthropy) scale, and self-rated personality attributes (sympathy, compassion, etc.) were completed by 41 residents and 183 medical students. Based on the results of factor analysis on item responses from the medical student sample, 20 items with the highest factor coefficients (>0.40) on the grand factor were retained. Mean score of the 20-item JSPE was 118 for both medical student and resident samples (SD = 11 and SD = 12, respectively). Women scored significantly higher than men. Scores on the 20-item JSPE correlated significantly with scores on perspective taking, empathic concern, and fantasy of the IRI, and with measures of compassion, sympathy, trust, tolerance, personal growth in resident and medical student samples; with scores on the NEO PI-R scales of warmth, and dutifulness, and with scores on the Faith-in-People scale in medical students. These findings provided evidence in support of convergent and discriminant validities of the JSPE. Cronbach's alpha coefficient was 0.87 for residents, and 0.89 for medical students.

Hsiao, C. Y., Tsai, Y. F., & Kao, Y. C. (2012). Psychometric properties of a Chinese version of the Jefferson Scale of Empathy–Health Professions Students. *Journal of Psychiatric and Mental Health Nursing, 20*, 866–873. doi: https://doi.org/10.1111/jpm.12024. Accessible from: http://onlinelibrary.wiley.com/doi/10.1111/jpm.12024/pdf.

Participants included 613 Taiwanese undergraduate (second-year and fourth-year) nursing students (546 women) who completed JSE HPS-Version. Content validity was confirmed by 11 experts with an agreement index of 89%. Corrected item-total score correlations ranged from 0.52 to 0.72 (all positive and statistically significant). The JSE mean score for men was 104.22 (SD = 16.07) and 108.57 (SD = 14.30) for women, a significant difference. Fourth-year students (*M* = 109.22, SD = 13.77) obtained significantly higher JSE mean score than second-year students (*M* = 105.57, SD = 15.91). Cronbach's alpha coefficient was 0.93 for the entire sample, and test–retest reliability was 0.92. Exploratory factor analysis resulted in three factors: Perspective Taking (Cronbach's alpha coefficient = 0.90), Compassionate Care (Cronbach's alpha coefficient = 0.87), and Standing in Patient's Shoes (Cronbach's alpha coefficient = 0.77).

Jumroonrojana, K., & Zartrungpak, S. (2012). Development of the Jefferson Scale of Physician Empathy-Student Version (Thai version). *Journal of the Psychiatric Association of Thailand, 57*, 213–224.

Participants included 708 medical students in all 6 years of their medical education at the Faculty of Medicine, Ramathibodi Hospital, and Mahidol University in Thailand, who completed a Thai translation of the JSE. Results showed that all item-total score correlations were positive and statistically significant, ranging from 0.26 to 0.57. Factor analysis of data resulted in three factors of Compassionate Care, Perspective Taking, and Standing in Patient's Shoes, similar to those that emerged in most other factor analytic studies, although in a different order. Cronbach's alpha coefficient was 0.79. The JSE mean score for this sample of Thai medical students was 111.31 (SD = 10.41). Women outscored men, and the JSE mean score declined significantly as students progressed from preclinical to the clinical phase of medical education in this cross-sectional study.

Karimi, F. Z., & Abdollahi, M. (2019). Factors affecting empathy with patient among healthcare provider students: A Structural Equation Modeling Study. *Indian Journal of Critical Care Medicine: Peer-Reviewed, Official Publication of Indian Society of Critical Care Medicine, 23*(9), 396–399. https://doi.org/10.5005/jp-journals-10071-23232.

This study was designed to investigate the factors affecting clinical empathy among healthcare provider students using a structural equation model. Participants included 398 students of the School of Nursing and Midwifery at the Mashhad University of Medical Sciences in Iran, who completed the JSE-HPS. Results of factor analysis showed three factors of "Perspective-Taking," "Compassionate Care," and "Standing in Patient's Shoes" that emerged in a number of other studies. The results of this study showed improvements in students' clinical empathy.

*Kataoka, H., Koide, N., Ochi, K., Hojat, M., & Gonnella, J. S. (2009). Measurement of empathy among Japanese medical students: psychometrics and score differences by gender and level of medical education. *Academic Medicine, 84*, 1192–1197.

Participants included 400 Japanese medical students (103 women) from all 6 years at the Okayama University Medical School in Japan, who completed a Japanese translation of the JSE. Results showed that the corrected item-total score correlations were all positive and statistically significant, ranging from 0.16 to 0.55 with a median of 0.42. Mean score for the total sample was 104.3 (SD=13.1). Women obtained a significantly higher mean score than men. Cronbach's alpha coefficient was 0.74. The JSE mean score increased from 98.5 in the first year to 107.8 in the last year of medical school in this cross-sectional study. Exploratory factor analysis showed five factors: "perspective taking," "compassionate care," "empathic understanding," and two additional factors of "difficulties in taking patient's perspective," and "standing in patient's shoes."

Kliszcz, J., Nowicka-Sauer, K., Trzeciak, B., Nowak, P., & Sadowska, A. (2006). Empathy in health care providers–validation study of the Polish version of the Jefferson Scale of Empathy. *Advances in Medical Sciences, 51*, 219–225. Accessible from: http://www.advms.pl/ms_2006/Kliszcz_J_et%20al_Empathy%20in%20health%20care%20providers.pdf.

Participants included 405 (324 women) health professional students and practitioners: 118 physicians (95 women), 76 nurses (all women), 149 medical students (91 women), 33 midwifery students (all women), and 29 nursing students (all women) who completed the Polish translation of the JSE (S- and HP-Versions), the IRI, and an Emotional Intelligence Scale. Results showed that the mean scores on the JSE were 112.40 (SD=11.40) and 111.30 (SD=16.01) for students and practicing health professionals, respectively; Cronbach's alpha coefficients were 0.72 and 0.79, respectively. No statistically significant gender difference was observed on the JSE, nor was there a significant difference among the five study samples. In the total sample, statistically significant correlations, although low in magnitude, were found between scores on the JSE and those of the Empathic Concern scale of the IRI (r=0.25); and the Perspective Taking scale of the IRI (r=0.26). However, no statistically significant correlation was found between the JSE scores, and Personal Distress and Fantasy scales of the IRI. Significant correlation was also observed between scores on the JSE and those on the emotional intelligence scale (r=0.30) in the total sample.

Kožený, J., Tišanská, L., & Hoschl, C. (2013). Assessing empathy among Czech medical students: A cross-sectional study. *Československá Psychologie, 57*, 246–254.

Participants included 725 medical students (457 women) at Charles University in Prague, and 871 students (624 women) at Dentistry Palacky University Olomouc in Czech Republic, who completed a Czech translation of the JSE. Results showed that all corrected item-total score correlations were positive and statistically significant, ranging from 0.05 to 0.51. The JSE mean score for the total sample ($n = 1596$) was 99.5 (SD = 13.08). No gender difference was observed on the JSE scores. The JSE mean score in this cross-sectional study declined significantly from 106.42 (SD = 10.42) in the first year to 98.20 (SD = 14.22) in the sixth year of training. Exploratory factor analysis of the JSE resulted in three factors of Perspective Taking, Compassionate Care, and Empathic Understanding. Cronbach's alpha coefficient for the total sample was 0.76.

Leombruni, P., Di Lillo, M., Miniotti, M., Picardi, A., Alessandri, G., Sica, C., Zizzi, F., Castelli, L., & Torta, R. (2014). Measurement properties and confirmatory factor analysis of the Jefferson Scale of Empathy in Italian medical students. *Perspectives on Medical Education*. Published online: 08 Aug 2014. doi: https://doi.org/10.1007/s40037-014-0137-9.

Participants included 257 medical students (114 men and 143 women) at the University of Turin Medical School, who completed an Italian translation of the JSE-S version. Results showed that the JSE mean score for the entire sample was 108.7 (SD = 10.60). Women scored significantly higher than men ($M = 110.21$, SD = 11.47 for women, $M = 106.83$, SD = 9.10 for men) on the total scores on the JSE; however, when compared on the JSE factor scores, women scored significantly higher than men only on the Compassionate Care factor, but not on the Perspective Taking, or Standing in Patient's Shoes factors. Cronbach's alpha coefficient was 0.76 for the entire sample (0.73 for men, and 0.79 for women). Test–retest reliability (2-weeks interval) was 0.72. Confirmatory factor analysis provided support for the three-factor model.

Li, L., Wang, J., Hu, X., & Xu, C. (2015). Empathy in Chinese pharmacy undergraduates: Implication for integrated humanities into professional pharmacy education. *Indian Journal of Pharmaceutical Education and Research, 49*, 31–39. doi: https://doi.org/10.5530/ijper.49.1.5.

Participants included 263 Chinese pharmacy students at the Wuhan University of Science and Technology, who completed the JSE (HPS-version). Results showed a mean score of 112.58 (SD = 11.64), and Cronbach's alpha coefficient of 0.81. No significant gender difference was observed. Exploratory factor analysis resulted in three factors of "perspective taking," "compassionate care," and "standing in patient shoes," which emerged in most of other factor analytic studies of the JSE. The JSE mean score for fourth-year students in this cross-sectional study was significantly higher ($M = 117.59$) than those for the previous years of pharmacy education. Social activities and humanistic education were the models most frequently suggested by pharmacy students for promoting empathy.

Li, D., Xu, H., Kang, M., & Ma, S. (2018). Empathy in Chinese eight-year medical program students: Differences by school year, educational stage, and future career preference. *BMC Medical Education, 18*(1), 241. https://doi.org/10.1186/s12909-018-1348-2.

The purpose of this study was to examine the psychometric properties of a Chinese translation of the JSE (Student-version, JSE-S), and to study differences in empathy scores among undergraduate medical students across gender, year of study, and future career preference. Research participants included first- to seventh-year students on an eight-year medical education course at Fudan University, who completed the Chinese translation of the JSE-S. Four factors emerged in factor analysis of the instrument: "perspective taking," "compassionate care," "standing in patient's shoes," and "difficulties in adopting patient's perspective." While a decline in empathy was observed across school years, the lowest empathy score was found in the seventh-year students. No gender difference was found in empathy scores. The findings support aspects of psychometrics of the Chinese translation of the JSE-S in Chinese medical students.

Magalhäes, E., Salgueira A. P., Costa, P., & Costa M. J. (2011). Empathy in senior year and first year medical students: A cross-sectional study. *BMC Medical Education, 11*, 52. doi: https://doi.org/10.1186/1472-6920-11-52. Accessible from: http://www.biomedcentral.com/1472-6920/11/52.

Participants included 476 medical students (321 women) at the School of Health Sciences, University of Minho in Portugal, who completed the Portuguese translation of the JSE-S version. The construct validity of the JSE was cross-validated by using exploratory and confirmatory factor analysis. Exploratory factor analysis resulted in three factors in the Portuguese original model: "compassionate care," "perspective-taking," and "standing in patients' shoes." Empathy scores of students in the final year of medical school were higher than those at the beginning of medical school. Female students scored significantly higher ($M=112.86$, SD = 10.81) than male students ($M=110.32$, SD = 10.69). No significant difference was observed on the JSE scores among students with different specialty preferences. Cronbach's alpha coefficient was 0.77 for this sample.

McMillan, L. R., & Shannon, D. M. (2011). Psychometric analysis of the JSPE nursing student version R: Comparison of senior BSN students and medical students' attitudes toward empathy in patient care. *International Scholarly Research Network Nursing*, Article ID 726063. doi: https://doi.org/10.5402/2011/726063. Accessible from: https://doi.org/10.5402/2011/726063.

Participants included 598 senior nursing students (88% women) at the Auburn University College of Nursing, who completed the JSE. Results showed a JSE mean score of 114.57 (SD = 10.94) and a Cronbach's alpha coefficient of 0.77 for the entire sample. Exploratory factor analysis initially resulted in five factors; however, two of them marginally met the Kaiser's criterion. Thus, three factors were retained which were very similar to those that emerged from most other studies with US medical students. Confirmatory factor analysis provided marginal support for the three-factor model.

Mostafa, A., Hoque, R., Mosrafa, M., Rana M., & Mostafa, F. (2014). Empathy in undergraduate medical students of Bangladesh: Psychometric analysis and differences by gender, academic year, and specialty preference. *International Scholarly Research Notices Psychiatry*, Article ID 375439. Accessible from: https://doi.org/10.1155/2014/375439.

Participants included 348 first- through fifth-year medical students (291 women) at Chattagram Maa-O-Shishu Hospital Medical College, who completed a Bengali translation of the JSE. Exploratory factor analysis resulted in three factors of "perspective taking," "compassionate care," and "standing in patent's shoes." Corrected item-total score correlations ranged from 0.33 to 0.66; all were statistically significant. Cronbach's alpha coefficient was 0.88. Women obtained higher JSE scores (M = 111.99, SD = 12.97) than men (M = 106.72, SD = 14.33). No significant association was found between scores on the JSE and specialty interests. In this cross-sectional study, JSE scores increased significantly as students progressed through medical school during the clinical years of medical education.

Osim, J. H.; Essien, E.A., Aniekan; Okegbe, J.; & Udofia, O. (2019) The Jefferson Scale of Physician Empathy: A preliminary study of validity and reliability among physicians in Nigerian tertiary hospital. *Acta Medica International* 6(1), 22–27. doi: https://doi.org/10.4103/ami.ami_70_18.

This purpose of this study was to investigate the validity and reliability of the JSE HP-Version among Nigerian physicians. The JSE HP-Version and the Emotional intelligence scale (EIS) were administered to 120 physicians in Nigeria. Exploratory factor analysis yielded three factors that were not quite consistent with previous reports. Statistical findings suggested that age, sex, and administrative roles were significant predictors of physician empathy. The JSE-HP had fairly strong reliability coefficients and an acceptable convergent validity with the EIS, which measures a related construct.

Paro, H. B. M. S., Daud-Gallotti, R. M., Pinto, I. C., Tiberio, L. F. L. C., & Martins, M. A. (2012). Brazilian version of the Jefferson Scale of Empathy: Psychometric properties and factor analysis. *BMC Medical Education, 12*, 73. doi: https://doi.org/10.1186/1472-6920-12-73.

Participants included 319 students in their fifth and sixth medical school years at the Sao Paulo University School of Medicine in Brazil, who completed a Brazilian translation of the JSE. Results showed that the JSE mean score was 114.95 (SD = 12.41). Women obtained a higher mean score (M = 116.54, SD = 12.81) than did men (M = 113.84, SD = 12.68), although the difference was not statistically significant. Cronbach's alpha coefficient was 0.84. Three factors of "compassionate care," "standing in patient's shoes," and "perspective taking" emerged in that order in an exploratory factor analysis. (Cronbach's alpha coefficients for these three factors were 0.83, 0.73, and 0.74, respectively.)

Piumatti, G., Costa, M. J., Ardenghi, S., Baroffio, A., Elorduy, M., Gerbase, M. W., Gustin, M. P., Palés, J., Quince, T., Rampoldi, G., Strepparava, M. G., Thiemann, P., Virumbrales, M., & Costa, P. S. (Published online, October 2024). Cross-national psychometric evaluation of the Jefferson Scale of Empathy-Medical Student Version. *Evaluation & the Health Professions*. https://doi.org/10.1177/01632787241296540.

The purpose of this study was to examine the factorial structure of the JSE-Medical Student Version (JSE-S) and assess items' discriminatory ability at higher and lower empathy levels in medical student populations from different countries and languages. JSE-S data were retrieved from previous studies of 4113 first- and/or second-year medical students from Switzerland, Portugal, Italy, Brazil, France, Spain, New Zealand, UK, Ireland, Mexico, and Peru. The "Compassionate Care" factor emerged in five samples (Switzerland, Portugal, Italy, France, and UK/Ireland), "Perspective Taking" factor in three (Switzerland, Portugal, and UK/Ireland), and "Walking in Patient's Shoes" in five (Switzerland, Portugal, Spain, UK/Ireland, and Mexico/Peru). There was no consistent support across countries for the JSE-S three-factorial structure. Items provided redundant information and discriminatory power decreased when aiming to differentiate students at high empathy levels.

Preusche, I., & Wagner-Menghin, M. (2013). Rising to the challenge: Cross-cultural adaptation and psychometric evaluation of the adapted German version of the Jefferson Scale of Physician Empathy for students (JSPE-S). *Advances in Health Science Education: Theory and Practice, 18*, 573–587. doi: https://doi.org/10.1007/s10459-012-9393-9.

Participants included 516 second-year medical students at the Medical University of Vienna in Austria, who completed a German translation of the JSE. Results showed that the JSE mean score was 110.52 (SD = 12.49). Item-total score correlations were all positive (ranged from 0.13 to 0.68). Cronbach's alpha coefficient was 0.82, and test–retest reliability for 96 students in a 6–7 week interval was 0.45. An exploratory factor analysis resulted in four factors: "perspective taking," "compassionate care," "standing in patient's shoes," and a residual factor.

Rahimi-Madiseh, M., Tavakol, M., Dennick, R., & Nasiri, J. (2010). Empathy in Iranian medical students: A preliminary psychometric analysis and differences by gender and year of medical school. *Medical Teacher, 32*, e471–e478.

Participants included 181 medical students (127 women) at the Shahrekord University of Medical Sciences in Iran, who completed the JSE (S-Version). Results showed that the JSE mean score for the sample was 105.1 (SD = 12.9). Cronbach's alpha coefficient was 0.74. Exploratory factor analysis resulted in three factors: Compassionate Care, Perspective Taking, and Walking in Patient's Shoes, similar to those found in US medical students, although in a different order. Women scored higher than men ($M = 105.6$ and $M = 103.7$, respectively) but the difference was not statistically significant. No significant change in empathy scores was observed in five medical school years in this cross-sectional study.

Roh, M. S., Hahm, B. J., Lee, D. H., & Suh, D. H. (2010). Evaluation of empathy among Korean medical students: A cross-sectional study using Korean version of the Jefferson Scale of Physician Empathy. *Teaching and Learning in Medicine: An International Journal, 22*, 167–171. doi: https://doi.org/10.1080/10401334.2010.488191.

Participants included 493 medical students (159 women) at the Seoul National University College of Medicine in Korea, who completed the JSE. Item-total score correlations were all positive and statistically significant, ranging from 0.28 to 0.68 with a median of 0.42. Cronbach's alpha coefficient was 0.84. Cross-sectional comparisons of students in different years of medical school showed that fourth-year students obtained a significantly higher JSE mean score than other students. Exploratory factor analysis of the JSE resulted in the three factors: "perspective taking," "compassionate care," and "standing in patient's shoes" which emerged in the US samples, and in some other international studies. No significant difference was observed between men and women on the JSE mean scores.

Shariat, S. V., Eshtad, E., & Ansari, S. (2010). Empathy and its correlates in Iranian physicians: A preliminary psychometric study of the Jefferson Scale of Physician Empathy. *Medical Teacher, 32*, e417–e421 (web paper). doi: https://doi.org/10.3109/0142159X.2010.498488.

Participants included 207 general practitioners in Iran who completed the JSE. Results showed that Cronbach's alpha coefficient was 0.78. Exploratory factor analysis resulted in three factors: "perspective taking," "compassionate care," and "standing in patient's shoes." Women scored higher than men, but place of practice and practice setting did not show significant association with scores on the JSE. Regression analysis indicated that practice experiences could significantly predict JSE scores beyond the effect of physicians' ages.

Comparisons of mean scores of each item of the JSE in Iran, Japan, the USA showed a similar pattern of findings, with items 2 and 19 showing the highest and items 3 and 18 the lowest mean scores in all three countries. The rank order correlations of the item mean scores were 0.90 (between Iran and the USA), 0.88 (between Japan and the USA), and 0.69 (between Iran and Japan).

Shariat, S. V., & Habibi, M. (2013). Empathy in Iranian medical students: Measurement model of the Jefferson Scale of Empathy. *Medical Teacher, 35*, e913–e918. doi: https://doi.org/10.3109/0142159x.2012.714881.

Participants included 1187 medical students (759 women) from 17 Iranian medical schools who completed the JSE. Results showed that the mean score for the total sample was 101.4 (SD = 14.5). Female students scored significantly higher than men (*M*= 102.75, SD = 13.94 and *M*= 98.94, SD = 15.23, respectively). Cronbach's alpha coefficient was 0.79, and test–retest reliability was 0.95 (2 weeks interval between testing, *n*= 31). A decline in empathy scores was observed as students progressed through medical school in this cross-sectional study. Students in larger medical schools obtained higher JSE mean scores than others in smaller universities. Confirmatory factor analysis provided a satisfactory fitness for the three-factor model (Perspective Taking, Compassionate Care, and Standing in the Patient's Shoes).

Sherman, J. J., & Cramer, A. (2005). Measurement of changes in empathy during dental school. *Journal of Dental Education, 69*, 338–345.

Participants included 130 dental students (45 women) at the University of Washington School of Dentistry, who completed the JSE. Results showed the mean score for total sample was 117.7 (SD=14.06). Women scored (*M*=122.29, SD=12.76) significantly higher than did men (*M*=115.28, SD=14.17). No significant association was observed between scores on the JSE and students' race, age, or marital status. Scores on the JSE declined after the first year and remained low throughout the fourth year of dental school. Cronbach's alpha coefficient was 0.90, and the split-half reliability coefficient was 0.87. Scores on the JSE were significantly correlated with 18 out of 26 clinical competency ratings. The largest correlation was obtained between JSE scores and ratings on applying the principles of behavioral sciences that pertain to patient-centered oral health care, and the lowest correlation was obtained with ratings on utilizing business and management skills to conduct an efficient and effective clinical practice. Exploratory factor analysis resulted in four factors of Perspective Taking, Patient's Experiences and Feelings, and Ignoring Emotions in Patient Care.

Stansfield, R.B., Schwartz, A., O'Brien, C.L., Dekhtar, M., Dunham, L., Quirk, M. (2016). Development of a metacognitive effort construct of empathy during clinical training: A longitudinal study of the factor structure of the Jefferson Scale of Empathy. *Advances in Heath Science Education, 21*, 5–17. doi: https://doi.org/10.1007/s10459-015-9605-1.

Participants included 4,797 students from 28 medical schools in the United States, who complete the JSE. They were divided into two groups. One group included students in the preclinical years, and the other included those in clinical years of medical school. Within each group, students were randomly assigned for exploratory factor analysis (EFA) and confirmatory factor analysis (CFA) of the JSE. Despite an unexplained departure from standard scoring of the JSE, results of EFA in preclinical years were almost identical to most factor analytic findings of the JSE reported by others. However, four factors emerged in the clinical years of medical school. The first three factors were similar to those that emerged in preclinical years of medical school, but were renamed to avoid confusion with the original model (according to the authors), and the fourth factor was called Metacognition. Confirmatory factor analytic results indicated that the 3-factor model was an acceptable fit for the preclinical years, and the 4-factor model was a better fit than the other models for the clinical years of medical school.

Ster, M. P., Ster, B. Petek, D., & Gorup, E. C. (2014). Validation of Slovenian version of Jefferson Scale of Empathy for students. *Slovenian Journal of Public Health, 53*, 89–100. doi: https://doi.org/10.2478/sjph-2014-0010.

Participants included 234 first-year medical students (69% or 162 women) in Slovenia (Ljubljana Medical School), who completed the Slovenian translation of the JSE. Results showed the JSE mean score for this sample was 107.7 (SD = 12.6), and Cronbach's alpha coefficient was = 0.79. Test–retest reliability was 0.70 (n = 80, 2-week interval between testing). Exploratory factor analysis resulted in factors of Perspective Taking, Compassionate Care, Standing in Patient's Shoes, Interpersonal Relationship, and a residual factor.

*Suh, D. H., Hong, J. S., Lee, D. H., Gonnella, J. S., & Hojat. M. (2012). The Jefferson Scale of Physician Empathy: A preliminary psychometric study and group comparisons in Korean physicians. *Medical Teacher, 34*, e464–e468 (web paper). doi: https://doi.org/10.3109/0142159x.2012.668632.

Participants included 229 physicians (103 women) in Seoul National University Hospital in Korea, who completed a Korean translation of the JSE HP-Version. Results showed that the JSE mean score was 98.2 (SD = 12). Cronbach's alpha coefficient was 0.84. Women scored significantly higher than did men (M = 100.3, SD = 11.7 and M = 96.5, SD = 12.0, respectively). Exploratory factor analysis resulted in three factors of compassionate care, perspective taking, and a residual factor.

Tavakol, S., Dennick, R., & Tavakol, M. (2011). Psychometric properties and confirmatory factor analysis of the Jefferson Scale of Physician Empathy. *BMC Medical Education, 11*, 54. doi: https://doi.org/10.1186/1472-6920-11-54. Accessible from: http://www.biomedcentral.com/1472-6920/11/54.

Participants included 853 medical students (470 women) at the University of Nottingham in England, who completed the JSE. Cronbach's alpha coefficient was 0.76. Exploratory factor analysis resulted in three factors entitled "compassionate care," "perspective taking," and "emotional detachment." Confirmatory factor analysis showed that the three-factor model fit well across genders of medical students.

Vallabh, K. (2011). Psychometrics of the student version of the Jefferson Scale of Physician Empathy (JSPE-S) in final-year medical students in Johannesburg in 2008. *South African Journal of Bioethics and Law, 4*, 63–68. Accessible from: http://www.sajbl.org.za/index.php/sajbl/article/view/164/140.

Participants included 158 final year medical students (143 women) who completed the JSE-S at the Faculty of Health Sciences of the University of the Witwatersrand Medical School in South Africa. Results showed that the JSE mean score was 107 (SD = 10.9). Women (M = 109, SD = 9.8) scored higher than men (M = 104, SD = 12). Item-total score correlations were all positive and statistically significant. Cronbach's alpha coefficient was 0.79. Exploratory factor analysis resulted in three factors of Perspective Talking, Compassionate Care, and Standing in Patient's Shoes.

*Veloski, J., & Hojat, M. (2006). Measuring specific elements of professionalism: Empathy, teamwork, and lifelong learning. In D. T. Stern (Ed.). *Measuring medical professionalism* (pp. 117–145). Oxford: Oxford University Press.

In this book chapter, professionalism in medicine was described as personal qualities beyond acquisition of medical knowledge and procedural skills that have relevance to optimal patient outcomes. It was suggested that professionalism is a multifaceted concept, involving different elements. Three major elements of professionalism were recognized based on a review of relevant literature, such as: Empathy in patient care, interprofessional collaboration/teamwork, and lifelong learning. Operational definitions and measuring instruments for these three elements of professionalism in medicine were provided, and a brief summary of psychometrics support (validity and reliability) of these measuring instruments was reported. The JSE was described as a measure of choice for quantifying empathic orientation/engagement in patient care. The Jefferson Scale of Physician Lifelong Learning was described as the instrument of choice for measuring orientation/attitudes toward lifelong learning, and the Jefferson Scale of Attitudes toward Interprofessional Collaboration (e.g., physician-nurse) was described as a psychometrically sound instrument for measuring teamwork and interprofessional collaboration.

*Ward, J., Schaal, M., Sullivan, J., Bowen, M. E., Erdmann, J. B., & Hojat, M. (2009). Reliability and validity of the Jefferson Scale of Empathy in undergraduate nursing students. *Journal of Nursing Measurement, 17*, 73–88. doi: https://doi.org/10.1891/1061-3749.17.1.73.

Participants included 333 undergraduate nursing students (284 women) who completed a slightly modified version of the JSE for administration to nursing students. Exploratory factor analysis resulted in three factors "perspective taking," "compassionate care," and "standing in patient's shoes." The JSE mean score for the entire sample was 114.0 (SD = 11.5). Cronbach's alpha coefficients were 0.78, 0.83, and 0.72 for the three extracted factors, respectively. The alpha reliability coefficient for the entire sample was 0.77. Corrected item-total score correlations were all positive and statistically significant, ranging from 0.20 to 0.64, with a median correlation of 0.44. Female students obtained a significantly higher JSE mean score than did men. No statistically significant associations were observed between JSE scores and ethnicity (White, Black, and Asian), academic backgrounds (humanities, sciences, and business); or marital status. Students with more clinical experiences obtained the highest JSE mean score. A statistically significant correlation ($r = 0.38$, $p < 0.01$) was found between scores on the JSE and a validated measure of attitudes toward teamwork and interprofessional collaboration (Jefferson Scale of Attitudes Toward Physician-Nurse Collaboration).

Wen, D., Ma, X., Li, H., Liu, Z., Xian, B., & Liu, Y. (2013). Empathy in Chinese medical students: Psychometric characteristics and differences by gender and year of medical education. *BMC Medical Education, 13*, 130. doi: https://doi.org/10.1186/1472-6920-13-130.

Participants included 753 first- to fourth-year Chinese students (476 women) at China Medical University, who completed a Chinese translation of the JSE. Exploratory factor analysis resulted in three factors of Perspective Taking, Compassionate Care, and the Ability to Stand in Patient's Shoes, similar to those that emerged in a majority of factor analytic studies of the JSE. The JSE mean score for the total sample was 109.60 (SD = 12.09), and Cronbach's alpha coefficient was 0.83. Women obtained a significantly higher mean JSE scores ($M = 111.53$, SD = 10.72) than men ($M = 106.29$, SD = 13.53). No significant association was found between JSE scores and student's age. An upward trend in empathy scores was observed in this cross-sectional study as students progressed through medical school. However, only the difference between the JSE mean score for the fourth-year students was significantly higher ($M = 112.12$, SD = 13.55) than that for first-year students ($M = 107.36$, SD = 13.35).

Wen, D., Ma, X., Li, H., & Xian, B. (2013). Empathy in Chinese physicians: Preliminary psychometrics of the Jefferson Scale of Physician Empathy (JSE) [Letter to the editor]. *Medical Teacher*, *35*, 609–610.

Participants included 1200 Chinese physicians (521 women) who completed a Chinese translation of the JSE. Results showed a JSE mean score of 109.54 (SD = 11.85). Exploratory factor analysis resulted in three factors of Perspective Taking, Compassionate Care, and Ability to Stand in Patient's Shoes accounting for 66.2% of the total variance. Cronbach's alpha coefficient was 0.80.

Williams, B., & Beovich, B. (2020). A systematic review of psychometric assessment of the Jefferson Scale of Empathy using the COSMIN Risk of Bias checklist. *Journal of Evaluation in Clinical Practice*, *26*(4), 1302–1315. https://doi.org/10.1111/jep.13293.

The purpose of this study was to critically evaluate the current evidence on the measurement properties of the JSE. The search strategy resulted in the retrieval of 985 papers, 59 of which were included in this study. The majority of papers reported on assessments of construct validity and internal consistency, and in these areas the highest quality of reporting was demonstrated. Additionally, there was generally very good quality in reporting of convergent validity. Reliability, measurement error, and cross-cultural validity were reported with less than optimum quality. The JSE demonstrates robust construct validity, internal consistency, and convergent validity. These measurement properties are generally well reported in the literature in studies of good methodological quality, and thus may be interpreted with relative confidence when used in empathy research.

Williams, B., Brown, T., Boyle, M., & Dousek, S. (2013). Psychometric testing of the Jefferson Scale of Empathy Health Professions Students' version with Australian paramedic students. *Nursing and Health Sciences, 15*, 45–50. doi: https://doi.org/10.1111/j.1442-2018.2012.00719.x.

Participants included 330 paramedic students (215 women) at Monash University in Australia, who completed the JSE HPS-Version. Cronbach's alpha coefficient for this sample was 0.75. Exploratory factor analysis resulted in two factors: "compassionate care" and "perspective taking." The two-factor model was appraised in a confirmatory factor analysis for 17 items of the JSE.

Williams, B., Sifris, A., & Lynch, M. (2016). A psychometric appraisal of the Jefferson Scale of Empathy using law students. *Psychology Research and Behavior Management, 9*, 171–178. https://doi.org/10.2147/PRBM.S108036.

The aim of this study was to examine psychometric properties of the JSE-Law Students (JSE-LS). The 20-item JSE-Health Professions Students Version was adapted for a law context (e.g., the word "health care" was replaced by "legal"). The revised instrument was completed by 275 students at Monash University, Melbourne, Australia. Data were subjected to principal component analysis. Four factors emerged: "understanding the client's perspective," "responding to clients' experiences and emotions," "responding to clients' cues and behaviors," and "standing in clients' shoes." The reliability of the factors varied, but the overall 18-item JSE-LS yielded a Cronbach's alpha coefficient of 0.80. The JSE-LS appears to be a reliable measure of empathy among undergraduate law students. Additional evaluation of the JSE-LS is required to disambiguate some of the minor findings explored.

Studies on Correlates of the JSE Scores

Antinienė, D., & Kaklauskaitė, Z. (2018). Empathy and burnout among physicians providing reanimatological and surgical treatment. *Baltic Journal of Sport and Health Sciences, 3*(110), https://doi.org/10.33607/bjshs.v3i110.245.

The purpose of this study was to determine relationships between empathy and burnout among practicing physicians. A total of 185 practicing physicians participated in the study and completed the JSE and the Copenhagen Burnout Inventory. The study results showed no statistically significant relationship between empathy and burnout among physicians.

Assing Hvidt, E., Søndergaard, J., Wehberg, S., Hvidt, N. C., & Andersen, C. M. (2022). A cross-sectional study of student empathy across four medical schools in Denmark-associations between empathy level and age, sex, specialty preferences and motivation. *BMC Medical Education*, *22*(1), 489. https://doi.org/10.1186/s12909-022-03532-2.

The aim of this study was to examine the associations between empathy scores among Danish medical students and medical school year, age, sex, co-habitation, parental status, specialty preferences, and motivations for choosing medicine as a future profession. All medical students from four medical schools in Denmark were invited to participate in the study. The JSE-S was completed by 672 medical students. The overall mean score was 112.7. There were no statistically significant differences in empathy between medical schools; first, third-, and sixth-year of medical school education; age groups; or parental status. Female students and students living with a spouse or partner scored higher on JSE-S than male students or students living alone. Preference for future medical specialty was statistically significant, with a decrease in scores for students choosing surgery specialties. Motivational factors were not significantly associated with empathy. Overall, results showed neither decrease nor increase but instead rather stable empathy scores across years of curriculum.

Austin, E. J., Evans, P., Goldwater, R., & Potter, V. (2005). A preliminary study of emotional intelligence, empathy and exam performance in first year medical students. *Personality and Individual Differences, 39*, 1395–1405. doi: https://doi.org/10.1016/j.paid.2005.04.014.

Participants included 156 first-year medical students (103 women) who completed the JSE, an emotional intelligence (EI) scale, and a "talking with families" scale measuring skills in communicating with patients and their families. Statistically significant correlations that were moderate in magnitudes were found between scores on the JSE, EI scale ($r=0.35$), and talking with families scale ($r=0.39$). Women scored higher than men on the JSE, and Cronbach's alpha coefficient for the JSE in this sample was 0.85.

Aziz, A. B., & Ali, S. K. (2020). Relationship between level of empathy during residency training and perception of professionalism climate. *BMC Medical Education, 20*(1), 320. https://doi.org/10.1186/s12909-020-02231-0.

This study examined the relationship between empathy level and perception of professionalism environment. Study participants included 70 residents of Obstetrics & Gynecology and Pediatrics departments of a private sector tertiary care hospital in Karachi, Pakistan, who completed the JSE and "Professionalism Climate Instrument" (PCI). The internal consistency of each scale measured by Cronbach's coefficient alpha was 0.76 for the JSE. No significant difference was observed in the mean empathy scores between senior and junior residents of both specialties. Statistically significant gender difference in empathy scores was observed. Cronbach's coefficient alpha for the JSE was 0.76. Professionalism score was not found to vary with either the year of residency or gender. Empathy score and professionalism climate were not found to be correlated. The findings suggested that empathy is a relatively stable trait that remains unchanged during residency training programs.

Beckman, T. J., Reed, D. A., Shanafelt, T. D., & West, C. P. (2010). Impact of resident well-being and empathy on assessments of faculty physicians. *Journal of General Internal Medicine, 25*, 52–56. doi: https://doi.org/10.1007/s11606-009-1152-0.

Participants included 149 residents at Mayo Clinic enrolled in the Mayo Internal Medicine Well-Being Study, who completed the JSE, the Quality of Life (QOL) survey, a measure of depression, Maslach Burnout Inventory (MBI), and a clinical teaching assessment instrument. Results showed a mean JSE score of 115.46 (SD = 12.27) in this sample. It was found that residents' assessments of faculty teachers are not influenced by scores on well-being, including QOL, burnout, and depression scales. However, scores on the JSE were significantly associated with residents' assessments of faculty.

*Berg, K., Blatt, B., Lopreiato, J., Jung, J., Schaeffer, A., Heil, D., Owens, T., Carter-Nolan, P. L., Berg, D., Veloski, J., Darby, E., & Hojat, M. (2015). Standardized patient assessment of medical student empathy: Ethnicity and gender effects in a multi-institutional study. *Academic Medicine, 90*, 105–111. doi: https://doi.org/10.1097/ACM0000000000000052.

Participants included 577 students (287 women) from four medical schools in the USA, who completed the JSE and two subscales of the IRI. The sample included 373 White students (65%), 79 (14%) Black/African American students, and 125 (22%) Asian/Pacific Islander students. The students were assessed by 84 standardized patients (SPs) (45 women); 62 (74%) were White and 22 (26%) were Black/African American. SPs completed the Jefferson Scale of Patient Perceptions of Physician Empathy (JSPPPE) and Global Ratings of Empathy (GRE). A total of 2882 student-standardized patient encounters were analyzed to examine the effects of ethnicity and gender, which could introduce bias in SPs' assessments of students; and to examine concordance between students' self-reported empathy and SPs' assessments of students' empathy. A significant correlation ($r = 0.61$, $p < 0.001$) was found between scores on the JSE and the IRI. Statistical analyses of patient encounters showed significant interaction effects of gender and ethnicity. Female students, regardless of ethnicity, obtained significantly higher mean score than did men on the self-reported JSE (mean scores for women and men were 114.9 and 109.3, respectively); on SPs' assessments of students' empathy (JSPPPE mean scores were 25.6 and 24.1, respectively); and on the GRE (mean scores 7.4 and 6.9, respectively). Male Black/African American students obtained the lowest SPs' assessments of empathy regardless of the SPs' ethnicity. Black/African American students obtained the highest mean scores on self-reported empathy. It was concluded that the significant interaction effects of ethnicity and gender in clinical encounters and the inconsistencies observed between SPs' assessments of students' empathy and students' self-reported empathy may raise concerns about possible ethnicity and gender biases in the SPs' assessments of students' clinical skills, and thus about the testing fairness in the SPs' assessments of students' interpersonal skills.

*Berg, K., Majdan, J. F., Berg, D., Veloski, J, & Hojat, M. (2011a). A comparison of medical students' self-reported empathy with simulated patients' assessment of the students' empathy. *Medical Teacher, 33*, 388–391. doi: https://doi.org/10.3109/0142159x.2010.530319.

Participants included 248 third-year students (123 women) at Jefferson (now Sidney Kimmel) Medical College, who completed the JSE-S version, who were assessed by standardized patients (SPs) on empathic engagement using the Jefferson Scale of Patient Perceptions of Physician Empathy (JSPPPE) and a global rating of empathy (GRE) in ten Objective Structured Clinical Examination (OSCE) stations. Correlation between students' self-reported empathy (JSE) and SPs' assessments of student empathic engagement (JSPPPE) was statistically significant but low in magnitude ($r=0.19$), indicating that the two measures were not redundant. However, correlations between SPs' assessments of students' empathic engagement (JSPPPE), and their GRE for students were statistically significant and relatively large in magnitude ($r=0.87$). It was argued that SPs' assessments of well-defined clinical skills such as physical examination, history taking, and laboratory data in the artificial OSCE environment can be more reliable than their assessments of interpersonal and empathic attributes, which require a reasonable time to form.

*Berg, K., Majdan, J., Berg, D., Veloski, J., & Hojat, M. (2011b). Medical students' self-reported empathy and simulated patients' assessments of student empathy: An analysis by gender and ethnicity. *Academic Medicine, 86*, 984–988. doi: https://doi.org/10.1097/ACM.0b013e3182224f1f.

Participants included 248 third-year medical students (123 women) at Jefferson (now Sidney Kimmel) Medical College. In Objective Structured Clinical Examinations (OSCE), standardized patients (SPs) assessed students' empathy by completing the Jefferson Scale of Patient Perceptions of Physician Empathy (JSPPPE), and rated students on a two-item Global Ratings of Empathy (GRE). Results showed that women obtained a significantly higher JSE mean score ($M=110.4$, SD=11.8) than men ($M=106.4$, SD=13.3, effect size=0.32). No significant difference on the JSE scores was observed between White and Asian-American students. Consistent with their self-reported empathy (reflected in the JSE scores), women also received higher empathy assessments (reflected in the JSPPPE, effect size=0.46) and on global ratings of empathy (reflected in the GRE assessment, effect size=0.63) given by SPs. However, inconsistent with students' self-reported empathy (JSE scores), SPs' assessments on the JSPPPE and GRE were significantly lower for Asian American students, probably indicating an assessment bias against Asian American medical students (effect sizes were 0.56 and 0.43 for the JSPPPE and GRE, respectively).

Biswas, B., Haldar, A., Dasgupta, A., Mallick, N., & Karmakar, A. (2018). An epidemiological study on empathy and its correlates: A cross-sectional assessment among medical students of a government medical college of India. *Indian Journal of Psychological Medicine*, *40*(4), 364–369. https://doi.org/10.4103/IJPSYM.IJPSYM_109_18.

The purpose of the study was to assess empathy level of medical students and its correlates. Undergraduate medical students (n = 249) of a medical school in India completed the JSE. Third-semester students had higher empathy scores (102.4 ± 12.4) compared to fifth (97.2 ± 12.9) and seventh semester (95.0 ± 10.9) students. The difference between the mean scores of different semesters was statistically significant. Female students were more empathic than male students. Empathy eroded as students progressed through medical school.

Braga-Simões, J., Costa, P. S., & Yaphe, J. (2017). Placebo prescription and empathy of the physician: A cross-sectional study. *The European Journal of General Practice, 23(1)*, 98–104. https://doi.org/10.1080/13814788.2017.1291625.

The purpose of this study was to examine the frequency of placebo prescription, doctors' beliefs, motivation, and attitudes toward placebos in general practice and to explore the association between placebo prescription and physician empathy. Participants included 93 general practitioners in 14 health centers in a northern Portuguese health region. The study survey included the Portuguese version of the JSE and questions about placebo prescription. Placebos were prescribed by 73% ($n = 68$) of the respondents, Results indicated that favorable attitudes toward placebo prescription were associated with higher empathy scores ($r = 0.31$, $p < .01$).

Brazeau, C. M., Schroeder, R., Rovi, S., & Boyd, L. (2010). Relationship between medical student burnout, empathy, and professionalism climate. *Academic Medicine, 85*, s33–s36. doi: https://doi.org/10.1097/ACM.0b013e3181ed4c47.

Participants included 127 fourth-year students at the University of Medicine and Dentistry of New Jersey, who completed the JSE, Maslach Burnout Inventory (MBI), and the Professionalism Climate Instrument (PCI), which measures desirable professional behavior. The JSE mean score for the sample was 113.31 (SD=13.35). Scores on the JSE were significantly ($p<0.01$) and positively correlated with those from the Personal Accomplishment scale of the MBI ($r=0.44$), and negatively with scores on Depersonalization scale ($r=-0.41$) and Emotional Exhaustion scale ($r=-0.30$) of the MBI. Also, correlation between JSE and PCI scores (desirable professional behavior in medical students) was statistically significant ($r=0.30$).

Brockhouse, R., Msetfi, R. M., Cohen, K., & Joseph, S. (2011). Vicarious exposure to trauma and growth in therapists: The moderating effects of sense of coherence, organizational support, and empathy. *Journal of Traumatic Stress, 24*, 735–742. doi: https://doi.org/10.1002/jts.20704.

Participants included 118 therapists (38 women) in England, who completed the JSE plus a short form of the Sense of Coherence Scale, Perceived Organizational Scale, and the Post Traumatic Growth Inventory. The JSE mean score for the sample was 121.20 (SD=9.53). Results showed that the JSE scores positively predicted the therapists' psychological growth, organizational support did not predict growth, and a strong sense of cohesiveness negatively predicted growth.

Byrd, J., Knowles, H., Moore, S., Acker, V., Bell, S., Alanis, N., Zhou, Y., d'Etienne, J. P., Kline, J. A., & Wang, H. (2021). Synergistic effects of emergency physician empathy and burnout on patient satisfaction: a prospective observational study. *Emergency Medicine Journal: EMJ, 38*(4), 290–296. https://doi.org/10.1136/emermed-2019-209393.

This study aimed to examine correlations among empathy, burnout, and patient satisfaction, and further analyze interactions among these factors. A single-center prospective observational study was conducted. Emergency physician (EP) empathy and burnout were measured by the JSE and the Copenhagen Burnout Inventory (CBI). We assessed patient perception of physician empathy and patient satisfaction with their treating physician by the Jefferson Scale of Patient Perceptions of Physician Empathy (JSPPPE) and a patient-assessed satisfaction survey. A total of 28 EPs and 423 patients were enrolled. Patient satisfaction had a weak correlation with JSE ($r = 0.11$) but showed a strong correlation with patient-assessed physician empathy ($r = 0.60$). Patient-assessed physician empathy had a strong positive correlation with patient satisfaction. Moreover, higher patient satisfaction was achieved from EPs of high patient-assessed physician empathy, low CBI, and high JSE, indicating a positive synergistic effect.

*Calabrese, L. H., Bianco, J. A., Mann, D., Massello, D., & Hojat, M. (2013). Correlates and changes in empathy and attitudes toward interprofessional collaboration in osteopathic medical students. *The Journal of the American Osteopathic Association, 113*, 898–907. doi: https://doi.org/10.7556/jaoa.2013.068.

Participants included 373 first- to fourth-year osteopathic medical students (53 %, $n = 197$ women) who completed the JSE and Jefferson Scale of Attitudes Toward Physician-Nurse Collaboration (JSAPNC). A statistically significant correlation of 0.42 was found between scores on the two instruments. Women scored significantly higher than did men on both the JSE ($M = 117.1$ and $M = 111.9$ for women and men, respectively) and the JSAPNC ($M = 50.1$ and $M = 48.7$, respectively). In contrast to most findings in allopathic medical schools, no statistically significant decline in students' mean scores on the JSE (and JSAPNC) was observed in different medical school years in this cross-sectional study. Inconsistent with the findings in allopathic medical students, no statistically significant difference was found on JSE scores among students who planned to pursue "people-oriented" compared with those interested in "technology/procedure-oriented" specialties. Comparisons of the JSE scores from this study with those of allopathic medical students (reported in other studies) showed no significant difference in the first and second years, but osteopathic medical students had a higher JSE mean score than their allopathic counterparts in the third year and their scores remained relatively high in the fourth year of osteopathic medical school.

Carrard, V., Bourquin, C., Berney, S., Schlegel, K., Gaume, J., Bart, P. A., Preisig, M., Schmid Mast, M., & Berney, A. (2022). The relationship between medical students' empathy, mental health, and burnout: A cross-sectional study. *Medical Teacher*, *44*(12), 1392–1399. https://doi.org/10.1080/0142159X.2022.2098708.

The purpose of this study was to investigate how medical students' empathy is related to their mental health and burnout. Research participants included 886 medical students from curriculum years 1–6. Cognitive and behavioral empathy were significantly correlated with fewer mental health issues and less burnout. Conversely, affective empathy was correlated with more mental health issues and burnout.

Chaitoff, A., Sun, B., Windover, A., Bokar, D., Featherall, J., Rothberg, M. B., & Misra-Hebert, A. D. (2017). Associations between physician empathy, physician characteristics, and standardized measures of patient experience. *Academic Medicine: Journal of the Association of American Medical Colleges, 92(10)*, 1464–1471. https://doi.org/10.1097/ACM.0000000000001671.

The purpose of this study was to examine correlates of physician empathy and determine whether physician empathy is related to standardized measures of patient experience. Empathy was assessed using the JSE. Results showed that in bivariable analysis ($n = 847$ physicians), female sex ($p < .001$), specialty ($p < .01$), outpatient practice setting ($p < .05$), and DO degree ($p < .05$) were associated with higher empathy scores. In multivariable analysis, female sex ($p < .001$) and four specialties (obstetrics–gynecology, pediatrics, psychiatry, and thoracic surgery; all $p < .05$) were significantly associated with higher empathy scores. Of the seven CG-CAHPS (*Consumer Assessment of Healthcare Providers and Systems- Clinician and Group*) measures, scores on five for the 583 physicians with visit-specific data and on three for the 277 physicians with 12-month data were positively correlated with empathy. This study concluded that specialty and sex were independently associated with physician empathy. Empathy was correlated with higher scores on multiple CG-CAHPS items, suggesting improving physician empathy might play a role in improving patient experience.

Costa, P., Alves, R., Neto, I., Marvão, P., Portela, M., & Costa, M. J. (2014). Associations between medical student empathy and personality: A multi-institutional study. *PLoS One*, *9*(3), e89254. doi: https://doi.org/10.1371/journal.pone.0089254.

Participants included 472 students (312 women) from three medical schools in Portugal (University of Beira Interior, University of Algarve, and University of Minho), who completed a Portuguese translation of the JSE (S-version) and the NEO-FFI (a personality inventory for measuring the big five personality factors). A subsample of 334 students was selected with the highest and the lowest JSE mean scores ($M = 121.9$ and $M = 97.8$, respectively) for statistical analyses. Correlations between the JSE scores and personality factors of Agreeableness ($r = 0.31$), Openness to Experience ($r = 0.22$), Conscientiousness ($r = 0.19$), and Extraversion ($r = 0.18$) were all statistically significant but moderate in magnitude.

Crump W. J., Ziegler C. H., & Fricker R. (2022). Do medical residents with rural upbringing show less decline in empathy during training? A report from a rural family medicine residency. *Marshall Journal of Medicine, 8*(1) DOI: https://doi.org/10.33470/2379-9536.1350.

The purpose of this study was to examine if demographic variables, specifically interest and rural upbringing, showed any association with the JSE scores among family medicine residents at a rural site. Participants included 40 residents annually using the JSE from 2016 to 2020 and compared scores between residents with rural vs. urban home towns. There was no significant difference in JSE scores of rural vs. urban residents at baseline, and both groups showed a decline after the PG-1 year. However, the rural-raised residents showed a significantly different rebound after the PG-2 and PG-3 year, with the urban-raised residents actually showing a slightly continuing decline. These preliminary findings among family medicine residents at a rural site suggest that rural background residents might regain empathy better than urban background residents during the course of their training.

Cyrus, A., Salehi, B., Naziri, M., Sedeh, B.S., & Vosoulie, R. (2017). Empathic communication and essential instruction for medical students. *Journal of Biology and Today's World, 6(6),* 97–101. DOI: https://doi.org/10.15412/J.JBTW.01060601.

This study aimed to evaluate and investigate if gender, age, grade, marriage, and specialized field affected empathy scores among trainees, interns, and resident physicians. Research participants included 215 medical students in practical stage and resident physicians in the Iran/Arak University of Medical Sciences, who completed the JSE. Results confirmed that females and married participants had higher empathy scores.

Diaz-Perez, A., Aragón, S. P. F., Narváez, V. P. D., Beleño, A. F., Navarro-Quiroz, E., & Cataño, C. L. M. (2018). Empathy in the curriculum for patient care. *Global Journal of Health Science; 10*(4), 93–99. doi: https://doi.org/10.5539/gjhs.v10n4p93.

The aim of this study was to evaluate the levels of empathy among nursing students at a higher education institution located in Cartagena de Indias/Colombia. A sample of nursing students ($n = 320$) from first to fourth year of training completed the Spanish version of the JSE. Results showed that women scored significantly higher than men on the JSE.

Eom, S., Kim, & S. S. (2018). Factors associated with nurses' moral sensitivity. *Journal of Korean Academy of Psychiatric Mental Health Nursing, 27*(3), 199–207. https://doi.org/10.12934/jkpmhn.2018.27.3.199.

The purposes of this study were to examine the associations among moral reasoning, empathy, communication self-efficacy, and moral sensitivity; and to determine predictors of nurses' moral sensitivity. Data were collected from nurses (n = 194) in the Republic of Korea. Structured questionnaires consisted of the JSE, the Moral Sensitivity Questionnaire, Defining Issues Test, and Counseling Self-Estimate Inventory. Results showed nurses' moral sensitivities were significantly associated with empathy, frequency of ethical education, and communication self-efficacy. In hierarchical multiple regression models, the significant predictors of nurses' moral sensitivity were empathy, age, the frequency of experience in ethics education, and communication self-efficacy.

Fuertes, J. N., Boylan, L. S., & Fontanella, J. A. (2008). Behavioral indices in medical care outcomes: The working alliance, adherence, and related factors. *Journal of General Internal Medicine, 24*, 80–85. doi: https://doi.org/10.1007/s11606-008-0841-4.

Participants included 152 adult outpatients (71 women) from a neurology clinic at Bellevue Hospital in New York, who completed a modified version of the JSE, the Physician-Patient Working Alliance Scale, Treatment Adherence Scale, and selected items from the Perceived Utility Scale and the Medical Outcome Study. Results showed significant bivariate correlations between scores on the modified JSE and working alliance (r=0.73), perceived utility treatment (r=0.46), treatment adherence (r=0.40), patient adherence (r=0.28), and patient satisfaction scores (r=0.67). However, in a multivariate statistical model, only working alliance, physician multicultural competence, and treatment adherence could predict patient satisfaction; and physician multicultural competence and treatment adherence could predict patient adherence with treatment.

*Glaser, K. M., Markham, F. W., Adler, H. M., McManus R. P., & Hojat, M. (2007). Relationships between scores on the Jefferson scale of physician empathy, patient perceptions of physician empathy, and humanistic approaches to patient care: A validity study. *Medical Science Monitor, 13*, 291–294.

Participants included 36 family medicine residents (23 women) at Thomas Jefferson University Hospital, who completed the JSE, and their 90 patients who assessed the residents by completing the Jefferson Scale of Patient Perceptions of Physician Empathy (JSPPPE) and a survey about the physicians' humanistic approach to patient care. The mean and standard deviation of the JSE for participating physicians were 118.0 and 9.2, respectively. The mean and standard deviation for the JSPPPE for participating patients were 30.0 and 2.8, respectively. Correlational analyses showed a statistically significant correlation between physician's self-reported JSE scores and patients' assessments of physician empathy (r=0.48). Also, scores on the JSE were significantly and positively correlated with patient assessments of their physician's concern about their feelings (r=0.55) and taking their wishes into account in making treatment decisions (r=0.48); and negatively correlated with patient's perception that their doctor was in hurry (r=–0.50).

Gradiski, I. P., Borovecki, A., Ćurković, M., San-Martín, M., Delgado Bolton, R. C., & Vivanco, L. (2022). Burnout in International Medical Students: Characterization of Professionalism and Loneliness as Predictive Factors of Burnout. *International Journal of Environmental Research and Public Health, 19*(3), 1385. https://doi.org/10.3390/ijerph19031385.

This study was designed to test the following hypothesis that in medical students enrolled in medical programs abroad, abilities associated with professionalism and family support play a protective role in the prevention of burnout. The Maslach Burnout Inventory was used as a dependent variable, while JSE, Jefferson measures of teamwork and physician lifelong learning, and the measure of Social and Emotional Loneliness Scale for Adults were used as independent variables. Research participants included 188 medical students at the University of Zagreb (38 Croatians and 144 foreigners from 28 countries). Empathy and lifelong learning, two specific elements of medical professionalism, appear as protective factors in the prevention of burnout in international students.

*Grosseman, S., Novack, D. H., Duke, P. Mennin, S., Rosenzweig, S., Davis, T. J., & Hojat, M. (2014). Residents' and standardized patients' perspectives on empathy: Issues of agreement. *Patient Education and Counseling, 96*, 22–28. Accessible from: https://doi.org/10.1016/j.pec.2014.04.007.

Participants included 214 first-year residents in 13 internal medicine or family medicine residency programs, who completed the JSE. Each resident was also assessed by five standardized patients who completed the Jefferson Scale of Patient Perceptions of Physician Empathy (JSPPPE). Participating residents also completed the JSPPPE from their own point of view. The JSE mean score was 111.8 (SD = 11.14) for the sample. Although women obtained a higher JSE mean score than did men, the difference was not statistically significant. Cronbach's alpha coefficients were 0.80 (for the JSE), 0.91 (for the JSPPPE completed by the standardized patients), and 0.94 (for the JSPPPE completed by residents). A significant correlation was found between scores on the JSE and residents' own view of their empathic engagement with standardized patients ($r=0.43$). However, the obtained correlation between residents' self-reported scores on the JSE and standardized patients' perceptions of residents' empathy was negligible ($r=0.11$). The authors raised a question about the use of standardized patients in the assessment of residents' empathy and also about residents' ability to gauge the effectiveness of their empathic communications with patients.

Guilera, T., Batalla, I., Forné, C., & Soler-González, J. (2019). Empathy and big five personality model in medical students and its relationship to gender and specialty preference: A cross-sectional study. *BMC Medical Education, 19*(1), 57. https://doi.org/10.1186/s12909-019-1485-2.

This study explores the relationship between empathy and personality, using three different measures of empathy, and taking into account gender and specialty preference. Medical students (n = 110) completed the JSE, the Interpersonal Reactivity Index, the Empathy Quotient, and the NEO-FFI Big Five personality model. Empathy scales showed weak and moderate correlation with personality. The strongest correlations were observed between IRI-Fantasy and Openness, and between IRI-Personal Distress and Neuroticism. Gender and specialty preference can modify this relationship. The extreme groups of Empathy Quotient had significant differences in most personality traits. This study confirmed that empathy is related to personality. Using three empathy scales allows personalizing the evaluation of different empathy models and their relationship with personality.

Hajibabaee, F., A Farahani, M., Ameri, Z., Salehi, T., & Hosseini, F. (2018). The relationship between empathy and emotional intelligence among Iranian nursing students. *International Journal of Medical Education, 9*, 239–243. https://doi.org/10.5116/ijme.5b83.e2a5.

The purpose of this study was to examine the relationship between empathy and emotional intelligence among Iranian nursing students. Research participants included 328 nursing students at the Tehran University of Medical Sciences, who completed the JSE and the Schutte Self-Report Emotional Intelligence Test. Results showed a strong positive correlation between empathy and emotional intelligence ($r = 0.499$). Students in their fourth year had the highest score on empathy. Female students got higher empathy scores than male students. Nurses with higher emotional intelligence tend to be better in establishing productive relationships with patients and their families, and high empathy scorers could manage their emotions more effectively.

Hasan, S., Al-Sharqawi, N., Dashti, F., AbdulAziz, M., Abdullah, A., Shukkur, M., Bouhaimed, M., & Thalib, L. (2013). Level of empathy among medical students in Kuwait University, Kuwait. *Medical Principles and Practice.* Open Access. doi: https://doi.org/10.1159/000348300.

Participants were 264 medical students in the Faculty of Medicine at Kuwait University, who completed the JSE. Results showed that the JSE mean score was 104.6 (SD = 16.3) for this sample. Women obtained a higher JSE mean score than men. Scores on the JSE were positively correlated with students' mother's level of education, higher household income, higher level of satisfaction with early relationship with the mother, and higher levels of perceived stress. Factors such as academic GPAs, specialty interest, marital status of parents, father's education level, and perceived relationships with their father did not significantly correlate with JSE scores. In this cross-sectional study, fourth-year medical students obtained the highest and second-year students the lowest JSE mean scores. However, the difference was not statistically significant. No significant association was found between JSE scores and the five personality factors measured by the ZKPQ; however, a trend toward a significant but negative association was noticed between scores of JSE and those of the Aggression-Hostility factor of the ZKPQ.

Hegazi, I., Hennessy, A., & Wilson, I. (2017). Empathy levels in medical students: do they really change over time? In M. Kondo (Eds.), *Empathy-An Evidence-based Interdisciplinary Perspective.* InTechOpen. DOI: https://doi.org/10.5772/intechopen.69625.

This work reports on a cross-sectional study of all medical students enrolled at an Australian medical school. The JSE-S version was administered to 404 medical students. Empathy levels were compared while controlling for effects of age, gender, marital status, religious belief, ethnicity/cultural background, year of medical training, previous education, and level of completion of programs promoting altruism, in an attempt to identify their effect on the levels of empathy. Findings suggest that levels of empathy differ by gender, favoring female medical students, and that empathy levels may be preserved in medical school despite prior evidence that a decline is pervasive.

*Hojat, M., Bianco, J. A., Mann, D., Massello, D., & Calabrese, L. H. (2015). Overlap between empathy, teamwork and integrative approach to patient care. *Medical Teacher, 37*, 755–785. doi: https://doi.org/10.3109/0142159x.2014.971722.

Participants included 373 students (197 women) at the Ohio University Heritage College of Osteopathic Medicine, who completed the JSE-S, the Jefferson Scale of Attitudes Toward Physician-Nurse Collaboration (JSAPNC), and an 11-item survey on orientation toward integrative patient care (IPC) to test the hypothesis that empathy, teamwork, and interprofessional collaboration, and an integrative approach to patient care share common denominators. Significant correlations were found among the three measures regardless of participants' gender. Also, a significant multivariate R of 0.60 was obtained in a multivariate regression model in which scores on the JSAPNC, IPC, and gender were predictors of the JSE scores. Although both JSAPNC and IPC contributed significantly to predicting JSE scores, the unique contribution of IPC scores (after partialing out the effect of gender) was substantially higher than that for the JSAPNC. Research hypothesis was confirmed, and it was suggested that the implementation of an integrative patient care approach in medical education curriculum may enhance empathy and teamwork among physicians-in-training.

*Hojat, M., DeSantis, J., Cain, R. Speicher, M., Bragan, L., Shannon, S., & Calabrese, L. (2021). Attitudes toward osteopathic medicine scale: Development, psychometrics. *International Journal of Medical Education, 12,* 222–232. https://doi.org/10.5116/ijme.615c.2cfa.

The purpose of this study was to develop a valid and reliable instrument for measuring attitudes toward osteopathic medicine and examine its associations with a number of personality attributes including clinical empathy. Research participants included 5669 first-year students from 33 US colleges of osteopathic medicine in the USA, who completed the JSE S-Version online at the beginning of academic year. A 13-item instrument: Attitudes Toward Osteopathic Medicine Scale (ATOMS) was developed and supported by psychometric evidence. The social desirability response bias was controlled in statistical analyses. Cronbach's coefficient alpha reliability was 0.83. Construct validity, corroborating face and content validity of the ATOMS, was supported by three components, emerged from factor analysis: "Perspectives on Osteopathic Medicine," "Osteopathic Diagnosis and Treatment," and "Holistic-Integrative Care." Correlations between ATOMS scores and scores of cognitive empathy JSE-S version, $r = 0.58$), emotional empathy (scores on the IRI, $r = 0.17$), measures on orientation toward interprofessional collaboration ($r = 0.60$); lifelong learning ($r = 0.36$); and burnout ($r = -0.29$) were statistically significant in the expected direction, providing validity evidence for the ATOMS (see Chapter 14 of the book for more detailed analysis).

*Hojat, M., Gonnella, J. S., Mangione, S., Nasca, T. J., Veloski, J. J., Erdmann, J. B., Callahan, C. A., & Magee, M. (2002). Empathy in medical students as related to academic performance, clinical competence and gender. *Medical Education, 36,* 522–527. doi: https://doi.org/10.1046/j.1365-2923.2002.01234.x.

Participants included 371 third-year medical students (173 women) at Jefferson (now Sidney Kimmel) Medical College, who completed the JSE. Women obtained a significantly higher JSE mean score (M=122, SD=10) than did men (M=119, SD=11). Statistically significant associations were observed between scores on the JSE and medical school faculty's global ratings of students' clinical competence in six third-year core clerkships (family medicine, internal medicine, obstetrics and gynecology, pediatrics, psychiatry, and surgery). No significant association was found between JSE scores and performance measures on objective examinations of acquisition of factual knowledge.

*Hojat, M., Louis, D. Z., Maxwell, K., Markham, F., Wender, R., & Gonnella, J. S. (2010). Patient perceptions of physician empathy, satisfaction with physician, interpersonal trust, and compliance. *International Journal of Medical Education, 1,* 83–87. doi: https://doi.org/10.5116/ijme.4d00.b701.

Participants included 535 outpatients (355 women) treated by family physicians in the Department of Family and Community Medicine, Jefferson (now Sidney Kimmel) Medical College, who completed the Jefferson Scale of Patient Perceptions of Physician Empathy (JSPPPE) and a 10-item scale of Patient Overall Satisfaction with Primary Care Physician. These patients were selected based on the following three criteria: (1) age between 18 and

75 years; (2) had at least two office visits with their primary care physicians during the past 36 months; and (3) spent at least two-thirds of the total office visits with the identified primary care physicians. Exploratory factor analysis of the JSPPPE resulted in one prominent component. Corrected item-total score correlations of the JSPPPE ranged from 0.88 to 0.94. Correlation between scores on the JSPPPE and scores on the patient satisfaction scale was 0.93. Scores on the JSPPPE were highly correlated with measures of physician–patient trust ($r=0.73$). Higher scores on the JSPPPE were significantly associated with patients' compliance with physician's recommendations for preventive tests (colonoscopy, mammogram for female patients, and PSA [prostate specific antigen] for male patients) (compliance rates > 80%). Cronbach's alpha coefficients for the JSPPPE ranged from 0.97 to 0.99 for the total sample, and for patients in different gender and age groups. Findings provide strong evidence in support of the psychometrics of the JSPPPE, and confirmed the link between patient perceptions of physician empathy, satisfaction with care, interpersonal trust, and compliance with physician's recommendations.

*Hojat, M., Mangione, S., Kane, G. C., & Gonnella, J. S. (2005). Relationships between scores of the Jefferson Scale of Physician Empathy (JSPE) and the Interpersonal Reactivity Index (IRI). *Medical Teacher, 27*, 625–628. doi: https://doi.org/10.1080/01421590500069744.

Participants included 93 first-year internal medicine residents at Thomas Jefferson University Hospital in Philadelphia, who completed the JSE and the Interpersonal Reactivity Index (IRI, a measure of cognitive and affective empathy developed for administration to the general population). Results showed a statistically significant correlation between JSE scores and total score on the IRI ($r=0.45$). Higher statistically significant correlations were observed between JSE scores and scores on those scales of the IRI that were relevant to patient care, such as Empathic Concern ($r=0.48$) and Perspective Taking ($r=0.40$). However, correlation between JSE scores and those on the IRI's Personal Distress scale (which is a measure of affective or emotional empathy, or sympathy) was negligible ($r=0.02$). Similarly, no significant correlation was observed between scores on the Personal Distress scale of the IRI and the JSE factor scores of Perspective Taking ($r=0.01$), Compassionate Care ($r=0.02$), and Standing in Patient's Shoes ($r=0.13$). Findings provided support for the validity of the JSE as a measure of cognitive empathy as opposed to sympathy or the so-called affective/emotional empathy.

*Hojat, M., Michalec, B., Veloski, J., & Tykocinski, M. L. (2015). Can empathy, other personality attributes, and level of positive social influence in medical school identify potential leaders in medicine? *Academic Medicine, 90*, 505–510.

Participants included 666 fourth-year students (338 women) at Sidney Kimmel (formerly Jefferson) Medical College, who completed the JSE, the Zuckerman–Kuhlman Personality Questionnaire (ZKPQ), Rosenberg Self-Esteem Scale, and the UCLA Loneliness Scale. They were also asked to identify their classmates (from a class list) who had a positive influence on their professional and personal development by using a peer nomination method. Students with the most nominations (top 25%) were compared to their classmates with the least number of nominations (bottom 25%) on personality measures. Results showed that top positive influencers obtained statistically significant higher mean scores on engaging personal qualities that were conducive to relationship building (such as JSE scores, Sociability, and Activity scales of the ZKPQ, and Self-Esteem scale). On the contrary, top positive influencers scored significantly lower on disengaging personal qualities that were detrimental to interpersonal relationships such as Neuroticism-Anxiety, Aggression-Hostility, Impulsive Sensation Seeking scales of the ZKPQ, and the UCLA Loneliness Scale.

*Hojat, M., Spandorfer, J., Louis, D. Z., & Gonnella, J. S. (2011). Empathic and sympathetic orientations toward patient care: Conceptualization, measurement, and psychometrics. *Academic Medicine, 86*, 989–995. doi: https://doi.org/10.1097/ACM.0b013e31822203d8.

Participants included 201 third-year medical students at Jefferson (now Sidney Kimmel) Medical College, who completed the JSE and the IRI; and responded to four vignettes developed for this study involving a diabetic patient with complications, a rape victim, a patient who had undergone radical prostatectomy and developed complications, and a 16-year-old girl who was pregnant. Students reviewed the vignettes and logged their responses to each scenario on two given Likert scales. One scale pertained to empathic orientation quantifying the student's inclination toward "understanding" the patient's pain or suffering. The other scale pertained to sympathetic orientation quantifying the student's tendency to "feel" the patient's pain or suffering. A factor analytic study confirmed the construct validity of the empathic and sympathetic orientations. Cronbach's alpha coefficients were 0.79 and 0.84 for measures of empathic and sympathetic orientations, respectively. Scores on empathic orientation were significantly associated with scores on the JSE (a measure of cognitive empathy to understand patient's suffering), but not with scores on the IRI (presumably a measure of sympathy or affective empathy to feel patient's pain and suffering). In contrast, scores on sympathetic orientation were significantly associated with scores on the IRI (feeling a patient's pain and suffering), but not with scores on the JSE. Quantifying empathic and sympathetic orientations in patient care is important for understanding their different consequences in patient care.

*Hojat, M., Vergare, M., Isenberg, G., Cohen, M., & Spandorfer, J. (2015). Underlying construct of empathy, optimism, and burnout in medical students. *International Journal of Medical Education, 6,*12–16. doi: https://doi.org/10.5116/ijme.54c3.60cd.

Participants included 265 third-year medical students (130 women) at Sidney Kimmel (formerly Jefferson) Medical College, who completed the JSE, the Life Orientation Test-Revised (LOT-R), and the Maslach Burnout Inventory (MBI, which includes three scales of Emotional Exhaustion, Depersonalization, and Personal Accomplishment). Mean and standard deviation of the JSE for this sample were 119.9 and 11.2, respectively. The JSE scores were significantly and positively correlated with scores on the Personal Accomplishment scale of the MBI ($r=0.36$), but inversely correlated with scores on the Depersonalization scale of the MBI ($r=-0.25$). Factor analysis resulted in two factors: "positive personality attributes" that are conducive to relationship building (involving empathy, optimism, and personal accomplishment) and "negative personality attributes" that are detrimental to interpersonal relationships (involving emotional exhaustion and depersonalization).

*Hojat, M., Zuckerman, M., Gonnella, J. S., Mangione, S., Nasca, T., Vergare, M., & Magee, M. (2005). Empathy in medical students as related to specialty interest, personality, and perception of mother and father. *Personality and Individual Differences, 39*, 1205–1215. doi: https://doi.org/10.1016/j.paid.2005.04.007.

Participants included 422 first-year medical students (207 women) enrolled at Jefferson (now Sidney Kimmel) Medical College in 2003 and 2004, who completed the JSE and the Zuckerman–Kuhlman Personality Questionnaire (ZKPQ); reported their satisfaction with early relationships with parents; and expressed their interest in a specialty they planned to pursue. Results showed that women obtained a statistically significantly higher JSE mean score than men ($M=115.9$, $SD=8.9$ for women; $M=111.6$, $SD=10.4$ for men, effect size$=0.43$). Those who were highly satisfied with their childhood relationships with their mother obtained a significantly higher JSE mean scorer than others. No significant association was observed between reported satisfaction with childhood relationships with the father and JSE scores. The JSE mean score was significantly higher for students interested in pursuing primary care specialties such as general internal medicine, family medicine, and general pediatrics ($M=116.6$, SD=8.6) than for those interested in pursuing technology-oriented specialties, such as orthopedic surgery, neurosurgery, or ophthalmology ($M=112.0$, SD=10.3), and hospital-based procedure-oriented specialties, such as radiology, pathology, or anesthesiology ($M=108.4$, SD=10.1). Scores on the JSE were significantly but moderately and positively correlated with measures of sociability ($r=0.15$, $p<0.01$), and negatively correlated with aggression-hostility scores ($r=-0.13$, $p<0.01$). No significant correlation was found between JSE scores and personality measures such as neuroticism-anxiety, impulsive sensation seeking, and activity. The effects of gender were controlled in all statistical analyses, and data for 4.9% of the total study sample with invalid and careless responses to the personality questionnaire (indicated by a high score on a social desirability scale in the ZKPQ) were discarded from final statistical analyses.

Huang, L., Thai, J., Zhong, Y., Peng, H., Koran, J., & Zhao, X. D. (2019). The positive association between empathy and self-esteem in Chinese medical students: A multi-institutional study. *Frontiers in Psychology, 10*, 1921. https://doi.org/10.3389/fpsyg.2019.01921.

This study examined the relationship between empathy and self-esteem to explore other possible methods to improve medical students' empathy. Study participants included 1690 medical students (n = 1690) in Shanghai, China, who completed the JSE-S version and the Rosenberg Self-esteem Scale (RSES). Results showed the JSE mean score of 102.73 (SD = 12.64). Multiple regression analysis revealed that significant predictors of empathy were "age," "perception of the importance of empathy," "academic pressure," "desire to be a doctor after graduation," and "self-esteem." Self-esteem explained 15.5% of the variation of empathy in the final regression model.

Iqbal, M. Z., AlBuraikan, A. R., AlQarni, A. A., AlQahtani, H. A., AlOhail, A. M., & AlMusaileem, M. M. (2022). Measuring empathy in medical students: A cross-sectional study. *JPMA. The Journal of the Pakistan Medical Association, 72*(6), 1101–1105. https://doi.org/10.47391/JPMA.3226.

The purpose of this study was to measure the empathy levels of undergraduate medical students and explore whether the empathy level has any significant association with gender, academic year, and academic achievement. The cross-sectional study was conducted using 391 medical students, at the College of Medicine, Imam Abdulrahman Bin Faisal University, Saudi Arabia; 251 (64%) were women, and 140 (36%) were men. The overall mean empathy score was 105.18 ± 12.51. Second-year medical students showed the highest empathy score. Empathy scores were significantly higher among female students and students with higher grade point averages.

Jacoby, J. L., Smith, A. B., Barraco, R. D., Greenberg, M. R., Donoghue, E. A., Kane, B. G., Macfarlan, J. E., Crowley, L. M., Weaver, K. R., & Quinn, J. F. (2022). Do incoming residents vary in measures of emotional status even prior to residency training? *International Journal of Medical Education, 13*, 198–204. https://doi.org/10.5116/ijme.62cb.f308.

This study examined whether Empathy, Emotional Intelligence, and Burnout scores differ by specialty in incoming residents. Study participants included 229 residents, of which 121 (53%) women who completed the JSE, Maslach Burnout Inventory, and Emotional and

Social Competency Inventory. Family Medicine residents had a higher median score on the JSE compared to Emergency Medicine. Differences were found among specialties even prior to the start of residency training in the Maslach Burnout Inventory subtests of Depersonalization and Personal Accomplishment.

*Kane, G. C., Gotto, J. L., Mangione, S., West, S., & Hojat, M. (2007). Jefferson Scale of Patient Perceptions of Physician Empathy: Preliminary psychometric data. *Croatian Medicine Journal, 48*, 81–86.

Participants included 225 patients seen by 166 residents in the internal medicine residency program at Jefferson Hospital Ambulatory Clinic at Thomas Jefferson University Hospital. Patients completed the 5-item Jefferson Scale of Patient Perceptions of Physician Empathy (JSPPPE) to assess their physician's empathic engagement in patient care, and also a patient rating form developed by the American Board of Internal Medicine (ABIM) to measure aspects of physician communication skills, humanistic qualities, and professionalism. A subsample of participating residents ($n = 27$) also completed the JSE. Factor analysis of the JSPPPE resulted in only one reliable factor indicating that the JSPPPE is a unidimensional scale. The mean score of the JSPPPE was 23.8, SD = 2.54, possible range 5–25, and actual range in the study sample 10–25. Cronbach's alpha coefficient was 0.58, which was relatively low, probably due to a small number of items. Corrected item-total score correlations were all positive and statistically significant, ranging from 0.77 to 0.90, with a median of 0.85. Correlation between JSPPPE scores and assessment on the ABIM patient rating form was 0.75, which was statistically significant, supporting criterion-related validity of the JSPPPE. Correlations between JSPPPE and responses to the following questions were all statistically significant, providing evidence for construct validity of the JSPPPE: "Physician shows concerns for my feelings and needs" ($r = 0.86$), "Asks me how I feel about my problems" ($r = 0.79$), "Takes my wishes into account" ($r = 0.76$), "Arranges for adequate privacy" ($r = 0.61$), and "is always in a hurry" ($r = -0.50$).

Kerr, N., & Tegge, A. M. (2017). Levels of empathy in undergraduate health-care-professions students. *International Journal of Human Caring*, 21(1), 41–45. doi: https://doi.org/10.20467/1091-5710.21.1.41.

The aim of this study was to compare empathy scores between health professions students (pharmacy and nursing) and non-health professions (law) students and between first-and third-year students. The JSE-Student Version was completed by 282 nursing, pharmacy, and law students. The results indicated that pharmacy students obtained significantly higher empathy scores than did law students. Third-year pharmacy students scored higher on empathy than did first-year pharmacy students, whereas the converse was true for nurses. There was no significant difference in empathy between first- and third-year law students. Empathy increased among pharmacy students, decreased among nurses, and remained the same among law students. Women scored higher on empathy than did men. Empathy scores among university students were found to vary depending on discipline and year of study.

Kiersma, M. E., Chen, A. M. H., Yehle, K. S., & Plake, K. S. (2013). Validation of an Empathy Scale in Pharmacy and Nursing Students. *American Journal of Pharmaceutical Education*, *77*. Article 94. doi: https://doi.org/10.5688/ajpe77594.

Participants included pharmacy ($n = 158$) and nursing ($n = 58$) students (146 women) who participated in a simulation game (Geriatric Medication Game) in which the challenges of elderly patients were addressed. Participants completed the JSE and another empathy-measuring instrument developed by two of the study authors (the Kiersma–Chen Empathy Scale, KCES) before and after participation in the simulation game. Before participation in the simulation game, Cronbach's alpha coefficients for the JSE were 0.82, 0.79, and 0.82 in pharmacy, nursing, and total samples, respectively. After the simulation game, these reliability coefficients were 0.80, 0.90, and 0.89, respectively. Correlations between scores on the JSE and the KCES were 0.59 and 0.77 before and after participation in the simulation game.

King, S., & Holosko, M. J. (2012). The development and initial validation of the empathy scale for social workers. *Research on Social Work Practice*, *22*, 174–185. doi: https://doi.org/10.1177/1049731511417136.

Participants included 271 students (81% women) in the Master of Social Work program at the University of Georgia, who completed the JSE and a newly developed instrument "Empathy Scale for Social Workers." As part of the validity study, the correlation between scores on the JSE and the newly developed instrument for measuring empathy in social workers was examined, and a statistically significant correlation was obtained ($r=0.34$).

Krasner, M. S., Epstein, R. M., Beckman, H., Suchman, A. L., Chapman, B., Mooney, C. J., & Quill, T. E. (2009). Association of an educational program in mindful communication with burnout, empathy, and attitudes among primary care physicians. *Journal of the American Medical Association*, *302*, 1284–1293. doi: https://doi.org/10.1001/jama.2009.1384.

Participants included 70 primary care physicians in Rochester, New York, who participated in a continuing medical education course in mindfulness meditation, self-awareness, reflective writing about clinical experiences, and didactic teaching and discussion. Before and after participation in the program, participants completed a survey which included the JSE, Maslach Burnout Inventory (MBI), Mindfulness Scale, the Profile of Mood State (POMS), a measure of the big five personality factors, and other scales. Results showed a significant enhancement in the total scores on the JSE as a result of participation in the program (effect size=0.45) and in factor scores on the JSE such as Perspective Taking (effect size=0.38) and Standing in Patient's Shoes (effect size=0.36). Improvements in mindfulness were significantly correlated with improvements in the Perspective-Taking factor scores on the JSE. Also, participation in the program was associated with improvements in personality measures such as Conscientiousness and Emotional Stability.

Lal, A., Tharyan, A., & Tharyan, P. (2020). The prevalence, determinants, and the role of empathy and religious or spiritual beliefs on job stress, job satisfaction, coping, burnout, and mental health in medical and surgical faculty of a teaching hospital: A cross-sectional survey. *La Revue de Medecine Interne*, *41*(4), 232–240. https://doi.org/10.1016/j.revmed.2019.12.005.

This study examined relationships among job stress and burnout and their mediators in health professionals from low- and middle-income countries. Consenting medical and surgical faculty of a large, charitable, teaching hospital ($n = 345$) were surveyed to evaluate: (1) the prevalence and sources of job stress and job satisfaction, and the ways used to cope with stress; (2) the prevalence of burnout and mental distress; and (3) the influence of age, gender, empathy, and religious or spiritual beliefs on job stress, satisfaction, mental health, and burnout. High job stress on the Physician Stress and Satisfaction questionnaire was reported by 23%. However, 98% of faculty reported high levels of job satisfaction with important contributory sources identified as deriving intellectual stimulation from teaching and a high level of responsibility. Significantly more respondents aged <45 years compared to older faculty achieved moderate or high scores on Emotional Exhaustion and Depersonalization. General Health Questionnaire-12 scores suggested psychiatric morbidity in 21%, particularly in younger faculty. High job stress was associated with high scores for Emotional Exhaustion and Depersonalization. High scores on the JSE correlated with high scores of Emotional Exhaustion. Religious or spiritual beliefs strongly influencing attitudes to work were significantly associated with high levels of Personal Accomplishment.

Lamothe, M., Boujut, E., Zenasni, F., & Sultan, S. (2014). To be or not to be empathic: The combined role of empathic concern and perspective taking in understanding burnout in general practice. *BMC Family Practice, 15*, 15. doi: https://doi.org/10.1186/1471-2296-15-15.

Participants included 294 general practitioners in France, who completed the JSE to assess cognitive empathy; the Toronto Empathy Questionnaire (TEQ) to assess emotional empathy; and the Maslach Burnout Inventory (MBI). Results showed a JSE mean score of 111.81 (SD = 10.60) in this sample of French physicians. Scores on the Standing in Patient's Shoes factor of the JSE were negatively but significantly correlated with scores on the Emotional Exhaustion scale of the MBI ($r = -0.14$). Scores on the Depersonalization scale of the MBI were negatively and significantly correlated with cognitive and emotional empathy. In multiple regression analysis models, lower empathy scores predicted higher burnout scores. Although the correlations were statistically significant, all were low in magnitude. The authors suggested that professionals need to regulate emotional empathy in order to minimize personal distress, compassion fatigue, and burnout.

Lelorain, S., Brédart, A., Dolbeault, S., Cano, A., Bonnaud-Antignac, A., Cousson-Gélie, F., & Sultan, S. (2014). How can we explain physician accuracy in assessing patient distress? A multilevel analysis in patients with advanced cancer. *Patient Education and Counseling, 94*, 322–327. doi: https://doi.org/10.1016/j.pec.2013.10.029.

Participants included 28 physicians (64% women) mostly medical oncologists (75%), who completed the JSE, and responded to the following single item to measure their self-efficacy in empathic skills: "In general, I feel competent to detect my patients' emotional distress and needs." In addition, physicians assessed their perceived quality of rapport with their patients. Patients assessed their own emotional distress by using a visual analog scale. Physicians, independent from the patient, also subjectively assessed the degree of patient's distress. An index of empathic accuracy was generated by calculating the absolute value of the difference between patients' and physicians' assessments of patient distress. Results showed that neither physicians' self-reported empathy (JSE scores) nor self-reported efficacy in empathic skills could significantly predict an empathic accuracy index. However, physician's self-reported quality of rapport with their patients was associated with better empathic accuracy.

Lelorian, S., Brédart, A., Dolbeault, S., Cano, A., Bonnaud-Antignac, A., Cousson-Gélie, F., & Sultan, S. (2015). How does a physician's accurate understanding of a cancer patient's unmet needs contribute to patient perception of physician empathy? *Patient Education and Counseling, 98*, 734–741. Accessible from: https://doi.org/10.1016/j.pec.2015.03.002.

Participants included 28 physicians, who completed the JSE, and their 201 metastatic cancer patients, who completed a survey of physical, psychological, sexual, informational, and support needs. Physicians completed the same survey from the patient perspective. Results showed that physicians' self-reported perspective taking but not compassionate care factor of the JSE was positively related to their understanding of patient's unmet needs.

Lelorain, S., Sultan, S., Zenasni, F., Catu-Pinault, A., Juar, P., Boujut, E., & Rigal, L. (2013). Empathic concern and professional characteristics associated with clinical empathy in French general practitioners. *European Journal of General Practice, 19*, 23–28. doi: https://doi.org/10.3109/13814788.2012.709842.

Participants included 295 French general practitioners who completed a French translation of the JSE and the Toronto Empathy Questionnaire (TEQ). Results showed that empathic concern (measured by the TEQ) was an important component of clinical empathy (measured by the JSE). However, in multiple regression statistical analysis, it was found that physician practice characteristics such as consultation length, and attending Balint group could uniquely predict clinical empathy. Clinical experiences did not make a significant contribution to predicting clinical empathy beyond empathic concern.

Li, C. Q., Ma, Q., Liu, Y. Y., & Jing, K. J. (2018). Are parental rearing patterns and learning burnout correlated with empathy amongst undergraduate nursing students? *International Journal of Nursing Sciences, 5*(4), 409–413. https://doi.org/10.1016/j.ijnss.2018.07.005.

This study aimed to explore the relationship between learning burnout, parental rearing patterns, and empathy amongst nursing students. Research participants included 562 nursing students who completed JSE, the Learning Burnout Scale, and the Short-Form Egna Minnen av Barndoms Uppfostran (s-EMBU) to assess parental styles and behavior. Results showed that clinical empathy was negatively correlated with learning burnout, parental rejection, and overprotection. Positive parental rearing patterns also helped to cultivate empathy.

Liang, A., Gao, C., Xu, W., Shen, Y., Liu, C., Lu, Z., & Yang, Y. (2022). Individual factors in dignified care: A cross-sectional study of critical care nurses. *Journal of Nursing Management, 30*(7), 3286–3294. https://doi.org/10.1111/jonm.13765.

This study aimed to determine the level of dignified care provided by critical care nurses and to explore the associated individual factors. Research participants included 526 critical care nurses working at intensive care units for adults in Zhejiang Province, China, who completed the JSE-Health Professions, the Intensive Care Unit Dignified Care Questionnaire, and Wong and Law Emotional Intelligence Scale. Findings suggest that emotional intelligence, empathy, professional values, age, and training in dignified care were predictors of dignified care.

Libert, Y., Canivet, D., Ménard, C., Van Achte, L., Farvacques, C., Merckaert, I., Liénard, A., Klastersky, J., Reynaert, C., Slachmuylder, J. L., Durieux, J. F., Delvaux, N., & Razavi, D. (2017). Predictors of physicians' communication performance in a decision-making encounter with a simulated advanced-stage cancer patient: A longitudinal study. *Patient Education and Counseling, 100*(9), 1672–1679. https://doi.org/10.1016/j.pec.2017.02.025.

In this longitudinal study, predictors of physicians' communication performance (CP) were investigated with a simulated advanced-stage cancer patient. Physicians ($n = 85$) performed a decision-making encounter with a simulated patient (SP). Their CP was calculated by analyzing encounter transcripts with validated interaction analysis systems. Potential specific psychological predictors were physicians' empathy toward the SP (JSE) and their decisional conflict about the treatment (Decisional Conflict Scale, DCS). Potential general psychological predictors were physicians' empathy toward cancer patients, their decisional conflict about cancer patients' treatments (DCS), and their affective reactions to uncertainty

(Physicians' Reactions to Uncertainty, PRU). During encounters with advanced-stage cancer patients, physicians' awareness of uncertainty about which treatments to consider may facilitate their communication performance, whereas physicians' affective reactions to uncertainty may inhibit their performance.

Lin, C., Li, L., Wan, D., Wu, Z., & Yan, Z. (2012). Empathy and avoidance in treating patients living with HIV/AIDS (PLWHA) among service providers in China . *AIDS Care, 24*, 1341–1348. doi: https://doi.org/10.1080/09540121.2011.648602.

Participants included 1760 health service providers from 40 county hospitals in China, who completed a brief (11-item) version of a Chinese translation of the JSE. Results showed that nurses, younger providers, and providers with lower education were more likely to avoid contact with HIV/AIDS patients. Multiple regression analysis showed that higher scores on the JSE were associated significantly and inversely with avoidance attitudes toward HIV/AIDS patients. Findings confirmed that the health providers' empathy (reflected in the JSE scores) plays an important role in providing quality care to HIV-infected and AIDS patients.

Magalhäes, E., Costa P., & Costa, M. (2012). Empathy of medical students and personality: Evidence from the Five-Factor Model. *Medical Teacher, 34*, 807–812.

Participants included 350 medical students (244 women) from six classes at the School of Health Sciences of the University of Minho in Portugal, who completed a Portuguese translation of the JSE and the big five personality factor survey (NEO-FFI). Correlations between scores on the JSE and those of the big five personality factors were examined: $r=-0.01$ (with Neuroticism), $r=0.04$ (with Extraversion), $r=0.22$, $p<0.01$ (with Openness), $r=0.24$, $p<0.01$ (with Agreeableness), and $r=0.14$, $p<0.05$ (with Conscientiousness).

*Michalec, B., Veloski, J. J., Hojat, M., & Tykocinski, M. (2015). Identifying potential engaging leaders within medical education: The role of positive influence on peers. *Medical Teacher, 37,* 677–683. doi: https://doi.org/10.3109/0142159X.2014.947933.

Participants included 630 fourth-year medical students in three graduating classes at Sidney Kimmel (formerly Jefferson) Medical College at Thomas Jefferson University, who were asked to think back to their medical school experiences and respond to the question, "Which of your classmates had significant positive influence on your professional and personal development?" Students who were selected most (top 10 %) were compared to the rest of the class on scores on the JSE and on selected performance measures. High positive influencers obtained a significantly higher score on the JSE ($M=117.1$, SD=9.0) than did the other students ($M=113.5$, SD=11.0). Also, high influencers compared to the rest of their classmates obtained higher clinical competence ratings on six core clerkships in the third year of medical school, and on simulated patients' assessments of their communication and interpersonal skills. No significant difference was found between top influencers and the rest on scores on the MCAT and medical licensing examinations (Steps 1 and 2 of the USMLE).

Miniotti M. (2022). Empathy for patient care in medical students: new evidence on the importance of self-transcendence. *Psychology, Health & Medicine*, *27*(5), 1035–1041. https://doi.org/10.1080/13548506.2020.1842897.

This study aimed to explore the associations between clinical empathy, temperament and character in a sample of medical students. Participants included 299 second-year Italian medical students who completed the Italian versions of the JSE for medical students (JSE-S) and the Temperament and Character Inventory (TCI-140). Results showed significant positive low correlations between clinical empathy and Reward Dependence, Cooperativeness, and Self-transcendence. Female medical students scored higher than their male counterparts on clinical empathy.

Ogle, J., Bushnell, J., & Caputi, P. (2013). Empathy is related to clinical competence in medical care. *Medical Education, 47*, 824–831. doi: https://doi.org/10.1111/medu.12232.

Participants included 57 (20 women) third-year medical students in Australia, who completed the JSE. The clinical competence of these students was assessed by Objective Structured Clinical Examinations (OSCE) by medical professionals. Also, students' empathic engagement was rated by an independent observer of the clinical interaction in OSCE stations. Results showed that observers' assessments of clinical competence in OSCE stations were significantly correlated with observers' assessment of students' empathic engagement in OSCE stations. However, no significant association was found between students' self-reported empathy (JSE scores) and observers' assessments of students' empathy in OSCE stations. Significant associations were also observed between observers' assessments of students' empathy and ratings of students' clinical performance. The JSE mean score for this sample was 111.98 (SD = 11.22).

O'Sullivan, J., & Whelan, T. A. (2011). Adversarial growth in telephone counsellors: Psychological and environmental influences. *British Journal of Guidance & Counselling, 39*, 307–323. doi: https://doi.org/10.1080/03069885.2011.567326.

Participants included 64 telephone counselors who completed the JSE, Posttraumatic Growth Inventory, and other surveys to examine the level of adversarial growth among these counselors. Results showed that scores on the JSE were not significant predictors of growth. However, compassion fatigue was significantly associated with posttraumatic growth.

Ozturk, M., & Demirci, H. (2020). Turkish validation of the Jefferson Scale of Empathy for nurses seeking kidney donations in intensive care units. *The Aging Male: The Official Journal of the International Society for the Study of the Aging Male, 23*(5), 564–570. https://doi.org/10.1080/13685538.2018.1544238.

The aim of this study was to find if a high level of empathy of intensive care nurses is effective in increasing organ donation. Research participants included 355 intensive care nurses in Turkey, who completed the Turkish translation of the JSE. Results showed a positive but weak correlation between donor declaration and empathy score. An increase was observed in empathy score as donor declaration increased.

Piumatti, G., Abbiati, M., Baroffio, A., & Gerbase, M. W. (2020). Empathy trajectories throughout medical school: Relationships with personality and motives for studying medicine. *Advances in Health Sciences Education: Theory and Practice, 25*(5), 1227–1242. https://doi.org/10.1007/s10459-020-09965-y.

The purpose of this study was to examine associations of clinical empathy with personality and motives for studying medicine. Study participants included 201 medical students who completed the JSE at entry year (year 1) and during the first two clinical years (years 4 and 5). Two empathy trajectory groups were identified: lower and decreasing ($n = 59$; 29%) and higher and stable ($n = 142$; 71%). The NEO-Five Factor Inventory was used for the assessment of personality. Results suggested that empathy remains stable in most medical students and declines in fewer; openness facet of personality and patients-oriented motives for studying medicine was associated with higher and stable clinical empathy. Encouraging medical students' patients-oriented motives from preclinical throughout clinical years may prevent empathy decline.

Podhorecka, M., Pyszora, A., Woźniewicz, A., Husejko, J., & Kędziora-Kornatowska, K. (2022). Empathy as a Factor Conditioning Attitudes towards the Elderly among Physiotherapists-Results from Poland. *International Journal of Environmental Research and Public Health*, *19*(7), 3994. https://doi.org/10.3390/ijerph19073994.

The purpose of this study was to assess attitudes toward the elderly in Polish physiotherapists. Research participants included 252 physiotherapists (189 women and 63 men) who completed the Jefferson Empathy Scale (JSE)and the Kogan Attitudes toward the Elderly (KAOP). Results showed that scores on the JSE scale were positively, but weakly associated with the KOAP scores. Empathy and own experience of health care providers may protect against negative attitudes toward the elderly, meaning empathy in healthcare professionals is crucial.

*Pohl, C. A., Hojat. M., & Arnold, L. (2011). Peer nominations as related to academic attainment, empathy, personality, and specialty interest. *Academic Medicine, 86*, 747–751. doi: https://doi.org/10.1097/ACM.0b013e318217e464.

Participants included 255 third-year medical students (125 women) at Jefferson (now Sidney Kimmel) Medical College, who completed the JSE and the Zuckerman–Kuhlman Personality Questionnaire (ZKPQ). Students were asked to nominate classmates whom they considered to be the best in six given areas of clinical and humanistic excellence. Results of comparing those who received at least one peer nomination ($n=155$) with those who received none ($n=100$) showed no significant difference in objective examination grades; however, nominated students obtained a statistically significant higher JSE mean score ($M=115.5$, SD=9.0) than their classmates who were not nominated ($M=112.4$, SD=11.2, effect size=0.32). Also, nominated students received higher faculty ratings on clinical competence and expressed more interest in pursuing "people-oriented" (rather than "technology- or procedure-oriented") specialties. On personality factors, nominated students obtained higher mean score on the Activity factor of the ZKPQ. No statistically significant difference was found between the nominated and not nominated students on other personality factors such as Sociability, Aggression-Hostility, Neuroticism-Anxiety, or Impulsive Sensation Seeking.

Rafaqat, W., Sami, A., Ibrahim, M. T., Ibad, H., Awais, S., Memon, A., Shahbaz, F. F., Ahmed, D., Zindani, S., Leghari, A. L., & Saleem, S. (2022). Impact of Perfectionism and Resilience on Empathy in Medical Students: A Cross-Sectional Study. *Journal of Patient Experience*, *9*, 23743735221106603. https://doi.org/10.1177/23743735221106603.

The purpose of this study was to determine the correlations of perfectionism and resilience with clinical empathy in medical students. Research participants included 320 medical students who completed the JSE, a measure of resilience, and a measure of perfectionism. Results showed a positive correlation between resilience and academic year with empathy, and a negative correlation between empathy and maladaptive perfectionism. Mean empathy scores were lowest in fifth-year students (96.8 ± 12.5) and highest in third-year students (107.8 ± 13.2).

Reisetter, B. C., Bently, J. P., & Wilkin, N. E. (2005). Relationship between psychosocial physician characteristics and physician price awareness. *Journal of Pharmaceutical Marketing & Management, 17*, 51–76. doi: https://doi.org/10.1300/j058v17n01_05.

Participants included 200 primary care and internal medicine physicians (32 women) who completed the JSE and the Physician Belief Scale (PBS). Physicians were also asked to estimate the cash price for 20 commonly prescribed prescription drugs at the usual quantities dispensed. Results showed that on average, physicians were able to estimate cash price for eight out of 20 sample drugs within ±20%. Scores on the JSE and PBS did not significantly predict physician price awareness. In a multivariate hierarchical regression analysis, variables such as gender and time spent with patients could significantly explain the variance in accuracy of physicians' awareness of drug costs.

Richards, H. L., Fortune, D. G., Weildmann, A., Sweeney, S. K. T., & Griffiths, C. E. M. (2004). Detection of psychological distress in patients with psoriasis: Low consensus between dermatologist and patient. *British Journal of Dermatology, 151*, 1227–1233. doi: https://doi.org/10.1111/j.1365-2133.2004.06221.x.

Participants included five dermatologists (three women) who completed the JSE, and their 43 patients (22 women) with psoriasis who completed the Hospital Anxiety and Depression Scale following their consultations with the dermatologists at the Psoriasis Clinic, Hope Hospital, Salford, Manchester, England. Participating dermatologists also assessed their patient's psychological distress level following the visit by using a 10-point visual analog scale. Results showed that the JSE mean score for participating dermatologists was 114 (SD = 14.2). The concordance rates between patient's self-reported depression and anxiety and the dermatologists' assessment of the patients' psychological distress was at a lower end of a fair agreement. Dermatologists' JSE scores did not appear to influence their identification of patients' psychological distress.

Román-Sánchez, D., Paramio-Cuevas, J. C., Paloma-Castro, O., Palazón-Fernández, J. L., Lepiani-Díaz, I., de la Fuente Rodríguez, J. M., & López-Millán, M. R. (2022). Empathy, burnout, and attitudes towards mental illness among Spanish mental health nurses. *International Journal of Environmental Research and Public Health, 19*(2), 692. https://doi.org/10.3390/ijerph19020692.

The aim of this study was to examine the association between empathy, burnout, and attitudes toward patients with mental disorders among mental health nurses in Spain. Research participants included 750 specialist nurses working in mental health facilities in Spain, who completed the JSE, the Maslach Burnout Inventory, and the Community Attitudes toward Mental Illness Inventory. Results showed that higher empathy was associated with an increase in positive attitudes toward patients with mental disorders, but it did not act as a protective factor against burnout.

Ruiz-Hernández, J. A., López-García, C., Llor-Esteban, B., Galián-Muñoz, I., & Benavente-Reche, A. P. (2016). Evaluation of the users violence in primary health care: Adaptation of an instrument. *International Journal of Clinical and Health Psychology, 16*(3), 295–305. https://doi.org/10.1016/j.ijchp.2016.06.001.

The aims of the study are to study the prevalence of workplace violence in primary healthcare professionals by adapting, to establish the frequency of exposure to hostile indicators and to determine which professional group is most exposed. Study participants included 574 professionals from 39 primary healthcare centers in Spain, who completed the JSE and a measure of aggressive behavior. The results showed that the JSE has excellent psychometric properties and correlates significantly with job satisfaction and psychological well-being.

San-Martín, M., Delgado-Bolton, R., & Vivanco, L. (2017). Professionalism and occupational well-being: Similarities and differences among Latin American health professionals. *Frontiers in Psychology*, *8*, 63. https://doi.org/10.3389/fpsyg.2017.00063.

The purpose of this study was to examine the influence that empathy, teamwork, and lifelong learning play in the occupational well-being of physicians and nurses working in Latin American healthcare institutions. Study participants included 353 physicians and nurses working in healthcare institutions in Mexico, Colombia, Ecuador, and Argentina, who completed the JSE, the Jefferson Scale of Attitudes toward Physician-Nurse Collaboration, the Jefferson Scale of Physicians Lifelong Learning, and the Scale of Collateral Effects (somatization, exhaustion, and work alienation). Results confirmed adequate reliability in all instruments. Correlation analyses confirmed in physicians an inverse association between empathy and collateral effects ($r = -0.16$; $p < 0.05$), and between collateral effects and lifelong learning ($r = -0.18$; $p < 0.01$). In nurses, this association was confirmed only for empathy. An inverse correlation between age and collateral effects was confirmed in physicians. Comparison by gender confirmed higher somatization in women physicians and nurses than in men groups ($p < 0.001$). On the other hand, comparison by discipline confirmed higher exhaustion and alienation in physicians than in nurses ($p < 0.01$). The findings support the importance of empathy, teamwork, and lifelong learning in practitioners' health and welfare, and the role that cultural behaviors, associated to work professional models and social stereotypes, play in the interaction between professionalism and occupational well-being.

Seo, J. W., Kyung H. P., Ha Y. P., Kyung H. S., Song Y. P., Tae H. K., HyeRin R., & Junho C. "Empathy and quality of life in Korean emergency physicians." *Journal of The Korean Society of Emergency Medicine* 27, no. 2 (April 30, 2016): 150–56. http://www.jksem.org/journal/view.php?number=2020.

The relationships between empathy, quality of life, and other factors among Korean emergency physicians were explored. Research participants completed the JSE and the brief version of the World Health Organization Quality of Life assessment instrument. Participants included 180 emergency medicine physicians. Empathy was positively correlated with quality of life, age, and work experience in men. Only work experience showed correlation with empathy in females. The more experienced the emergency physicians were, and the better quality of life they had, the higher level of empathy scale they had. Therefore, good quality of life could lead to good empathy, and vice versa.

Sharma, R., Sapkota, A., Acharya, A., Luintel, P., Paudel, L., Sharma, S., & Pradhan, S. N. (2022). A cross-sectional study on empathy and its association with stress in medical students. *International Journal of Occupational Safety and Health*, *12*(3), 224–229. https://doi.org/10.3126/ijosh.v12i3.44432.

The purpose of this study was to assess the level of empathy and its association with the level of stress in 3rd and 4th year medical students. Research participants included 255 medical students in Nepal who completed the JSE-S version. Findings showed that the mean empathy score was 101.79 ($SD = 11.26$). There was a statistically significant negative correlation between empathy and stress ($p < 0.01$), and similar negative correlations were seen in sub-group analysis. Female students had higher empathy scores compared to their male counterparts ($p < 0.01$). Fourth-year students reported lower empathy scores than third-year students (p-value < 0.05). Stress was found to be a significant determinant of empathy among medical students. Medical educators must be aware of this and should try to incorporate means to alleviate stress in medical education. Furthermore, effective stress management techniques to preserve empathy in medical students need to be studied with a view to improve clinical competency and achieve optimum patient care.

Soler-Gonzalez, J., San-Martín, M., Delgado-Bolton, R., & Vivanco, L. (2017). Human connections and their roles in the occupational well-being of healthcare professionals: A study on loneliness and empathy. *Frontiers in Psychology, 8*, 1475. https://doi.org/10.3389/fpsyg.2017.01475.

The purpose of this study was to assess the relationship between absence (loneliness) and presence (empathy) of human connections with the occupational well-being of healthcare professionals. The JSE as well as other scales was administered to 433 healthcare professionals working in Spanish public healthcare institutions. The JSE and the Scale of Collateral Effects were included in the study survey. Findings showed an inverse correlation between empathy scores and collateral effects such as somatization, exhaustion, and work alienation. Also, loneliness was found to be positively associated with collateral effects. These findings support an important role for empathy in the prevention of work stress in healthcare professionals. They also confirm that loneliness, as a multidimensional and domain-specific experience, is detrimental to occupational well-being.

Wang, C., Wu, Q., Feng, M., Wan, Q., & Wu, X. (2017). International Nursing: Research on the correlation between empathy and China's Big Five Personality Theory: Implications for nursing leaders. *Nursing Administration Quarterly, 41*(2), E1–E10. https://doi.org/10.1097/NAQ.0000000000000219.

The study purpose was to investigate the characteristics of nurses' empathy and explore the correlation between nurses' empathy and personality. Research participants included 250 nurses from a general hospital in China, who completed the JSE-HP version and the Chinese Big Five Personality Inventory. Results showed that the total score of the JSE-HP was 110.60 (*SD* = 11.71). Multiple hierarchical regression analysis indicated that the JSE-HP score was positively correlated with conscientiousness and agreeableness of the Big Five Personality Inventory, and the Big Five Personality model is a significant predictor of nurses' empathy.

Weng, H. C., Steed, J. F., Yu, S. W., Liu, Y. T., Hsu, C. C., Yu, T. J., & Chen, W. (2011). The effect of surgeon empathy and emotional intelligence on patient satisfaction. *Advances in Health Sciences Education, 16*, 591–600. doi: https://doi.org/10.1007/s10459-011-9278-3.

Participants included 50 surgeons and their 896 outpatients who were scheduled to undergo surgery in Taiwan. A Chinese translation of the JSE and an emotional intelligence test was completed by the surgeons. Patients completed a survey about their satisfaction with their surgeons, and their perception of their relationship with the surgeon. In a follow-up telephone interview after surgery, patients were asked to rate their health status on a 7-point scale. Results showed that surgeons' scores on the JSE were significantly correlated with higher ratings on self-reported patient health status two weeks after surgery ($r=0.25$, $p<0.05$). Patients' satisfaction with their surgeons was also correlated significantly with their self-reported health status after surgery ($r=0.26$, $p<0.05$). No significant association was observed between JSE scores and dimensions of the Chinese test of emotional intelligence. The authors reported that a patient's long-term satisfaction with their physicians is influenced more by their physician's empathy than by physician's emotional intelligence.

Xia, L., Hongyu, S., & Xinwei, F. (2011). Study on correlation between empathy ability and personality characteristics of undergraduate nursing students. *Chinese Nursing Research, 32*.

Participants included 229 undergraduate nursing students from six nursing schools in China, who completed a Chinese translation of the JSE and the Eysenck Personality Questionnaire (EPQ). Correlational analyses showed statistically significant but negative correlations between scores on the Neuroticism scale of the EPQ with total scores on the JSE, as well as with factor scores on Perspective Taking, and Compassionate Care of the JSE.

Yu, H., Jiang, A., & Shen, J. (2016). Prevalence and predictors of compassion fatigue, burnout, and compassion satisfaction among oncology nurses: A cross-sectional survey, *International Journal of Nursing Studies, 57,* 28–38. doi:https://doi.org/10.1016/j.ijnurstu.2016.01.012.

The purpose of this study was to describe and explore the prevalence of predictors of professional quality of life (compassion, fatigue, burnout, and satisfaction) among Chinese oncology nurses under the guidance of two theoretical models. Participants included 669 oncology nurses who completed Chinese versions of the JSE, the Professional Quality of Life Scale for Nurses, the Simplified Coping Style Questionnaire, the Perceived Social Support Scale, and the Big Five Personality Inventory. Results showed that cognitive empathy, training, and support from organizations were identified as significant protectors, and "perspective taking" was the strongest predictor of compassion satisfaction. Personality traits of openness and conscientiousness were positively associated with compassion satisfaction, while neuroticism was a negative predictor of the variance in compassion fatigue and burnout, respectively.

Yuguero, O., Forné, C., Esquerda, M., Pifarré, J., Abadías, M. J., & Viñas, J. (2017). Empathy and burnout of emergency professionals of a health region: A cross-sectional study. *Medicine, 96*(37), e8030. https://doi.org/10.1097/MD.0000000000008030.

The objective of this study was to assess the association between levels of empathy and burnout of emergency room professionals. Study participants included 100 professionals from the emergency room in the health region of Lleida and the Pyrenees, who completed Spanish versions of the JSE and Maslach Burnout Inventory. Professionals with high burnout showed the lowest levels of empathy. The highest levels of empathy were associated with the lowest levels of burnout, especially in depersonalization factor of the burnout, and to a lesser extent in personal accomplishment.

Yuguero, O., Melnick, E. R., Marsal, J. R., Esquerda, M., & Soler-Gonzalez, J. (2018). Cross-sectional study of the association between healthcare professionals' empathy and burnout and the number of annual primary care visits per patient under their care in Spain. *BMJ open, 8*(7), e020949. https://doi.org/10.1136/bmjopen-2017-020949.

The purpose of this study was to evaluate the association between physician and nurse empathy and burnout and the number of annual primary care visits per patient under their care. In the Lleida Health Region in Spain, 22 primary care centers were surveyed. The number of visits and the number of diagnoses coded per visit were obtained through the Region's electronic health record. Healthcare professionals ($n = 267$) participated and completed the JSE and the Maslach Burnout Inventory. Results showed that healthcare professionals' scores on empathy and burnout were associated with the number of annual visits per patient under their care. Those with higher burnout scores received fewer visits. More empathic physicians received more visits per patient and documented more diagnoses per visit. Less burned out and less empathic nurses documented more diagnoses per visit. It was concluded that these results should serve to promote empathic skills and establish organizational changes that promote efficiency in the practice and, in turn, reduce the degree of burnout of healthcare professionals.

Zenasni, F., Boujut, E., de Vaure, C. B., Catu-Pinault, A., Tavani, J. L., Rigal, L., Juary, P., Magnier, A.M., Falcoff, H., & Sultan, S, (2012). Development of a French-language version of the Jefferson Scale of Physician Empathy and association with practice characteristics and burnout in a sample of general practitioners. *The International Journal of Person Centered Medicine, 2*, 759–766. Accessible from: http://www.ijpcm.org/index.php/IJPCM/article/view/295.

Participants included 308 general practitioners (150 women) attending a national congress of family medicine in France, who completed a French translation of the JSE and the Maslach Burnout Inventory (MBI). Confirmatory factor analysis of the JSE showed an acceptable fit for the three-factor model of the JSE (Perspective Taking, Compassionate Care, and Standing in the Patient's Shoes). Scores on the Perspective-Taking factor of the JSE were significantly associated with personal experience with psychotherapy and duration of consultation. Scores on the Compassionate Care factor of the JSE were significantly associated with being female and living in a coupled relationship. Scores on the Depersonalization scale of the MBI were inversely and significantly correlated with factor scores on the JSE: $r=-0.30$ with the Standing in Patient's Shoes factor scores; $r=-0.26$ with Compassionate Care factor scores; and $r=-0.18$ with Perspective-Taking factor scores. Conversely, scores on the Personal Accomplishment scale of the MBI were positively and significantly correlated with factor scores on the JSE: $r=0.36$ with Perspective Taking, $r=0.18$ with Compassionate Care, and $r=0.21$ with Standing in Patient's Shoes. Also, scores on the Exhaustion scale of the MBI were significantly and inversely correlated with Standing in the Patient's Shoes factor scores on the JSE ($r=-0.15$).

Studies on Group Comparisons on the JSE Scores

Aggarwal, R. (2007). Empathy: Do psychiatrists and patients agree? *The American Journal of Psychiatry Resident's Journal*, *2*, 2–3.

Participants included ten psychiatrists who completed the JSE and 50 of their patients who completed a modified version of the JSE to reflect their views of their psychiatrist's empathic engagement. Psychiatrists' self-reported JSE mean score was 119.7 (SD=8.65), which was significantly higher than that reported by their patients ($M=104.4$, SD=11.3). The self-reported JSE mean score was higher for female psychiatrists compared to their male counterparts. Also, patients' assessments of the empathy of the female psychiatrists were higher than for male psychiatrists, regardless of the patient's gender.

Boyle, M. J., Williams, B., Brown, T., Molloy, A., McKenna, L., Molloy, L., & Lewis, B. (2009). Levels of empathy in undergraduate health science students. *The Internet Journal of Medical Education, 1*. doi: https://doi.org/10.5580/1b15.

Participants included 459 students (81% women) from six health-related disciplines: paramedics, nursing, midwifery, occupational therapy, physiotherapy, and health sciences, who completed the JSE. Results showed that women obtained a significantly higher JSE mean score ($M=109.78$, SD=14.73) than men ($M=104.76$, SD=12.21). No statistically significant difference on JSE scores was found among students in different disciplines. Cronbach's alpha coefficient for the entire sample was 0.85.

*Bucher, J. T., Vu, D. M., & Hojat, M. (2013). Psychostimulant drug abuse and personality factors in medical students. *Medical Teacher, 35*, 53–57.

Participants included 321 first- to fourth-year students (148 women) at Jefferson (now Sidney Kimmel) Medical College, who anonymously completed the JSE, the Zuckerman–Kuhlman Personality Questionnaire (ZKPQ) and responded to a question about whether they had used psychostimulant medications (e.g., Adderall, Ritalin, dextroamphetamine, and methamphetamine) for medical or non-medical purposes before or during medical school. Those who had used psychostimulant medications for medical reasons ($n=34$) were excluded from statistical analyses. Results for the rest of the sample showed that 14% had abused psychostimulant drugs for non-medical reasons. Comparisons of psychostimulant drug abusers and the rest showed no statistically significant difference on the JSE scores between the two groups. However, drug abusers obtained a significantly higher mean score on the Aggression-Hostility scale of the ZKPQ. No other statistically significant difference was observed between the two groups on other scales of the ZKPQ.

Dehning, S., Reiß, E., Krause, D., Gasperi, S., Meyer, S., Dargel, S., Müller N., & Siebeck, M. (2014). Empathy in high-tech and high-touch medicine. *Patient Education and Counseling. 95*, 259–264. Accessible from: https://doi.org/10.1016/j.pec.2014.01.013.

Participants included 56 surgeons (14 women) and 50 psychiatrists (25 women) in the departments of surgery, and psychiatry and psychotherapy at the Ludwig Maximilian University in Munich, Germany, who completed the JSE, a short version of the Balanced Emotional Empathy Scale (BEES), and a short version of the Reading the Mind in the Eye Test (RME-R6). Results showed that male psychiatrists scored significantly higher on the JSE ($M=118.0$, SD=9.86) than male surgeons ($M=107.5$, SD=13.84). The gender difference was not statistically significant between female psychiatrists ($M=115.4$, SD=14.19) and female surgeons ($M=114.1$, SD=7.16). No statistically significant gender difference was observed on the BEES and RME-R6 results. In addition, analytically trained psychiatrists obtained a significantly higher mean score on the JSE than their behaviorally trained counterparts. Significant correlations were observed between scores on the JSE and the BEES ($r=0.46$) and the RME-R6 ($r=0.31$).

Delgado-Bolton, R., San-Martin, M., Alcorta-Garza, A., & Vivanco, L. (in press). Medical empathy of physicians-in-training who are enrolled in professional training program: A comparative intercultural study in Spain. *Atención Primaria*. Accessible from: https://doi.org/10.1016/j.aprim.2015.10.005.

Participants included 67 residents from Spain and 32 from Latin America, who completed a Spanish translation of the JSE-HP version. Results showed that the JSE mean score was higher for the Spanish (M = 116, SD = 13) than the Latin American group (M = 109, SD = 14). Cronbach's alpha coefficients were 0.82, and 0.81 for the Spanish and the Latin American groups, respectively.

Diaz-Narvaez, V.P., Calzadilla-Nunez, A., Carrasco, D., Bustos, A., Zamorano, A., Silva, H., Lopez Tagle, E., Hubermann, J. (2016). Levels of empathy among dental students in five Chilean universities. *Health, 8*, 32–41. Accessible from: https://doi.org/10.4236/health.2016.81005.

Participants included 1722 students from five dental schools in Chile, who completed the JSE. Results showed that women scores higher (M = 114.21) than men (M = 111.42) on the JSE, mean scores varied from 110.63 to 115.56 in different universities, and empathy scores tended to increase as students progressed through dental school in this cross-sectional study.

Diaz-Narvaez, V. P., Coronado, A. M.E., Bilbao, J.L., Gonzalez, F., Padilla, M., Howard, M., Silva, G., Alboleda, J., Bullen, M., Utsman, R., Fajardo, E., Alonso, L.M., & Cervantes, M. (2015). Empathy levels of dental students of Central America and the Caribbean. Health, 7, 1678–1686. Accessible from: https://doi.org/10.4236/health.2015.712182.

Participants included 1834 students from nine dental schools in Colombia, Panama, Costa Rica, and Dominican Republic who completed a Spanish translation of the JSE. The JSE mean scores for students from different dental schools ranged from a high of 111.89 to a low of 100.99. Differences were statistically significant among some of the schools. Cronbach's alpha coefficient for the entire sample was 0.77 (ranged from 0.75 to 0.78 for different dental schools).

Diaz-Narvaez, V. P., Gutierrez-Ventura, F.G., de Villalba, T.V., Salcedo-Rioja, M., Galzadilla-Nunez, A., Hamdan-Rodriguiz, M. (2015). Empathy levels of dentistry students in Peru and Argentina. *Health, 7*, 1268–1274. Accessible from: https://doi.org/10.4236/health.2015.710141.

Participants included 647 students from three dental schools in Peru and Argentina, who completed translated versions of the JSE. Results showed that with a few exceptions, women generally scored a higher mean scores (ranged from 96.5 to 118.6) than men (92.4–120.1) in different universities and in different years of training. Also, empathy scores generally tended to increase as students progressed through dental school in this cross-sectional study. However, none of the differences were considered practically important.

*Fields, S. K., Hojat, M., Gonnella, J. S., Mangione, S., Kane, G., & Magee, M. (2004). Comparisons of nurses and physicians on an operational measure of empathy. *Evaluation & The Health Professions, 27*, 80–94. doi: https://doi.org/10.1177/0163278703261206.

Participants included 56 female registered nurses and 42 female physicians at Thomas Jefferson University Hospital, who completed the JSE. Comparison of physicians and nurses on the total JSE scores showed no statistically significant differences ($M=115.7$, $SD=13.60$ in physicians; $M=117.2$, $SD=14.05$ in nurses). However, comparisons of the two groups on their responses to the individual items of the JSE showed statistically significant differences between physicians and nurses on five out of 20 items of the JSE (physicians scored higher on two; and nurses scored higher on three items). Cronbach's alpha coefficients were 0.89 and 0.87 for physicians and nurses, respectively.

*Grosseman, S., Hojat, M., Duke, P. M., Mennin, S., Rosenzweig, S., & Novack, D. (2014). Empathy, self-reflection, and curriculum choice. *The Interdisciplinary Journal of Problem-Based Learning, 8*, 35–41. Accessible from: http:/dx.doi.org/10.7771/1541-5015.1429.

Participants included 223 first-year medical students at the Drexel University College of Medicine, who completed the JSE and the Groningen Reflection Ability Scale. Of this sample, 60 (30 women) self-selected a problem-based learning curriculum track, and 163 (79 women) self-selected a lecture-based curriculum track. Those who chose the problem-based learning curriculum track scored significantly higher on the JSE ($M=118.0$, $SD=8.9$) than their classmates who chose the lecture-based track ($M=114.0$, $SD=11.1$). A similar pattern of findings was observed on the Groningen Reflection Ability Scale ($M=94.6$, $SD=7.5$; and $M=92.0$, $SD=8.2$, respectively). Women scored significantly higher than men on both scales.

*Hojat, M., DeSantis, J., Shannon, S. C., Speicher, M. R., Bragan, L., & Calabrese, L. H. (2020). Empathy as related to gender, age, race/ethnicity, academic background, and career interest: Results of a nationwide study of medical students. *Medical Education, 54*(6), 571–581. https://doi.org/10.1111/medu.14138.

This study was designed to examine associations between clinical empathy and gender, age, race and ethnicity, academic background and career interest in nationwide, multi-institutional samples of medical students in the United States. Four nationwide samples participated in this study (n = 10 751). Samples 1, 2, 3, and 4 included 3616 first-year, 2764 second-year, 2413 third-year, and 1958 fourth-year students who completed the JSE-S and the Infrequency Scale of the Zuckerman–Kuhlman Personality Questionnaire to control for the effect of "good impression" response bias. Results showed statistically significant and practically important associations between empathy scores and gender (in favor of women), race and ethnicity (in favor of African-American and Hispanic/Latino/Spanish), academic background (in favor of "Social and Behavioral Sciences" and "Arts and Humanities" in Samples 1 and 2) and career interest (in favor of "People-Oriented" and "Psychiatry" specialties).

*Hojat, M., Fields, S. K., & Gonnella, J. S. (2003). Empathy: An NP/MD comparison. *The Nurse Practitioner, 28*, 45–47.

Participants included 32 female nurse practitioners, 37 female pediatricians, and 33 female physicians in hospital-based specialties (anesthesiology, radiology, and pathology), who completed the JSE. Results showed no statistically significant difference on JSE mean scores between nurse practitioners (M=124.0, SD=12.3) and pediatricians (M=124.0, SD=9.3); however, physicians in hospital-based specialties scored significantly lower (M=118.0, SD=13.1) than nurse practitioners and pediatricians. Cronbach's alpha coefficient for nurse practitioners was 0.85.

*Hojat, M., Mangione, S., Gonnella, J. S., Nasca, T., Veloski, J. J., & Kane, G. (2001). Empathy in medical education and patient care [Letter to the editor]. *Academic Medicine, 76*, 669.

Participants included 704 physicians affiliated with the Jefferson Health Care System, who completed the JSE. Those who were practicing medicine in "people-oriented" specialties (e.g., general internal medicine, family medicine, pediatrics, obstetrics and gynecology, emergency medicine, psychiatry, and medical subspecialties) obtained a significantly higher JSE mean score (M=121.0, SD=11.6) than their counterparts in "technology-oriented" specialties (e.g., anesthesiology, pathology, radiology, surgery, and surgical subspecialties) (M=117.2, SD=12.1). Results remained unchanged when the effect of physicians' gender was controlled.

*Kataoka, H. U., Koide, N., Hojat, M., & Gonnella, J. S. (2012). Measurement and correlates of empathy among female Japanese physicians. *BMC Medical Education, 12*, 48. doi: https://doi.org/10.1186/1472-6920-12-48. Accessible from: http://www.biomedcentral.com/1472-6920/12/48.

Participants included 285 female Japanese physicians who graduated from Okayama University Medical School or were practicing medicine in Okayama University Hospital. They completed a Japanese translation of the JSE (HP-Version). Results showed that the JSE mean score for this sample was 110.4 (SD=11.9). Corrected item-total score correlations were all positive and statistically significant, ranging from 0.20 to 0.54 with a median of 0.41. Cronbach's alpha coefficient was 0.80. Physicians who were practicing in "people-oriented" specialties obtained a significantly higher JSE mean score than their counterparts in "procedure or technology-oriented" specialties. Physicians who reported living with their parents in an extended family or living close to their parents scored higher on the JSE than those who were living alone or were living in a small nuclear family.

Kerr, N., & Tegge, A. M. (2017). Levels of empathy in undergraduate health-care-professions students. *International Journal of Human Caring*, 21(1), 41–45. DOI: https://doi.org/10.20467/1091-5710.21.1.41.

The aim of this study was to compare empathy scores between health professions students (pharmacy and nursing) and non-health professions (law) students and between first-and third-year students. The JSE-S version was completed by 282 nursing, pharmacy, and law students. The results indicated that pharmacy students obtained significantly higher empathy scores than did law students. Third-year pharmacy students scored higher on empathy than did first-year pharmacy students, whereas the converse was true for nurses. There was no significant difference in empathy between first- and third-year law students. Empathy increased among pharmacy students, decreased among nurses, and remained the same among law students. Women scored higher on empathy than did men. Empathy scores among university students were found to vary depending on discipline and year of study.

McKenna, L., Boyle, M., Brown, T., Williams, B., Molloy, A., Lewis, B., & Molloy, L. (2012). Levels of empathy in undergraduate nursing students. *International Journal of Nursing Practice*, *18*, 246–251. doi: https://doi.org/10.1111/j.1440-172X.2012.02035.x.

Participants included 106 nursing students (93% women) at Monash University, Australia, who completed the JSE. Results showed a JSE mean score of 107.34 (SD = 13.74). No statistically significant association was observed between JSE scores and students' gender, age, and year of training in this cross-sectional study.

Ouzouni, C., & Nakakis, K. (2012). An exploratory study of student nurses' empathy. *Health Science Journal, 6*, 534–552.

Participants included 279 nursing students (239 women) in the first-, third-, fourth-, and sixth-semester of their nursing education at the Nursing School of the Technological Educational Institute of Lamia in Greece, who completed a Greek translation of the JSE. Results showed that women outscored their male classmates. The following groups of students obtained significantly higher JSE mean scores than their other classmates: those who expressed a plan to work as nurses after graduation, those who reported that they were able to understand feelings of others, those who reported receiving emotional support from their nuclear families, those who reported being exposed to training in understanding patient's perspective, those who observed their clinical faculty displaying emotional understanding of the patients, older students, and students who were in higher stages of training.

*Park, K. H., Roh, H., Suh, D. H., & Hojat, M. (2015). Empathy in Korean medical students: Findings from a nationwide survey. *Medical Teacher, 37*, 943–948. doi: https://doi.org/10.3109/0142159X.2014.956058.

Participants included 5343 first- to fourth-year Korean medical students (2056 women) across the country from two types of medical school admission systems: undergraduate admission system ($n = 2624$) and post-baccalaureate admission system ($n = 2719$). Students completed a Korean translation of the JSE. Results showed a JSE mean score of 105.90 (SD = 12.80) for the total sample. Women's JSE mean score ($M = 106.95$, SD = 11.74) was significantly higher than men ($M = 105.25$, SD = 13.73). A similar pattern of gender difference was observed in students of both medical school systems. Controlling for gender, significant difference on the JSE was found between students from the two medical school systems in favor of students in the post-baccalaureate system. No significant association was observed between JSE scores and students' age in both medical school systems. In both systems, students in higher years of medical education scored lower on the JSE.

Shariat, S. V., & Kaykhavoni, A. (2010). Empathy in medical residents at Iran University of Medical Sciences. *Iranian Journal of Psychiatry and Clinical Psychology*, *16*, 248–256.

Participants included 251 residents (41% women) who were pursuing their residency training in hospitals affiliated with the Iran University of Medical Sciences in Tehran, Iran. They completed a Persian (Farsi) translation of the JSE. Results showed no significant gender difference (for men: $M=100.4$, SD = 13.1; for women: $M=100.9$, SD = 13.3). Psychiatry residents obtained the highest JSE mean score ($M=114.2$, SD = 14.1) compared to other residents. No significant association was found between scores on the JSE and residents' age and level of training.

Soncini, F., Silvestrini, G., Poscia, A., Clorba. V., Conti, A., Murru, C., Rinaldi, A., Zoccali, A., Azzolini, E., & Ziglio, A. (2013). Public health physicians and empathy: Are we really empathic? The Jefferson Scale applied to Italian resident doctors in public health. *European Journal of Public Health, 23*(Suppl. 1), 264–265.

Participants included 352 Italian resident physicians from residency programs in Italian schools of hygiene and public health, who completed an Italian translation of the JSE sent to them by mail (87% response rate). Results showed an overall mean score of 118.5 (SD = 13.4, $M=120$, score range 54–120) for this sample. Women obtained a significantly higher JSE mean score ($M=120.3$) than men ($M=114.9$), and physicians who had healthcare administrative experiences scored significantly higher than those who were only involved in research ($M=120.4$ and $M=117.1$, respectively). No significant association was found between the JSE scores and physicians' age or level of residency training.

Tavakol, S., Dennick, R., & Tavakol, M. (2011). Empathy in UK medical students: Differences by gender, medical year and specialty interest. *Education for Primary Care*, *22*, 297–303.

Participants included 853 medical students (470 women) at the University of Nottingham Medical School, who completed the JSE-S. Three hypotheses were tested: (1) Women would score higher than men on the JSE, (2) Scores on the JSE would decline as students progressed through medical school in this cross-sectional study, and (3) Students interested in "people-oriented" specialties would score higher on the JSE than students interested in "technology-oriented" specialties. The first and third hypotheses were confirmed, but the second hypothesis was not.

Voinescu, B. I., Szentagotai, A., & Coogan, A. (2009). Residents' clinical empathy: Gender and specialty comparisons—A Romanian study. *Acta Medica Academica, 38*, 11–15. doi: https://doi.org/10.5644/ama.v38i1.50.

Participants included 112 residents (74% women) in Cluj-Napoca, Romania, who completed a Romanian translation of the JSE. Results showed that the JSE mean score for the sample was 113.4 (SD = 14.4). Women's JSE mean score ($M=114.9$, SD = 14.75) was significantly higher than men's ($M=107.2$, SD = 11.5). Residents in the psychiatry program ($n=60$) obtained a significantly higher JSE mean score ($M=115.8$, SD = 15.7) than other residents ($M=110.4$, SD = 12.3). Corrected item-total score correlations for the JSE ranged from 0.21 to 0.67 with a median of 0.42. Cronbach's alpha coefficient was 0.84.

Williams, B., Brown, T., Boyle, M., McKenna, L., Palermo, C., & Etherington, J. (2014). Levels of empathy in undergraduate emergency health, nursing, and midwifery students: A longitudinal study. *Advances in Medical Education and Practice, 5*, 299–306. Accessible from: https://doi.org/10.2147/AMEP.S66681.

Participants included 948 first-, second-, and third-year paramedic, nursing, and midwifery students (798 women) at Monash University in Australia, who completed the JSE. Midwifery students scored significantly higher on the JSE (M = 109.0, SD = 17.2) than those in nursing (M = 104.0, SD = 14.4) and paramedics (M = 104.4, SD = 14.9). No statistically significant difference was observed on JSE scores of students in different years of training. Although women obtained a higher JSE mean score (M = 106.6, SD = 14.83) than did men (M = 100.6, SD = 14.41), the difference was not statistically significant. Older students scored higher on the JSE than younger students.

Williams, B., Brown, T., McKenna, L., Boyle, M. J., Palermo, C., Nestel, D., Brightwell, R., McCall, L., & Russo, V. (2014). Empathy levels among health professional students: A cross-sectional study at two universities in Australia. *Advances in Medical Education and Practice, 5*, 107–113. doi: https://doi.org/10.2147/AMEP.S57569.

Participants included 1111 first- to fourth-year health professional students (907 women) studying in disciplines such as medicine, nursing, paramedics, midwifery, occupational therapy, physiotherapy, and nutrition and dietetics from Monash University and Edith Cowan University in Australia, who completed the JSE. Exploratory factor analysis of data resulted in three factors of Perspective Taking, Patient Perceptions, and Compassionate Care, somewhat similar to those that emerged in most other factor analytic studies of the JSE. No significant difference was observed on JSE scores between the two universities: The mean score for students from Monash University was 110.06 (SD = 11.76) and for students from Edith Cowan University was 109.18 (SD = 13.31). Cronbach's alpha coefficient for the total sample was 0.78. Women obtained a significantly higher JSE mean score (M = 110.86, SD = 11.67) than did men (M = 105.31, SD = 13.47). Paramedic students had significantly lower JSE mean score (M = 106.37, SD = 12.73) than all other students with the exception of nursing students. A significant increase in the JSE mean score was observed from the first-year (M = 108.71, SD = 12.52) to second-year (M = 111.01, SD = 11.94) in this cross-sectional study, but no significant change was found afterward. Students' age was positively associated with JSE scores.

Wilson, S. E., Prescott, J., & Becket, G. (2012). Empathy levels in first- and third-year students in health and non-health disciplines. *American Journal of Pharmaceutical Education, 76*(2), Article 24. Accessible from: http://www.ncbi.nlm.nih.gov/pmc/articles/PMC3305933/.

Participants included 282 first- and third-year students (190 women) in nursing, pharmacy, and law, who completed the JSE at the University of Central Lancashire in England. Results showed that women scored higher than men (M = 103 and M = 97, respectively). No significant difference was found between students in nursing and pharmacy programs; however, students in both of these health-related professions obtained significantly higher JSE mean scores than did the law students in both the first- and third-year of their education. In this cross-sectional study, a significant decline was observed in the JSE mean scores from the first- to third-year nursing students (M = 107.9, SD = 11.9; M = 101.9, SD = 14.2, respectively); however, an increase in the JSE mean score was found in pharmacy students between the first year (M = 100.3, SD = 11.8) and third year (M = 110.4, SD = 10.5); no significant change was noticed on the empathy scores between first (M = 95.3, SD = 11.1) and third year (M = 94.2, SD = 13.4) in law students.

Studies on Changes in Clinical Empathy

Aye, S.Z., Sein, H.H., Nyunt, M.K., & Min Y. (2022). Comparative study of Malaysian medical students' empathy scores between preclinical and clinical training. *Education in Medicine Journal, 4*(1):27–38. https://doi.org/10.21315/eimj2022.14.1.3.

The purpose of this study was to compare the empathy scores of Malaysian medical students. Research participants included 242 Malaysian medical students who completed the JSE-S in preclinical and clinical phases of medical school training. Results showed that compared to medical students in preclinical training, clinical students had statistically significant higher empathy scores in the compassionate care factor of clinical empathy, but their perspective-taking factor of clinical empathy remained unchanged.

Beattie, A., Durham, J., Harvey, J., Steele, J., & McHanwell, S. (2012). Does empathy change in first-year dental students? *European Journal of Dental Education, 16*, e111–e116. doi: https://doi.org/10.1111/j.1600-0579.2011.00683.x.

Participants included 66 first-year students (46 women) at the School of Dental Sciences, Newcastle University in England, who completed the JSE and the Patient-Practitioner Orientation Scale (PPOS, a measure of patient-centered care), before and after a behavioral science course. Results showed a significant increase in the JSE mean score after completion of the behavioral science course. No significant pre–post-course change was observed in PPOS scores. A statistically significant correlation was found between scores on the JSE and the PPOS caring scale ($r=0.36$) in pre-course, but not in post-course testing.

Brown, T., Williams, B., Boyle, M., Molloy, A., McKenna, L., Molloy, L., & Lewis, B. (2010). Levels of empathy in undergraduate occupational therapy students. *Occupational Therapy International, 17*, 135–141. doi: https://doi.org/10.1002/oti.297.

Participants included 92 occupational therapy students (91% women) at Monash University in Australia, who completed the JSE. The median JSE score for this sample was 115. No statistically significant association was observed between JSE scores and students' gender, age, or year of training in this cross-sectional study.

Chatterjee, A., Ravikumar, R., Singh, S., Chauhan, P. S., & Goel, M. (2017). Clinical empathy in medical students in India measured using the JSE-Student Version. *Journal of Educational Evaluation for Health Professions, 14*, 33. https://doi.org/10.3352/jeehp.2017.14.33.

The purpose of this study was to assess the clinical empathy of a cohort of medical students spanning 4 years of undergraduate study and to identify factors associated with empathy in India. Research participants (n = 418) completed the JSE. The mean empathy score was 96.01 (of a maximum of 140), with a standard deviation of 14.56. The empathy scores decreased from the first to the third semester, plateaued at the fifth semester, and rose again in the seventh semester. Empathy was found to be significantly associated with the gender of the participant, with females having higher scores. The age of the participant, place of residence, and the choice of future specialty were not significantly associated with students' empathy scores. The empathy scores tended to decline initially and then rebound over time. The mean empathy levels found in this study were lower than those reported in most similar studies around the world.

Chen, D., Lew, R., Hershman, W., & Orlander, J. (2007). A cross-sectional measurement of medical student empathy. *Journal of General Internal Medicine, 22*, 1434–1438. doi: https://doi.org/10.1007/s11606-007-0298-x.

Participants included 658 students at the Boston University School of Medicine, who completed the JSE S-Version. In this cross-sectional study, the JSE mean score was 118.5 in the first year but significantly declined in the third (M=112.7) and remained low in the fourth year of medical school (M=106.6). Women obtained a significantly higher JSE mean score (M=116.5) than men (M=112.1). Students who were interested in pursuing people-oriented specialties scored higher on the JSE than others who were interested in pursuing technology-oriented specialties (M=114.6 and M=111.4, respectively). No substantial association was found between scores on the JSE and students' ages.

Chen, D. C. R., Kirshenbaum, D. S., Yan, J., Kirshenbaum, E., & Aseltine, R. H. (2012). Characterizing changes in student empathy throughout medical school. *Medical Teacher, 34*, 305–311. doi: https://doi.org/10.3109/0142159X.2012.644600.

Participants included 1162 students (622 women) at the Boston University School of Medicine, who completed the JSE at the beginning of medical school and approximately at the end of each academic year. Results showed an upward trend in mean scores on the JSE in preclinical years but a downward trend in clinical years (e.g., JSE mean score in the second year=116.02, SD=12.42; declined to 113.29, SD=12.59 in the fourth year). Women scored higher than men on the JSE. Those interested in technology-oriented specialties (pathology, radiology, anesthesiology, and surgery) obtained a significantly lower JSE mean score than others. Higher level of educational debt was associated with higher empathy scores after adjustment for specialty interest. It was noticed that the decline in empathy was less for students with higher JSE scores at the beginning of medical school than for students with lower baseline empathy scores.

Chen, D. C. R., Pahilan, M. E., & Orlander, J. D. (2010). Comparing a self-administered measure of empathy with observed behavior among medical students. *Journal of General Internal Medicine, 25*, 200–202. doi: https://doi.org/10.1007/s11606-009-1193-4.

Participants in this cross-sectional study included 167 second-year and 162 third-year students at the Boston University School of Medicine, who completed the JSE. Their clinical skills, including interactions with patients, were assessed by standardized patients in the Objective Structured Clinical Examinations (OSCE). A statistically significant decline in the JSE mean score was noticed when comparing the second-year (M=118.68) and third-year students (M=116.08). However, a statistically significant increase in the average ratings of clinical competence given by standardized patients in the OSCE setting was observed (M=3.96 in the second-year, M=4.15 in the third-year). The overall correlation between JSE scores and the OSCE assessment was statistically significant but moderate in magnitude (r=0.22).

Costa, P., Magalhães, E., & Costa, M. J. (2013). A latent growth model suggests that empathy of medical students does not decline over time. *Advances in Health Sciences Education, 18*, 509–522. doi: https://doi.org/10.1007/s10459-012-9390-z. Accessible from: http://link.springer.com/article/10.1007/s10459-012-9390-z?null.

Participants included 77 medical students (53 women) at the School of Health Sciences, University of Minho in Portugal, who completed a Portuguese translation of the JSE S-Version three times: upon admission, upon completion of the preclinical phase of medical education (third year), and at the start of the clinical phase of medical education (beginning of the fourth year). Students also completed the NEO-FFI (a personality inventory for measuring the big five personality factors). Results for the total sample showed no significant decline in empathy scores prior to the clinical phase of medical education. For example, the JSE mean scores taken during preclinical was 111.21 (SD = 10.80), and at beginning of the clinical phase of medical education it was 110 (SD = 10.85). However, the JSE mean score declined significantly for women from preclinical phase (M = 113.41, SD = 10.57) to the beginning of clinical phase (M = 110.77, SD = 10.84). Such significant decline was not observed for men. Although JSE mean score was higher for women as compared to men in all three test administrations, the gender difference was statistically significant only at the end of the preclinical phase of medical education. Scores on the JSE were significantly and positively correlated with those of Openness to Experiences and Agreeableness personality factors at admission to medical school.

Diaz-Narváez, V. P. D., Palacio, L. M. A., Caro, S. E., Silva, M. G., Castillo, J. A., Bilbao, J. L., & Acosta, J. I. (2014). Empathic orientation among medical students from three universities in Barranquilla, Colombia and one university in the Dominican Republic. *Archivos Argentinos de Pediatria, 112*, 41–49. Accessible from: https://doi.org/10.5546/aap.2014.eng.41.

Participants included 1838 medical students from the School of Medicine of Universidad del Norte (n = 345), Universidad San Martin (n = 283), and Universidad Libre (n = 695) in the city of Barranquilla in Colombia, and Universidad Central del Este (n = 515) in the Dominican Republic, who completed the JSE. Mean scores on the JSE for students in different years (years 1–5) within each medical school ranged from a low of 98.2 to a high of 110.7. Differences in JSE scores were observed among medical schools. Empathy scores declined for both men and women as students progressed through medical school in this cross-sectional study, but the decline was not substantial.

Gabard, D. L., Lowe, D. L., Deusinger, S. S., Stelzner, D. M., & Crandall, S. J. (2013). Analysis of empathy in doctor of physical therapy students: A multi-site study. *Journal of Allied Health*, *42*, 10–16.

Participants included two cohorts (classes of 2009 and 2010) of students enrolled in the doctor of physical therapy program in five academic institutions (Chapman University, Mount St. Mary's College, University of Colorado, University of Nebraska, and Washington University), who completed a slightly modified version of the JSE (changing "physician" to "physical therapist") in the first, second, and third years of training. The face validity of the modified version was confirmed in a pilot study, and a test–retest reliability coefficient of 0.58 was obtained within a 2-week interval between testing in a sample of 20 physical therapy students. Results of comparisons by institution showed significant differences on the JSE among entering classes in the five participating institutions, ranging from 111.0 (SD = 9.9) to 120.1 (SD = 8.0). Within-institution comparisons on the JSE scores in the 3 years of training in this cross-sectional study showed mixed results. Comparisons of the JSE scores in the 3 years of study, in the two cohorts, within each institution either did not change significantly or declined in some students and increased in others.

Hall, M., Hanna, L.A., Hanna, A., & McDevitt, C. (2015). Empathy in UK pharmacy students: Assessing differences by gender, level in the degree programme, part-time employment and medical status. *Pharmacy Education, 15*, 241–247.

Participants included 318 undergraduate pharmacy students at the Queen's University Belfast, who completed the JSE HPS-Version. Results showed a mean score of 106.19 (SD = 11.81) and a Cronbach's alpha coefficient of 0.81. Although women scored higher than men on the JSE, the difference was not statistically significant. Students in the fourth year of training obtained a significantly higher JSE mean score (M = 110.26, SD = 10.93) than those in the first year (M = 104.96, SD = 12.39) in this cross-sectional study. No significant difference on the JSE scores was found among those who had a part-time job compared to their counterparts without a job; those who reported chronic health problems compared to others without such problems; and those who were taking medication compared to the rest.

*Hojat, M., Mangione, S., Nasca, T. J., Rattner, S., Erdmann, J. B., Gonnella, J. S., & Magee, M. (2004). An empirical study of decline in empathy in medical school. *Medical Education, 38*, 934–941. doi: https://doi.org/10.1111/j.1365-2929.2004.01911.x.

Participants included 125 medical students (61 women) who completed the JSE at the beginning and at the end of the third year of medical school. In this first longitudinal study of change in the JSE scores during medical school, a statistically significant decline in JSE mean score was found when scores at the beginning (M = 123.1, SD = 9.9) and the end of third-year (M=120.6, SD=13.9) were compared (effect size of the change=0.29). Analysis of differences at item level showed significant decline on five of the 20 items of the JSE (effect size estimates ranged from 0.34 to 0.55). Correlation coefficient of scores on the JSE administered at the beginning and end of the academic year was 0.51.

*Hojat, M., Shannon, S. C., DeSantis, J., Speicher, M., Braga, L., & Calabrese, L. (2020). Does empathy decline in the Clinical phase of medical education? A nationwide, multi-institutional, cross-sectional study of students at DO granting medical schools. *Academic Medicine, 95*(6), 911–918. https://doi.org/10.1097/ACM.0000000000003175.

The purpose of this study was to examine differences in students' empathy in different years of medical school in a nationwide study of students of US DO-granting medical schools. Research participants in this cross-sectional study included 10,751 students enrolled in 41 of 48 campuses of DO-granting medical schools in the United States (3616 first-year, 2764 second-year, 2413 third-year, and 1958 fourth-year students). They completed a web-based survey at the end of the academic year, which included the Jefferson Scale of Empathy (S-version) and the Infrequency Scale of the Zuckerman–Kuhlman Personality Questionnaire for controlling "good impression" response bias. Comparisons were made on empathy scores among students in different years of medical school using analysis of covariance, controlling for the effect of "good impression" response bias. Also, comparisons were made with preexisting data from students of US MD-granting medical schools. Results showed a statistically significant decline in clinical empathy scores when comparing students in the preclinical (years 1 and 2) and the clinical (years 3 and 4) phases of medical school ($P < .001$); however, the magnitude of the decline was negligible (effect size = 0.13). Comparison of findings with MD students showed that while the pattern of empathy decline was similar, the magnitude of the decline was less pronounced in DO students.

*Hojat, M., Vergare, M., Maxwell, K., Brainard, G., Herrine, S. K., Isenberg, G. A., Veloski, J. J., & Gonnella, J. S. (2009). The devil is in the third year: A longitudinal study of erosion of empathy in medical school. *Academic Medicine, 84*, 1182–1191.

Participants in this longitudinal study included 456 students (226 women) in two entering classes at Jefferson (now Sidney Kimmel) Medical College, who completed the JSE five times during their medical school education: at the beginning of medical school and at the end of the fist-, second-, third-, and fourth-year of medical school. Results showed the mean scores on the JSE for both cohorts did not change significantly during the first 2 years of medical school. However, a significant decline in the JSE mean score was observed at the end of the third-year (from $M = 115.7$ at the end of the second year to $M = 108.5$ at the end of the third year in the matched cohorts), which persisted until graduation from medical school. Patterns of decline in JSE scores were similar for men and women, and for students interested in pursuing "people-oriented" or "technology- or procedure-oriented" specialties. Possible reasons for erosion of empathy in medical school were described based on students' own reports.

Hong, M., Lee, W. H., Park, J. H., Yoon, T. Y., Moon, D. S., & Lee, S. M. (2012). Changes of empathy in medical college and medical school students: One-year follow up study. *BMC Medical Education, 12*, 122. doi: https://doi.org/10.1186/1472-6920-12-122. Accessible from: http://www.biomedcentral.com/1472-6920/12/122.

Participants included 113 students (24% women) in medical college (6-year curriculum including two years of premedical education) and 113 students (26% women) in medical school (4-year curriculum after completing undergraduate education) at Kyung Hee University. Participants completed a Korean translation of the JSE in 2007 and 2008. They were in the first, second, and third years of medical education. Medical school students' JSE mean score ($M = 109.23$, SD = 11.06) in the first test administration was significantly higher than those in medical college ($M = 106.96$, SD = 10.50); however, no significant difference was found between medical school and medical college students in the second test administration one year later. Also, no significant change in empathy scores was observed in the two groups of students from the first to the second test administration, and no significant gender difference was noticed.

Igde, F. A., & Sahin, M. K. (2017). Changes in Empathy during Medical Education: An Example from Turkey. *Pakistan Journal of Medical Sciences, 33*(5), 1177–1181. https://doi.org/10.12669/pjms.335.13074.

The purpose of this study was to explore change of clinical empathy in Turkish medical students. Turkish adapted form of the medical student version of JSE was administered to medical students. Results showed significant differences in the empathy scores during the first three years of medical school and gender variation.

Khademalhosseini, M., Khademalhosseini, Z., & Mahmoodian, F. (2014). Comparison of empathy score among medical students in both basic and clinical levels. *Journal of Advances in Medical Education & Professionalism, 2*, 88–91.

Participants included 260 students (140 women) at the Shiraz University of Medical Sciences in Iran, who completed a Persian translation of the JSE. Findings of this cross-sectional study showed that students' JSE mean score declined as they progressed from the basic science to clinical science component of medical education. Also, women obtained a significantly higher JSE mean score than men, and younger students scored higher than their older counterparts.

Kimmelman, M., Giacobbe, J., Faden, J., Kumar, G., Pinckney, C. C., & Steer, R. (2012). Empathy in osteopathic medical students: A cross-sectional analysis. *Journal of the American Osteopathic Association, 112*, 347–355.

Participants included 405 (218 women) osteopathic medical students enrolled in the first year ($n=127$), second year ($n=105$), third year ($n=88$), and fourth year ($n=85$) at the University of Medicine and Dentistry of New Jersey, School of Osteopathic Medicine, who completed the JSE. Results of comparisons of JSE scores at different years of medical education in this cross-sectional study showed no statistically significant difference. The JSE mean scores were 108.6 (SD = 15.0), 111.2 (SD = 12.6), 109.4 (SD = 10.8), and 107.0 (SD = 15.2) for the first, second, third, and fourth years, respectively. No statistically significant association was found between the JSE scores, on the one hand, and gender, ethnicity, and specialty interest, on the other hand. Comparisons of students' JSE scores from this study sample of osteopathic medical students with published data from allopathic medical students showed that osteopathic students had significantly lower JSE mean scores in the first 2 years, but no significant difference was observed in the last 2 years of medical education.

Lim, B. T., Moriarty, H., Huthwaite, M., Gray, L., Pullon, S., & Gallagher, P. (2013). How well do medical students rate and communicate clinical empathy? *Medical Teacher*, *35*, e946–e951. doi: https://doi.org/10.3109/0142159X.2012.715783.

Participants included 72 medical students (39 women) at the University of Otago, Wellington School of Medicine and Health Sciences in New Zealand, who completed the JSE at the beginning and end of the fifth year in which students spend half of their time in clinical setting under supervision. Students also completed the JSE in the sixth year, in which they spend the majority of their time in clinical settings with and without direct supervision. Results of this longitudinal study showed no significant change in JSE scores in the fifth year, but a significant decline in mean JSE scores in the sixth year of medical school education ($M=114.21$, SD = 9.46 at the beginning of the fifth year; $M=113.55$, SD = 10.50 at the end of the fifth year; $M=82.52$, SD = 17.87 in the sixth year). No gender difference on the JSE scores was observed in this sample.

*Mangione, S. Kane, G. C., Caruso, J. W., Gonnella, J. S., Nasca, T. J., & Hojat, M. (2002). Assessment of empathy in different years of internal medicine training. *Medical Teacher, 24*, 370–373.

Participants included 98 internal medicine residents in the first ($n=40$), second ($n=27$), and third ($n=31$) years of residency training, who completed the JSE. Results of this cross-sectional study showed that the JSE mean score declined as residents progressed through training in this cross-sectional study ($M=117.5$, SD = 12.4 in the first year; $M=114.0$, SD = 14.3 in the second year, and $M=113.5$, SD = 10.8 in the third year of training), but the differences did not reach the level of statistical significance. Results remained unchanged when gender was taken into consideration. A test–retest reliability of 0.72 was obtained for residents who completed the JSE twice within a year of training.

McKenna, L., Boyle, M., Brown, T., Williams, B., Molloy, A., Lewis, B., & Molloy, L. (2011). Levels of empathy in undergraduate midwifery students: An Australian cross-sectional study. *Women and Birth: Journal of the Australian College of Midwives*, *24*, 80–84. doi: https://doi.org/10.1016/j.wombi.2011.02.003.

Participants included 52 undergraduate female midwifery students in three years of training at Monash University, Australia, who completed the JSE. Results showed a JSE mean score of 109.9 (SD = 20.9) for the sample. A steady increase in the mean JSE scores was observed in this cross-sectional study as students progressed from the first to the third year of training.

Michalec, B. (2010). As assessment of medical student school stressors on preclinical students' level of clinical empathy. *Current Psychology, 29*, 210–221.

Participants were 329 first-, second-, and third-year US medical students who completed the JSE at the beginning and at the end of the academic year to examine the impact of medical school-specific stressors (e.g., financial worries, lack of time, fear of academic failure, competition, mistreatment by faculty, and interaction with patients) on changes in empathy during the academic year. Results showed that female students outscored their male counterparts, empathy declined in each year, and those who scored high on the JSE were more likely to report that medical school stressors had more negative impact on their lives. Also, changes in scores on the Conscientiousness and Extroversion factors of the NEO-PI-R were found to have unique and significant effects on the JSE scores. It is suggested that while medical school stress may not be the cause of the decline in empathy in medical school, students may be adapting to the stressful medical school environment by "shedding" empathy in order to become less vulnerable to the negative impact of the stressors.

Nunes, P., Williams, S., Sa, B., & Stevenson, K. (2011). A study of empathy decline in students from five health disciplines during their first year of training. *International Journal of Medical Education, 2*, 12–17. doi: https://doi.org/10.5116/ijme.4d47.ddb0.

Participants included 355 students (259 women) enrolled in schools of medicine, nursing, dentistry, pharmacy, and veterinary medicine, who completed the JSE at the beginning of their professional education and at the end of the academic year. Women scored higher than men, and older students scored higher than their younger counterparts. The highest JSE mean scores were obtained by nursing and dental students. Empathy declined to some extent in all five groups; however, the decline in medical, nursing, and dental students was statistically significant.

Rosenthal, S., Howard, B., Schlussel, Y. R., Herrigel, D., Smolarz, B. G., Gable, B., Vassquez, J., Grigo, H., & Kaufman, M. (2011). Humanism at heart: Preserving empathy in third-year medical students. *Academic Medicine, 86*, 350–358.

Participants included 209 medical students at Robert Wood Johnson Medical School, who completed the JSE. In a pretest–posttest design, no significant decline in JSE scores was observed in students who were exposed in their clerkship to a mandatory "humanism and professionalism" component of the curriculum. The authors concluded that the erosion of empathy in medical school can be prevented by targeted educational programs.

Schwartz, B., & Bohay, R. (2012). Can patient help teach professionalism and empathy to dental students? Adding patient video to lecture course. *Journal of Dental Education, 76*, 174–184.

Participants included 31 second-year and 54 third-year dental students at the Schulich School of Medicine and Dentistry, University of Western Ontario in Canada, who completed the JSE. Students viewed videos on patient management and participated in discussion and reflective writing about their experiences. Despite these activities, a statistically significant decline in the JSE mean scores was found between the second (M=117.13, SD=7.64) and third-year students (M=110.28, SD=16.58).

Smith, K. E., Norman, G. J., & Decety, J. (2017). The complexity of empathy during medical school training: evidence for positive changes. *Medical Education, 51*(11), 1146–1159. https://doi.org/10.1111/medu.13398.

In this longitudinal study, 129 medical students completed a series of self-report and behavioral measures twice per year during the first 3 years of their study, including the JSE for the assessment of clinical empathy and the Questionnaire of Cognitive and Affective Empathy (QCAE) for the assessment of cognitive and affective empathy. Results showed that students' empathy, assessed by the JSE, decreased over training. However, on the QCAE, overall cognitive empathy, its subcomponent perspective taking, and the emotion contagion subcomponent of affective empathy all improved. Students also exhibited comparable growth in their understanding of others' emotions and increased sensitivity to others' pain. Aspects of empathy thought to be valuable in positive physician–patient interactions improve during training. Overall, this study points to the importance of assessing the distinct components of empathy using multiple forms of measurement in order to better understand the mechanisms involved in empathy changes in medical practice.

Sng, G., Tung, J., Ping, Y. S., Lee, S. S., Win, M. T., Hooi, S. C., & Samarasekera, D. D. (2016). Complex and novel determinants of empathy change in medical students. *Korean Journal of Medical Education, 28*(1), 67–78. https://doi.org/10.3946/kjme.2016.11.

This study explored the empathy changes in Korean medical students in Singapore. Research participants included 881 students in years 1 to 5, who completed the JSE-S version. Results showed that empathy declined significantly between preclinical and clinical years. High workload and inappropriate learning environments were the most relevant stressors. Time spent with family, arts, and community service correlated with higher empathy scores.

Wahjudi, J. W., Findyartini, A., & Kaligis, F. (2019). The relationship between empathy and stress: a cross-sectional study among undergraduate medical students. *Korean Journal of Medical Education, 31*(3), 215–226. https://doi.org/10.3946/kjme.2019.132.

The purpose of this study was to identify whether the empathy of medical students is associated with their perceived stress. Research participants included 464 medical students in Indonesia, who completed the JSE and the Perceived Stress Scale. Results showed that the students' empathy levels increased during their first 3 years, declined significantly upon entering the first clinical year, and increased during the second clinical year. However, no correlations were found between stress level and empathy level.

*Ward, J., Cody, J., Schaal, M., & Hojat, M. (2012). The empathy enigma: An empirical study of decline in empathy among undergraduate nursing students. *Journal of Professional Nursing, 28*, 34–40. doi: https://doi.org/10.1016/j.profnurs.2011.10.007.

Participants included 214 undergraduate nursing students (179 women) at the Jefferson School of Nursing, Thomas Jefferson University, who completed the JSE twice: at the beginning and at the end of the academic year. The JSE mean score for total participants was 114.6 (SD = 11.8) at the beginning of the academic year, which declined significantly to 112.7 (SD = 12.1) at the end of the academic year. The magnitude of decline during the study period was significantly greater among nursing students who were exposed to patient encounters more than for their counterparts with limited clinical experiences. Gender did not significantly contribute to the decline in empathy; however, the magnitude of the decline was significantly larger for Asian students, for those with prior work experiences in clinical settings, and for students with undergraduate major in business.

Williams, B., Boyle, M., & Earl, T. (2013). Measurement of empathy levels in undergraduate parametric students. *Prehospital and Disaster Medicine, 28*, 145–149. doi: https://doi.org/10.1017/S1049023X1300006X.

Participants included 94 paramedic students (63% women) at Monash University, Australia, who completed the JSE. Results showed that men obtained a higher JSE mean score ($M = 113.25$) than women ($M = 107.05$) which was inconsistent with most other findings on gender difference. No statistically significant difference was observed in this cross-sectional study among students in the first-, second-, and third-year of training. Students' age was not associated with the JSE scores.

Yeo S. (2019). Differences and changes in the empathy of Korean medical students according to gender and vocational aptitude, before and after clerkship. *Korean Journal of Medical Education, 31*(4), 343–355. https://doi.org/10.3946/kjme.2019.144.

The purpose of this study was to determine whether there is any change in the empathy scores of third-year medical students after they have taken a clerkship and have begun gaining more opportunities to meet patients through the clerkship. Research participants included 109 third-year students and 110 fourth-year students in Korea, who completed the Korean version of the JSE. Results showed that male students in their third year exhibited higher JSE scores. The empathy score increased slightly from third to fourth-year; however, the difference was not statistically significant. There were no statistically significant changes in the JSE scores between the 2 years.

Youssef, F. F., Nunes, P., Sa, B., & Williams S. (2014). An exploration of changes in cognitive and emotional empathy among medical students in the Caribbean . *International Journal of Medical Education, 5*, 185–192. doi: https://doi.org/10.5116/ijme.5412.e641.

Participants included 669 first- to seventh-year students (438 women) of the Faculty of Medical Sciences at the University of West Indies, St. Augustine, Trinidad and Tobago. The JSE S-Version, Toronto Empathy Questionnaire, and the Reading the Mind in the Eye Test (this test involves 36 photographs that show the eye region, asking participants to identify the emotion being expressed in the photos) were administered. In this cross-sectional study, a significant decline in the JSE mean scores was found in year 3 compared to years 1 and 2. Women obtained a significantly higher JSE mean score ($M = 106.9$, SD = 11.59) than men ($M = 104.3$, SD = 11.778). Correlation coefficient between scores on the JSE and Toronto Empathy Questionnaire was statistically significant ($r = 0.48$, $p < 0.001$); however, correlation between scores on the JSE and the Reading the Mind in the Eye Test was statistically significant but negligible in magnitude ($r = 0.08$, $p = 0.04$).

Studies on Interventions to Enhance Clinical Empathy

Ahmadzadeh, H., Isfahani, M.N., Ahmadzad-Ast, M., Shalbafan, M., Shariat, S.V. (2019). Does watching a movie improve empathy? A cluster randomized controlled trial. *Canadian Medical Education Journal. 10*(4), e4–e12, available at: http://www.cmej.ca.

The purpose was to examine enhancement of clinical empathy. Research participants included 133 medical students in Iran, divided into 4 groups. Group A participated in a 3-hour communication skills training workshop; Group B watched a movie, "The Doctor," based on a real story of a heart surgeon who become sick and was treated in his own hospital; Group C included students who watched "The Doctor" movie and also participated in the communication skills training workshop; Group D, the control group, neither participated in a communication training workshop nor watched "The Doctor" movie. Results of pretest–posttest comparisons showed that the JSE scores increased significantly in the three intervention Groups A, B, and C, but not in the control group (Group D). A one-month follow-up assessment indicated that enhancement in the JSE scores remained significant only in Groups A and C.

Avlogiari, E., Maria Karagiannaki, S., Panteris, E., Konsta, A., & Diakogiannis, I. (2021). Improvement of Medical Students' Empathy Levels After an Intensive Experiential Training on Empathy Skills. *Psychiatry and Clinical Psychopharmacology*, *31*(4), 392–400. https://doi.org/10.5152/pcp.2021.21098.

The link between training and enhancement of empathy was explored in this study undertaken in Greece. Research participants included 50 medical students (25 men and 25 women) who voluntarily participated in the course and completed the Greek version of the JSE-S version before and after the 20-hour training, in a 6-month follow-up. Gender, age, preferred medical specialty, and baseline empathy score were explored as possible moderator variables of the training effect. Empathy increased after training. After 6 months, the mean JSE-S score maintained a difference of 6.5 points. No differences were observed with regard to gender, age group, or medical specialty. Women in the 22–24 year-old age group had a 5-point mean difference (p = .05), and higher post-training scores than men. Lower initial scorers, compared to high scorers, were the ones who mostly improved their empathy scores and also showed a smaller decline in empathy levels 6 months after the training. Results showed that intensive experiential training can improve clinical empathy in the patient care setting.

Bazarko, D., Cate, R. A., Azocar, F., & Kreitzer, M. J. (2013). The Impact of an innovative mindfulness-based stress reduction program on the health and well-being of nurses employed in a corporate setting. *Journal of Workplace Behavioral Health*, *28*, 107–133. doi: https://doi.org/10.1080/15555240.2013.779518.

Participants included 36 nurses (all women) who participated in an 8-week Mindfulness-Based Stress Reduction (MBSR) program and completed the JSE and five other tests, three times: prior to participation in the MBSR program (Time 1), immediately after completing the program (Time 2), and 4 months after completing the program (Time 3). Results showed a significant improvement in the JSE scores from Time 1 (M=116.59, SD=8.98) to Time 2 (M=123.59, SD=9.31), which was sustained to Time 3 (M=123.0, SD=10.48). A Cronbach's alpha coefficient of 0.78 was obtained for the JSE in this study sample. Participation in the program also contributed to improvement in scores measuring burnout, general health, serenity, mindfulness, and self-compassion.

Beverly, E. A., Love, M., & Love, C. (2022). Fully Immersive Virtual Reality Improves Empathy towards People with Diabetes. *Diabetes Education*, *71*(Supplement 1), 495-P, https://doi.org/10.2337/db22-495-P.

The purpose of this study was to compare fully-immersive and semi-immersive virtual reality (VR) in diabetes training. Research participants included 69 trainees in the fully-immersive arm and 46 in the semi-immersive arm, who completed the JSE. Results showed that the fully-immersive participants' empathy improved significantly. Such improvement was not observed in the other group. The findings suggest that fully-immersive VR is more effective in improving clinical empathy than semi-immersive VR training.

Bombeke, K., Van Roosbroeck, S., De Winter, B., Debaene, L., Schol, S., Van Hal, G., & Van Royen, P. (2011). Medical students trained in communication skills show a decline in patient-centred attitudes: An observational study comparing two cohorts during clinical clerkships. *Patient Education and Counseling, 84*, 310–318. doi: https://doi.org/10.1016/j.pec.2011.03.007.

Participants included 85 medical students; 37 received preclinical communication skills training, and 48 did not. Participants completed the JSE and a set of other measures on attitudes toward patient-centered care and communication skills learning before and after the training. Results showed no statistically significant change in JSE scores in those who participated in the communication skills training and their counterparts who did not.

Bond, A. R., Mason, H. F., Lemaster, C. M., Shaw, S. E., Mullin, C. S., Hollick, E. A., & Saper, R. B. (2013). Embodied health: The effects of mind-body course for medical students. *Medical Education Online, 18.*doi: https://doi.org/10.3402/meo.v18i0.20699.

Participants included 27 first- and second-year medical students at the Boston University School of Medicine, who participated in an 11-week elective embodied health course to enhance their well-being and mindfulness. They completed the JSE, and a few other tests before and after course. Although an increase in the JSE mean score was observed after completion of the course, the difference did not reach the conventional level of statistical significance. Significant improvements were observed in measures of self-regulation and self-compassion used in the study.

Brazeau, C. M. L. R., Schroeder, R., Rovi, S., & Boyd, L. (2011). Relationship between medical student service and empathy. *Academic Medicine, 86*, s42–s45. doi: https://doi.org/10.1097/ACM.0b013e31822a6ae0.

Participants included 462 medical students (51% women) from four classes at the UMDNJ-New Jersey Medical School, who completed the JSE at graduation. For two classes, the JSE was also administered at the beginning of medical school. Comparison of students who participated in service activities (such as a student-run free clinic to render patient care services) and those who did not showed that the former group obtained a significantly higher JSE mean score ($M=115.18$) than did the latter group ($M=107.97$) at graduation. It was also found that students who did not participate in any service activities had lower JSE scores both at the beginning and at the end of medical school. Women were more likely than men to participate in service activities (93% versus 78%, respectively), and women outscored men on the JSE ($M=116.12$ and $M=111.14$, respectively).

Buck, E., Holden, M. & Szauter, K. (2017). Changes in humanism during medical school: A synthesis of the evidence. *Medical Science Educator, 27,* 1–7. https://doi.org/10.1007/s40670-017-0438-9.

This review focused on longitudinal studies of medical students to answer two research questions: (1) Do components of humanism change over time in medical students? and (2) Do components of humanism respond to intervention? A systematic review of the literature for English language articles published between 2000 and 2014 was undertaken. Data extracted included the type of intervention included (deliberate programming vs. standard curriculum), and direction of change of the construct was assessed. Forty-eight studies from 22 journals were reviewed. Empathy was assessed in 37 (77%), humanism in 16 (33%), and altruism in 1 study.

Cataldo, K. P., Peeden, K., Geesey, M. E., & Dickerson, L. (2005). Association between Balint training and physician empathy and work satisfaction. *Family Medicine, 37*, 328–331. Accessible from: http://www.stfm.org/fmhub/fm2005/may/kari328.pdf.

Participants included 182 family physicians who graduated from the Medical University of South Carolina Family Medicine Residency Program. One group of residents voluntarily participated in the Balint training program (n=113), and another group did not (n=69). Mean score of the JSE for residents who participated in the Balint training program was higher (M=119.4, SD=8.9) than that for nonparticipants (M=116.7, SD=13.2), but the difference was not statistically significant. Also, no significant differences were found between the two groups on overall work satisfaction.

Chen, A., Hanna, J. J., Manohar, A., & Tobia, A. (2018). Teaching Empathy: The Implementation of a Video Game into a Psychiatry Clerkship Curriculum. *Academic Psychiatry: The Journal of the American Association of Directors of Psychiatric Residency Training and the Association for Academic Psychiatry*, *42*(3), 362–365. https://doi.org/10.1007/s40596-017-0862-6.

The purpose of this study was to investigate the use of the interactive video game, "That Dragon, Cancer," as a tool to teach empathy to third-year medical students. A modified JSE was administered to 84 third-year medical students in their psychiatry clerkship before and after they played and completed "That Dragon, Cancer." The majority of students agreed that learning empathy through video games was preferable and more effective than traditional didactics.

Chen, P. J., Huang, C. D., & Yeh, S. J. (2017). Impact of a narrative medicine program on healthcare providers' empathy scores over time. *BMC Medical Education*, *17*(1), 108. https://doi.org/10.1186/s12909-017-0952-x.

The purpose of this study was to investigate whether a narrative medicine (NM) program can improve healthcare providers' empathy. Research participants included 142 participants who attended the NM program, were divided into single (n = 58) and team groups (n = 84). Clinical empathy was measured by the Chinese version of JSE-Healthcare Providers Version (JSE-HP)—at three time points: prior to (Time 1), immediately after (T2), and 1.5 years (T3) after the program. Results showed an enhancement of empathy. Empathy scores increased after the NM program and were sustainable for 1.5 years. Further research is needed to examine gender difference as it might be that males and females respond differently to NM program intervention.

Chen, J. T., LaLopa, J., & Dang, D. K. (2008). Impact of patient empathy modeling on pharmacy students caring for the underserved. *American Journal of Pharmaceutical Education, 72*(2), Article 40.

Participants included 25 students at the School of Pharmacy and Pharmaceutical Sciences, Purdue University, and the University of Connecticut School of Pharmacy, who completed the JSE. They completed the patient empathy modeling assignment to enhance their attitudes toward caring for underserved patients. Comparisons of the JSE scores before and after completing the assignment showed statistically significant improvements in 16 out of 20 items of the JSE. The increase in the mean score of the JSE before (M=114, SD=9) and after completing the patient empathy modeling assignment (M=119.6, SD=10.5) was statistically significant. The pretest–posttest increase in the JSE mean score was 6.5 points for students at Purdue University, and it was 5.0 points for those at the University of Connecticut.

Croft, R. L., Byrd, C. T., & Kelly, E. M. (2022). The influence of active listening on parents' perceptions of clinical empathy in a stuttering assessment: A preliminary study. *Journal of Communication Disorders, 100*, 106274. https://doi.org/10.1016/j.jcomdis.2022.106274.

The purpose of this study was to explore whether a clinician's use of active listening skills (i.e., client-directed eye gaze and paraphrasing) influenced parents' perceptions of clinical empathy in a stuttering assessment. Research participants included 51 parents/guardians of children who stutter; they watched two counter-balanced videos of a clinician demonstrating either high or low frequency use of active listening skills during the clinician's initial assessment with a standardized patient actor portraying a parent of a child who stutters. After each video, parents rated the clinician's empathy and active listening skills via the Jefferson Scale of Physician Empathy for Observers (JSPEO; Hojat et al., 2017). Results demonstrated significantly higher ratings of perceived clinical empathy in the high frequency active listening condition compared to the low frequency ($d = 0.548$). Results of this study showed that the clinician was viewed as significantly more understanding, concerned, and caring (i.e., perceived as empathic) when they used active listening skills.

de Oliveira, R., Montagna, E., Zaia, V., Torres, B. B., & Barbosa, C. P. (2019). The Development of Cognitive and Affective Skills Through a Sexual and Reproductive Health Medical Education Unit. *Sexual Medicine, 7*(3), 326–336. https://doi.org/10.1016/j.esxm.2019.06.008.

The purpose of this study was to examine the structure and evaluation of a curricular unit that used an active teaching and learning strategy, and to evaluate both the cognitive and affective student learning outcomes. The JSE showed a high index of self-reported general empathy, with a significantly higher index for female students than male students; however, this gender difference disappeared after the intervention.

Dean, S., Foureur, M., Zaslawski, C., Newton-John, T., Yu, N., & Pappas, E. (2017). The effects of a structured mindfulness program on the development of empathy in healthcare students. *NursingPlus Open, 3,* 1–5. https://doi.org/10.1016/j.npls.2017.02.001.

The purpose of this study was to examine the effect of the Mindfulness-Based Empathy Training (MBET) program on nursing students' empathy and age discrimination. Research participants included 123 nursing students who were randomly assigned to two groups and completed the JSE. Experimental group received the MBET and the control group received no interventions. Results showed significant increase in the JSE scores in the experimental compared to the control group. This study indicated that empathy can be enhanced over an 8-week duration when mindfulness practices are integrated into a curriculum.

D'souza, P. C., Rasquinha, S. L., D'souza, T. L., Jain, A., Kulkarni, V., & Pai, K. (2020). Effect of a single-session communication skills training on empathy in medical students. *Academic Psychiatry: The Journal of the American Association of Directors of Psychiatric Residency Training and the Association for Academic Psychiatry, 44*(3), 289–294. https://doi.org/10.1007/s40596-019-01158-z.

The purpose of this study was to evaluate the change in empathy levels in medical students following a single-session communication skills training. Second-year medical students ($n = 82$) were randomized into intervention and control groups. The intervention consisted of a single-session empathetic communication skills training using PowerPoint, video clips, and roleplay. Empathy was assessed using the JSE S-Version at baseline, post-intervention (for the intervention group), and at follow-up after 3 weeks. Significant improvement post-intervention was observed. However, the score declined at the 3-week follow-up. The mean baseline JSE score of the control group declined at the follow-up. Though both groups showed a decline in the JSE score at follow-up, the decline was significant only for the control group, who did not receive the training. The study showed significant improvement immediately, and lower decline at follow-up, in empathy levels following a communication skills training.

du Vaure, C.B., Lemogne, C., Bunge, L., Catu-Pinault, A., Hoertel, N., Ghasarossian, C., Vincens, M. E., Galam, E., & Jaury, P. (2017). Promoting empathy among medical students: A two-site randomized controlled study. *Journal of Psychosomatic Research, 103*, 102–107. https://doi.org/10.1016/j.jpsychores.2017.10.008.

The purpose of this study was to assess the effects of Balint groups on empathy measured by the Consultation and Relational Empathy Measure (CARE) scale and self-rated JSE-Medical Student Version. A two-site randomized controlled trial was planned at Paris Diderot and Paris Descartes University, France. Research participants included fourth-year students, allocated in equal proportion to the intervention group (n = 155) or to the control group (n = 144). Participants in the intervention group received a training of 7 sessions of 1.5-hour Balint groups, over 3 months. The intervention group displayed significantly higher JSE score at follow-up than the control group. The JSE mean score increased from baseline to follow-up in the intervention group, whereas it decreased in the control group. It was concluded that Balint groups may contribute to promoting clinical empathy among medical students.

Duke, P., Grosseman, S., Novack, D. H., & Rosenzweig, S. (2015). Preserving third-year medical students' empathy and enhancing self-reflection using small group "virtual hangout" technology. *Medical Teacher, 37*, 566–571. doi: https://doi.org/10.3109/0142159X.2014.956057.

Participants included 259 third-year students (123 women) at the Drexel University College of Medicine, who were invited to participate in a faculty-facilitated, peer small group course of creating virtual classrooms by using social networking and online learning involving narrative self-reflection, group inquiry and discussion, and peer support. Participants completed the JSE and the Groningen Reflection Ability Scale (GRAS) before and after participation in the course. Results showed that empathy can be sustained after the course (reflected in the JSE scores), and self-reflection can be improved (reflected in the GRAS scores), suggesting that the course could prevent the erosion of empathy that has been observed in some other studies with third-year medical students, and can foster reflective ability.

Fernandez-Olano, C., Montoya-Fernandez, J., & Salinas-Sanchez, A. S. (2008). Impact of clinical interview training on the empathy level of medical students and medical residents. *Medical Teacher, 30*, 322–324. doi: https://doi.org/10.1080/01421590701802299.

Participants (203 total) included 137 second-year medical students at the University of Castilla-La Mancha, and 66 medical residents at the Family and Community Medicine Teaching Unit of Albacete, Spain. Participants were divided into experimental (82 students and 46 residents) and control groups (55 students and 20 residents). The experimental group participated in a 5-day (25 hours) communication skill training workshop. In the experimental group, significant increase in the JSE pretest–posttest mean scores was observed (from 119.5 to 125.1, effect size estimate = 0.78) among students and residents regardless of their gender. In the control group, no significant change in JSE mean scores was observed in residents; however, a slight increase in scores (from 118.4 to 119.1) was found in students in the control group.

*Forstater, A. T., Chauhan, N., Allen, A., Hojat, M., & Lopez, B. L. (2011). An emergency department shadowing experience for emergency medicine residents: Can it prevent the erosion of empathy? (Abstract). *Academic Emergency Medicine, 18*(10), s2.

Participants included 12 first-year emergency medicine residents at Thomas Jefferson University Hospital, who were randomly divided into experimental and control groups. Each resident in the experimental group shadowed one patient in the emergency department in the first month of residency training. The control group did not participate in shadowing and followed a routine training schedule. The JSE was completed by all residents 2 and 9 months after the shadowing experiment. No substantial difference was observed on the JSE scores between the two groups 2 months after the experiment; however, a larger decline in empathy scores was noticed in the control group (−7.2 points, effect size = 1.2) than in the experimental group (−2.7 points, effect size = 0.22), suggesting that the erosion of empathy may be prevented by shadowing experiences.

Fraiman, Y. S., Cheston, C., Michelson, C. D., & Sox, C. M. (2017). Pilot of a novel facilitator-friendly six-month mindfulness curriculum for interns. *Academic Pediatrics, 17*(5), e45. https://doi.org/10.1016/j.acap.2017.04.129.

The purpose of this study was to design and pilot a 6-month mindfulness curriculum during pediatric internship in order to assess feasibility and acceptability. This study implemented a 7-session mindfulness curriculum during the first 6 months of internship in a large pediatric residency program. Interns were invited to complete surveys that included the JSE, Maslach Burnout Inventory, 5-Facet Mindfulness Questionnaire, and items assessing resident knowledge, attitudes, and behaviors about mindfulness practice. Data were analyzed using chi-square and t-tests. All 50 interns participated in the curriculum, representing 100% response rate at baseline, and 6 months later response rate was 84%. Results showed 1) Improved attitudes toward mindfulness (69%); 2) Increased knowledge on how mindfulness impacts well-being (67%); 3) Increased knowledge on how to apply mindfulness in real-life (62%); and 4) Mindfulness training positively benefited their lives (62%). This novel 6-month mindfulness curriculum targeting physician trainees was feasible to implement during a busy pediatric internship.

Friedrich, B., Evans-Lacko, S., London, J., Rhydderch, D., & Henderson, C. (2013). Anti-stigma training for medical students: The Education not Discrimination project. *British Journal of Psychiatry, 202*, s89–s94. doi: https://doi.org/10.1192/bjp.bp.112.114017.

Participants included 1452 medical students (1066 in intervention group, 587 women; 386 in the control group, 216 women) in England. Students in the intervention group participated in an anti-stigma training called "Education not Discrimination" (END). Students completed JSE (four items), The Mental Health Knowledge Schedule (measuring stigma-related mental health knowledge), the Community Attitudes toward the Mentally Ill, and a measure of changes in behavior at the beginning of the program, immediate follow-up, and 6-month follow-up subsequent to the completion of the program. Results showed significant improvements immediately after the END training in the intervention group as compared to the control group, on measures of empathy, mental health knowledge, attitudes toward mentally ill, and the assessment of intended behavior. However, the improvement was not sustained for a longer time, measured 6 months following the intervention.

Ghetti, C., Chang, J., & Gosman, G. (2009). Burnout, psychological skills, and empathy: Balint training in obstetric and gynecology residents. *Journal of Graduate Medical Education, 1*, 231–235. doi: https://doi.org/10.4300/JGME-D-09-00049.1.

Participants included 17 obstetrics and gynecology residents who participated in a Balint training program and completed the JSE, the Maslach Burnout Inventory (MBI), and the Psychological Medicine Inventory before and after completing the program. Results showed no significant change in scores on the JSE and MBI; however, overall scores on the Psychological Medicine Inventory improved as a result of participation in the Balint program.

Gholamzadeh, S., Khastavaneh, M., Khademian, Z., & Ghadakpour, S. (2018). The effects of empathy skills training on nursing students' empathy and attitudes toward elderly people. *BMC Medical Education, 18*(1), 198. https://doi.org/10.1186/s12909-018-1297-9.

The purpose of this study was to investigate the effects of empathy skills training on nursing students' empathy and attitudes toward older adults. Research participants included 63 students at Nursing and Midwifery School in Yasuj, Iran, who were randomly divided into intervention and control groups. The intervention group attended an 8-hour workshop on empathy skills training that was presented through lectures, demonstration, group discussions, scenarios, and questioning. The data were collected using the Persian Jefferson Scale of Physician Empathy-Health Professional Version and the Kogan's Attitudes toward Old People Scale. The results showed that the empathy skills training program had a significant impact on the students' mean scores of empathy and attitudes toward older adults. Additionally, the empathy and attitude scores of the intervention group remained significantly higher than those in the control group immediately and 2 months after the intervention.

Graham, K. L., Green, S., Kurlan, R., & Pelosi, J. S. (2014). A patient-led educational program on Tourette Syndrome: Impact and implications for patient-centered medical education. *Teaching and Learning in Medicine*, *26*, 34–39. doi: https://doi.org/10.1080/10401334.2013.857339.

Participants included 79 medical residents (56 women) in five New Jersey hospitals, who completed the JSE (ten items of the Perspective-Taking factor) before and after participation in a patient-centered educational program by patient educators involving young patients with Tourette syndrome who were accompanied by their parent(s). Results of pretest–posttest comparison on the JSE scores showed a statistically significant increase in empathic perspective taking.

Gross, N., Nicolas, M., Neigher, S., McPartland, S., Heyes, M., Wrigley, S., & Kurlan, R. (2014). Planning a patient-centered Parkinson's disease support program: Insights from narrative medicine. *Advances in Parkinson's Disease*, *3*, 35–39. doi: https://doi.org/10.4236/apd.2014.34006. Accessible from: https://doi.org/10.4236/apd.2014.34006.

Participants included six health professionals (internist, neurologist, nurses, and speech therapist), six patients with Parkinson disease, and four of their caregivers. Health professionals participated in seven monthly sessions on improving their narrative skills, and completed the JSE before and after completing the narrative skill training sessions. Pretest–posttest scores on the JSE showed an improvement from $M = 120.67$ to $M = 126.00$. No inferential analysis was reported to test the significance of the difference due to a small sample size.

Harz, D., Begin, A. S., Alansari, R., Esparza, R., Zimmermann, C., Evans, B. D., Eisenberg, S., & Katz, J. T. (2023). The art of empathy: Teaching empathy through art. *The Clinical Teacher, 20*(5), e13643. https://doi.org/10.1111/tct.13643.

The aim of this study was to design and implement a virtual art-based curriculum focused on fostering empathy-The Art of Empathy. This novel curriculum used diverse art-based education methodologies to promote meticulous and collaborative observation and reflection, building on constructivism. Participants included 21 interns at the Brigham and Women's Hospital, who participated in the curriculum, while 34 served as control. Two instruments were used to measure empathy: the JSE and the Toronto Empathy Questionnaire (TEQ). Results showed The Art of Empathy curriculum promoted interns' reflections and actions toward empathy. This was partially supported by the quantitative data showing significantly higher scores on the "Compassionate Care" factor of the JSE, when compared with interns in the control group. The program participants appreciated the curriculum and valued its benefits.

Hogan, R., Rossiter, C., & Catling, C. (2018). Cultural empathy in midwifery students: Assessment of an education program. *Nurse Education Today, 70*, 103–108. https://doi.org/10.1016/j.nedt.2018.08.023.

The purpose of this study was to evaluate the effectiveness of an education program for midwifery students. Research participants included 55 students from all three years of an undergraduate midwifery program, who completed the JSE for health professions students, before and immediately after the education program, and also after 4 weeks subsequent to completion of the program. Results showed that midwifery students tended to have higher empathy scores than students in other health disciplines. The education workshop further increased participant's scores.

*Hojat, M., Axelrod, D., Spandorfer, J., & Mangione, S. (2013). Enhancing and sustaining empathy in medical students. *Medical Teacher, 35*, 996–1001. doi: https://doi.org/10.3109/0142159X.2013.802300.

Participants included 248 second-year medical students (126 women) at Jefferson (now Sidney Kimmel) Medical College, who were divided into experimental and control groups and participated in this two-phase study. In phase 1, students in the experimental group watched and discussed video clips of patient encounters meant to enhance empathic understanding; those in the control group watched a documentary film. Ten weeks later in phase 2 of the study, students who were in the experimental group were divided into two groups. One group attended a lecture on the importance of empathy in patient care, and the other plus those in the control group watched a movie about racism. The JSE was administered pre-test in phase 1 and posttest in phase 2. Results showed a statistically significant increase in the JSE mean scores for the experimental group in phase 1, from $M = 113.0$ (SD = 11.4) in pretest to $M = 115.2$ (SD = 12.3) in posttest. No significant change in the JSE scores was found in the control group. In phase 2 of the study, the JSE mean score improvement was sustained in the experimental group who attended the lecture on the importance of empathy in patient care, but not in the experimental group who watched a movie about racism in this phase of the study. Also, no significant change of empathy was observed in the control group in the second phase of the study. It is concluded that enhancement of empathy in medical students can be sustained by additional educational reinforcement.

Hsieh, N. K., Herzig, K., Gansky, S. A., & Danley, D. (2006). Changing dentists' knowledge, attitudes and behavior regarding domestic violence through an interactive multimedia tutorial. *Journal of American Dental Association, 137*, 596, 603.

Participants included 174 (40% women) practicing dentists (86 in the experimental and 88 in the control groups) who completed a slightly modified version of the JSE (adapted for dentists) and a survey of attitudes toward domestic violence in a randomized controlled trial. An educational tutorial was developed to help dentists with their roles in addressing domestic violence experienced by their patients. The experimental group completed the pretest JSE and the domestic violence survey at the baseline; was exposed to the tutorial; and subsequently completed the posttests to examine the impact of the tutorial. The control group completed the pretests, then the posttests, and was exposed to the tutorial after completing the posttests. Findings suggest that the tutorial could significantly improve dentists' knowledge of how to help patients affected by domestic violence, but had less effect on questions pertaining to their attitudes toward domestic violence. Scores on the JSE were significantly correlated with those from the domestic violence survey ($r=0.34$ in pretest; $r=0.40$ in posttest). Although women scored ($M=117.28$, SD = 11.02) higher than men ($M=114.33$, SD = 12.32), the difference was not statistically significant. The mean JSE score for total participants in pretest was 115.5 (SD = 11.87). No significant changes in the JSE pretest–posttest mean scores were found in the experimental and control groups.

Hu, S., & Lai, B. W. P. (2022). Increasing empathy for children in dental students using virtual reality. *International Journal of Paediatric Dentistry*, *32*(6), 793–800. https://doi.org/10.1111/ipd.12957.

The aim of this study was to evaluate the effect of virtual reality (VR) simulation on empathy and comfort managing children among dental students. Research participants included 60 dental students who completed the JSE and who experienced a VR scenario created for the study. Results indicated that all participants felt that the VR scenarios helped them better empathize with children. It is concluded that VR could be used to improve empathy, self-perceived comfort and ability at managing children in dental students.

Kazanowski, M., Perrin, K., Potter, M., & Sheehan, C. (2007). The silence of suffering: Breaking the sound barriers. *Journal of Holistic Nursing*, *25*, 195–203. doi: https://doi.org/10.1177/0898010107305501.

Participants included 30 nursing students who completed the JSE before and after a course on understanding suffering. Results showed a statistically significant increase in the JSE mean scores from $M=118.6$ (pretest) to $M=124.9$ (posttest).

Kelly, Cavanaugh. (2022). Improving Empathy of Occupational Therapy Students Through Reading Literary Narratives. *Journal of Occupational Therapy Education, 6*(4). https://doi.org/10.26681/jote.2022.060404.

This study explored the impact of teaching empathy to occupational therapy students through the reading of literary narratives. Study participants included 31 graduate-level rehabilitation students; it involved close reading and critical reflection of literary narratives course to improve their clinical empathy; and completion of the JSE (JSE) and the Reading the Mind in the Eyes Test (RMET). The pre and post-test comparison showed statistically significant improvement on the JSE. However, no differences were found between pre and post-test on the RMET.

Krishna Bahadur G. C., Arjyal, A., Douglas, A. H., Subedi, M., & Gongal, R. (2022). A quantitative evaluation of empathy using JSE-S Tool, before and after a Medical

Humanities Module, amongst first-year medical students in Nepal. *BMC Medical Education*, *22*(1), 159. https://doi.org/10.1186/s12909-022-03188-y.

This study was a quantitative evaluation of empathy before and after a Medical Humanities Module. Participants included 62 first-year medical students in Nepal, who completed the JSE-S prior to completion of a 6-week Medical Humanities Module. Findings showed that women were more likely to obtain higher empathy scores than men, and those who preferred people-oriented specialities scored higher than those preferring procedure and technology-oriented specialities. There was a significant increase in mean score for the entire class from pre-module to post-module (increase from $M = 105$ to $M = 116$, $p < 0.001$). This study provides evidence of the impact of a Medical Humanities course in increasing medical student clinical empathy in Nepal.

Lemogne, C., Buffel du Vaure, C., Hoertel, N., Catu-Pinault, A., Limosin, F., Ghasarossian, C., Le Jeunne, C., & Jaury, P. (2020). Balint groups and narrative medicine compared to a control condition in promoting students' empathy. *BMC Medical Education*, *20*(1), 412. https://doi.org/10.1186/s12909-020-02316-w.

This study aimed to assess the effects of Balint groups and narrative medicine training on clinical empathy. Research participants included 392 medical students who completed the JSE-S. Participants were randomly assigned into a Balint group, a narrative medicine group, and a control group. The change in JSE mean score from baseline to follow-up was significantly higher in the Balint group than in narrative and control groups. The change in JSE mean score in the narrative medicine group did not significantly differ from the changes in the control group or the Balint group. Balint groups remained associated with better outcomes compared to the control group. It was concluded that the Balint group may promote clinical empathy to some extent among medical students, at least in the short run.

Lim, B. T., Moriarty, H., & Huthwaite, M. (2011). "Being-in-role": A teaching innovation to enhance empathy communication skills in medical students. *Medical Teacher, 33*, e663–e669. doi: https://doi.org/10.3109/0142159X2011.611193.

Participants included 149 medical students (84 women) at the University of Otago, Wellington School of Medicine and Health Sciences in New Zealand. They were divided into an intervention ($n=77$) and a control group ($n=72$). All students participated in seminars and workshops in the Psychological Medicine course. The intervention group participated in an additional one-hour actor-facilitated teaching innovation, i.e., a "how to act-in-role" workshop, focusing on enhancing the participants' capacity to connect with the patients. The JSE was completed by students before and after the course. The Behavioral Change Counselling Index (BECCI) to assess students' competence in consultation was completed by students and tutors. Also, assessments were made using the Objective Structured Clinical Examination (OSCE) by tutors and students. Results showed no significant difference on the JSE pretest scores between the intervention and control groups; however, a statistically significant difference in posttest was observed on the JSE between the two groups in favor of the intervention group. The intervention group obtained significantly higher tutor ratings on the BECCI and in overall OSCE performances. Findings suggest that teaching "how to act-in-role" was effective not only in increasing medical students' self-reported empathy but also their competence in consultation skills.

Lin, I. H., Wang, C. Y., Lin, Y. N., Chen, H. C., & Lin, L. F. (2022). Simulation-based holistic education in physiotherapy interns to increase empathy toward older adults and individuals with disabilities. *BMC Geriatrics*, *22*(1), 795. https://doi.org/10.1186/s12877-022-03500-x.

This study investigated the effect of simulation-based, holistic health-care education on physiotherapy interns' empathy, attitudes, and knowledge. Participants included 30 physiotherapy interns (15 in experimental group and 15 in control group). Both groups received standard clinical training. However, the experimental group received an additional simulation-based holistic health-care education. The JSE was administered pretest and posttest. Results showed substantial between-group differences on the JSE. Simulation-based, holistic health-care education can significantly improve empathy.

Logan, A., Yule, E., Hughes, J., Peters, D., Hadley, M., Betts, B., Jones, L., & Froude, E. (2022). The impact of face-to-face mental health consumer-led teaching on occupational therapy student empathy levels: Two-group comparison design. *Australian Occupational Therapy Journal, 69*(6), 703–713. https://doi.org/10.1111/1440-1630.12833.

The aim of this study was to investigate if occupational therapy students who received teaching from a mental health consumer demonstrated higher levels of empathy compared with students who received teaching delivered by occupational therapy academics. Research participants included 217 occupational therapy students randomly assigned into two groups ("consumer-led teaching tutorial" and "usual teaching"). The JSE was used to measure student empathy. Little difference in empathy scales was detected between groups. The challenge for future research is to identify appropriate ways to measure the impact of mental health consumer involvement on occupational therapy curriculum and students.

Lwow, M., Canetti, L., & Muszkat, M. (2020). Gender differences in the effect of medical humanities program on medical students' empathy: a prospective longitudinal study. *BMC Medical Education, 20*(1), 413. https://doi.org/10.1186/s12909-020-02333-9.

The aim of this study was to examine changes in medical students' empathy during their first clinical experience, and to determine the impact of gender and humanities curriculum on empathy changes. Research participants included 262 fourth-year students who completed the JSE-S. Results showed that female students showed no decline in empathy during the fourth year of medical school, regardless of the type of humanities program they were exposed to.

MacLean, H., Braschi, E., Archibald, D., Sanchez-Campos, M., Jebanesan, D., Koszycki, D., & Gonsalves, C. (2020). A pilot study of a longitudinal mindfulness curriculum in undergraduate medical education. *Canadian Medical Education Journal, 11*(4), e5–e18. https://doi.org/10.36834/cmej.56726.

The purpose of this study was to assess outcomes of a mindfulness program for medical students, who completed the JSE, the Freiburg Mindfulness Inventory, the Connor–Davidson Resilience Scale, and the Perceived Stress Scale. Results indicated that scores of mindfulness correlated positively with those for empathy ($r = 0.22$, $p < 0.01$) and resilience ($r = 0.549$, $p < 0.01$), and negatively with stress scores ($r = -0.38$, $p < 0.01$). Statistically significant increases were observed in empathy, mindfulness, and resilience scores with a trend toward lower stress scores in students who felt they applied the curriculum principles. Findings suggest that a mindfulness curriculum integrated into formal undergraduate medical education is feasible; however, benefits may be confined to those students who apply curriculum principles and practice regularly.

*Magee, M., & Hojat, M. (2010). Rocking chair and empathy: A pilot study [Letter to the editor]. *Family Medicine, 42*, 466–467.

Participants included 57 residents from 16 family medicine residency programs, who completed the pretest JSE; 18 of them completed the JSE posttest. Residents were given the opportunity in the second year of their training to choose one of their indigent pregnant patients who was in the second trimester of pregnancy to receive the free gift of a glider rocking chair. Shortly after the baby was born, in postpartum period, ten of the residents made a prearranged home visit to the mother of the newborn to assist in assembling the chair while talking with the mother in a friendly manner about child care and well-being. Compared to the residents who did not make such a home visit, the simple home visit experience contributed to an impressive increase of about one standard deviation unit in posttest JSE scores among those residents who made such a home visit.

Mathad, M. D., Pradhan, B., & Sasidharan, R. K. (2017). "Effect of Yoga on Psychological Functioning of Nursing Students: A Randomized Wait List Control Trial." *Journal of Clinical and Diagnostic Research: JCDR, 11*(5), KC01–KC05. https://doi.org/10.7860/JCDR/2017/26517.9833.

The purpose of this study was to evaluate the effectiveness of an 8-week yoga intervention on psychological functioning of nursing students. Research participants included 100 nursing students who completed the JSE-HPS. The results showed that the intervention was significantly effective in improving self-compassion and mindfulness among study participants.

McManus, S., Killeen, D., Hartnett, Y., Fitzgerald, G., & Murphy, K. C. (2020). Establishing and evaluating a Balint group for fourth-year medical students at an Irish University. *Irish Journal of Psychological Medicine, 37*(2), 99–105. https://doi.org/10.1017/ipm.2019.28.

The purpose of this study was to evaluate the impact of a Balint group on empathy and resilience in fourth-year medical students during their psychiatry rotation. The JSE-Student Version and the Brief Resilience Scale were completed by research participants pre-post participation in the Balint groups. Participating students also completed a qualitative assessment of their experience. Results showed that the implementation of the Balint group for fourth-year medical students was successful in increasing empathy. Students also reported a positive view of Balint and its beneficial role.

*Misra-Hebert, A. D., Isaacson, J. H., Kohn, M., Hull, A. L., Hojat, M., Papp, K. K., & Calabrese, L. (2012). Improving empathy of physicians through guided reflective writing. *International Journal of Medical Education, 3*, 71–77. doi: https://doi.org/10.5116/ijme.4f7e.e332.

Participants included 40 staff physicians at the Cleveland Clinic, who completed the JSE. Twenty physicians were assigned to participate in a six-session program on narrative medicine and engagement in guided reflective writing (intervention group). Ten physicians received the assigned course reading materials but did not participate in the course sessions (control group 1), and ten physicians neither received the reading materials nor participated in the course sessions. Quantitative and qualitative analyses showed improvements in the intervention group compared to the two control groups. Mean scores on the JSE, which was administered three times—at the beginning, at session four of the program, and at the completion of the program—showed steady improvement in the intervention group (117.0, 120.7, and 124.6, respectively) compared to control group 1 (114.6, 116.2, and 110.8, respectively) and control group 2 (118.7, 116.2, and 118.9, respectively). Qualitative analyses of physicians' reflective writings in the intervention group showed compassionate solidarity and empathic concern and more exploration of negative rather than positive emotions.

Potash, J. S., Chen, J. Y., Lam, C. L., & Chau, V. T. (2014). Art-making in a family medicine clerkship: How does it affect medical student empathy? *BMC Medical Education*, *14*, 247. doi: https://doi.org/10.1186/s12909-014-0247-4. Accessible from: www.biomedcentral.com/1472-6920/14/247.

Participants included 161 third-year medical students at the University of Hong Kong, who were randomly divided into experimental and control groups in their family medicine clerkship. Students in the experimental group participated in a workshop on arts-making, involving in writing poems, creating art works, and writing reflective essays. Those in the control group were involved with clinical problem-solving. Students in both groups completed the JSE before and after the workshops. Results showed a decrease in the mean scores on the JSE in both groups. For students in the experimental group, the difference between pretest ($M=106.6$, SD = 12.4) and posttest ($M=102.2$, SD = 14.3) was statistically significant. However, in the control group, the pretest ($M=107.2$, SD = 11.5) posttest ($M=106.6$, SD = 14.7) difference did not reach the level of statistical significance. No significant association was found between JSE scores and students' gender and age.

Pratiwi, H., Kristina, S. A., Widayanti, A. W., & Prabandari, Y. S. (2022). Educational Interventions to Improve Pharmacy Students' Empathy Towards Geriatrics: A Systematic Review. *Indonesian Journal of Pharmacy*, *33*(2), 174–185. https://doi.org/10.22146/ijp.3837.

The purpose of this systematic review was to evaluate and synthesize studies about educational interventions that improve the empathy of pharmacy students toward geriatrics. Three databases, PubMed, Science Direct, and Google Scholar, were searched for articles that included educational interventions and focused on outcome measures related to improving empathy toward geriatrics. The Medical Education Research Study Quality Instrument (MERSQI) was used to assess the possibility of bias. The Preferred Reporting Items for Systematic Reviews and Meta-Analyses (PRISMA) guidelines were also used in this review. Of the nine included studies, eight studies had quasi-experimental pretest–posttest measurement design. Eight studies reported a statistically significant increase in empathy toward geriatrics. It was concluded that educational intervention could help pharmacy students develop empathy for older adults.

Quail, M., Brundage, S. B., Spitalnick, J., Allen, P. J., & Beilby, J. (2016). Student self-reported communication skills, knowledge and confidence across standardised patient, virtual and traditional clinical learning environments. *BMC Medical Education*, *16*, 73. https://doi.org/10.1186/s12909-016-0577-5.

This study investigated students' communication skills, knowledge, confidence, and empathy across simulated and traditional learning environments. Undergraduate speech pathology students were randomly allocated to one of three communication partners with whom they engaged conversationally for up to 30 mins: a patient in a nursing home ($n = 21$), an older adult trained patient actor ($n = 22$), or a virtual patient ($n = 21$). One week prior to, and again following the conversational interaction, participants completed the JSE-HPS. Results showed that students interacting with a nursing home resident reported higher empathy. Students reported that conversing with the virtual patient was more challenging than conversing with a nursing home patient or actor.

Riess, H., Kelley, J., Bailey, R., Dunn, E., & Phillips, M. (2012). Empathy training for resident physicians: A randomized controlled trial of a neuroscience-informed curriculum. *Journal of General Internal Medicine, 27*, 1280–1286. doi: https://doi.org/10.1007/s11606-012.2063-z.

Participants included 99 residents and fellows (52% women) in surgery, medicine, anesthesiology, psychiatry, ophthalmology, and orthopedics, who were randomly assigned to the intervention ($n=54$) and control groups ($n=45$). Physicians in the intervention group participated in a postgraduate medical education program grounded in the neurobiology of empathy, and those in the control group followed the standard residency or fellowship training. Participants completed the JSE, the Ekman Facial Decoding Test, and the Balanced Emotional Empathy Scale (BEES). Each participating physician was assessed by multiple patients using the Consultation and Relational Empathy (CARE) scale, measuring empathy in the context of medical consultation. Results showed statistically significant differences in favor of the intervention group on CARE scale and Ekman Facial Decoding Test. Changes observed on the JSE and BEES in the intervention and control groups were not statistically significant.

Riess, H., Kelley, J. M., Bailey, R., Konowitz, P. M., & Gray, S. T. (2011). Improving empathy and relational skills in otolaryngology residents: A pilot study. *Otolaryngology-Head and Neck Surgery, 144*, 120–122. doi: https://doi.org/10.1177/0194599810390897.

Participants included 11 otolaryngology residents (43% women) who completed the JSE, the Balanced Emotional Empathy Scale (BEES), the Ekman Facial Decoding Test, and the Consultation and Relational Empathy (CARE). They participated in a brief series of empathy training sessions to increase their knowledge of the neurology and physiology of empathy as well as their self-reported empathy. Patients also rated physicians on the CARE at the baseline and completion of training. Pretest–posttest scores on all measures showed an increase in the expected direction. The change of the JSE mean scores before training was 110.1 (SD = 10.8), and after training it increased to 114.3 (SD = 10.7). However, the difference was not statistically significant. Also, increases in mean scores on the BEES and Ekman Facial Decoding Test were not significant. Pretest–posttest difference on physician-reported CARE mean scores reached the level of statistical significance ($p<0.01$). However, no statistically significant increase was obtained in patient-reported CARE scores.

Robertson, A. D., Moore, M., McFadden, L., Steere, E. L., Barnes, J., & Shrader, S. (2022). Implementation and evaluation of simulations in a required course to improve empathy of pharmacy students. *Currents in Pharmacy Teaching & Learning, 14*(11), 1404–1410. https://doi.org/10.1016/j.cptl.2022.09.021.

The purpose of this study was to examine the effect of a course enhancement consisting of formal instruction and application-based simulations on empathy in pharmacy students. The JSE-HPS was administered at the start of the semester and again at the end of the 16-week required course for third-year pharmacy students. A combination of didactic and skills-based training led to an improvement in empathy in pharmacy students. Student comments highlighted the value of practicing empathy skills in a simulated environment.

Rosenzweig, J., Blaizot, A., Cougot, N., Pegon-Machat, E., Hamel, O., Apelian, N., Bedos, C., Munoz-Sastre, M. T., & Vergnes, J. N. (2016). Effect of a Person-Centered Course on the Empathic Ability of Dental Students. *Journal of Dental Education, 80*(11), 1337–1348. https://doi.org/10.1002/j.0022-0337.2016.80.11.tb06219.x.

A controlled study was conducted with fourth-year dental students in four dental faculties in France. The experimental group (n = 63) received 20 hours of person-centered care

(PCC) training, including arts-based approaches, narrative dentistry activities, and workshops on communication. There was no change in the curriculum of the control group ($n = 217$). Pretest and posttest measures with the JSE, and Toronto Empathy Questionnaire (TEQ) were compared for the two groups. The results showed no significant differences on the TEQ or JSE. Findings suggest that PCC training constitutes a promising approach to developing dental students' empathic ability, but there is a need to assess the effects of such training over longer periods.

Runyan, C., Savageau, J. A., Potts, S., & Weinreb, L. (2016). Impact of a family medicine resident wellness curriculum: a feasibility study. *Medical Education Online*, *21*, 30648. https://doi.org/10.3402/meo.v21.30648.

The purpose of this study was to evaluate the impact of a new, 1-month wellness curriculum for 12 second-year family medicine residents on burnout, empathy, stress, and self-compassion. Cultivation of mindfulness and self-compassion in order to enhance empathy and reduce stress was the focus. Pre-test and 3-month follow-up post-test on measures of burnout, empathy, self-compassion, and perceived stress were used to evaluate the impact of the curriculum. Results showed positive trends using measures applied in the study, including the JSE.

San-Martín, M., Delgado-Bolton, R., & Vivanco, L. (2017). Role of a Semiotics-Based Curriculum in Empathy Enhancement: A Longitudinal Study in Three Dominican Medical Schools. *Frontiers in Psychology*, *8*, 2018. https://doi.org/10.3389/fpsyg.2017.02018.

The purpose of this study was to determine if in medical schools the empathic orientation of medical students improves as a consequence of the acquisition and development of students' communication skills that are required in clinician–patient encounters. This quasi-experimental study was undertaken in three medical schools in the Dominican Republic, which offer three different medical curricula: (i) a theoretical and practical semiotic-based curriculum; (ii) a theoretical semiotic-based curriculum; and (iii) a curriculum without semiotic courses. The JSE was administered in two different times to students enrolled in preclinical phase of medical school education. Results confirmed that gender, age, and a semiotic-based curriculum contributed toward the enhancement of empathy.

Schwartz, B. D., Horst, A., Fisher, J. A., Michels, N., & Van Winkle, L. J. (2020). Fostering Empathy, Implicit Bias Mitigation, and Compassionate Behavior in a Medical Humanities Course. *International Journal of Environmental Research and Public Health*, *17*(7), 2169. https://doi.org/10.3390/ijerph17072169.

It was hypothesized that selecting and performing service-learning projects by teams of prospective medical students in a Medical Humanities course would foster students' compassion by raising their reflective capacity, empathy, and unconscious bias mitigation. In this study, teams wrote individual and team critical reflections on these class discussions and their service-learning experiences. Research participants included 32 students who completed the JSE and Reflective Practice Questionnaire before and after the course. The students reported changes in their behavior to mitigate biases and become more compassionate, and their reflective capacity and empathy grew in association with discussions and team service-learning experiences in the course.

Schweller, M., Costa, F. O., Antônio, M. Â., Amaral, E. M., & de Carvalho-Filho, M. A. (2014). The impact of simulated medical consultations on the empathy levels of students at one medical school. *Academic Medicine*, *89*, 632–637.

Participants included 124 fourth-year and 123 sixth-year medical students at the State University of Campinas in Brazil, who participated in a simulated medical consultation involving simulated patients in four clinical situations followed by debriefing discussions. Participants completed a Brazilian translation of the JSE and the Interpersonal Reactivity Index (IRI) before and after simulated medical consultation experiences. Results of comparing pre–post simulated medical consultations experiences showed statistically significant increases in scores on the JSE in fourth-year students ($M = 115.8$, SD = 8.8 pretest, and $M = 121.1$, SD = 8.6 posttest, effect size = 0.61) and in sixth-year students ($M = 117.1$, SD = 10.0 pretest, and $M = 123.5$, SD = 9.9 posttest, effect size = 0.64). Also, statistically significant pretest–posttest improvements were observed in the IRI scores, but with smaller effect sizes (effect size for the fourth-year students was 0.19, and for sixth-year students was 0.20).

Sheehan, C. A., Perrin, K. O., Potter, M. L., Kazanowski, M. K., & Bennett, L. A. (2013). Engendering empathy in baccalaureate nursing students. *International Journal of Caring Sciences, 6*, 456–464.

Participants included 99 baccalaureate nursing students who participated in an elective course on understanding suffering and completed the JSE before and after participating in the course. Results showed a significant increase in the JSE mean score (from $M = 116.96$ in pretest to $M = 123.97$ in posttest) for the total participants.

Souror, Y. R., Aljehani, D. K., & Alshaikh, M. H. (2020). Empathy of dental students towards children after behaviour guidance lectures and clinical experience. *European Journal of Dental Education: Official Journal of the Association for Dental Education in Europe*, *24*(3), 458–464. https://doi.org/10.1111/eje.12523.

A modified form of the JSE-HPS was administered to 65 dental students in two rounds: (R1) before and (R2) after introducing behavior guidance course and exposure to 3 clinical experiences with children to measure changes in empathy of dental students toward child patients. The modifications include replacing the "patient" words with "child patients" and translation into Arabic. Results showed a significant decrease in the empathy of dental students in R2 compared to R1. The level of empathy for men was lower than women in both rounds. It is suggested that a specific training course is needed to improve dental students' empathy toward children.

Srivastava, A. K., Tiwari, K., Vyas, S., Semwal, J., & Kandpal, S. D. (2017). Teaching clinical empathy to undergraduate medical students of Dehradun: A quasi-experimental study. *Indian Journal of Community Health*, *29*(3), 258–263. https://doi.org/10.47203/IJCH.2017.v29i03.008.

The purpose of this study was to evaluate any change in empathy level of undergraduate medical students after an interactive audio-visual teaching session on clinical empathy, using a pretest–posttest quasi-experimental design. Research participants included 328 undergraduate medical students who completed the JSE-S before and one month after an interactive audio-visual teaching session on clinical empathy. Results showed a statistically significant improvement in overall mean empathy scores with a large effect size (Cohen's d = 1.1).Statistically significant improvement in empathy level was seen irrespective of gender, age, year, and area of interest for future specialty with large effect sizes. Clinical empathy can be improved during the years of medical education by specifically designed interventions.

Tamayo, C. A., Rizkalla, M. N., & Henderson, K. K. (2016). Cognitive, behavioral and emotional empathy in pharmacy students: targeting programs for curriculum modification. *Frontiers in Pharmacology*, 7, 96. https://doi.org/10.3389/fphar.2016.00096.

The purpose of this study was to parse the underlying components of empathy and correlate them to psychosocial attributes, with the overall goal of identifying curriculum modifications to enhance levels of empathy in pharmacy students. The study survey included the JSE and questions regarding demographics and personality traits. Overall, empathy levels in pharmacy students were similar to prior studies with women scoring higher than men. It was concluded that targeted educational programs that promote volunteerism and activities that foster responsiveness to patient needs may attenuate self-serving behavior and medical authoritarianism and, therefore, improve empathy levels in pharmacy students.

Van Winkle, L. J., Bjork, B. C., Chandar, N., Cornell, S., Fjortoft, N., Green, J. M., La Salle, S., Lynch, S. M., Viselli, S. M., & Burdick, P. (2012). Interprofessional workshop to improve mutual understanding between pharmacy and medical students. *American Journal of Pharmaceutical Education*, *76*(8), Article 150. Accessible from: http://www.ncbi.nlm.nih.gov/pmc/articles/PMC3475779/.

Participants included 215 first-year pharmacy students and 205 first-year osteopathic medical students at Midwestern University, who completed the JSE and the Scale of Empathy Toward Physician-Pharmacist Collaboration and participated in an interprofessional development workshop. Results showed that interprofessional collaboration scores of pharmacy students who participated in the workshop increased significantly, and medical students' scores increased on the factor of shared education of interprofessional collaboration. The collaboration scores of pharmacy students exceeded those of medical students. Statistically significant correlations between scores on the JSE and the Scale of Physician-Pharmacy Collaboration were found in pharmacy students ($r=0.42$) as well as medical students ($r=0.38$).

Van Winkle, L. J., Burdick, P., Bjork, B. C., Chandar, N., Green, J. M., Lynch, S. M., La Salle, S., Viselli, S. M., & Robson, C. (2014). Critical thinking and reflection on community service for a medical biochemistry course raise students' empathy, patient-centered orientation, and examination scores. *Medical Science Educator, 24*, 279–290. doi: https://doi.org/10.1007/s40670-014-0049-7.

Participants included 204 first-year osteopathic medical students (45% women) at Midwestern University, who were required to complete a team community project (such as visiting elderly patients with heart failure, diabetes, etc.) and prepare written reports for group discussion. The JSE and Patient-Practitioner Orientation Scale (PPOS) were administered to the students before and after their community service project was completed. Statistical analyses of pretest–posttest data showed a significant increase in the JSE scores, and the PPOS total and Caring subscale scores as a result of participation in the community service program.

*Van Winkle, L. J., Fjortoft, N., & Hojat, M. (2012). Impact of a workshop about aging on the empathy scores of pharmacy and medical students. *American Journal of Pharmaceutical Education, 76*(1), Article 9. doi: https://doi.org/10.5688/ajpe7619. Accessible from: http://www.ncbi.nlm.nih.gov/pmc/articles/PMC3298407/.

Participants included 370 first-year pharmacy students ($n=187$) at the Chicago College of Pharmacy, Midwestern University, and medical students ($n=183$) at the Chicago College of Osteopathic Medicine, Midwestern University, who completed the JSE and participated in a workshop in which they observed and discussed a 10-min theatrical performance by their classmates who were coached to enact problems and concerns of elderly patients. Comparisons of the JSE scores before and immediately after the workshop showed a significant increase in medical students (from $M=112.9$, SD=10.9 to $M=115.0$, SD=11.9) and pharmacy students (from $M = 110.9$, SD = 12.2 to $M = 113.2$, SD = 13.5). However, follow-up assessments showed that the improvement in empathy scores did not sustain for a longer time after the workshop (26 days after the workshop for medical students: $M = 112.7$, SD = 13.9; and 7 days after the workshop for pharmacy students: $M = 110.5$, SD = 17.3). Pattern of findings was similar for men and women.

Van Winkle, L. J., La Salle, S., Richardson, L., Bjork, B. C., Burdick, P., Chandar, N., Green, J. M., Lynch, S. M., Robson, C., & Viselli, S. M. (2013). Challenging medical students to confront their biases: A case study simulation approach. *Medical Science Educator, 23*, 217–224.

Study participants included 205 first-year osteopathic medical students (47% women) at Midwestern University, who completed the JSE on five occasions. Students watched a play of a simulated patient in prison during a 50-min workshop of a case of biochemical fatigue. Students were expected to relate this patient with a book, "The Immoral Life of Henrietta Lacks," as a required reading at the beginning of medical school to identify biases through critical reflection. No statistically significant differences on the total scores on the JSE were found before or after students' participation in the workshop; however, statistically significant increase in the score of one item of the JSE (on attention to patients' emotions in history taking) was observed after participation in the workshop, which was sustained through the study time period.

Verweij, H., Waumans, R. C., Smeijers, D., Lucassen, P. L., Donders, A. R., van der Horst, H. E., & Speckens, A. E. (2016). Mindfulness-based stress reduction for GPs: results of a controlled mixed methods pilot study in Dutch primary care. *The British Journal of General Practice: The Journal of the Royal College of General Practitioners*, 66(643), e99–e105. https://doi.org/10.3399/bjgp16X683497.

The purpose of this study was to gain insight into the feasibility and effectiveness of the Mindfulness-Based Stress Reduction (MBSR) program on burnout, empathy, and (work-related) well-being in GPs in the Netherlands. Participants included 50 Dutch GPs; empathy was measured by the JSE in a pretest–posttest design. Experimental group participated in the MBSR program and control group in the waiting list. Results showed that the MBSR group had a greater decrease in depersonalization than the control group. There was no significant change in empathy. The MBSR course increased their well-being and compassion toward themselves and others, including their patients. The study showed that MBSR for GPs is feasible and might result in fewer burnout symptoms and increased work engagement and well-being.

Weisse, C. S., Melekis, K., & Hutchins, B. (2019). Providing end-of-life care: increased empathy and self-efficacy among student caregivers in residential homes for the dying. *The American Journal of Hospice & Palliative Care, 36*(6), 538–545. https://doi.org/10.1177/1049909118820844.

The study purpose was to evaluate the effectiveness of a Community Action, Research, and Education (CARE) program for promoting empathy and self-efficacy communicating with and caring for terminally ill patients. This study collected pre-post data from 18 undergraduates in an 8-week immersive program where they served as primary caregivers in residential homes for the dying, providing 200 hours of bedside care to hospice patients during their final days. The JSE-HP was completed by research participants. Results revealed significant increases in empathy and self-efficacy to provide end-of-life care. It was concluded that community-run residential homes for the dying offer a unique opportunity for skills training in end-of-life care.

West, C. P., Dyrbye, L. N., Rabatin, J. T., Call, T. G., Davidson, J. H., Multari, A., Romanski, S. A., Henriksen Hellyer, J. M., Sloan, J. A., & Shanafelt, T. D. (2014). Intervention to promote physician well-being, job satisfaction, and professionalism: A randomized clinical trial. *JAMA Internal Medicine, 174*, 527–533. doi: https://doi.org/10.1001/jamainternmed.2013.14387.

Participants included 74 physicians in this clinical trial in the Department of Medicine at the Mayo Clinic in Rochester, Minnesota; 37 were assigned to the intervention arm, and 37 to the control arm. There were also 350 nontrial physicians who responded to annual surveys timed to coincide with the trial surveys. Physicians in the intervention arm of the clinical trial group participated in 19 biweekly facilitated physician discussions incorporating elements of mindfulness, reflection, and shared experiences. The JSE and a set of other instruments were administered to the physicians before starting, during, and after the trial. No statistically significant change was observed in the JSE scores, or measures of stress, symptoms of depression, overall quality of life, job satisfaction, fatigue, and mental and physical well-being. Comparisons on physicians who volunteered to participate in the trail with the nontrial cohort showed that rates of burnout dropped substantially in the trial intervention arm, declined slightly in the trial control arm, but increased in the nontrial cohort. No other significant changes were observed between trial and nontrial physicians.

Williams, B., Brown, T., & McKenna, L. (2013). DVD empathy simulations: An interventional study. *Medical Education, 47*, 1142–1143.

Participants included 293 health professions students (226 women) from four Australian universities, who participated in empathy-oriented DVD simulation workshops. Participants completed the JSE before and after the workshops. Results showed a statistically significant increase in the JSE (from 114.34 before to 120.32 after participation in the workshops).

Williams, B., Brown, T., McKenna, L., Palermo, C., Morgan, P., … Wright, C. (2015). Student empathy levels across 12 medical and health professions: An interventional study. *Journal of Compassionate Health Care, 2*, 4 (open access). doi: https://doi.org/10.1186/s40639-015-0013-4.

Participants included 239 students from 12 different medical and healthcare professions from four universities in Australia, who completed the JSE pretest–posttest intervention. Intervention included watching a 20-min DVD simulation showing a teenager with Asperger syndrome, a young pregnant woman suffering from stroke, and an elderly indigenous woman suffering from a suspected neck of femur fracture. Results showed a statistically significant improvement in the JSE scores as a result of participation in the workshop from a mean scores of 114.39 (SD = 14.56) in pretest to 120.56 (SD = 12.48) in posttest (effect size = 0.22). Women outscored men in pretest and posttest.

Williams, B., Sadasivan, S., Kadirvelu, A., & Olaussen, A. (2014). Empathy level among first year Malaysian medical students: An observational study. *Advances in Medical Education and Practice, 5*,149–156. doi: https://doi.org/10.2147/AMEP.S58094.

Participants included 122 first-year students (56% women) at the Jeffrey Cheah School of Medicine and Health Sciences in Malaysia, who participated in a workshop to enhance empathic awareness by watching and discussing a video involving a pregnant patient suffering from a stroke. The JSE was completed by participants before and five weeks after the workshop. Results showed a statistically significant improvement in mean score of the JSE from 112.08 (SD = 10.76) before to 117.93 (SD = 13.13) after the workshop (effect size = 0.48). Women were influenced by the workshop more than men (effect size = 0.54). Cronbach's alpha coefficient for this Malaysian sample was 0.70 before and 0.83 after the workshop.

Worly, B. (2013). Professionalism education of OB/GYN resident physicians: What makes a difference? *Open Journal of Obstetrics and Gynecology*, *3*, 137–141. doi: https://doi.org/10.4236/ojog.2013.31A026.

Participants included 32 obstetrics and gynecology residents at Thomas Jefferson University Hospital, who participated in a new professionalism program involving narrative medicine training and a professional development/support group. Twenty residents completed the JSE, the Jefferson Scale of Attitudes Toward Physician-Nurse Collaboration, and the Barry Challenges to Professionalism Questionnaire. Comparisons of scores pre and post program showed no statistically significant changes on the JSE and on the Barry Questionnaire. A significant decline in scores on attitudes toward physician-nurse collaboration was observed.

Yaghmaei, M., Monajemi, A., & Soltani-Arabshahi, K. (2014). The effect of storytelling course on medical students' empathy toward patients. *International Journal of Body, Mind & Culture, 1*, 127–134.

Study participants included 41 medical students at the Zahedan University of Medical Sciences in Iran (16 in the experimental and 25 in the control group). Students in the experimental group participated in ten sessions of storytelling, each lasting two hours in which stories from books and literature about human illness, pain, and suffering, selected by the researchers were described and discussed. Students in both groups completed the JSE before and after the experiment. Those in the experimental groups gained less than one point on the JSE (pretest mean score = 106.7, SD = 12.78; posttest mean score = 107.6, SD = 11.32); but the JSE mean score declined 5.68 points in the control group (pretest mean score = 105.8, SD = 15.24; posttest mean score = 100.12, SD = 14.04). However, the pretest–posttest changes in empathy scores were not statistically significant.

Yamada, Y., Fujimori, M., Shirai, Y., Ninomiya, H., Oka, T., & Uchitomi, Y. (2018). Changes in physicians' intrapersonal empathy after a communication skills training in Japan. *Academic Medicine: Journal of the Association of American Medical Colleges, 93*(12), 1821–1826. https://doi.org/10.1097/ACM.0000000000002426.

The purpose of this study was to investigate whether physicians' empathy increased after a communication skills training (CST) workshop. Participants were oncologists from across Japan with three or more years of clinical experience in oncology. Participants attended two-day CST workshops. Prior to the workshop (baseline/T1), participants completed a survey with demographic questions, the JSE, and the Interpersonal Reactivity Index (IRI). The JSE was administered again immediately after completion of the workshop (follow-up/T2). Then the JSE and IRI were administered as part of a three-month follow-up (T3) survey. Changes in participants' mean total JSE scores, JSE subscale scores, and IRI subscale scores were compared using multivariate analysis of variance. Of the workshop participants, 383 responded to the three-month follow-up survey. Total JSE scores and JSE subscale scores at T2 and T3 were significantly higher than those at T1 ($p < .01$). IRI-Perspective Taking and IRI-Empathic Concern subscale scores increased significantly from T1 to T3 ($p < .01$), whereas IRI-Fantasy and IRI-Personal Distress subscale scores showed no significant changes. The JSE scores of palliative care physician participants were significantly higher than those of medical oncologist participants at T1 and T3. It was concluded that empathy in oncologists in Japan can increase after a two-day CST workshop.

Yang, K. T., & Yang, J. H. (2013). A study of the effect of a visual arts-based program on the scores of Jefferson Scale of Physician Empathy . *BMC Medical Education, 13*, 142. Accessible from: http://www.biomedcentral.com/1472-6920/13/142.

Participants included 110 (92 medical students, clerks and 18 first-year residents; 33 women) who completed the JSE. The intervention program in this pretest–posttest study design included exposing participants to visual arts for appreciation of paintings related to human suffering and discussion of related arts, such as novels, poems, music, and films. The purpose was to help participants use visual art as a tool for physician competency development and improvement of their interest in the arts. Psychometric findings, using pretest data, supported the three-factor model (exploratory factor analysis). Cronbach's coefficient alpha was 0.81, and the mean score was 110.92 (SD = 10.3). The pretest JSE mean score was significantly lower for residents compared to medical students. The JSE mean score increase in the posttest (M = 111.30, SD = 11.57) was not significantly different from that of pretest scores.

Zhang, X., Pang H., Duan, Z. (2023). Educational efficacy of medical humanities in empathy of medical students and health professionals: A systematic review and meta-analysis. *BMC Medical Education, 23*, 925. Accessible from: https://doi.org/10.1186/s12909-023-04932-8.

This review article included 15 published studies on effectiveness of medical humanities in improving empathy among medical students and healthcare professionals. The JSE was used in 12 of the reviewed studies. Results of meta-analysis showed that medical humanities programs can improve the empathy of medical students and health professionals. However, different intervention durations and different intervention methods produce different intervention effects. Also, it was observed that women can benefit more from medical humanities programs than men.

Studies on Patient Outcomes of Clinical Empathy

Chaitoff A, Rothberg MB, Windover AK, Calabrese L, Misra-Hebert A, Martinez K. (2018). Physician empathy is not associated with laboratory outcomes in diabetes: a cross-sectional study. *Journal of General Intern Medicine*, *34*(1), 75-81. https:// doi. org/ 10. 1007/ s11606- 018- 4731-0.

This study was an attempt to replicate our original study on physicians clinical empathy and tangible patient outcomes (Hojat, Louis, Markham, Wender et al., 2011) at the Cleveland Clinic. Study participants included 51 physicians who completed the SE and their 4176 diabetic patients. The authors, however, failed to reproduce our findings. In our rebuttal (Hojat, M., Maio, V., Markham. F. W., Louis, D., Z. L, Gonnella, J. S. (2019). Physician empathy and diabetes outcomes. *Journal of General Internal Medicine, 34(10, 1966.* https:// doi. org/ 10. 1007/ s11606- 019- 05187-0), we attributed such failure to several factors including technical dissimilarities, incompatibility in physician samples, differences in the case mix of patients, and confounding institutional factors.

*Del Canale, S., Louis, D. Z., Maio, V., Wang, X., Rossi, G., Hojat, M., & Gonnella, J. S. (2012). The relationship between physician empathy and disease complications: An empirical study of primary care physicians and their diabetic patients in

Parma, Italy. *Academic Medicine, 87*, 1243–1249. doi: https://doi.org/10.1097/ACM.0b013e3182628fbf.

Participants included 242 primary care physicians in Parma, Italy, who completed an Italian translation of the JSE. From electronic records of 20,961 adult patients with type 1 or type 2 diabetes mellitus who were treated by one of these physicians, information was extracted on acute metabolic complications that required hospitalization (e.g., diabetic ketoacidosis, coma, and hyperosmolar) and demographic data. Results showed statistically significant associations between physicians' scores on the JSE and rates of hospitalization due to metabolic complications in their diabetic patients. Rates of disease complication in diabetic patients of physicians who scored high on the JSE (≥112), compared to other physicians with moderate scores (111–97) or low JSE scores (<97), were 4.0, 7.1, and 6.5 per 1000, respectively. The association remained statistically significant after controlling for physicians' gender, age, type of practice (solo or group), geographical location of practice (pain, hills, and mountain); and also patients' gender, age, and duration of time enrolled with the physician.

*Hojat, M., Louis, D. Z., Markham, F. W., Wender, R., Rabinowitz, C., & Gonnella, J. S. (2011). Physicians' empathy and clinical outcomes in diabetic patients. *Academic Medicine*, 86, 359–364. doi: https://doi.org/10.1097/ACM.0b013e3182086fe1.

Participants included 29 family physicians in the Department of Family and Community Medicine at Jefferson (now Sidney Kimmel) Medical College, who completed the JSE. From electronic records of 891 adult patients with diabetes mellitus who were treated by one of these physicians, information was extracted on the most recent results of hemoglobin A1c and low-density lipoprotein cholesterol (LDL-C), and selected demographic data. Positive clinical outcomes were defined as good control of the disease reflected in A1c test results <7.0 % and LDL-C <100. Results showed that physicians' scores on the JSE could significantly predict clinical outcomes in their diabetic patients. Patients of physicians with high JSE scores were significantly more likely to have good control of their disease (56% had A1c < 7.0, and LDL-C < 100), compared to patients of physicians with low JSE scores (40% had A1c < 7.0 and LDL-C < 100). The association between physicians' scores on the JSE and patient outcomes remained statistically significant after controlling for physicians' gender and age; and also patients' gender, age, and type of health insurance.

Miscellaneous

Arora, S., Ashrafian, H..,Davis, R., Athanasiou, T., Darzi, A., & Sevdalis, N. (2010). Emotional intelligence in medicine: A systematic review through the context of the ACGME competencies. *Medical Education, 44*, 749–764. doi: https://doi.org/10.1111/j.1365-2923.2010.03709.x.

In this article, 485 citations were identified from a review of relevant literature in the English language published between January 1980 and March 2009 about measures used to assess emotional intelligence (EI) and its outcomes, as related to the six core competencies that constitute the hallmarks of graduate medical education proposed by the Accreditation Council for Graduate Medical Education (ACGME): Patient care, professionalism, system-based practice, interpersonal and communication skills, medical knowledge, and practice-based learning. The final collection that met the inclusion criteria included 16 articles. Four of these studies examined relationships between EI and empathy (measured by the JSE and the IRI). Results generally suggested that women obtained higher empathy and EI scores than men, and that EI was positively associated with compassionate care, empathic patient care, communication and interpersonal skills, and teamwork and collaboration.

Austin, E. J., Evans, P., Magnus, B., & O'Hanlon, K. N. (2007). A preliminary study of empathy, emotional intelligence, and examination performance in MBChB students. *Medical Education, 41*, 684–689. doi: https://doi.org/10.1111/j.1365-2923.2007.02795.x.

Participants included 273 medical students (85 women) in years 1, 2, and 5 of the MBChB program at the University of Edinburgh, who completed the JSE and an emotional intelligence (EI) scale. Results showed that women scored significantly higher than did men on the JSE and EI scales. A declining trend in the JSE mean score was observed between years 1 and 2 in women, but an increasing trend in the JSE scores was noticed in men. Cronbach's alpha coefficient for the JSE in this sample was 0.88.

Babar, M. G., Omar, H., Lim, L. P., Khan, S. A., Mitha, S., & Ahmad, S. F. B. (1013). An assessment of dental students' empathy levels in Malaysia. *International Journal of Medical Education, 4*, 223–229. doi: https://doi.org/10.5116/ijme.5259.4513.

Participants included 582 (141 women) first- to fifth-year dental students at two public universities, the University of Malaya and University Technology Mara; and one private university, International Medical University. They completed the JSE HPS-Version. Results of exploratory factor analysis (principal component factor analysis) showed three factors of "perspective-taking," "compassionate care," and "standing in patient's shoes," similar to most other findings with US health professions students. The overall Cronbach's alpha coefficient was 0.70. Students enrolled at public universities obtained significantly higher mean JSE scores than their counterparts in the private university. Third-year students obtained the lowest mean empathy scores than those in other years. Students of Indian origin enrolled at public universities and students of Chinese origin enrolled at the private university obtained higher JSE mean scores than other ethnic groups.

Beovich, B., & Williams, B. (2021). Empathy in Japanese paramedicine students: A cross-sectional study. *Nursing & Health Sciences, 23*(1), 176–182. https://doi.org/10.1111/nhs.12795.

This study aimed to examine self-reported empathy in Japanese paramedic students using the JSE, and compare results with similar international students. Research participants included 455 Japanese paramedicine students. Results showed that the JSE-HPS scores in the Japanese cohort were higher among women compared to men. In addition, there was a decrease in empathy with each subsequent year of the paramedic program, and a general decrease as age increased. This contrasts with comparable Australian cohorts which demonstrated no significant change in empathy levels during the undergraduate program. Empathy levels measured in the Japanese paramedic students were generally lower than for Australian students.

Brown, T., Boyle, M., Williams, B., Molloy, A., Palermo, C., McKenna, L., & Molloy, L. (2011). Predictors of empathy in health science students. *Journal of Allied Health, 40*, 143–149.

Participants included 860 undergraduate health science students (750 women) at Monash University in Australia, who completed the JSE, the Listening Style Profile, and the Communication Style Profile. Results showed that the JSE mean score for the sample was 115.5 (SD = 13.1). Women scored a significantly higher JSE mean score ($M = 116.4$,

SD = 12.3) than did men (M = 109.5, SD = 15.8). In multiple regression statistical analyses, gender and factors such as People and Time (of the Listening Style Profile) and Friendly and Relaxed Style of communication (of the Communication Style Profile) predicted the JSE scores.

Bruggi, F., & Falaschi, F. (2022). Correlation between attending physicians' empathy and readmission rate in internal medicine. *American Journal of Biomedical Science & Research, 16*(4). doi: https://doi.org/10.34297/AJBSR.2022.16.002254.

The purpose of this study was to examine the association between empathy of internal medicine ward physicians with readmission rates of their patients. The readmission data was extracted for all patients discharged from internal medicine wards between January 1, 2011, and May 31, 2017. The 30-day readmission rate was recorded for each doctor. The clinical empathy of physicians who discharged more than 100 patients during that period was measured by the JSE. A total of 4280 index discharge events were identified, 383 of which (8.9%) were readmitted within 30 days. JSE scores were found to be inversely correlated with readmission rates. Clinical empathy scores of internal medicine physicians correlated with readmission rates of the patients they cared for, especially heart failure patients for whom this is a relevant outcome.

Bukowski, H., Sweeney, C., Bennett, D., Rizzo, G., & O'Tuathaigh, C. M. P. (2022). Medical student empathy and breaking bad news communication in a simulated consultation. *Patient Education and Counseling, 105*(5), 1342–1345. https://doi.org/10.1016/j.pec.2021.09.017.

This study examined the relationship between self-reported empathy and breaking bad news (BBN) communication skills performance in a sample of undergraduate medical students (n = 100) in the clinical years of their program. Correlational and regression analysis examined the relationship between JSE-S and Empathy Quotient (EQ) scores. Higher BBN communication skills performance was positively correlated with scores on the "Social Skills" EQ subscale (r = 0.31, p = 0.002), which measures spontaneous and context-independent use of social skills. Multiple regression confirmed that "Social Skills" subscale variation predicted BBN score variation ($p < 0.01$). A weak positive association was also observed between BBN score and the "Standing in Patient's Shoes" JSE subscale (r = 0.22, p = 0.03). Findings suggest that specific aspects of dispositional empathy may moderate BBN communications skills competence in medical students.

Catlow, R., Aikins-Snyper, F., Carson, M., Jaggi, A., & Bench, S. (2020). Empathy in Action in Healthcare (EACH): A mixed methods study of nurses' and therapists' empathy. *International Journal of Orthopaedic and Trauma Nursing, 39*, 100777. https://doi.org/10.1016/j.ijotn.2020.100777.

The aim of this single-center mixed methods study was to investigate nurses' and therapists' empathy levels and explore their views regarding the impact of empathy on clinical decision-making at a national specialist orthopedic center. Data were collected from respondents (n = 126) using the JSE, supplemented by interviews with a convenience sample of 20 respondents. There was a statistically significant difference in empathy levels between nurses and therapists, with nurses scoring lower than therapists. Interview findings identified four key themes: displaying empathy, therapeutic use of self, influences and impacts, and learning. Differences between empathy scores and participants' subjective accounts of empathy were apparent. Authors concluded empathy is an important construct built upon personal and professional experiences.

Colliver, J. A., Conlee, M. J., Verhulst, S. J., & Dorsey, J. K. (2010). Reports of the decline of empathy during medical education are greatly exaggerated: A reexamination of the research. *Academic Medicine, 85*, 588–593.

This study reviews findings on 11 published studies in which a decline in empathy in medical and dental schools was reported. The JSE was used in five of these studies. Concern was raised about the validity of the empathy-measuring instruments used in these studies, and about practical significance of these findings on the grounds that response rates in most of these studies were low, and the effect size estimates were not large enough to warrant a strong conclusion that empathy erodes during training (These critics were not left unchallenged by five researchers, including myself; see *Academic Medicine*, 2010, 85, pp. 1812–1813).

Colliver, J. A., Conlee, M. J., Verhulst, S. J., & Dorsey, J. K. (2010). Rebuttals to critics on studies of the decline of empathy [Letter to the editor]. *Academic Medicine, 85*, 1813–1814.

This is a response to the rebuttals (*Academic Medicine*, 2010, *85*, 1812–1813) by the authors, whose studies were reviewed by Colliver et al. (*Academic Medicine*, 2010, *85*, 588–593). Colliver and colleagues confirmed that the JSE was developed "on an extensive research base and had a solid psychometric foundation—possibly the most researched and widely used instrument in medical education" (p. 1913) [which defies their own criticism about the validity of empathy-measuring instruments]. The authors did not recognize the empirical evidence presented in other rebuttals (Hojat et al., *Academic Medicine, 85*, 1812–1813) on the link between physicians' scores on the JSE and patient outcomes or physicians' self-reported JSE scores and patients' assessments of physician empathy; neither did Colliver et al. provide evidence to substantiate criticisms that the decline in empathy in physicians-in-training reported in several empirical studies was exaggerated.

Consorti, F., Notarangelo, M. A., Potasso, L. A., & Toscano, E. (2012). Developing professionalism in Italian medical students: An educational framework. *Advances in Medical Education and Practice, 3*, 55–60. doi: https://doi.org/10.2147/AMEP.S31228.

The study by researchers at the Faculty of Medicine and Dentistry of the University Sapienza of Rome, Italy, summarizes the main issues and experiences in development of professionalism among Italian medical students. The JSE was chosen by investigators as one of the three instruments, validated in Italy, for the overall assessment of professionalism in the context of health professions education.

Crandall, S. J., & Marion, G. S. (2009). Commentary: Identifying attitudes towards empathy: An essential feature of professionalism. *Academic Medicine, 84*, 1174–1176.

In this commentary, the authors comment on three empirical studies published in the same issue of the journal with samples of medical students and physicians from the USA, Japan, and Italy in which the JSE was used. They proposed that decline in empathy in medical education and the practice of medicine can be remedied through the promotion of relationship-centered patient care and interprofessional education and practice.

Di Lorenzo, R., Venturelli, G., Spiga, G., & Ferri, P. (2019). Emotional intelligence, empathy, and alexithymia: a cross-sectional survey on emotional competence in a group of nursing students. *Acta Bio-Medica: Atenei Parmensis, 90*(4-S), 32–43. https://doi.org/10.23750/abm.v90i4-S.8273.

The aim of the study was to analyze emotional intelligence (EI), empathy, and alexithymia in nursing students. Research participants included 237 nursing students (53 men and 184 women), attending both the 1st and 3rd year of the University Nursing Course in Modena, who completed the Italian versions of the JSE-HPS, Schutte Self-Report Emotional Intelligence Test (SSEIT), and Toronto Alexithymia Scale (TAS). Results showed statistically significant differences between the 1st and 3rd year students on SSEIT, JSE-HPS, and the TAS scores. Among 3rd year students, females obtained significantly different scores than males on the SSEIT. Furthermore, the findings highlighted a good level of emotional skills among students at the beginning of nursing training, that increased by the last year of the course, suggesting that emotional competences can be learned, and confirmed that empathy, but not alexithymia, is a dimension of EI.

Díaz-Narváez, V. P., Amezaga-Avitia, A. C., Sarabia-Alvarez, P. A., Lagos-Elgueta, M., Saavedra-Madrid, M., Silva-Reyes, P., Padilla, M., & Rodríguez-Hopp, M. P. (2018). Chilean Dentistry students, levels of empathy and empathic erosion: Necessary evaluation before a planned intervention: Levels of empathy, evaluation and intervention. *The Saudi Dental Journal*, *30*(2), 117–124. https://doi.org/10.1016/j.sdentj.2017.11.004.

The study purpose was to estimate the general empathy levels and the potential for empathic growth in Dentistry students. Research participants included 534 first- to fifth-year dentistry students at Universidad San Sebastián, Santiago Campus (Chile), who completed the Spanish version of the JSE. Results of statistical analyses showed significant differences in mean scores between academic years and by gender on empathy and some if its components. Findings suggest a considerable growth potential for empathy and its components.

Dohrenwend A. M. (2018). Defining empathy to better teach, measure, and understand its impact. *Academic medicine, 93*(12), 1754–1756. https://doi.org/10.1097/ACM.0000000000002427.

No consensus on the definition of empathy exists. The authors of the Interpersonal Reactivity Index see empathy as multidimensional, involving both emotional and cognitive aspects, while the authors of the Jefferson Scale of Physician Empathy see empathy as a predominately cognitive process. To address this problem, the author of this Invited Commentary proposed adopting the cognitive definition of empathy, noting that it allows physicians to distinguish between empathy and other communication skills and is the most consistent with counseling psychology descriptions. The author described four aspects of empathy that are rarely noted in the medical education literature but that are fundamental to understanding its practice: the "as if" condition, the use of soft interpretation, the primacy of cognition, and the relevance of reflection.

Dyrbye, L. N., Eacker, A. M., Harper, W., Power, D. V., Massie Jr., F. S., Satele, D., Thomas, M. R., Sloan, J. A., & Shanafelt, T. D. (2012). Distress and empathy do not drive changes in specialty preference among US medical students. *Medical Teacher, 34*, e116–e122. doi: https://doi.org/10.3109/0142159x.2012.644830.

Participants included 858 medical students (473 women) at the Mayo Clinic College of Medicine, University of Alabama School of Medicine, University of Minnesota Medical School, and University of Washington School of Medicine; to measure symptoms of depression and quality of life, participants completed the JSE and the Maslach Burnout Inventory (MBI) plus a survey. Results showed no significant change of JSE scores in those who did change their specialty interest during medical school ($M = 1186$, SD = 10.53) and their counterparts who did not change their interest ($M = 117.6$, SD = 11.31). Scores on the

Depersonalization scale of the MBI declined among those who changed their specialty preference. In a multivariate logistic regression analysis, it was found that being male, being a third-year student, and scores on the Depersonalization scale of the MBI independently predicted a change in specialty preference in medical students.

Foreback, J., Kusz, H., Lepisto, B. L., & Pawlaczyk, B. (2018). Empathy in internal medicine residents at community-based hospitals: A cross-sectional study. *Journal of Medical Education and Curricular Development, 5*. https://doi.org/10.1177/2382120518771352.

The aim of this study was to examine the self-reported empathy levels of internal medicine (IM) residents in 3 community-based teaching hospitals. The JSE was completed by 45 residents at 1 osteopathic and 2 allopathic IM training programs in Flint, Michigan. Results showed an increase in empathy score from the beginning level of training, postgraduate year 0 (PGY0), to the PGY1 level; and a noticeable, although statistically non-significant, decrease in empathy score for both PGY2 and PGY3 residents. The graduating residents' scores were higher compared with incoming residents. The cumulative mean empathy score in community-based IM residents showed an increase in the beginning of residents' training and decrease in empathy score by the end of training. There were significant differences in empathy scores by level of training at individual hospitals.

Galam, E., Vauloup Soupault, C., Bunge, L., Buffel du Vaure, C., Boujut, E., & Jaury, P. (2017). 'Intern life': a longitudinal study of burnout, empathy, and coping strategies used by French GPs in training. *BJGP Open, 1*(2). bjgpopen17X100773. https://doi.org/10.3399/bjgpopen17X100773.

The aim of this study was to define and follow the evolution of factors, such as empathy and coping strategies, associated with burnout. Self-reported anonymous online questionnaires were sent three times every 6 months to research participants, French GPs in training. Empathy was measured by the JSE, stress was measured using the Intern-Life Scale, burnout was measured using the Maslach Inventory, and anxiety and depression measured using the Hospital Anxiety and Depression Scale. Data included 104 paired samples analyzed between T0 and T1, and between T1 and T2. Social support, problem-centered coping, perspective taking empathy, and professional support improved the sense of personal accomplishment.

Giménez-Espert, M. D. C., Valero-Moreno, S., & Prado-Gascó, V. J. (2019). Evaluation of emotional skills in nursing using regression and QCA models: A transversal study. *Nurse Education Today, 74*, 31–37. https://doi.org/10.1016/j.nedt.2018.11.019.

This study aimed to compare linear relationship models (linear regressions) and models based on comparative qualitative analysis in the analysis of the possible influence of sociodemographic variables (age and sex), working conditions (type of contract and seniority), and academic training (type of degree and specific training) on emotional abilities (emotional intelligence and empathy) in nursing. The sample of this study consisted of direct patient care nursing professionals ($n = 217$) from 7 public hospitals in Valencia, Spain. The JSE was used to measure empathy, and the Trait of Meta-Mood Scale 24 to measure emotional intelligence. The results of the regression model suggest that only sex (negatively in the case of predicting perspective taking) and positively (in predicting compassionate care and thinking like the patient) of empathy, but not in emotional intelligence.

Gonçalves-Pereira, M., Trancas, B., Loureiro, J., Papoila, A., & Caldas-De-Almeida, J. M. (2013). Empathy as related to motivations for medicine in a sample of first-year medical students. *Psychological Reports*, *11*, 73–88. doi: https://doi.org/10.2466/17.13.PR0.112.1.73-88.

Participants included 202 medical students (136 women) at the Faculty of Medical Sciences, Nova University in Lisbon, Portugal, who completed a Portuguese translation of the JSE, plus other instruments for measuring motivation to pursue medicine and specialty interest. Results showed a mean score of 110 (SD = 11) for the total sample. Although women obtained a JSE mean score which was higher than that for men (M = 110.74, SD = 10.50 for women; M = 107.79, SD = 10.12 for men), the difference was not statistically significant. Cronbach's alpha coefficient was 0.75. Those who scored high on the people orientation index, as opposed to status/security index of motivation measure, tended to score higher on the JSE. Although the JSE mean score was higher for students who expressed an interest to pursue medical specialties (M = 110.3, SD = 9.3) and those interested in medico-surgical specialties (M = 109.72, SD = 10.92) than for others who were unsure about their specialty interest (M = 106.69, SD = 9.96), the difference was not statistically significant.

*Gonnella, J. S., Hojat, M., & Veloski, J. J. (2011). AM last page: The Jefferson longitudinal study of medical education. *Academic Medicine, 86*, 404.

In this one-page snapshot of the Jefferson Longitudinal Study of Medical Education, the history, goals, and scope of the study were briefly described. The JSE was described among the major medical education outcomes of the Jefferson Longitudinal Study, which contains over 10,600 students and graduates of Jefferson (now Sidney Kimmel) Medical College at Thomas Jefferson University. The study garnered data from more than 573 postgraduate programs, and inspired over 179 publications in peer-reviewed journals, including a considerable number of publications on empathy in medical education and patient care.

Gonzalez A, Kortlever J, Rijk L, Ring D, Brown L, Reichel L. (2020) Is there a correlation between the patient-doctor relationship questionnaire and other patient-reported experience measures? *Patient Experience Journal; 7*(1):44-50. doi: https://doi.org/10.35680/2372-0247.1399.

Patient-reported experience measures (PREMs) can quantify the quality of the patient–clinician relationship, which is associated with adherence and improved health. This study assessed the correlation of four PREMs, using the patient–doctor relationship questionnaire (PDRQ). This study prospectively enrolled 103 new and return patients. Patients completed the Jefferson Scale of Patient Perceptions on Physician Empathy (JSPPPE), the PDRQ, and four questions assessing communication effectiveness from the Clinician and Group Consumer Assessment of Healthcare Providers and Systems (CG-CAHPS). Results showed the PDRQ had large correlations with measures of perceived empathy ($r = 0.58, p < 0.001$), satisfaction ($r = 0.59, p < 0.001$), and communication effectiveness.

Håkansson Eklund, J., Holmström, I. K., Ollén Lindqvist, A., Sundler, A. J., Hochwälder, J., & Marmstål Hammar, L. (2019). Empathy levels among nursing students: A comparative cross-sectional study. *Nursing Open*, *6*(3), 983–989. https://doi.org/10.1002/nop2.280.

The aim of the study was to compare empathy levels at different stages of undergraduate nursing education and different master's nursing programs. Participants in Sweden, composed of nursing students in their second and sixth semesters in an undergraduate nursing program as well as master's nursing students (n = 329), rated their own empathy using the JSE. Students in their sixth semester in an undergraduate nursing program expressed more empathy than did students in their second semester and master's nursing students. Among the five master's programs, public-health nursing students expressed the most empathy and intensive-care nursing students the least.

Hasan, S. H., Babar, M. G., Chen, K. K., Ahmed, S. I., & Mitha, S. (2013). An assessment of pharmacy students' empathy levels in Malaysia. *Journal of Advanced Pharmacy Education & Research, 3*, 531–540.

Participants included 719 first- to fourth-year pharmacy students (596 women) in a public university (University of Kebangsaan Malaysia, $n=313$) and a private university (International Medical University, $n=406$) in Malaysia who completed the JSE HPS-Version. Exploratory factor analysis of data resulted in three factors of Perspective Taking, Compassionate Care, and Standing in Patient's Shoes, consistent with most other factor analytic studies of the JSE. Inconsistent with most other studies, men scored higher than women in this Malaysian sample. Students in the private university scored higher on the JSE than did those in the public university. No statistically significant association was observed between the JSE scores and students' ages. A statistically significant decline in empathy mean score was found between second- and fourth-year students in this cross-sectional study. Cronbach's alpha coefficient was 0.70.

Hemmerdinger, H. M., Stoddart, A. D. R., & Lilford, R. J. (2007). A systematic review of tests of empathy in medicine. *BMC Medical Education, 7*, 24. doi: https://doi.org/10.1186/1472-6920-7-24.

Based on their systematic review of the literature (using Medline, EMBASE, and PsycINFO data bases) on reliability and validity of empathy-measuring instruments in medical students and physicians, the authors identified 50 relevant papers among 1147 citations in the English language. The identified studies used 36 instruments; 8 instruments (including the JSE) demonstrated evidence in support of their validity, internal consistency, and reliability. The authors concluded that no empathy measures were found with sufficient evidence of predictive validity for use in medical school admissions.

*Hojat, M. (2009). Ten approaches for enhancing empathy in health and human services cultures. *Journal of Health and Human Services Administration, 31*, 412–450.

In this article, conceptualization and measurement of empathy in medicine and other health professions are discussed, and emphasis is placed on the usefulness of the JSE in quantifying empathy in the context of health professions education and the practice of medicine. The following ten approaches for enhancing empathy in health professions students and practitioners are described: improving interpersonal skills; using audio- or video-recording of encounters with patients; exposure to positive role models; role playing; shadowing a patient; hospitalization experiences; studying literature and the arts; improving narrative skills; theatrical performances; and the Balint method.

*Hojat, M. (2014). Assessments of empathy in medical school admissions: What additional evidence is needed? *International Journal of Medical Education, 5*, 7–10. doi: https://doi.org/10.5116/ijme.52b7.5294.

In this invited editorial, it was argued that personality plays an unquestionable role in human behavior and in the care of the patient. The crucial question was which personality attributes are more credible for the assessment of professional development of doctors-in-training and for consideration in the admission of applicants to medical schools. Three requirements were proposed: (1) Conceptual relevancy of personality attributes to clinical competence and patient outcomes, (2) Availability of a psychometrically sound instrument to measure the desirable attribute, and (3) Empirical link of the personality attribute to clinical competence and patient outcomes. Evidence was presented in support of the idea that empathy, as measured by the JSE, seems to be a unique personality attribute that can meet all three requirements. It was suggested that for rendering more optimal care, for regaining the lost reputation of the profession of medicine, and for reclaiming a compassionate image of doctors, bold actions must be taken to break free from lingering doubts, persistent skepticism, and a lack of enthusiasm to include in medical school admission decisions assessments of pertinent personality attributes, including empathy, measured by the JSE.

*Hojat, M., Erdmann, J. B., & Gonnella, J. S. (2014). *Personality assessments and outcomes in medical education and the practice of medicine-AMEE Guide 79.* Dundee, UK: Association for Medical Education in Europe (AMEE). First published in 2013 in *Medical Teacher, 35*, e1267–e1301.

In a paradigm of physician performance, it was proposed that both "cognitive" (academic performance), and "noncognitive" (personal qualities) components contribute to performance of physicians-in-training and physicians-in-practice. Personality as an important factor of the "noncognitive" component plays a significant role in academic and professional performance outcomes. In this article, 14 personality instruments frequently used in medical education research were described, their strengths and shortcomings, and their major findings relevant to health professions education and practice. It was suggested that two conditions, including personality measures, must be met for the assessment of applicants to medical school, candidates for postgraduate medical education, and professional development of physicians-in-training or in-practice. These include: (1) conceptual relevance to clinical performance and patient outcomes, and (2) strong psychometric support for the instrument's validity (particularly predictive validity) and reliability. It was argued that among the selected personality instruments, the JSE can successfully meet the two aforementioned conditions. It was suggested that another conceptually relevant personality attribute with reasonable support for its psychometrics is "conscientiousness." It was concluded that the lingering doubts and hesitation to use personality assessments in the selection and professional development of trainees in medicine can result in a futile and never-ending search for additional evidence which would be counterproductive. Leaders, admission officers, and faculty in medical and other health professions education were encouraged to take bold action to incorporate personality assessments as complementary measures in admissions and in professional development of students for the sake of medicine to regain its well-deserved reputation, and to reclaim the altruistic image that physicians used to embody.

*Hojat, M., Gonnella, J. S., Mangione, S., Nasca, T. J., & Magee, M. (2003). Physician empathy in medical education and practice: Experience with the Jefferson Scale of Physician Empathy. *Seminars in Integrative Medicine, 1*, 25–41.

This was a report summarizing experiences in the development and psychometrics of the JSE. Starting with conceptualization and definition of empathy in the context of medical education and patient care, a distinction was made between empathy and sympathy, and their different consequences in patient outcomes. Then we briefly described the step-by-step development of the JSE, and provided evidence in support of its validity and reliability. We reported our findings at the time of writing this article about gender and specialty differences in the JSE scores. We proposed that empathy is amenable to change and described a few approaches that could help to enhance empathy in physicians-in-training.

*Hojat, M., Gonnella, J. S., & Veloski, J. (2010). Rebuttals to critics of studies of the decline of empathy [Letters to the editor]. *Academic Medicine, 85*, 1812.

This was a rebuttal in response to criticism by Colliver and his colleagues (2010) about findings of 11 studies in which a decline of empathy during health professions education had been reported. It was argued that Colliver and colleagues failed to recognize the extensive literature on psychometrics of the JSE, used in five of their reviewed studies, and also overlooked the findings that reported a significant association between physicians' empathy and clinical outcomes. Furthermore, it was argued that Colliver and colleagues' suggestion to transform scores on each scale back to the unit of the original Likert scale for addressing the clinical or practical significance of the findings did not make sense as the three instruments used in the reviewed studies used three different types of 4-, 7-, and 9-point Likert scales, which could not lead to a "scale free" measure to examine the practical importance of the findings. Instead, it was suggested that a widely used approach for examining the practical or clinical significance of the findings is to calculate the effect size of the differences which yields a "scale free" and an operationally defined index (ranged from 0.29 to 0.64 in the Jefferson studies). It concluded that the concerns raised by Colliver and colleagues were mostly baseless.

*Hojat, M., Louis, D. Z., Maio, V., & Gonnella, J. S. (2013). Empathy and health care quality [Editorial]. *American Journal of Medical Quality, 28*, 6–7. doi: https://doi.org/10.1177/1062860612464731.

In this editorial, it was suggested that empathic engagement in patient care revolves around reciprocity and mutual understanding, which evokes "psychosocial" and "bioneurological" responses, providing plausible explanations for the significant associations reported in two empirical studies between physician empathy (measured by the JSE) and clinical outcomes in diabetic patients. It described that at the psychosocial level, empathic engagement lays the foundation for a trusting relationship, prompting the patient to tell the tale of his or her illness without concealment. This leads to a more accurate diagnosis and greater compliance. At the bioneurological level, empathic engagement was described as analogous to a synchronized dance between patient and caregiver, orchestrated by bioneurological markers. Also, a set of neurons, known as the mirror neuron system, is discharged by observing actions or emotions of another person, which is believed to play a crucial role in understanding the experiences of other human beings, a key ingredient of empathic engagement. Such bioneurological interaction has also been highlighted in the perception-action theory, suggesting that perceptions of another person's cognitive, affective, or somatosensory states automatically activate representations of those states in the observer, unless inhibited. The combined effects of these psychosocial and bioneurological mechanisms provide plausible explanation for the findings that physician's empathic engagement in patient care (reflected in higher JSE scores) paves the road to more optimal clinical outcomes.

*Hojat, M., Louis, D. Z., Maxwell, K., & Gonnella, J. S. (2011). The Jefferson Scale of Empathy (JSE): An update. *Health Policy Newsletter, 24*, 5–6.

This brief article highlighted some of the empirical findings from studies using the JSE, including associations of JSE scores with gender, clinical competence, long-term predictive validity, specialty choice, peer nomination, objective structured clinical examinations (OSCE), erosion of empathy during medical education, enhancement of empathy by targeted educational programs, patient perceptions of physician empathy, and patient outcomes.

*Hojat, M., Shannon, S., DeSantis, J., Speicher, M., Bragan, L., & Calabrese, L. (2019). National norms for the Jefferson Scale of Empathy: A nationwide project in osteopathic medical education and empathy (POMEE). *Journal of American Osteopathic Association, 119*(8), 520–532. https://doi.org/10.7556/jaoa.2019.091.

The study purpose was to develop national norms for the assessments of osteopathic medical students' clinical empathy scores on the broadly used and well-validated Jefferson Scale of Empathy (JSE S-Version) at all levels of osteopathic medical school education. Research participants included 16149 students from 41 of 48 participating campuses of osteopathic medical schools in USA, who completed the JSE. Three national norm tables were developed for first-year matriculants and for students in preclinical (years 1 and 2) and clinical (years 3 and 4) phases of medical school. The norm tables allow any raw score on the JSE S-Version for male and female osteopathic medical students from matriculation to graduation to be converted to a percentile rank to assess an individual's score against national data.

Hong, M., Bahn, G. H., Lee, W. H., & Moon, S. J. (2011). Empathy in Korean psychiatric residents. *Asia-Pacific Psychiatry, 3*, 83–90. doi: https://doi.org/10.1111/j.1758-5872.2011.00123x.

Participants included 316 residents (133 women) in 82 psychiatric residency training programs in Korea, who completed the JSE and the Cloninger's Temperament and Character Inventory (TCI). Results showed that married residents scored higher on the JSE ($M=105.2$, $SD=11.1$) than unmarried residents ($M=102.0$, $SD=11.8$). In this cross-sectional study, steady increase in the JSE scores was observed as residents progressed through residency training. It was found that mean scores on the JSE in the third year ($M=105.2$, $SD=9.3$) and fourth year ($M=106.0$, $SD=13.8$) were higher than those in the first year ($M=100.7$, $SD=11.6$) and second year ($M=101.2$, $SD=11.1$) of residency training. Statistically significant positive correlations were found between scores on the JSE and the TCI's personality attributes such as Cooperativeness ($r=0.39$), Persistence ($r=0.31$), Self-Directedness ($r=0.29$), and Reward Dependence ($r=0.28$). Also, a significantly negative correlation was observed between the JSE and Harm and Avoidance scores on the TCI ($r=-0.26$).

Kristensen, T., Ejersted, C., Ahnfeldt-Mollerup, P., Søndergaard, J., & Charles, J. A. (2022). Profiles of GPs with high and low self-reported physician empathy-personal, professional, and antibiotic-prescribing characteristics. *BMC Primary Care, 23*(1), 243. https://doi.org/10.1186/s12875-022-01847-z.

The purpose of this study was to compare profiles of personal, professional, and antibiotic-prescribing characteristics of GPs with high and low empathy. The study participants included 464 Danish GPs who completed the JSE-HP. The top and bottom decile on empathy scores were compared and results showed that top empathy scorers were mostly women, and it reported the following person-centered factors as more important for their job satisfaction than the bottom decile: The patient–physician relationship, interaction with colleagues, and intellectual stimulation. Also, high-empathy scoring GPs prescribed significantly less penicillin than the low-empathy GPs.

Lee, B. K., Bahn, G. H., Lee, W. H., Park, J. H., Yoon, T. Y., & Baek, S. B. (2009). The relationship between empathy and medical education system, grades, and personality in medical college students and medical school students. *Korean Journal of Medical Education, 21*, 117–124. doi: https://doi.org/10.3946/kjme.2009.21.2.117.

Participants included 155 (36 women) medical college and 137 (83 women) medical school students who completed a Korean translation of the JSE and the Temperament and Character Inventory (TCI). Results showed no significant gender difference on the JSE scores ($M=106.8$, $SD=11.6$ for men and $M=109.2$, $SD=11.0$ for women). Also, no significant association was observed between the JSE scores and internal or external motivation to pursue medicine; and JSE scores and interest in the people-oriented and technology-oriented specialties. Students in the medical school system obtained a statistically significant higher JSE mean score ($M = 109.2$, SD = 11.1) than their counterparts in the medical college system ($M = 106.6$, $SD = 11.6$). Significant correlations in the 0.30s were found between JSE and Cooperativeness, Self-Directedness, and Reward Dependence scale scores on the TCI.

Liu, Q., Tao, J., Gao, L., He, X., Wang, Y., Xia, W., & Huang, L. (2021). Attitudes of front-line nurses toward hospice care during the COVID-19 pandemic. *The American Journal of Hospice & Palliative Care, 38*(2), 204–210. https://doi.org/10.1177/1049909120968533.

The aim of this study was to understand the attitudes of front-line clinical nurses toward hospice care in the fight against the COVID-19 pandemic, and to provide a source of reference for hospice care education and training in hospitals treating patients with COVID-19. Research participants included 149 front-line nurses from a designated COVID-19 hospital in Wuhan, China. Participants completed the Chinese versions of the JSE, the General Information Questionnaire, the Frommelt Attitudes Toward Care of the Dying Scale, and the General Self-Efficacy Scale. Results showed that the nurses' attitudes toward hospice care were significantly associated with their level of clinical empathy, age, knowledge of hospice care, and self-efficacy.

Mandel, E. D., & Schweinle, W. E. (2012). A study of empathy decline in physician assistant students at completion of first didactic year. *The Journal of Physician Assistant Education, 23*, 16–24.

Participants included 328 (270 women) physician assistant students at Seton Hall University, who completed the JSE within 4 weeks of matriculation, one year later, and approximately one year through their clinical training. Because data were collected anonymously, no one-to-one matching in different time points was possible for inferential statistical analyses. The findings showed women obtained a higher JSE mean score than men. Cronbach's alpha coefficient was 0.80. Although a declining trend was observed in empathy scores as students progressed through the physician assistant program, the trend was not substantial. No significant association was found between scores on the JSE and specialty preferences, or with health care experiences prior to matriculating in the physician assistant program.

Moreto, G. , Santos, I. S., Blasco, P. G., Pessini, L., & Lotufo, P. A. (2018). "Assessing Empathy among Medical Students: A Comparative Analysis Using Two Different Scales in a Brazilian Medical School." *Educación Médica, 19,* 162–170.

The aim of this study was to compare two different empathy scales across the 6-year medical course, among undergraduate medical students in Brazil. Research participants included 296 medical students who completed the the Brazilian translation of JSE and the Interpersonal Reactivity Index (IRI-Brazilian version). The students were divided into three groups, according to their year in the medical school course: Basic Group (1st and 2nd years), Clinical Group (3rd and 4th years), and Clerkship Group (5th and 6th years). Results showed that the JSE scores were similar among the students from the Basic, Clinical, and Clerkship groups. On the other hand, the affective dimension of IRI-Brazilian version revealed a significantly lower score in the Clerkship Group. The authors suggest that the level of empathy can change, and in this case, the affective dimension was most affected during medical school.

Mizobe, M., Kataoka, H., Yamagami, H., Ito, C., Koyama, Y., Yawata, E., & Shiga, T. (2019). A night on call or an overnight shift does not reduce residents' empathy: a randomized crossover multicenter survey. *BMC Medical Education, 19*(1), 391. https://doi.org/10.1186/s12909-019-1822-5.

This study aimed to examine whether a night on call or an overnight shift reduced physicians' empathy. A multicenter randomized crossover survey was undertaken using the Japanese version of the JSE-HP. Participants included 229 physicians who worked at academic hospitals and community hospitals in Japan, randomly assigned into two groups. Group A first completed the JSE prior to a night on call or an overnight shift; then, 8 weeks later, Group A ($n = 117$) completed the JSE after a night on call or an overnight shift. Group B ($n = 112$) first completed the JSE after a night on call or an overnight shift; then, 8 weeks later, Group B completed the JSE prior to a night on call or an overnight shift. There was no significant difference in the JSE scores between pre- and post-night on call or overnight shift in either group. A night on call or an overnight shift did not reduce the Japanese physicians' clinical empathy.

Mocny-Pachońska, K., Łanowy, P., Trzcionka, A., Skaba, D., & Tanasiewicz, M. (2020). Gender related changes of empathy level among Polish dental students over the course of training. *Medicine, 99*(1), e18470. https://doi.org/10.1097/MD.0000000000018470.

This study aimed to determine the levels of empathy among students of dentistry at different stages in their training. Research participants included 100 dental students (66 female and 34 male), ranging from first to fifth years of training, who completed the JSE-Health Professions Students Version. Results showed that the level of clinical empathy among dentistry students increased from the first and second to fourth years, where it reached its maximum. During the fifth year, a decrease in levels of empathy was observed. The increase in empathy during the dental course may be correlated with the growth of clinical practice during the subsequent years of study. A slight decrease in empathy in the fifth-year students may be due to the curricular focus on performing procedures, with students having to meet a set target in order to finish the course.

Naguib, G. H., Sindi, A. M., Attar, M. H., Alshouibi, E. N., & Hamed, M. T. (2020). A cross-sectional study of empathy among dental students at King Abdulaziz University. *Journal of Dental Education, 84*(1), 22–26. https://doi.org/10.21815/JDE.019.160.

The aim of this study was to assess the level of empathy among dental students at King Abdulaziz University with an emphasis on the effect of gender and study level. A cross-sectional study was carried out among third- to sixth-year dental students of King Abdulaziz University in Saudi Arabia. Participants included 300 students in their third to sixth years of dental school training, who completed the JSE-HPS. The results showed that the fifth- and sixth-year students obtained higher scores than the third- and fourth-year students, although the differences were not statistically significant. The mean empathy scores for women was significantly higher than that of men, and the women demonstrated significantly better perspective taking ($p < 0.001$) than their male counterparts.

Neumann, M., Edehäuser, F., Tauschel, D., Fischer M. R., Wirtz, M., Woopen, C., Haramati, A., & Scheffer, C. (2011). Empathy decline and its reasons: A systematic review of studies with medical students and residents. *Academic Medicine, 86*, 996–1009.

In this review study, the authors searched the PubMed, EMBASE, and PsycINFO electronic databases, and identified 669 studies in English, each with a sample size of 30 or greater, published from January 1990 through January 2010 by using keywords "empathy," "medical education," and "change," of which 18 articles were selected which met their selection criteria. None of the articles documented an increase in self-assessed empathy; two reported increased empathy only during early years of medical school but significant declines on entering the clinical phase of medical school. The authors reported that the most valid and reliable measures of self-assessed empathy used most frequently in these studies were the JSE and the Interpersonal Reactivity Index (IRI). The authors concluded that their review of eligible studies, especially those with longitudinal data, suggests that empathy declines during medical education, particularly in the clinical phase of medical education and among those who are interested in patient-remote specialties (e.g., procedure-oriented).

Neumann, M., Scheffer, C., Tauschel, D., Lutz, G., Wirtz, M., & Edelhäuser, F. (2012). Physician empathy: Definition, outcome-relevance and its measurement in patient care and medical education. *GMS Zeitschrift Für Medizinische Ausbildung, 29*, 11–21. Accessible from: http://www.ncbi.nlm.nih.gov/pmc/articles/PMC3296095/.

Participants included 44 medical students (20 women) and 63 from other disciplines (38 women) at the University of Cologne in Germany, who completed German translations of the JSE and the Interpersonal Reactivity Index (IRI). Results of psychometric analyses of both the JSE and IRI showed that they are promising tools to evaluate achievement of educational objectives and to assess empathy in German medical students.

Nguyen, V. P., & Newton, B. W. (2019). Anecdote or reality: Are people from the south and/or rural areas of the USA more empathetic? *Medical Science Educator, 29*(1), 277–284. https://doi.org/10.1007/s40670-019-00693-6.

This study looked at demographic data from first- and second-year students at a southeastern US osteopathic medical school. Study participants included 567 medical students who completed the JSE and the Balanced Emotional Empathy Scale (BEES) for measuring cognitive and affective empathy, respectively. Results showed a statistically significant difference in the first year of osteopathic medical students (OMS-I) on the JSE scores: those from towns with <10,000 population had higher JSE scores in comparison to students coming from towns with 50,000–99,999 population. The findings also revealed OMS-I students from the southern U.S. had a slightly lower BEES scores than OMS-I students from the northeastern states. The JSE scores were nearly identical across all four US census bureau regions. Additionally, OMS-I students coming from an urban background had a higher BEES score than those coming from a rural background. Combined OMS-I JSE scores were below the population norm at the 37th percentile, and combined OMS-II JSE scores were also at the 37th percentile, except for students from the western region at the 44th percentile. This study provides initial insights into whether demographic information (i.e., USA census bureau regions, town/city sizes, and rural vs. urban areas) has an impact on clinical empathy scores for osteopathic medical students. The data do not support the anecdotal evidence that individuals raised in the South and/or from rural areas have higher empathy scores than those raised in other regions of the USA or in urban areas.

Pedersen, R. (2009). Empirical research on empathy in medicine: A critical review. *Patient Education and Counseling, 76*, 307–322. doi: https://doi.org/10.1016/j.pec.2009.06.012.

This was a review article on measures of empathy used in health education research. The authors identified 200 publications for their critical review. The JSE and the Jefferson Scale of Patient Perceptions of Physician Empathy (JSPPPE) were among the reviewed instruments. It was concluded that empirical research on empathy in medicine was dominated by relatively narrow quantitative research, including physicians' and patients' cognitive understanding and affective experiences to a limited degree.

Raja B, A. J., K, S., Khandhadiya, K., Guru S, C. S., & Mahajan, U. (2022). Physician empathy during crisis: A survey of doctors in COVID-19 pandemic (COPE study). *Medical Journal, Armed Forces India*, *80*(3), 335–345. Advance online publication. https://doi.org/10.1016/j.mjafi.2022.08.012.

This study aimed at assessing physician clinical empathy during a crisis like the COVID-19 pandemic. A cross-sectional online-based survey was conducted among 409 practicing doctors from varied healthcare roles during the pandemic, who completed the Jefferson Physician's Empathy HP-Version. Results showed that physicians' empathy scores during the COVID pandemic were relatively high. Middle-aged physicians involved in outpatient consultation and those working in government healthcare gained high scores. However, findings regarding lower empathy scores when the patient load increased highlights the need for administrative and medical education interventions.

Rezayat, A. A., Shahini, N., Asl, H. T., Jarahi, L., Behdani, F., Shojaei, S. R. H., & Abadi, J. S. A. (2018). Empathy score among medical students in Mashhad, Iran: Study of the Jefferson Scale of Physician Empathy. *Electronic Physician, 10*(7), 7101–7106. https://doi.org/10.19082/7101.

The aim of this study was to assess the empathy scores among medical students in Iran. Participants included 624 students at the Mashhad University of Medical Sciences, who completed the JSE. Results showed that women outscored men on the JSE, and students' empathy declined as they progressed in medical school from preclinical to clinical phase of medical education. The mean of the JSE for this sample was 103.67 (SD = 15.34).

Seo, H. Y., Lee, D. W., Nam, S., Cho, S. J., Yoon, J. Y., Hong, Y. C., & Lee, N. (2020). Burnout as a mediator in the relationship between work-life balance and empathy in Healthcare Professionals. *Psychiatry Investigation*, *17*(9), 951–959. https://doi.org/10.30773/pi.2020.0147.

The purpose of this study was to: 1) explore the relationships among work–life balance (WLB), empathy, and burnout; and 2) investigate the roles of the subtypes of burnout relating to WLB and empathy. Research participants included 105 healthcare professionals from a general hospital in Seoul, who completed the JSE, the Maslach Burnout Inventory, and a single question on subjective WLB. Results showed that personal achievement was a potential mediating variable between empathy and WLB. The direct effect and indirect effects of WLB on empathy were also significant. Personal achievement was considered as a potential mediating variable between WLB and empathy.

Spiro, H. (2009). Commentary: The practice of empathy. *Academic Medicine, 84*, 1177–1179.

In this commentary, the author made some remarks about three empirical studies published in the same issue of the journal, with samples of medical students and physicians from the USA, Japan, and Italy in which the JSE was used. The author maintained that in patient care, the eye is for accuracy to discern diseases, but the ear is for truth to hear patients' complaints. With regard to the findings on decline of the JSE scores in physicians-in-training, the author explained that there is a risk of losing humanities in the crusade for "evidence-based" certainty in medicine than can lead to a loss of empathy. It was suggested that in this protocol-based era, selecting medical students as much for their character as their knowledge may be one approach to promote empathy, ensuring that faculty and preceptors serve as reliable role models of empathic understanding for physicians-in-training.

Starr, J. A., Holmes, M. B., Riley, E., McDonnell, B., Driscoll, L., Camarinos, J., Grabowska, W., & Harbaugh, A. G. (2020). A Quantitative Measurement of Physical Therapists' Empathy and Exploration of the Relationship with Practice Setting and Work Engagement. *Evaluation & the Health Professions, 43*(4), 255–263. https://doi.org/10.1177/0163278719864687.

The aim of this study was to investigate the level of clinical empathy in physical therapists and its relationship to practice environment and workplace engagement. Research participants included 123 physical therapists working full time at either an acute care setting, a rehabilitation hospital, or an outpatient clinic. The JSE-HP and the Oldenburg Burnout Inventory (OLBI) were administered. These physical therapists obtained a mean JSE-HP score of 118.5 ($SD = 9.1$), and a mean OLBI score of 15.63 ($SD = 3.5$). Practice setting was not found to be a significant factor regarding empathy levels in physical therapists. There was a positive correlation between being female and having higher empathy. A negative correlation between empathy and work disengagement was confirmed, suggesting that workplace disengagement may diminish a physical therapist's empathy.

Sulzer, S. H., Feinstein, N. W., & Wendland, C. L. (2016). Assessing empathy development in medical education: a systematic review. *Medical Education, 50*(3), 300–310. https://doi.org/10.1111/medu.12806.

A systematic review was performed to examine how researchers conceptualize the construct of empathy, identify what instruments were used to measure empathy in medical education, and explore how well conceptualization and operationalization match. It was found that the JSE was the most frequently used instrument to measure empathy in medical education research. Among the 109 studies that met the search inclusion criteria, 20% failed to define the central construct of empathy, and 13% used an operationalization that was matched to the definition provided. The results of this review found that the methods most commonly used to measure empathy in medical education relied heavily on self-report and cognition, not behavior and action, and may therefore have limited power to predict the presence or absence of empathy in clinical settings.

Sundling, V., Dulmen, S. & Eide, H. (2016). Communication self-efficacy in optometry: The mediating role of mindfulness. *Scandinavian Journal of Optometry and Visual Science, 9(2)*, 8-12. https://doi.org/10.5384/sjovs.vol9i2p8-12.

The aim of this study was to examine the relationship between optometry students' communication self-efficacy and their level of empathy and mindfulness. The study participants included 33 qualified optometrists in their first year of the master's degree program. The students reported level of communication self-efficacy, empathy, and mindfulness by responding to the following three questionnaires: Ammentorp's Clear-Cut Communication with Patients, JSE, and Mindful Attention Awareness Scale. Results showed a significant positive correlation between communication self-efficacy and mindfulness but not between communication self-efficacy and empathy. Mindfulness correlated with communication self-efficacy.

Tisdale, C. E., Black, A. C., Jr, Jain, S., Lowther, E., Madeline, L., Troup, C., Nathaniel, T., & Fowler, L. A. (2020). The impact of meeting patients with neurological disorders on medical student empathy. *Medical Science Educator, 30*(4), 1561–1568. https://doi.org/10.1007/s40670-020-01102-z.

The purpose of this study was to examine if first-year medical student empathy is affected by small group interactions with patients with neurological disorders, and to investigate if empathy changes over time. Research participants included 71 first-year medical students participating in a Neuroscience Module, who interacted with a variety of neurological patients in a small group informational session. Students completed the JSE before and immediately after participation in the program, and finally 5 weeks after completion of the program. Results showed a significant increase in the JSE scores immediately after the program that was sustained during the 5 weeks following.

Wang, C. X. Y., Pavlova, A., Boggiss, A. L., O'Callaghan, A., & Consedine, N. S. (2023). Predictors of Medical Students' Compassion and Related Constructs: A Systematic Review. *Teaching and Learning in Medicine*, *35*(5), 502–513. https://doi.org/10.1080/10401334.2022.2103816.

The purpose of this review article was to investigate the predictors of compassion and related constructs among medical students, allowing for a better understanding of the factors that both positively and negatively contribute to the development of compassionate future physicians. Of 14,060 retrieved articles, 222 studies were included. Of these, 95% studied student factors, but only 25% studied environmental, 9% studied patient, and 6% studied clinical factors. Predictors of greater compassion included maturity; work and life experiences; personality traits of openness to experience and agreeableness; skills such as perspective taking, reflection, and mindfulness; and positive role modeling. Conversely, negative attitudes/emotions, burnout, stress, detachment, operating in cultures prioritizing knowledge and efficiency over humanistic care, negative role models, time constraints, and heavy workloads predicted lower compassion. Patient-related factors included "difficult" and "noncompliant" patients or those perceived as responsible for their illness. Overall, 60% of studies had a serious risk of bias, particularly confounding and participant selection biases.

Williams, B., Boyle, M., Brightwell, R., Devenish, S., Hartley, P., McCall, M., McMullen, P., Munro, G., O'Meara, P., & Webb, V. (2012). Paramedic empathy levels: Results from seven Australian universities. *International Journal of Emergency Services*, *1*, 111–121. Accessible from: www.emeraldinsight.com/doi/abs/10.1108/20470891211275902.

Participants included 784 paramedic students (449 women) from seven Australian universities, who completed the JSE (HPS-Version). Results showed an overall JSE mean score of 106.74 (SD = 14.8) for this sample. A statistically significant gender difference was found in favor of women (M = 108.69, SD = 14.65 for women; M = 103.81, SD = 14.17 for men). The lowest JSE mean score was obtained by the first-year students (M = 106.29, SD = 15.40) and the highest by fourth-year students (M = 110.60, SD = 13.71), but the differences by level of training were not statistically significant. Cronbach's alpha coefficient was 0.83.

Williams, B., Boyle, M., Tozer-Jones, J., Devenish, S., Hartley, P., McCall, M., McMullen, P., Munro, G., & O'Meara, P. (2015). Undergraduate paramedic students' empathy levels: A 2-year longitudinal study. *Journal of Nursing Education and Practice*, *5*, 58–64. doi: https://doi.org/10.5430/jnep.v5n1p58. Accessible from: https://doi.org/10.5430/jnep.v5n1p58.

Participants included 1719 undergraduate first-, second-, and third-year paramedic students (979 women) from six Australian universities, who completed the JSE (HPS-Version). The overall JSE mean score was 105.92 (SD = 12.85). Women obtained a significantly higher JSE mean score than did men (M = 107.45 and M = 103.86 for women and men, respectively, effect size = 0.28). The JSE scores did not change by level of training in this cross-sectional study. No significant association was found between JSE scores and students' ages.

Yu, J., & Kirk, M. (2009). Evaluation of empathy measurement tools in nursing: Systematic review. *Journal of Advanced Nursing, 65*, 1790–1806. doi: https://doi.org/10.1111/j.1365-2648.2009.05071.x.

Based on an extensive literature review of empathy-measuring instruments in nursing samples published in 20 years (between 1987 and 2007), this review article identified 20 tools, of which 12 were selected that met the inclusion criteria (e.g., full description of the original development, reported psychometrics properties including validity and reliability, and publication in English language).The JSE was one of the selected tools. However, because only a few early publications (between 2001 and 2003) about the JSE were reviewed, some specific features of the JSE (e.g., confirmation of the latent variable structure, utility in the assessment of changes, and applicability to students as well as practitioners in all health professions disciplines and specialties) could not be captured in this review.

Yu, J., Lee, S., Kim, M., Lim, K., Chang, K., & Lee, M. (2020). Relationships between perspective-taking, empathic concern, and self-rating of empathy as a physician among medical students. *Academic Psychiatry*, 44(3), 316–319. https://doi.org/10.1007/s40596-019-01114-x.

The purpose of this study was to examine the relationships between perspective taking, empathic concern, and self-rating of empathy as a physician among medical students. The study participants included 152 medical students in the Republic of Korea, who completed the Korean versions of the JSE and the Interpersonal Reactivity Index (IRI). Results showed that medical students with clinical clerkship experience demonstrated higher levels of perspective taking and empathy than did students without such experience. Moreover, perspective taking and empathic concern were significant predictors of medical students' clinical empathy in a multivariable regression model.

Doctoral Dissertations in Which the JSE Was Used

1. Adams, S. (2016). *An exploration of applied liberal education competencies and empathic decision-making in BSN nurses.* (Publication No. 10470836). [Doctoral dissertation, University of Illinois at Chicago]. ProQuest Dissertations & Theses Global. DAI-B 78/07(E).
2. Attiogbe, K. (2024). *The influence of prosocial and leadership traits on work engagement in a social work setting.* (Publication No. 31147787). [Doctoral dissertation, City University of Seattle]. ProQuest Dissertations & Theses Global. DAI-A 85/10(E).
3. Austin, G. M. (2012). *The relationship between work stressors and clinical empathy for hospital based physicians and nurses.* (Publication No. 3548885). [Doctoral dissertation, Capella University]. ProQuest Dissertations & Theses Global. DAI-B 74/05(E).
4. Bergstresser, K. (2017). *Empathy in medical students: Exploring the impact of a longitudinal integrated clerkship model.* (Publication No. 10596918). [Doctoral dissertation, Marywood University]. ProQuest Dissertations & Theses Global. DAI-A 81/1(E).
5. Berry, K R. (2019). *Storytelling and how it aids empathy for providers of the trauma patient population.* (Publication No. 27666925). [Doctoral dissertation, The University of Arizona]. ProQuest Dissertations & Theses Global. DAI-B 81/7(E).

6. Biswas, A. (2024). *Exploring the impact of empathic communication on stress among students in higher education institutions.* (Publication No. 30993968). [Doctoral dissertation, Northeastern University]. ProQuest Dissertations & Theses Global. DAI-A 85/9(E).
7. Bonuso, C. F. (2013). *Empathy in the clinical encounter: a study of situational and dispositional empathy levels as associated with clinical training and practice.* (Publication No. 3570197). [Doctoral dissertation, Pace University]. ProQuest Dissertations & Theses Global. DAI-B 74/09(E).
8. Bristow, P. M. (2014). *Reel influence: video as an instructional strategy in addressing the affective domain in instructional design.* (Publication No. 3625747). [Doctoral dissertation, Capella University]. ProQuest Dissertations & Theses Global. DAI-A 75/10(E).
9. Burkhard, S. (2023). *The relationship of medical provider humility, empathy, and competency on patient satisfaction.* (Publication No. 30316452). [Doctoral dissertation, George Fox University]. ProQuest Dissertations & Theses Global. DAI-A 84/10(E).
10. Carter, R. D. (2017). *Physician wellness: impact of stress, burnout, and depression on medical trainee empathy.* (Publication No. 13837064). [Doctoral dissertation, University of Houston]. ProQuest Dissertations & Theses Global. DAI-A 77/09(E).
11. Chandler, C. (2021). *Clinician empathy and alliance building with patients during clinician and patient interactions in a drug addiction treatment center in northeastern new jersey*. (Publication No. 28643746). [Doctoral dissertation, Grand Canyon University].ProQuest Dissertations & Theses Global. DAI-B 83/1(E).
12. Coles, B. A. (2015). *Compassion fatigue and empathy in nurses caring for clients with HIV/AIDS.* (Publication No. 3730826). [Doctoral dissertation, University of Phoenix]. ProQuest Dissertations & Theses Global. DAI-B 77/03(E).
13. Coulmas, M. C. (2006).*A study of the effect of clinical experience on nursing empathy.* (Publication No. 3226809). [Doctoral dissertation, Capella University]. ProQuest Dissertations & Theses Global. DAI-B 67/07.
14. Courtenay, T. M. (2016). *Improving inpatient experience utilizing an empathy enhancement program.* (Publication No. 10295869). [Doctoral dissertation, University of Hawai'i at Manoa]. ProQuest Dissertations & Theses Global. DAI-A 81/1(E).
15. Delano Holden, J. (2017). *A toolkit to support nurse-patient communication through nurse-expressed empathy*. Publication No. 10271796). [Doctoral dissertation, Widener University]. ProQuest Dissertations & Theses Global. DAI-B 78/09(E).
16. Dorough, R. J. M. (2022). *The medicalization of communication: an analysis of the policies and educational practices surrounding patient and physician interaction.* (Publication No. 29331342). [Doctoral dissertation, The University of Texas at Arlington]. ProQuest Dissertations & Theses Global. DAI-A 83/12(E).
17. Eaton, D. (2018). *The effect of participation in a dementia simulation on participants empathy.* (Publication No. 13421992). [Doctoral dissertation, Clarion University of Pennsylvania and Edinboro University]. ProQuest Dissertations & Theses Global. DAI-B 80/06(E).

18. Garza, J. M. (2015). *Physician assistant students' perceptions of mental illness: a correlational study of empathy, attitudes, and stigma levels.* (Publication No. 3728874). [Doctoral dissertation, The University of Texas - Pan American]. ProQuest Dissertations & Theses Global. DAI-B 77/03(E).
19. Gurfein, E. G. (2017). *Enhancing empathy and emotion regulation to decrease burnout: a pilot study of compassion cultivation for physicians in training.* (Publication No. 10193576). [Doctoral dissertation, Palo Alto University]. ProQuest Dissertations & Theses Global. DAI-A 81/1(E).
20. Holub, P. G. (2011). *The influence of narrative in fostering affective development of medical professionalism in an online class.* (Publication No 3439139). [Doctoral dissertation, Nova Southeastern University]. ProQuest Dissertations & Theses Global. DAI-A 72/03.
21. Juan, S. (2023). *The application of virtual simulation to promoting empathy in undergraduate nursing students.* (Publication No. 30420283). [Doctoral dissertation, Teachers College, Columbia University]. ProQuest Dissertations & Theses Global. DAI-A 84/11(E).
22. Kane, S. E. (2018).*The effects of a longitudinal patient experience on the enhancement of empathy in first and second year medical students.* (Publication No. 10809816). [Doctoral dissertation, City University of New York]. ProQuest Dissertations & Theses Global. DAI-A 79/10(E).
23. Kelly, C. P. (2021). *Empathic instruction through literary narratives: a quasi-experimental study of an occupational therapy course.* (Publication No. 28681265). [Doctoral dissertation, The University of Maine]. ProQuest Dissertations & Theses Global. DAI-A 83/3(E).
24. Kinney, S. (2022). *The effects of abbreviated mindfulness-based interventions on empathy growth of prelicensure BSN students.* (Publication No. 28970879). [Doctoral dissertation, Capella University]. ProQuest Dissertations & Theses Global. DAI-A 83/9(E).
25. Klim, G. (2019). *Social empathy and associated factors among nurses: a mixed method study.* (Publication No. 13901527). [Doctoral dissertation, Loma Linda University]. ProQuest Dissertations & Theses Global. DAI-B 81/11(E).
26. Komor, T. L. (2024). *Does baseline empathy level of undergraduate nursing students affect empathic responses and change in empathy following participation in a simulation? A mixed method study.* (Publication No. 31243640). [Doctoral dissertation, State University of New York at Binghamton]. ProQuest Dissertations & Theses Global. DAI-A85/12(E).
27. Lockett, J. M. (2021). *The effect of empathy training on associate degree nursing students' empathy.* (Publication No. 28316507). [Doctoral dissertation, Capella University]. ProQuest Dissertations & Theses Global. DAI-A 82/8(E).
28. Lombardi, M. J. (2016). *Fostering humanism in medicine: a mixed methods study on the influence of humanism in medicine workshops on medical student empathy.* (Publication No. 10132967). [Doctoral dissertation, Rowan University]. ProQuest Dissertations & Theses Global. DAI-A 81/1(E).

29. McKnight-Chelius, R. (2017). *The relationships among emergency nurses' perceptions of nurse empathy, compassion fatigue, compassion satisfaction, and emergency patients' perception of nurse empathy.* Publication No. 10282345). [Doctoral dissertation, Widener University]. ProQuest Dissertations & Theses Global. DAI-B 78/10(E).
30. McTighe, Adam J. (2014). *Effect of Medical Education on Empathy in Osteopathic Medical Students.* [Unpublished doctoral dissertation]. Philadelphia College of Osteopathic Medicine.
31. Miller, M. T. (2016). *Comparison of empathy scores in RN-BSN students before and after compassionate care course.* (Publication No. 10016589). [Doctoral dissertation, Carlow University]. ProQuest Dissertations & Theses Global. DAI-B 77/07(E).
32. Montanari, P. (2012). *Psychometric Analysis of the Jefferson Scale of Empathy (JSE) Health Professional Students (HPS) Version: An Italian Validation Study with Undergraduate Nursing Students.* [Unpublished doctoral dissertation]. University of L'Aquila, Italy.
33. Moreto, G. (2015) *Evaluating Empathy In Undergraduate Medical Students At São Paulo University Using Two Instruments.* [Unpublished doctoral dissertation]. São Paulo University, Brazil.
34. Nonnenkamp, D. J. (2013). *A quantitative study of the impact of an empirically validated empathy training program on pre-med students.* (Publication No. 3605751). [Doctoral dissertation, Saint Louis University]. ProQuest Dissertations & Theses Global. DAI-A 75/04(E).
35. Orr, F. (2017). *I know how it feels: a voice-hearing simulation to enhance nursing students' empathy and self-efficacy.* (Publication No. 31100612). [Doctoral dissertation, University of Technology Sydney, Australia]. ProQuest Dissertations & Theses Global. DAI-A 85/10(E).
36. Panizzi Woodley, K. T. C. (2012). *A repeated measures quantitative prospective inquiry into the change in medical student self-reported empathy in clinical rotations.* (Publication No. 3550376). [Doctoral dissertation, The University of Alabama at Birmingham]. ProQuest Dissertations & Theses Global. DAI-A 74/05(E).
37. Pietro, K. (2023). *Examining empathy during an initial nutrition counseling session through video-cued narrative reflection.* (Publication No. 30426358). [Doctoral dissertation, University of New Hampshire]. ProQuest Dissertations & Theses Global. DAI-A 84/12(E).
38. Pinkston, M. M. (2008). *Increasing empathy in medical school students towards individuals living with HIV/AIDS and medication adherence.* (Publication No. 3328710). [Doctoral dissertation, University of Missouri-Kansas City]. ProQuest Dissertations & Theses Global. DAI-A 81/1(E).
39. Reisetter, B. C. (2002). *Relationship between psychosocial physician characteristics and physician price awareness.* (Publication No. 3069120). [Doctoral dissertation, The University of Mississippi]. ProQuest Dissertations & Theses Global. DAI-B 63/10.

40. Riess, D. L. (2018). *Effects of simulated clinical experiences on empathy, self-confidence, and satisfaction in nursing students.* (Publication No. 10829752). [Doctoral dissertation, Walden University]. ProQuest Dissertations & Theses Global. DAI-A 81/1(E).
41. Rodewald, E. E. (2012). *Attachment style and empathy in health care counseling: is there an association?* (Publication No. 3491500). [Doctoral dissertation, Capella University]. ProQuest Dissertations & Theses Global. DAI-B 73/05.
42. Rohrer, J. (2021). *Teaching compassion skills to students of behavior analysis via telehealth.* (Publication No. 28493962). [Doctoral dissertation, Endicott College]. ProQuest Dissertations & Theses Global. DAI-A 82/11(E).
43. Ross, R. (2017). *"This will only hurt a bit" evaluating the usage of patient focused empathy amongst general surgery residents.* (Publication No. 10757883). [Doctoral dissertation, Rutgers The State University of New Jersey, Graduate School of Applied and Professional Psychology]. ProQuest Dissertations & Theses Global. DAI-A 79/04(E).
44. Sherrard, S. (2007). *Empathy in psychology interns and medical residents: An investigation of the cognitive and emotional components of empathy.* (Publication No. 3253152). [Doctoral dissertation, George Fox University]. ProQuest Dissertations & Theses Global. DAI-B 68/02.
45. Skogevall, S. (2023). *Telephone nurses' work with persons calling healthcare services frequently.* (Publication No. 30663515). [Doctoral dissertation, Malardalen University, Sweden]. ProQuest Dissertations & Theses Global. DAI-A 85/1(E).
46. Smolarz, B. G. (2005). *Determining the relationship between medical student empathy and undergraduate college major* (Publication No. 1459590).[Master's thesis, Albany Medical College] ProQuest Dissertations & Theses Global. MAI 47/02M.
47. Stebbins, C. A. (2005). *Enhancing empathy in medical students using FLEX Care™ communication training.* (Publication No. 3172245). [Doctoral dissertation, Iowa State University]. ProQuest Dissertations & Theses Global. DAI-A 81/1(E).
48. Suppiah Cavert, M. (2020). *Continuing medical education (CME): an exploration of method in teaching empathy to first year residents in a Singapore hospital.* (Publication No. 28018299). [Doctoral dissertation, The University of Liverpool, United Kingdom]. ProQuest Dissertations & Theses Global. DAI-A 81/12(E).
49. Tamsukhin, S. M. (2022). *Measuring empathy of undergraduate dietetics students at two southwestern Ohio universities.* (Publication No. 29704808). [Doctoral dissertation, University of Cincinnati]. ProQuest Dissertations & Theses Global. DAI-B 84/3(E).
50. Zhang, Y. (2021). *Empathy among nursing undergraduates at a Chinese private university.* (Publication No. 28714514). [Doctoral dissertation, Chapman University]. ProQuest Dissertations & Theses Global. DAI-A 83/2(E).

Appendix B: Jefferson Scale of Empathy, Health Professions Version (JSE HP-Version)

Jefferson
Thomas Jefferson University
HOME OF SIDNEY KIMMEL MEDICAL COLLEGE

Jefferson Scale of Empathy

Physician/Health Professions (HP-Version)

Use a ball-point pen.
Mark one response for each of the items below.

For *ID Code* and *Optional* fields, write numerals completely inside the boxes, one numeral to a box.

Name (optional) ______________________ **ID Code** ☐☐☐☐☐☐☐☐☐

Date ___/___/___

Age:
☐ <21 ☐ 21-30 ☐ 31-40 ☐ 41-50 ☐ 51-60 ☐ 61-70 ☐ >70

Gender:
☐ Male ☐ Female

Physician primary specialty: [Please choose only one]

☐ Anesthesiology	☐ Dermatology	☐ Emergency Medicine
☐ Family Med./General Prac.	☐ Internal Med./Med. specialties	☐ Neurology
☐ Neurosurgery	☐ Obstetrics/Gynecology	☐ Ophthalmology
☐ Otolaryngology	☐ Orthopaedic Surgery	☐ Pathology
☐ Pediatrics	☐ Physical Med./Rehabilitation	☐ Plastic Surgery
☐ Preventive Medicine	☐ Psychiatry	☐ Public Health
☐ Radiology	☐ Surgery/Surgical specialties	☐ Urology
☐ Other ___________		

Other health professions primary specialty: [Please choose only one]

☐ Community Healthcare Worker	☐ Dentistry	☐ Midwifery
☐ Nursing	☐ Nurse Practitioner	☐ Nutrition/Dietician
☐ Occupational Therapy	☐ Pharmacy	☐ Physician Assistant
☐ Physical Therapy/Physiotherapy	☐ Podiatry	☐ Psychology/Counseling
☐ Public Health Worker	☐ Speech Therapy/Audiology	☐ Social Worker
☐ Other ___________		

Optional field #1.. ☐☐☐☐

Optional field #2.. ☐☐☐☐

Please continue on the back --- Do not write below this line

SELF-SCORE

0E0 Page 1

 160106 (ver. 4.0)

Jefferson
Philadelphia University + Thomas Jefferson University

Jefferson Scale of Empathy

Physician/Health Professions (HP-Version)

Instructions: Using a ball-point pen, please indicate the extent of your agreement or disagreement with *each* of the following statements by marking the appropriate circle to the right of each statement.

Please use the following 7-point scale (*a higher number on the scale indicates more agreement):*
Mark one and only one response for each statement.

1-------2-------3-------4-------5-------6-------7
Strongly Disagree ***Strongly Agree***

	1	2	3	4	5	6	7
1. My understanding of how my patients and their families feel does not influence medical or surgical treatment.	○	○	○	○	○	○	○
2. My patients feel better when I understand their feelings.	○	○	○	○	○	○	○
3. It is difficult for me to view things from my patients' perspectives.	○	○	○	○	○	○	○
4. I consider understanding my patients' body language as important as verbal communication in caregiver-patient relationships.	○	○	○	○	○	○	○
5. I have a good sense of humor that I think contributes to a better clinical outcome.	○	○	○	○	○	○	○
6. Because people are different, it is difficult for me to see things from my patients' perspectives.	○	○	○	○	○	○	○
7. I try not to pay attention to my patients' emotions in history taking or in asking about their physical health.	○	○	○	○	○	○	○
8. Attentiveness to my patients' personal experiences does not influence treatment outcomes.	○	○	○	○	○	○	○
9. I try to imagine myself in my patients' shoes when providing care to them.	○	○	○	○	○	○	○
10. My patients value my understanding of their feelings which is therapeutic in its own right.	○	○	○	○	○	○	○
11. Patients' illnesses can be cured only by medical or surgical treatment; therefore, emotional ties to my patients do not have a significant influence on medical or surgical outcomes.	○	○	○	○	○	○	○
12. Asking patients about what is happening in their personal lives is not helpful in understanding their physical complaints.	○	○	○	○	○	○	○
13. I try to understand what is going on in my patients' minds by paying attention to their non-verbal cues and body language.	○	○	○	○	○	○	○
14. I believe that emotion has no place in the treatment of medical illness.	○	○	○	○	○	○	○
15. Empathy is a therapeutic skill without which success in treatment is limited.	○	○	○	○	○	○	○
16. An important component of the relationship with my patients is my understanding of their emotional status, as well as that of their families.	○	○	○	○	○	○	○
17. I try to think like my patients in order to render better care.	○	○	○	○	○	○	○
18. I do not allow myself to be influenced by strong personal bonds between my patients and their family members.	○	○	○	○	○	○	○
19. I do not enjoy reading non-medical literature or the arts.	○	○	○	○	○	○	○
20. I believe that empathy is an important therapeutic factor in medical or surgical treatment.	○	○	○	○	○	○	○

 160106 (ver. 4.0)

Appendix C: Jefferson Scale of Empathy, Medical Student Version (JSE S-Version)

Jefferson
Thomas Jefferson University
HOME OF SIDNEY KIMMEL MEDICAL COLLEGE

Jefferson Scale of Empathy

Medical Student version (S-Version)

Use a ball-point pen. Mark one response for each item below.
For *ID Code*, write numerals completely inside the boxes, one numeral to a box.
Leave *Optional* fields blank unless otherwise instructed.

Name ______________________________ **ID Code** .... ☐☐☐☐☐☐☐☐☐

Date ___/___/______

Age:

☐ <22 ☐ 22-24 ☐ 25-27 ☐ 28-30 ☐ 31-33 ☐ 34-36 ☐ >36

Gender:

☐ Male ☐ Female

Year of Medical School:

☐ 1st year ☐ 2nd year ☐ 3rd year ☐ 4th year ☐ > 4th year

Which specialty do you plan to pursue? [Please choose only one]

☐ Anesthesiology ☐ Dermatology ☐ Emergency Medicine
☐ Family Med./General Prac. ☐ Internal Med. (see below) ☐ Neurology
☐ Neurosurgery ☐ Obstetrics/Gynecology ☐ Ophthalmology
☐ Otolaryngology ☐ Orthopaedic Surgery ☐ Pathology
☐ Pediatrics ☐ Physical Med./Rehabilitation ☐ Plastic Surgery
☐ Preventive Medicine ☐ Psychiatry ☐ Public Health
☐ Radiology ☐ Surgery (see below) ☐ Urology
☐ Other ____________ ☐ Undecided

Medical Sub-specialty: [Please choose one if your primary specialty interest is Internal Medicine]

☐ Cardiology ☐ Critical Care/Pulmonary ☐ Endocrinology
☐ General Internal Medicine ☐ Gastroenterology ☐ Hematology/Oncology
☐ Infectious Disease ☐ Nephrology ☐ Rheumatology
☐ Other ____________ ☐ Undecided

Surgical Sub-specialty: [Please choose one if your primary specialty interest is Surgery]

☐ Cardiothoracic ☐ Colorectal ☐ General Surgery
☐ Transplant ☐ Trauma/Critical Care ☐ Vascular
☐ Other ____________ ☐ Undecided

Optional field #1 .... ☐☐☐☐

Optional field #2 .... ☐☐☐☐

Please continue on the back --- Do not write below this line

SELF-SCORE

B60 Page 1

Jefferson Scale of Empathy

Medical Student version (S-Version)

Instructions: Using a ball-point pen, please indicate the extent of your agreement or disagreement with *each* of the following statements by marking the appropriate circle to the right of each statement.

Please use the following 7-point scale (*a higher number on the scale indicates more agreement*):
Mark one and only one response for each statement.

1-------2-------3-------4-------5-------6-------7
Strongly Disagree ***Strongly Agree***

	1	2	3	4	5	6	7
1. Physicians' understanding of their patients' feelings and the feelings of their patients' families does not influence medical or surgical treatment.	O	O	O	O	O	O	O
2. Patients feel better when their physicians understand their feelings.	O	O	O	O	O	O	O
3. It is difficult for a physician to view things from patients' perspectives.	O	O	O	O	O	O	O
4. Understanding body language is as important as verbal communication in physician-patient relationships.	O	O	O	O	O	O	O
5. A physician's sense of humor contributes to a better clinical outcome.	O	O	O	O	O	O	O
6. Because people are different, it is difficult to see things from patients' perspectives.	O	O	O	O	O	O	O
7. Attention to patients' emotions is not important in history taking.	O	O	O	O	O	O	O
8. Attentiveness to patients' personal experiences does not influence treatment outcomes.	O	O	O	O	O	O	O
9. Physicians should try to stand in their patients' shoes when providing care to them.	O	O	O	O	O	O	O
10. Patients value a physician's understanding of their feelings which is therapeutic in its own right.	O	O	O	O	O	O	O
11. Patients' illnesses can be cured only by medical or surgical treatment; therefore, physicians' emotional ties with their patients do not have a significant influence in medical or surgical treatment.	O	O	O	O	O	O	O
12. Asking patients about what is happening in their personal lives is not helpful in understanding their physical complaints.	O	O	O	O	O	O	O
13. Physicians should try to understand what is going on in their patients' minds by paying attention to their non-verbal cues and body language.	O	O	O	O	O	O	O
14. I believe that emotion has no place in the treatment of medical illness.	O	O	O	O	O	O	O
15. Empathy is a therapeutic skill without which the physician's success is limited.	O	O	O	O	O	O	O
16. Physicians' understanding of the emotional status of their patients, as well as that of their families is one important component of the physician-patient relationship.	O	O	O	O	O	O	O
17. Physicians should try to think like their patients in order to render better care.	O	O	O	O	O	O	O
18. Physicians should not allow themselves to be influenced by strong personal bonds between their patients and their family members.	O	O	O	O	O	O	O
19. I do not enjoy reading non-medical literature or the arts.	O	O	O	O	O	O	O
20. I believe that empathy is an important therapeutic factor in medical treatment.	O	O	O	O	O	O	O

B60 Page 2

Appendix D: Jefferson Scale of Empathy, Health Professions Student Version (JSE HPS-Version)

Jefferson
Thomas Jefferson University
HOME OF SIDNEY KIMMEL MEDICAL COLLEGE

Jefferson Scale of Empathy

Health Professions Student version (HPS-Version)

Use a <u>ball-point pen</u>. Mark one response for each item below.
For *ID Code*, write numerals completely inside the boxes, one numeral to a box.

Name (optional) ____________________ **ID Code**........... ☐☐☐☐☐☐☐☐☐

Date ___/___/______

Age:
☐ < 19 ☐ 19 - 21 ☐ 22- 24 ☐ 25 - 27 ☐ 28 - 30 ☐ 31 - 33 ☐ 34 - 36
☐ 37 - 39 ☐ 40 - 42 ☐ 43 - 45 ☐ 46 - 48 ☐ 49 - 51 ☐ >51

Gender:
☐ Male ☐ Female

What is your degree program?
☐ Bioscience/Medical technology ☐ Counseling/Psychology ☐ Dentistry
☐ Diagnostic Imaging ☐ Nursing ☐ Nurse Practitioner
☐ Occupational Therapy ☐ Ophthalmology/Optometry ☐ Pharmacy
☐ Physical Therapy ☐ Physician Assistant ☐ Public Health
☐ Other ______________

Year in this program:
☐ 1st year ☐ 2nd year ☐ 3rd year ☐ 4th year ☐ > 4th year

Please leave *Optional* fields blank unless otherwise instructed.

Optional field #1 .... ☐☐☐☐

Optional field #2 .... ☐☐☐☐

PLEASE CONTINUE ⇨⇨⇨

SELF-SCORE

Jefferson
Philadelphia University + Thomas Jefferson University

Jefferson Scale of Empathy

Health Professions Student version (HPS-Version)

Instructions: Using a ball-point pen, please indicate the extent of your agreement or disagreement with *each* of the following statements by marking the appropriate circle to the right of each statement.

Please use the following 7-point scale (*a higher number on the scale indicates more agreement*):
Mark one and only one response for each statement.

1-------2-------3-------4-------5-------6-------7
Strongly Disagree ***Strongly Agree***

	1	2	3	4	5	6	7
1. Health care providers' understanding of their patients' feelings and the feelings of their patients' families does not influence treatment outcomes.	○	○	○	○	○	○	○
2. Patients feel better when their health care providers understand their feelings.	○	○	○	○	○	○	○
3. It is difficult for a health care provider to view things from patients' perspectives.	○	○	○	○	○	○	○
4. Understanding body language is as important as verbal communication in health care provider - patient relationships.	○	○	○	○	○	○	○
5. A health care provider's sense of humor contributes to a better clinical outcome.	○	○	○	○	○	○	○
6. Because people are different, it is difficult to see things from patients' perspectives.	○	○	○	○	○	○	○
7. Attention to patients' emotions is not important in patient interview.	○	○	○	○	○	○	○
8. Attentiveness to patients' personal experiences does not influence treatment outcomes.	○	○	○	○	○	○	○
9. Health care providers should try to stand in their patients' shoes when providing care to them.	○	○	○	○	○	○	○
10. Patients value a health care provider's understanding of their feelings which is therapeutic in its own right.	○	○	○	○	○	○	○
11. Patients' illnesses can be cured only by targeted treatment; therefore, health care providers' emotional ties with their patients do not have a significant influence in treatment outcomes.	○	○	○	○	○	○	○
12. Asking patients about what is happening in their personal lives is not helpful in understanding their physical complaints.	○	○	○	○	○	○	○
13. Health care providers should try to understand what is going on in their patients' minds by paying attention to their non-verbal cues and body language.	○	○	○	○	○	○	○
14. I believe that emotion has no place in the treatment of medical illness.	○	○	○	○	○	○	○
15. Empathy is a therapeutic skill without which a health care provider's success is limited.	○	○	○	○	○	○	○
16. Health care providers' understanding of the emotional status of their patients, as well as that of their families is one important component of the health care provider - patient relationship.	○	○	○	○	○	○	○
17. Health care providers should try to think like their patients in order to render better care.	○	○	○	○	○	○	○
18. Health care providers should not allow themselves to be influenced by strong personal bonds between their patients and their family members.	○	○	○	○	○	○	○
19. I do not enjoy reading non-medical literature or the arts.	○	○	○	○	○	○	○
20. I believe that empathy is an important factor in patients' treatment.	○	○	○	○	○	○	○

THANK YOU!

206 Page 2

 140716 (ver. 1.2.1)

Appendix E: Jefferson Scale of Patient Perceptions of Physician Empathy (JSPPPE)

Jefferson
Thomas Jefferson University
HOME OF SIDNEY KIMMEL MEDICAL COLLEGE

Jefferson Scale of Patient Perceptions of Physician Empathy (JSPPPE)

Instructions: We would like to know the extent of your agreement or disagreement with *each* of the following statements *about your physician named below*. Please use the following 7-point scale and write your rating number from 1 to 7 on the underlined space before each statement (1 means that you Strongly Disagree, and 7 means you Strongly Agree with the statement, a higher number indicates more agreement).

1-------2-------3-------4-------5-------6-------7
Strongly Disagree ***Strongly Agree***

***Dr.(Name of the physician in here)*____**

1. __ Can view things from my perspective (see things as I see them).
2. __ Asks about what is happening in my daily life.
3. __ Seems concerned about me and my family.
4. __ Understands my emotions, feelings, and concerns.
5. __ Is an understanding doctor.

References

AAMC (Association of American Medical Colleges). (2004). *Medical School Objectives Project.* http://www.aamc.org/meded/msop

Abbott, L. C. (1983). A study of humanism in family physicians. *The Journal of Family Practice, 16*, 1141–1146.

Abe, K., Niwa, M., Fujisaki, K., & Suzuki, Y. (2018). Associations between emotional intelligence, empathy and personality in Japanese medical students. *BMC Medical Education, 18*, 47. https://doi.org/10.1186/s12909-018-1165-7

Abele, A. E., & Wojciszke, B. (2007). Agency and communion from perspective of self versus others. *Journal of Personality and Social Psychology, 93*(5), 751–763. https://doi.org/10.1037/0022-3514.93.5.751

ABIM (American Board of Internal Medicine). (1983). Evaluation of humanistic qualities in the internist. *Annals of Internal Medicine, 99*, 720–724.

Abramson, L., Uzefovsky, F., Toccaceli, V., & Knafo-Noam, A. (2020). The genetic and environmental origins of emotional and cognitive empathy: Review and meta-analyses of twin studies. *Neuroscience & Biobehavioral Reviews, 114*, 113–133. https://doi.org/10.1016/j.neubiorev.2020.03.023

Ackoff, R. L., & Emery, F. E. (1981). *On purposeful systems*. Intersystems.

Acuna, L. E. (2000). Don't cry for us Argentinians: Two decades of teaching medical humanities. *Journal of Medical Ethics: Medical Humanities, 26*, 66–70.

Adams, S. (2016). *An exploration of applied liberal education competencies and empathic decision-making in BSN nurses.* (Publication No. 10470836). [Doctoral dissertation, University of Illinois at Chicago]. ProQuest Dissertations & Theses Global. DAI-B 78/07(E).

Adams, G. R., Jones, R. M., Schvaneveldt, J. D., & Jenson, G. O. (1982). Antecedents of affective role-taking behaviour: Adolescent perceptions of parental socialization styles. *Journal of Adolescence, 5*, 259–265.

Adib, S. M., & Hamadeh, G. N. (1999). Attitudes of the Lebanese public regarding disclosure of serious illness. *Journal of Medical Ethics, 25*, 399–403.

Adler, H. M. (1997). The history of the present illness as treatment: Who's listening, and why does it matter? *The Journal of the American Board of Family Practice, 10*, 28–35.

Adler, H. M. (2002). The sociophysiology of caring in the doctor-patient relationship. *Journal of General Internal Medicine, 17*, 874–882.

Adler, H. M., & Hammett, V. B. O. (1973). The doctor-patient relationship revisited: An analysis of the placebo effect. *Annals of Internal Medicine, 78*, 595–598.

Adolphs, R., Damasio, H., Tranel, D., Cooper, G., & Damasio, A. R. (2000). A role for somatosensory cortices in the visual recognition of emotion as revealed by three-dimensional lesion mapping. *Journal of Neuroscience, 20*, 2683–2690.

M. Hojat, *Clinical Empathy*, https://doi.org/10.1007/978-3-031-87413-0

Adolphs, R., Tranel, D., Damasio, H., & Damasio, A. R. (1994). Impaired recognition of emotion in facial expression following bilateral damage to human amygdala. *Nature, 372*, 669–672.

Aggarwal, R. (2007). Empathy: Do psychiatrists and patients agree? *The American Journal of Psychiatry Resident's Journal, 2*, 2–3.

Agosta, C. (1984). Empathy and intersubjectivity. In J. Lichtenberg, M. Borenstein, & D. Silver (Eds.), *Empathy II* (pp. 43–61). Analytic Press.

Ahlgren, A., & Johnson, D. W. (1979). Sex differences in cooperative and competitive attitudes from the 2nd to the 12th grades. *Developmental Psychology, 15*, 45–49.

Ahmadzadeh, H., Esfahani, M. N., Ahmadzad-Ast, M., Shalbafan, M., & Shariat, S. V. (2019). Does watching a movie improve empathy? A cluster randomized controlled trial. *Canadian Medical Education Journal., 10*(4), e4–e12. https://doi.org/10.36834/cmej.56979

Ainsworth, M. D. S. (1985a). Attachment across the life span. *Bulletin of the New York Academy of Medicine, 61*, 792–812.

Ainsworth, M. D. S. (1985b). Patterns of infant-mother attachment: Antecedents and effects on development. *Bulletin of the New York Academy of Medicine, 61*, 771–791.

Ainsworth, M. D. S., Blehar, M. C., Waters, E., & Wall, S. (1978). *Patterns of attachment: A psychological study of the strange situation*. Erlbaum.r.

Albanese, M. A., Snow, M. H., Skochelak, S. E., Huggett, K. N., & Farrell, P. M. (2003). Assessing personal qualities in medical school admissions. *Academic Medicine, 78*, 313–321.

Alcorta-Garza, A., Gonzalez-Guerrero, J. F., Tavitas-Herrera, S. E., Rodrigues-Lara, F. J., & Hojat, M. (2005). Validación de la escala de empatia medica de Jefferson en estudiantes de medicina Mexicanos [Validity of the Jefferson Scale of Physician Empathy among Mexican medical students]. *Salud Mental [Mental Health], 28*, 57–63.

Ali, N. S., Khalil, H. Z., & Yousef, W. (1993). A comparison of American and Egyptian cancer patients' attitudes and unmet needs. *Cancer Nursing, 16*, 193–203.

Allport, F. H. (1924). *Social psychology*. Houghton Mifflin.

Allport, G. W. (1960). The open system in personality theory. *Journal of Abnormal and Social Psychology, 61*, 301–310.

Ameh, P. O., Uti, O. G., & Daramola, O. O. (2019). Empathy among dental students in a Nigerian institution. *European Journal of Dental Education: Official Journal of the Association for Dental Education in Europe, 23*(2), 135–142. https://doi.org/10.1111/eje.12412

Amini, F., Lewis, T., Lannon, R., Louie, A., Baumbacher, G., McGuinness, T., & Schiff, E. Z. (1996). Affect, attachment, memory: Contributions toward psychobiologic integration. *Psychiatry, 59*, 213–239.

Anastasi, A. (1976). *Psychological testing*. Macmillan.

Anderson, S. W., Bechara, A., Damasio, H., Tranel, D., & Damasio, A. R. (1999). Impairment of social and moral behavior related to early damage in human prefrontal cortex. *Nature Neuroscience, 2*, 1032–1037.

Anthony, A. A., & Wain, H. J. (1971). An investigation of the outcome of empathy training for medical corpsmen. *Psychological Aspects of Disability, 18*, 86–88.

Antinienė, D., & Kaklauskaitė, Z. (2018). Empathy and Burnout Among Physicians Providing Reanimatological and Surgical Treatment. *Baltic Journal of Sport and Health Sciences, 3*(110). https://doi.org/10.33607/bjshs.v3i110.245

Antonovsky, A., Anson, O., & Bernstein, J. (1979). Interviewing and the selection of medical students: The experience of five years of Beersheba. *Innovation in Education & Training International, 16*, 328–334.

Arbuckle, J. J., & Wothke, W. (1999). *Amos 4.0 user's guide*. SPSS.

Archer, J. (1988). *The behavioural biology of aggression*. Cambridge University Press.

Archer, J. (2004). Sex differences in aggression in real-world settings: A meta-analytic review. *Review of General Psychology, 8*, 291–322.

Aring, C. D. (1958). Sympathy and empathy. *Journal of the American Medical Association, 167*, 448–452.

Arnkoff, D. B., Glass, C. R., & Shapiro, S. (2002). Expectations and preferences. In J. C. Norcross (Ed.), *Psychotherapy relationships at work: Therapist contributions and responsiveness to patients* (pp. 335–356). Oxford University Press.

Arnold, L. (2002). Assessing professional behavior: Yesterday, today, and tomorrow. *Academic Medicine, 77*, 28–37.

Arnold, L., Calkins, E. V., & Willoughby, T. L. (1997). Antecedent and concurrent correlates of primary care practice. *Teaching and Learning in Medicine, 9*, 192–199.

Aronfreed, J. (1970). The socialization of altruistic and sympathetic behavior: Some theoretical and experimental analyses. In J. Macauley & L. Berkowitz (Eds.), *Altruistic and helping behavior* (pp. 103–126). Academic Press.

Aronson, E., & Patnoe, S. (1997). *Jigsaw classroom.* Longman.

Arora, S., Ashrafian, H., Davis, R., Athanasiou, T., Darzi, A., & Sevdalis, N. (2010). Emotional intelligence in medicine: A systematic review through the context of the ACGME competencies. *Medical Education, 44*(8), 749–764. https://doi.org/10.1111/j.1365-2923.2010.03709.x

Ashcroft, J., & Straus, A. (1993). *Families first: Report of the National Commission on America's Urban Families.* National Commission on America's Urban Families.

Ashworth, C. D., Williamson, P., & Montano, D. (1984). A scale to measure physician beliefs about psychosocial aspects of patient care. *Social Science & Medicine, 19*, 1235–1238.

Astin, H. S. (1967). Assessment of empathic ability by means of a situational test. *Journal of Counseling Psychology, 14*, 57–60.

Attiogbe, K. (2024). *The influence of prosocial and leadership traits on work engagement in a social work setting.* (Publication No. 31147787). [Doctoral dissertation, City University of Seattle]. ProQuest Dissertations & Theses Global. DAI-A 85/10(E).

Austin, G. M. (2012). *The relationship between work stressors and clinical empathy for hospital based physicians and nurses.* (Publication No. 3548885). [Doctoral dissertation, Capella University]. ProQuest Dissertations & Theses Global. DAI-B 74/05(E).

Austin, E. J., Evans, P., Goldwater, R., & Potter, V. (2005). A preliminary study of emotional intelligence, empathy and exam performance in first year medical students. *Personality and Individual Differences, 39*, 1395–1405. https://doi.org/10.1016/j.paid.2005.04.014

Austin, E. J., Evans, P., Magnus, B., & O'Hanlon, K. N. (2007). A preliminary study of empathy, emotional intelligence and examination performance in MBChB students. *Medical Education, 41*(7), 684–689. https://doi.org/10.1111/j.1365-2923.2007.02795.x

Avenanti, A., Bueti, D., Galati, G., & Aglioti, S. (2005). Transcranial magnetic stimulation highlights the sensorimotor side of empathy for pain. *Nature, Neuroscience, 8*, 955–960. https://doi.org/10.1038/nn1481

Avery, J. K. (1985). Lawyers tell what turns some patients litigious. *Medical Malpractice Review, 2*, 35–37.

Ax, A. F. (1964). Goals and methods of psychophysiology. *Psychophysiology, 1*, 8–25.

Aye, S. Z., Sein, H. H., Nyunt, M. K., & Min, Y. (2022). Comparative study of Malaysian medical students' empathy scores between preclinical and clinical training. *Education in Medicine Journal, 4*(1), 27–38. https://doi.org/10.21315/eimj2022.14.1.3

Ayers, J. W., Poliak, A., Dredze, M., Leas, E. C., Zhu, Z., Kelley, J. B., Faix, D. J., Goodman, A. M., Longhurst, C. A., Hogarth, M., & Smith, D. M. (2023). Comparing physician and artificial intelligence chatbot responses to patient questions posted to a public social media forum. *JAMA Internal Medicine, 183(6)*, 589–596. https://doi.org/10.1001/jamainternmed.2023.1838

Ayra, D. K. (1993). To empathize or to dissociate-A physician's dilemma. *Journal of the Royal Society of Medicine, 86*, 3.

Aziz, A. B., & Ali, S. K. (2020). Relationship between level of empathy during residency training and perception of professionalism climate. *BMC Medical Education, 20*(1), 320. https://doi.org/10.1186/s12909-020-02231-0

Babar, M. G., Omar, H., Lim, L. P., Khan, S. A., Mitha, S., & Ahmad, S. F. B. (2013). An assessment of dental students' empathy levels in Malaysia. *International Journal of Medical Education, 4*, 223–229. https://doi.org/10.5116/ijme.5259.4513

Bacharach, M. H. (1976). Empathy: We know what we mean, but what do we measure? *Archives of General Psychiatry, 33*, 35–38.

Baggaley, A. R. (1983). Deciding on the ratio of number of subjects to number of variables in factor analysis. *Multivariate Experimental Clinical Research, 6*, 81–86.

Bailey, B. A. (2001). Empathy in medical students: Assessment and relationship to specialty choice. *Dissertation Abstracts International, 62*(6-A), 2024.

Bakan, D. (1966). *The duality of human existence*. Addison-Wesley.

Baldwin, D. A., & Baird, J. A. (2001). Discerning intentions in dynamic human action. *Trends in Cognitive Science, 5*, 171–178.

Balint, M. (1957). *The doctor, his patient and the illness*. International Universities Press.

Ballou, J. W. (1978). *The psychology of pregnancy*. Lexington Books.

Bandura, A. (1977). *Social learning theory*. Prentice Hall.

Banks, J. A. (1997). *Educating citizens in a multicultural society*. Teachers College Press.

Bargh, J. A., Chen, M., & Burrows, L. (1996). Automaticity of social behavior: Direct effects of trait construct and stereotype-activation on action. *Journal of Personality and Social Psychology, 71*, 230–244.

Barnett, M. A. (1987). Empathy and related responses to children. In N. Eisenberg & J. Strayer (Eds.), *Empathy and its development* (pp. 146–162). Cambridge University Press.

Barnett, M. A., Feighny, K. M., & Esper, J. A. (1983). Effect of anticipated victim responsiveness and empathy upon volunteering. *The Journal of Social Psychology, 119*, 211–218.

Barnett, M. A., Howard, J. A., King, L. M., & Dino, G. A. (1980). Antecedents of empathy: Retrospective accounts of early socialization. *Personality & Social Psychology Bulletin, 6*, 361–365.

Barnett, R. C., Biener, L., & Baruch, G. K. (1987). *Gender and stress*. Free Press.

Barnsley, J., Williams, A. P., Cockerill, R., & Tanner, J. (1999). Physician characteristics and the physician-patient relationship: Impact of sex, year of graduation, and specialty. *Canadian Family Physician, 45*, 935–942.

Baron-Cohen, S. (2003). *The essential difference: The truth about the male and female brain*. Basic Books.

Baron-Cohen, S., & Wheelwright, S. (2004). The empathy quotient: An investigation of adults with Asperger syndrome or high functioning autism, and normal sex differences. *Journal of Autism and Developmental Disorders, 34*, 163–175. https://doi.org/10.1023/B:JADD.0000022607.19833.00

Baron-Cohen, S., Wheelwright, S., Hill, J., Raste, Y., & Plumb, I. (2001). The "Reading the Mind in the Eye" test, revised version: A study with adults, and adults with Asperger syndrome or high functioning autism. *Journal of Child Psychology and Psychiatry, 42*, 241–251.

Barondess, J. A. (2003). Medicine and professionalism. *Archives of Internal Medicine, 163*, 145–149.

Barrett-Lennard, G. T. (1962). Dimensions of therapist response as causal factors in therapeutic change. *Psychological Monographs, 76*, 1–36.

Barrett-Lennard, G. T. (1986). The relationship inventory now: Issues and advances in theory, method and use. In L. S. Greenberg & W. M. Pinsof (Eds.), *The psychotherapeutic process: A research handbook* (pp. 439–476). Guilford.

Barsky, A. J. (1981). Hidden reasons some patients visit doctors. *Annals of Internal Medicine, 94*, 492–498.

Bartholomew, K., & Horowitz, L. (1991). Attachment styles among adults: A test of four-category model. *Journal of Personality and Social Psychology, 61*, 226–244.

Basch, M. F. (1983). Empathic understanding: A review of the concept and some theoretical considerations. *Journal of the American Psychoanalytic Association, 31*, 101–126.

Basch, M. F. (1996). Affect and defense. In D. L. Nathanson (Ed.), *Knowing feeling: Affect, script, and psychotherapy* (pp. 257–269). W.W. Norton.

Bateson, G. (1971). A systems approach. *International Journal of Psychiatry, 9*, 242–244.

Batson, C. D. (1991). *The altruism question: Toward a social psychological answer*. Erlbaum.

Batson, C. D., Batson, J. G., Singlsby, J. K., Harrell, K. L., Peeka, H. M., & Todd, R. M. (1991). Empathic joy and the empathy-altruism hypothesis. *Journal of Personality and Social Psychology, 61*, 413–426.

Batson, C. D., & Coke, J. S. (1981). Empathy: A source of altruistic motivation for helping? In J. P. Rushton & R. M. Sorrentino (Eds.), *Altruism and helping behavior: Social personality, and developmental perspectives* (pp. 167–211). Erlbaum.

Batson, C. D., Coke, J. S., & Pych, V. (1983). Limits on the two-stage model of empathic mediation of helping: A reply to Archer, Diaz-Loving, Gollwitzer, Davis, and Foushee. *Journal of Personality and Social Psychology, 45*, 895–898.

Batson, C. D., Early, S., & Salvarini, G. (1997a). Perspective taking: Imagining how another feels versus imagining how you would feel. *Personality and Social Personality Bulletin, 23*, 751–758.

Batson, C. D., Fultz, J., & Schoenrade, P. A. (1987). Distress and empathy: Two qualitatively distinct vicarious emotions with different motivational consequences. *Journal of Personality, 55*, 19–39.

Batson, C. D., Lishner, D. A., Carpenter, A., Dulin, L., Harjusola-Webb, S., Stocks, E. L., Gale, S., Hassan, O., & Sampat, B. (2003). As you would have them do unto you: Does imagining yourself in the other's place stimulate moral action? *Personality and Social Psychology Bulletin, 29*, 1190–1201.

Batson, C. D., Polycarpou, M. P., Harmon-Jones, E., Imhoff, H. J., Mitchener, E. C., Bednar, L. L., & Highberger, L. (1997b). Empathy and attitudes: Can feeling for a member of a stigmatized group improve feelings toward the group? *Journal of Personality and Social Psychology, 72*, 105–118.

Batson, C. D., Sager, K., Garst, E., Kang, M., Rubchinsky, K., & Dawson, K. (1997c). Is empathy-induced helping due to self-other merging? *Journal of Personality and Social Psychology, 73*, 495–509.

Baumann, A. O., Deber, R. B., Silverman, B. E., & Mallette, C. M. (1998). Who cares? Who cures? The ongoing debate in the provision of health care. *Journal of Advanced Nursing, 28*, 1040–1045.

Bavelas, J. B., Black, A., Lemery, C. R., & Mullett, J. (1986). "I show how you feel": Motor mimicry as a communicative act. *Journal of Personality and Social Psychology, 50*, 322–329.

Bayes, M. A. (1972). Behavioral cues of interpersonal warmth. *Journal of Consulting and Clinical Psychology, 39*, 333–339.

Bazarko, D., Cate, R. A., Azocar, F., & Kreitzer, M. J. (2013). The Impact of an innovative mindfulness-based stress reduction program on the health and well-being of nurses employed in a corporate setting. *Journal of Workplace Behavioral Health, 28*(2), 107–133. https://doi.org/10.1080/15555240.2013.779518

Beattie, A., Durham, J., Harvey, J., Steele, J., & McHanwell, S. (2012). Does empathy change in first-year dental students? *European Journal of Dental Education, 16*, e111–e116. https://doi.org/10.1111/j.1600-0579.2011.00683.x

Becker, H., & Sands, D. (1988). The relationship of empathy to clinical experience among male and female nursing students. *Journal of Nursing Education, 27*, 198–203.

Becker, H. S., & Geer, B. (1958). The fate of idealism in medical school. *American Sociological Review, 23*, 50–56.

Beckman, H. B., & Frankel, R. M. (1984). The effect of physician behavior on the collection of data. *Annals of Internal Medicine, 101*, 692–696.

Beckman, H. B., Markakis, K. M., Suchman, A. L., & Frankel, R. M. (1994). The doctor-patient relationship and malpractice: Lessons from plaintiff depositions. *Archives of Internal Medicine, 154*, 1365–1370.

Beckman, T. J., Reed, D. A., Shanafelt, T. D., & West, C. P. (2010). Impact of resident well-being and empathy on assessments of faculty physicians. *Journal of General Internal Medicine, 25*, 52–56. https://doi.org/10.1007/s11606-009-1152-0

Beddoe, A. E., & Murphy, S. O. (2004). Does mindfulness decrease stress and foster empathy among nursing students? *Journal of Nursing Education, 43*, 305–312. https://doi.org/10.3928/01484834-20040701-07

Beecher, H. K. (1955). The powerful placebo. *Journal of the American Medical Association, 159*, 1602–1606.

Beisecker, A. E., & Beisecker, T. D. (1990). Patient information-seeking behaviors when communicating with doctors. *Medical Care, 28*, 19–28.

Bellet, P. S., & Maloney, M. J. (1991). The importance of empathy as an interviewing skill in medicine. *Journal of the American Medical Association, 266*, 1831–1832.

Bellini, L. M., Baime, M., & Shea, J. A. (2002). Variation of mood and empathy during internship. *Journal of the American Medical Association, 287*, 3143–3146.

Bellini, L. M., & Shea, J. A. (2005). Mood change and empathy decline persist during three years of internal medicine training. *Academic Medicine, 80*(2), 164–167. https://doi.org/10.1097/00001888-200502000-00013

Belsky, J. (1988). The "effects" of infant day care reconsidered. *Childhood Research Quarterly, 3*, 235–272.

Bem, S. L. (1974). The measurement of psychological androgyny. *Journal of Consulting and Clinical Psychology, 42*, 155–162.

Benbassat, J., & Baumal, R. (2004). What is empathy, and how can it be promoted during clinical clerkships? *Academic Medicine, 79*(9), 832–839. https://doi.org/10.1097/00001888-200409000-00004

Benedict, R. H. B., Priore, R. L., Miller, C., Munschauser, F., & Jacobs, L. (2001). Personality disorder in multiple sclerosis correlates with cognitive impairment. *Journal of Neuropsychiatry & Clinical Neurosciences, 13*, 70–76.

Bennett, J. A. (1995). "Methodological notes on empathy": Further considerations. *Advances in Nursing Science, 18*, 36–50.

Bennett, M. J. (2001). *The empathic healer: An endangered species*. Academic Press.

Benton, A. L. (1991). The prefrontal region: Its early history. In H. Levin, H. M. Eisenberg, & A. L. Benton (Eds.), *Frontal lobe function and dysfunction* (pp. 3–32). Oxford University Press.

Beovich, B., & Williams, B. (2021). Empathy in Japanese paramedicine students: A cross-sectional study. *Nursing & Health Sciences, 23*(1), 176–182. https://doi.org/10.1111/nhs.12795

Beres, D., & Arlow, J. A. (1974). Fantasy and identification in empathy. *Psychoanalytic Quarterly, 43*, 26–40.

Berg, K., Blatt, B., Lopreiato, J., Jung, J., Schaeffer, A., Heil, D., Owens, T., Carter-Nolan, P. L., Berg, D., Veloski, J., Darby, E., & Hojat, M. (2015). Standardized patient assessment of medical students empathy: Ethnicity and gender effects in a multi-institutional study. *Academic Medicine, 90*(1), 105–111. https://doi.org/10.1097/ACM.0000000000000529

Berg, K., Majdan, J. F., Berg, D., Veloski, J., & Hojat, M. (2011a). A comparison of medical students' self-reported empathy with simulated patients' assessments of the students' empathy. *Medical Teacher, 33*(5), 388–391. https://doi.org/10.3109/0142159X.2010.530319

Berg, K., Majdan, J., Berg, D., Veloski, J., & Hojat, M. (2011b). Medical students' self-reported empathy and simulated patients' assessments of student empathy: An analysis by gender and ethnicity. *Academic Medicine, 86(8)*, 984–988. https://doi.org/10.1097/ACM.0b013e3182224f1f

Berg, S. J., & Wynne-Edwards, K. E. (2001). Changes in testosterone, cortisol, and estradiol levels in men becoming fathers. *Mayo Clinic Proceedings, 76*, 582–592.

Berger, D. M. (1987). *Clinical empathy*. Jason Aronson.

Berger, S. M. (1962). Conditioning through vicarious instigation. *Psychological Review, 69*, 450–466.

Bergstresser, K. (2017). *Empathy in medical students: Exploring the impact of a longitudinal integrated clerkship model.* (Publication No. 10596918). [Doctoral dissertation, Marywood University]. ProQuest Dissertations & Theses Global. DAI-A 81/1(E).

Berkman, L. F. (1995). The role of social relations in health promotion. *Psychosomatic Medicine, 57*, 245–254.

Berkman, L. F. (2000). Which influences cognitive function: Living alone or being alone? *Lancet, 355*, 1291–1292.

Berkman, L. F., Glass, T., Brissette, I., & Seeman, T. E. (2000). From social integration to health: Durkheim in the new millennium. *Social Science & Medicine, 51*, 843–857.

Berkman, L. F., Leo-Summers, L., & Horwitz, R. I. (1992). Emotional support and survival after myocardial infarction. *Annals of Internal Medicine, 117*, 1003–1009.

Berkman, L., & Syme, S. (1979). Social networks, host resistance, and mortality: A nine-year follow-up of Alameda County residents. *American Journal of Epidemiology, 109*, 186–204.

Berkowitz, L. (1984). Some effects of thoughts on anti and prosocial influences of media events: A cognitive-neoassociation analysis. *Psychological Bulletin, 95*, 410–427.

Berry, K. R. (2019). *Storytelling and how it aids empathy for providers of the trauma patient population.* (Publication No. 27666925). [Doctoral dissertation, The University of Arizona]. ProQuest Dissertations & Theses Global. DAI-B 81/7(E).

Bertakis, K. D., Helms, L. J., Callahan, E. J., Azari, R., & Robbins, J. A. (1995). The influence of gender on physician practice style. *Medical Care, 33*, 407–416.

Bertakis, K. D., Roter, D., & Putman, S. M. (1991). The relationship of physician medical interview style to patient satisfaction. *Journal of Family Practice, 32*, 175–181.

Beutler, L. E., Johnson, D. T., Neville, C. W., & Workman, S. N. (1973). Some sources of variance in "Accurate Empathy" ratings. *Journal of Consulting and Clinical Psychology, 40*, 167–169.

Beven, J. P., O'Brien-Malone, A., & Hall, G. (2004). Using the Interpersonal Reactivity Index to assess empathy in violent offenders. *International Journal of Forensic Psychology, 1*(2), 33–41.

Beverly, E. A., Love, M., & Love, C. (2022). Fully Immersive Virtual Reality Improves Empathy towards People with Diabetes. *Diabetes. Education, 71*(Supplement 1), 495. https://doi.org/10.2337/db22-495-P

Bickel, J. (1994). Special needs and affinities of women medical students. In E. S. More & M. A. Milligan (Eds.), *The empathic practitioner: Empathy, gender, and medicine* (pp. 237–249). Rutgers University Press.

Biswas, A. (2024). *Exploring the impact of empathic communication on stress among students in higher education institutions.* (Publication No. 30993968). [Doctoral dissertation, Northeastern University]. ProQuest Dissertations & Theses Global. DAI-A 85/9(E).

Biswas, B., Haldar, A., Dasgupta, A., Mallick, N., & Karmakar, A. (2018). An epidemiological study on empathy and its correlates: A Cross-sectional assessment among medical students of a government medical college of India. *Indian Journal of Psychological Medicine, 40*(4), 364–369. https://doi.org/10.4103/IJPSYM.IJPSYM_109_18

Bjorklund, D. F., & Kipp, K. (1996). Parental investment theory and gender differences in the evolution of inhibition mechanism. *Psychological Bulletin, 100*, 163–188.

Black, D. M. (2004). Sympathy reconfigured: Some reflections on sympathy, empathy and the discovery of values. *International Journal of Psychoanalysis, 85*(Pt 3), 579–595. https://doi.org/10.1516/002075704774200753

Black, H., & Phillips, S. (1982). An intervention program for the develop empathy in student teachers. *Journal of Psychology: Interdisciplinary & Applied, 112*, 159–168.

Blackman, N., Smith, K., Brokman, R., & Stern, J. (1958). The development of empathy in male schizophrenics. *Psychiatric Quarterly, 32*, 546–553.

Blackwell, B. (1973). Drug therapy, patient compliance. *New England Journal of Medicine, 289*, 249–252.

Blakemore, S. J., Bristow, D., Bird, G., Frith, C., & Ward, J. (2005). Somatosensory activations during the observation of touch and a case of vision-touch synaesthesia. *Brain, 128*(Pt 7), 1571–1583. https://doi.org/10.1093/brain/awh500

Blanco, J. M., Caballero, F., García, F. J., Lorenzo, F., & Monge, D. (2018). Validation of the Jefferson Scale of Physician Empathy in Spanish medical students who participated in an Early Clerkship Immersion programme. *BMC Medical Education, 18*(1), 209. https://doi.org/10.1186/s12909-018-1309-9

Bland, C. J., Meurer, L. N., & Maldonado, G. (1995). Determinants of primary care specialty choice: A non-statistical meta-analysis of the literature. *Academic Medicine, 70*, 620–641.

Blanton, S. (1960). *The healing power of poetry*. Crowell.

Blass, C. D., & Hech, E. J. (1975). Accuracy of accurate empathy ratings. *Journal of Counseling Psychology, 22*, 243–246.

Blazer, D. G. (1982). Social support and mortality in an elderly community population. *American Journal of Epidemiology, 115*, 684–694.

Block, J. H. (1976). Assessing sex differences: Issues, problems, and pitfalls. *Merrill-Palmer Quarterly, 22*, 283–308.

Bloom, B. L., Asher, S. J., & White, S. W. (1978). Marital disruption as a stressor: A review analysis. *Psychological Bulletin, 85*, 867–894.

Bloom, P. (2016). *Against empathy*. Harper Collins.

Blumenthal, J. A., Burg, M. M., Barefoot, J., Williams, R. B., Haney, T., & Zimet, G. (1987). Social support, Type A behavior, and coronary artery disease. *Psychosomatic Medicine, 49*, 331–340.

Blumgart, H. L. (1964). Caring for the patient. *New England Journal of Medicine, 270*, 449–456.

Bohart, A. C., Elliot, R., Greenberg, L. S., & Watson, J. C. (2002). Empathy. In J. C. Norcross (Ed.), *Psychotherapy relationships that work: Therapist contributions and responsiveness to patients* (pp. 89–108). Oxford University Press.

Bolognini, S. (1997). Empathy and "empathism". *International Journal of Psychoanalysis, 78*, 279–293.

Bombeke, K., Van Roosbroeck, S., De Winter, B., Debaene, L., Schol, S., Van Hal, G., & Van Royen, P. (2011). Medical students trained in communication skills show a decline in patient-centred attitudes: An observational study comparing two cohorts during clinical clerkships. *Patient Education and Counseling, 84*(3), 310–318. https://doi.org/10.1016/j.pec.2011.03.007

Bond, A. R., Mason, H. F., Lemaster, C. M., Shaw, S. E., Mullin, C. S., Hollick, E. A., & Saper, R. B. (2013). Embodied health: The effects of mind-body course for medical students. *Medical education online, 18, 1–8*. https://doi.org/10.3402/meo.v18i0.20699

Bonuso, C. F. (2013). *Empathy in the clinical encounter: a study of situational and dispositional empathy levels as associated with clinical training and practice*. (Publication No. 3570197). [Doctoral dissertation, Pace University]. ProQuest Dissertations & Theses Global. DAI-B 74/09(E).

Book, A. S., Starzyk, K. B., & Quinsey, V. L. (2001). The relationship between testosterone and aggression: A meta-analysis. *Aggression and Violent Behavior: A Review Journal, 6*, 579–599.

Book, H. E. (1988). Empathy: Misconceptions and misuses in psychotherapy. *American Journal of Psychiatry, 145*, 420–424.

Book, H. E. (1991). Is empathy cost efficient? *American Journal of Psychotherapy, 45*, 21–30.

Booth, A., Granger, D. A., Mazur, A., & Kivlighan, K. T. (2006). Testosterone and social behavior. *Social Forces, 85(1)*, 167–191. https://doi.org/10.1353/sof.2006.0116

Borgenicht, L. (1984). Richard Selzer and the problem of detached concern. *Annals of Internal Medicine, 100*, 923–934.

Borke, H. (1971). Interpersonal perception of young children: Ego-centrism or empathy. *Developmental Psychology, 5*, 263–269.

Boruch, R. F. (1982). Evidence and inference in research on mass psychogenic illness. In M. J. Colligan, J. W. Pennebaker, & L. R. Murphy (Eds.), *Mass psychogenic illness: A social psychological analysis* (pp. 101–125). Erlbaum.

Boscarino, J. A. (1995). Post-traumatic stress and associated disorders among Vietnam veterans. The significance of combat exposure and social support. *Journal of Trauma Stress, 8*, 317–336.

Botvinick, M., Jha, A. P., Bylsma, L. M., Fabian, S. A., Solomon, P. E., & Prkachin, K. M. (2005). Viewing facial expression of pain engages cortical areas involved in the direct experience of pain. *Neuroimage, 25*(1), 312–319. https://doi.org/10.1016/j.neuroimage.2004.11.043

Bowers, M. R., Swan, J. E., & Koehler, W. F. (1994). What attributes determine quality and satisfaction with health care delivery? *Health Care Management Review, 19*, 49–55.

Bowlby, J. (1973). *Attachment and loss (Vol. 2): Separation: Anxiety and anger*. Basic Books.

Bowlby, J. (1980). *Attachment and loss (Vol. 3): Loss: Sadness and depression*. Basic Books.

Bowlby, J. (1982). *Attachment and loss (Vol. 1): Attachment*. Basic Books.

Bowlby, J. (1988). *A secure base: Parent-child attachment and healthy human development*. Basic Books.

Boyd, R. W., & DiMascio, A. (1957). Social behavior and automatic physiology: A sociophysiological study. *Journal of Nervous and Mental Disease, 120*, 207–212.

Boyle, M. J., Williams, B., Brown, T., Molloy, A., McKenna, L., Molloy, L., & Lewis, B. (2009). Levels of empathy in undergraduate health science students. *The Internet Journal of Medical Education, 1*. https://ispub.com/IJME/1/1/9959

Braga-Simões, J., Costa, P. S., & Yaphe, J. (2017). Placebo prescription and empathy of the physician: A cross-sectional study. *The European Journal of General Practice, 23*(1), 98–104. https://doi.org/10.1080/13814788.2017.1291625

Branch, W. T. (2000). The ethics of caring and medical education. *Academic Medicine, 75*, 127–132.

Branch, W. T., & Malik, T. K. (1993). Using windows of opportunities in brief interviews to understand patients' concerns. *Journal of the American Medical Association, 169*, 1667–1668.

Branch, W. T., Pels, R. J., & Hafler, J. P. (1998). Medical students' empathic understanding of their patients. *Academic Medicine, 73*, 360–362.

Brazeau, C. M. L. R., Schroeder, R., Rovi, S., & Boyd, L. (2010). Relationship between medical student burnout, empathy, and professionalism climate. *Academic Medicine, 85*(10 Suppl), s33–s36. https://doi.org/10.1097/ACM.0b013e3181ed4c47

Brazeau, C. M. L. R., Schroeder, R., Rovi, S., & Boyd, L. (2011). Relationship between medical student service and empathy. *Academic Medicine, 86*(10 Suppl), S42–S45. https://doi.org/10.1097/ACM.0b013e31822a6ae0

Bretherton, I. (1987). New perspectives on attachment relations: Security, communication, and internal working models. In J. Osofsky (Ed.), *Handbook of infant development* (pp. 1061–1100). John Wiley & Sons.

Bridgman, D. L. (1981). Enhanced role taking through cooperative interdependence: A field study. *Child Development, 52*, 1231–1238.

Brislin, R. W. (1970). Back-translation for cross-cultural research. *Journal of Cross-Cultural Psychology, 1*, 185–216.

Bristow, P. M. (2014). *Reel influence: video as an instructional strategy in addressing the affective domain in instructional design.* (Publication No. 3625747). [Doctoral dissertation, Capella University]. ProQuest Dissertations & Theses Global. DAI-A 75/10(E).

Briton, N. J., & Hall, J. A. (1995). Beliefs about female and male nonverbal communication. *Sex Roles, 32*, 79–90.

Brock, C. D., & Salinsky, J. V. (1993). Empathy: An essential skill for understanding the physician-patient relationship in clinical practice. *Family Medicine, 25*, 245–248.

Brockhouse, R., Msetfi, R. M., Cohen, K., & Joseph, S. (2011). Vicarious exposure to trauma and growth in therapists: The moderating effects of sense of coherence, organizational support, and empathy. *Journal of Traumatic Stress, 24(6)*, 735–742. https://doi.org/10.1002/jts.20704

Brody, H. (1985). Placebo effect: An examination of Grunbaum's definition. In L. White, B. Tursky, & G. E. Schwartz (Eds.), *Placebo: Theory, Research, And Mechanisms* (pp. 37–58). Guilford Press.

Brody, H. (1997). Placebo response, sustained partnership, and emotional resilience in practice. *Journal of the American Board of Family Practice, 10*, 72–74.

Brody, L. R., & Hall, J. A. (2008). Gender and emotion in context. In M. Lewis & J. Haviland (Eds.), *Handbook of emotions* (3rd ed., pp. 395–408). Guilford.

Brothers, L. (1989). A biological perspective on empathy. *American Journal of Psychiatry, 146*, 10–19.

Brown, J., & Dunn, J. (1996). Continuities in emotional understanding from 3 to 6 years. *Child Development, 67*, 789–802.

Brown, T., Boyle, M., Williams, B., Molloy, A., Palermo, C., McKenna, L., & Molloy, L. (2011). Predictors of empathy in health science students. *Journal of Allied Health, 40*(3), 143–149.

Brown, T., Williams, B., Boyle, M., Molloy, A., McKenna, L., Molloy, L., & Lewis, B. (2010). Levels of empathy in undergraduate occupational therapy students. *Occupational Therapy International, 17*, 135–141. https://doi.org/10.1002/oti.297

Brownell, A. K., & Cote, L. (2001). Senior residents' views on the meaning of professionalism and how they learn about it. *Academic Medicine, 76*, 734–737.

Bruggi, F., & Falaschi, F. (2022). Correlation Between Attending Physicians' Empathy and Readmission Rate in Internal Medicine. *American Journal of Biomedical Science & Research, 16*(4). https://doi.org/10.34297/AJBSR.2022.16.002254

Bruner, J. (1990). *Acts of meaning*. Harvard University Press.

Bryant, B. K. (1982). An index of empathy for children and adolescents. *Child Development, 53*, 413–425.

Buccino, G., Binkofski, F., Fink, G. R., Fadiga, L., Fogassi, L., Gallese, V., Seitz, R. J., Zilles, K., Rizzolatti, G., & Freund, H. J. (2001). Action observation activates premotor and parietal areas in a somatotypic manner: An fMRI study. *European Journal of Neuroscience, 13*, 400–404.

Bucher, J. T., Vu, D. M., & Hojat, M. (2013). Psychostimulant drug abuse and personality factors in medical students. *Medical Teacher, 35*(*1*), 53–57. https://doi.org/10.3109/0142159X.2012.731099

Buchheimer, A. (1963). The development of ideas about empathy. *Journal of Counseling Psychology, 10*, 61–70.

Buck, E., Holden, M., & Szauter, K. (2017). Changes in humanism during medical school: A synthesis of the evidence. *Medical Science Educator, 27*, 1–7. https://doi.org/10.1007/s40670-017-0438-9

Buck, R. (1984). *The communication of emotion*. Guilford Press.

Buck, R., & Ginsburg, B. (1997a). Communicative genes and the evolution of empathy: Selfish and social emotions as voices of selfish and social genes. *Annals of the New York Academy of Sciences, 807*, 481–483.

Buck, R., & Ginsburg, B. (1997b). Communicative genes and the evolution of empathy. In W. Ickes (Ed.), *Empathic accuracy* (pp. 17–43). Guilford.

Buck, R., Miller, R. E., & Caul, W. F. (1974). Sex, personality, and physiological variables in the communication of affect via facial expression. *Journal of Personality and Social Psychology, 30*, 587–596.

Buck, R. W., Savin, V. J., Miller, R. E., & Caul, W. F. (1972). Communication of affect through facial expressions in humans. *Journal of Personality and Social Psychology, 23*, 362–371.

Burack, J. H., Irby, D. M., Carline, J. D., Ambrozy, D. M., Ellsbury, K. E., & Stritter, F. T. (1997). A study of medical students' specialty-choice pathways: Trying on possible selves. *Academic Medicine, 72*, 534–541.

Burdi, M. D., & Baker, L. C. (1999). Physicians' perceptions of autonomy and satisfaction in California. *Health Affairs, 18*, 134–145.

Burger, J. M. (2009). Replicating Milgram: Would people still obey today? *American Psychologist, 64*(1), 1–11. https://doi.org/10.1037/a0010932

Burkhard, S. (2023). *The relationship of medical provider humility, empathy, and competency on patient satisfaction.* (Publication No. 30316452). [Doctoral dissertation, George Fox University]. ProQuest Dissertations & Theses Global. DAI-A 84/10(E).

Burlingham, D. (1967). Empathy between infant and mother. *Journal of the American Psychoanalytic Association, 15*, 764–780.

Burns, D. D., & Nolen-Hoeksema, S. (1992). Therapeutic empathy and recovery from depression in cognitive-behavioral therapy: A structural equation model. *Journal of Consulting and Clinical Psychology, 60*, 441–449.

Burnstein, A. G., Loucks, S., Kobos, J., Johnson, G., Talbert, R. L., & Stanton, B. (1980). A longitudinal study of personality characteristics of medical students. *Journal of Medical Education, 55*, 786–787.

Bush, L. K., Barr, C. L., McHugo, G. J., & Lanzetta, J. T. (1989). The effects of facial control and facial mimicry on subjective reactions to comedy routines. *Motivation and Emotion, 13*, 31–52.
Bushnell, M. C., Duncan, G. H., Hofbauer, R. K., Ha, B., Chen, J. I., & Carrier, B. (1999). Pain perception: Is there a role for primary somatosensory cortex? *National Academy of Sciences, 96*, 7705–7709.
Buss, D. M. (1989). Sex differences in human mate preferences: Evolutionary hypotheses tested in 37 cultures. *Behavioral and Brain Sciences, 12*, 1–49.
Buss, D. M. (1995). Psychological sex differences: Origins through sexual selection. *American Psychologist, 50*, 164–168.
Buss, D. M. (2003). *The evolution of desire: Strategies of human mating*. Basic Books.
Buss, D. M., & Barnes, M. (1986). Preferences in human mate selection. *Journal of Personality and Social Psychology, 50*, 559–570.
Buss, D. M., & Schmitt, D. P. (1993). Sexual strategies theory: An evolutionary perspective on human mating. *Psychological Review, 100*, 204–232.
Butow, P. N., Maclean, M., Dunn, S. M., Tattersall, M. H. N., & Boyer, M. J. (1997). The dynamics of change: Cancer patients' preferences for information, involvement and support. *Annals of Oncology, 8*, 857–863.
Bylund, C. L., & Makoul, G. (2002). Empathic communication and gender in the physician-patient encounter. *Patient Education and Counseling, 48*, 207–216.
Bylund, C. L., & Makoul, G. (2005). Examining empathy in medical encounters: An observational study using the empathic communication coding system. *Health Communication, 18*(2), 123–140. https://doi.org/10.1207/s15327027hc1802_2
Byrd, J., Knowles, H., Moore, S., Acker, V., Bell, S., Alanis, N., Zhou, Y., d'Etienne, J. P., Kline, J. A., & Wang, H. (2021). Synergistic effects of emergency physician empathy and burnout on patient satisfaction: a prospective observational study. *Emergency Medicine Journal: EMJ, 38*(4), 290–296. https://doi.org/10.1136/emermed-2019-209393
Cacioppo, J. T., Hawkley, L. C., Crawford, E., Ernst, J. M., Burleson, M. H., Kowalewski, R. B., & Berntson, G. G. (2002). Loneliness and health: Potential mechanisms. *Psychosomatic Medicine, 64*, 401–417.
Cahill, L. (2005). His brain, her brain. *Scientific American, 292*(5), 40–47.
Calabrese, L. H., Bianco, J. A., Mann, D., Massello, D., & Hojat, M. (2013). Correlates and changes in empathy and attitudes toward interprofessional collaboration in osteopathic medical students. *The Journal of the American Osteopathic Association, 113*, 898–907. https://doi.org/10.7556/jaoa.2013.068
Calhoun, J. B. (1962). Population density and social pathology. *Scientific American, 206*, 3–10.
Calman, K. C., Downie, R. S., Duthie, M., & Sweeney, B. (1988). Literature and medicine: A short course for medical students. *Medical Education, 22*, 265–269.
Campbell, A. (2008). Attachment, aggression, and affiliation: The role of oxytocin in female social behavior. *Biological Psychology, 77*, 1–10. https://doi.org/10.1016/j.biopsycho.2007.09.001
Campbell, D. T., & Fiske, D. W. (1959). Convergent and discriminant validation by the multitrait-multimethod matrix. *Psychological Bulletin, 56*, 81–105.
Campos, J., & Sternberg, C. (1981). Perception, appraisal and emotion in the onset of social referencing. In M. E. Lamb & L. R. Sherrod (Eds.), *Infant social cognition* (pp. 273–314). Erlbaum.
Campus-Outcalt, D., Senf, J., Watkins, A. J., & Bastacky, S. (1995). The effects of medical school curricula, faculty role models, and biomedical research on choice of generalist physician career: A review and quality assessment of the literature. *Academic Medicine, 70*, 611–619.
Cannon, W. (1957). "Voodoo" death. *Psychosomatic Medicine, 19*, 182–190.
Carey, T. S., Motyka, T. M., Garret, J. M., & Keller, R. B. (2003). Do osteopathic physicians differ in patient interaction from allopathic physicians? An empirically derived approach. *Journal of American Osteopathic Association, 103*(7), 313–318.
Carkhuff, R. (1969). *Helping and human relations: Selection and training* (Vol. 1). Holt, Rinehart & Winston.

Carmel, S., & Glick, S. M. (1996). Compassionate-empathic physicians: Personality traits and social-organizational factors that enhance or inhibit this behavior pattern. *Social Science and Medicine, 43*, 1253–1261.

Carr, L., Iacoboni, M., Dubeau, M. C., Mazziotta, J. C., & Lenzi, G. L. (2003). Neural mechanisms of empathy in humans: A relay from neural systems for imitation to limbic areas. *Proceedings of the National Academy of Sciences of the United States of America, 100*, 5497–5502. https://doi.org/10.1073/pnas.0935845100

Carr, P. L., Ash, A. S., & Friedman, E. H. (1998). Relation of family responsibilities and gender to the productivity and career satisfaction of medical faculty. *Annals of Internal Medicine, 129*, 532–538.

Carrard, V., Bourquin, C., Berney, S., Schlegel, K., Gaume, J., Bart, P. A., Preisig, M., Schmid Mast, M., & Berney, A. (2022). The relationship between medical students' empathy, mental health, and burnout: A cross-sectional study. *Medical Teacher, 44*(12), 1392–1399. https://doi.org/10.1080/0142159X.2022.2098708

Carter, C. S. (2007). Sex differences in oxytocin and vasopressin: Implications for autism spectrum disorders? *Behavior and Brain Research, 176*, 170–186. https://doi.org/10.1016/j.bbr.2006.08.025

Carter, F. (1976). *The education of little tree*. University of New Mexico Press.

Carter, R. D. (2017). *Physician wellness: impact of stress, burnout, and depression on medical trainee empathy.* (Publication No. 13837064). [Doctoral dissertation, University of Houston]. ProQuest Dissertations & Theses Global. DAI-A 77/09(E).

Case, R. B., Moss, A. J., Case, N., McDermott, M., & Eberly, S. (1992). Living alone after myocardial infarction: Impact on prognosis. *Journal of the American Medical Association, 267*, 515–519.

Caspi, A., & Silva, P. A. (1995). Temperamental qualities at age three predict personality traits in young adulthood: Longitudinal evidence from a birth cohort. *Child Development, 66*, 486–492.

Castiello, U. (2003). Understanding other people's actions: Intention and attention. *Journal of Experimental Psychology, 29*, 416–430.

Castiello, U., Lusher, D., Mari, M., Edwards, M., & Humphreys, G. (2002). Observing a human or a robotic hand grasping an object: Differential motor priming effects. In W. Prinz & B. Hommel (Eds.), *Common mechanisms in perception and action: Attention and performance XIX* (pp. 315–333). Oxford University Press.

Castiglioni, A. (1941). *A history of medicine*. Knopf.

Cataldo, K. P., Peeden, K., Geesey, M. E., & Dickerson, L. (2005). Association between Balint training and physician empathy and work satisfaction. *Family Medicine, 37*(5), 328–331. http://www.stfm.org/fmhub/fm2005/may/kari328.pdf

Catlow, R., Aikins-Snyper, F., Carson, M., Jaggi, A., & Bench, S. (2020). Empathy in Action in Healthcare (EACH): A mixed methods study of nurses' and therapists' empathy. *International Journal of Orthopaedic and Trauma Nursing, 39*, 100777. https://doi.org/10.1016/j.ijotn.2020.100777

Cattle, R. B. (1966). The scree test for the number of factors. *Multivariate Behavioral Research, 1*, 245–276.

Chaitoff, A., Sun, B., Windover, A., Bokar, D., Featherall, J., Rothberg, M. B., & Misra-Hebert, A. D. (2017). Associations between physician empathy, physician characteristics, and standardized measures of patient experience. *Academic Medicine: Journal of the Association of American Medical Colleges, 92*(10), 1464–1471. https://doi.org/10.1097/ACM.0000000000001671

Chaitoff, A., Rothberg, M. B., Windover, A. K., Calabrese, L., Misra-Hebert, A., & Martinez, K. (2018). Physician empathy is not associated with laboratory outcomes in diabetes: a cross-sectional study. *Journal of General Intern Medicine, 34*(1), 75–81. https://doi.org/10.1007/s11606-018-4731-0

Chakrabarti, B., & BaronCohen, S. (2006). Empathizing: Neurocognitive developmental mechanisms and individual differences. *Progress in Brain Research, 156*, 403–417. https://doi.org/10.1016/S0079-6123(06)56022-4

Chamberlin, J. (2015). Social psychology on the silver screen. *Monitor on Psychology, 46*(3), 16–17.

Chaminade, T., Meltzoff, A., & Decety, J. (2002). Does the end justify the means? A PET exploration of the mechanisms involved in human imitation. *Neuroimage, 15*, 318–328.

Chandler, C. (2021). *Clinician empathy and alliance building with patients during clinician and patient interactions in a drug addiction treatment center in northeastern new jersey*. (Publication No. 28643746). [Doctoral dissertation, Grand Canyon University]. ProQuest Dissertations & Theses Global. DAI-B 83/1(E).

Charlesworth, W. R., & Dzur, C. (1987). Gender comparisons of preschoolers' behavior and resource utilization in group problem-solving. *Child Development, 58*, 191–200.

Charman, T., Swettenham, J., Baron-Cohen, S., Cox, A., Baird, G., & Drew, A. (1997). Infants with autism: An investigation of empathy, pretend play, joint attention, and imitation. *Developmental Psychology, 33*, 781–789.

Charon, R. (1993). The narrative road to empathy. In H. Spiro, M. G. McCrea Curnen, E. Peschel, & D. St. James (Eds.), *Empathy and the practice of medicine* (pp. 147–159). Yale University Press.

Charon, R. (2000). Medicine, the novel, and the passage of time. *Annals of Internal Medicine, 132*, 63–68.

Charon, R. (2001a). Narrative medicine: A model for empathy, reflection, profession, and trust. *Journal of the American Medical Association, 286*, 1897–1902.

Charon, R. (2001b). Narrative medicine: Form, function, and ethics. *Annals of Internal Medicine, 134*, 83–87.

Charon, R., Greene, M. G., & Adelman, R. (1994). Woman readers, woman doctors: A feminist reader-response theory of medicine. In E. S. More & M. A. Milligan (Eds.), *The empathic practitioner: Empathy, gender, and medicine* (pp. 205–221). Rutgers University Press.

Charon, R., & Montello, M. (2002). *Stories matter: The role of narrative in medical ethics*. Routledge.

Charon, R., Trautmann Banks, J., Connelly, J. E., Hawkins, A. H., Hunter, K. M., Jones, A. H., Montello, M., & Poirer, S. (1995). Literature in medicine: Contribution to clinical practice. *Annals of Internal Medicine, 122*(8), 599–606.

Chartrand, T. L., & Bargh, J. A. (1999). The chameleon effect: The perception-behavior link and social interaction. *Journal of Personality and Social Psychology, 76*, 893–910.

Chase-Lansdale, P. L., Wakschlag, L. S., & Brooks-Gunn, J. (1995). A psychological perspective on the development of caring in children and youth: The role of the family. *Journal of Adolescence, 18*, 515–556.

Chatterjee, A., Ravikumar, R., Singh, S., Chauhan, P. S., & Goel, M. (2017). Clinical empathy in medical students in India measured using the Jefferson Scale of Empathy-Student Version. *Journal of Educational Evaluation for Health Professions, 14*, 33. https://doi.org/10.3352/jeehp.2017.14.33

Chen, A., Hanna, J. J., Manohar, A., & Tobia, A. (2018). Teaching Empathy: The Implementation of a Video Game into a Psychiatry Clerkship Curriculum. *Academic Psychiatry : The Journal of the American Association of Directors of Psychiatric Residency Training and the Association for Academic Psychiatry, 42*(3), 362–365. https://doi.org/10.1007/s40596-017-0862-6

Chen, D., Lew, R., Hershman, W., & Orlander, J. (2007). A cross-sectional measurement of medical student empathy. *Journal of General Internal Medicine, 22(10)*, 1434–1438. https://doi.org/10.1007/s11606-007-0298-x

Chen, J. T., LaLopa, J., & Dang, D. K. (2008). Impact of patient empathy modeling on pharmacy students caring for the underserved. *American Journal of Pharmaceutical Education, 72*(2), Article 40.

Chen, D. C. R., Kirshenbaum, D. S., Yan, J., Kirshenbaum, E., & Aseltine, R. H. (2012). Characterizing changes in student empathy throughout medical school. *Medical Teacher, 34*(4), 305–311. https://doi.org/10.3109/0142159X.2012.644600

Chen, D. C. R., Pahilan, M. E., & Orlander, J. D. (2010). Comparing a self-administered measure of empathy with observed behavior among medical students. *Journal of General Internal Medicine, 25*(3), 200–202. https://doi.org/10.1007/s11606-009-1193-4

Chen, P. J., Huang, C. D., & Yeh, S. J. (2017). Impact of a narrative medicine program on healthcare providers' empathy scores over time. *BMC Medical Education, 17*(1), 108. https://doi.org/10.1186/s12909-017-0952-x

Cheng, Y., Lin, C. P., Liu, H. L., Hsu, Y. Y., Lim, K. E., Hung, D., & Decety, J. (2007). Expertise modulates the perception of pain in others. *Current Biology, 17*(19), 1708–1713. https://doi.org/10.1016/j.cub.2007.09.020

Chessick, R. D. (1992). *What constitutes the patient in psychotherapy: Alternative approaches to understanding humans*. Jason Aronson.

Chinsky, J. M., & Rappaport, J. (1970). Brief critique of the meaning and reliability of "Accurate Empathy" ratings. *Psychological Bulletin, 73*, 379–382.

Chismar, D. (1988). Empathy and sympathy: The important difference. *Journal of Value Inquiry, 22*, 257–266.

Chlopan, B. E., McCain, M. L., Carbonell, J. L., & Hagen, R. L. (1985). Empathy: Review of available measures. *Journal of Personality and Social Psychology, 48*, 635–653.

Cho, E., & Jeon, S. (2019). The role of empathy and psychological need satisfaction in pharmacy students' burnout and well-being. *BMC Medical Education, 19*, 43. https://doi.org/10.1186/s12909-019-1477-2

Chochinov, H. (2007). Dignity and the essence of medicine: The A, B, C, and D of Dignity conserving care. *British Medical Journal, 335*, 184–187. https://doi.org/10.1136/bmj.39244.650926.47

Chodorow, N. (1978). *The reproduction of mothering: Psychoanalysis and sociology of gender*. University of California Press.

Chow, K. L., Riesen, A. H., & Newell, F. W. (1957). Degeneration of retinal ganglion cells in infant chimpanzees reared in darkness. *Journal of Comparative Neurology, 107*, 27–42.

Christenfeld, N., & Gerin, W. (2000). Social support and cardiovascular reactivity. *Biomedicine and Pharmacotherapy, 54*, 251–257.

Christodoulou, G. N., Lykousras, L. P., Mountaokalakis, T., Voulgari, A., & Stefanis, C. N. (1995). Personalities of psychiatric versus other medical trainers. *Journal of Nervous and Mental Disease, 183*, 330–340.

Ciechanowski, P. S., Russo, J. E., Katon, W. J., & Walker, F. A. (2004). Attachment theory in health care: The influence of relationship style on medical students' specialty choice. *Medical Education, 38*(*3*), 262–270. https://doi.org/10.1046/j.1365-2923.2004.01767.x

Clark, K. B. (1980). Empathy—A neglected topic in psychological research. *American Psychologist, 35*, 187–190.

Clearly, P. D., & McNeil, B. J. (1988). Patient satisfaction as an indicator of quality care. *Inquiry, 25*, 25–36.

Cleghorn, S. M. (1978). Empathy: Listening with the third ear. *Tennessee Education, 8*, 7–11.

Cliffordson, C. (2002). The hierarchical structure of empathy: Dimensional organization and elations to social functioning. *Scandinavian Journal of Psychology, 43*, 49–59.

Cloninger, C. R., Svrakic, D. M., & Przybeck, D. M. (1993). A psychobiological model of temperament and character. *Archives of General Psychiatry, 50*, 975–990.

Clouser, K. D. (1990). Humanities in medical education: Some contributions. *Journal of Medical Philosophy, 15*, 289–301.

Cohen, J. (1987). *Statistical power analysis for the behavioral sciences*. Erlbaum.

Cohen, S. (1988). Psychological models for the role of social support in the etiology of physical disease. *Health Psychology, 7*, 269–297.

Cohen, S. (2004). Social relationship and health. *American Psychologist, 59*(*8*), 676–684. https://doi.org/10.1037/0003-066X.59.8.676

Cohen, E. L., & Hoffner, C. (2013). Gifts of giving: The role of empathy and perceived benefits to others and self in young adults' decisions to become organ donors. *Journal of Health Psychology, 18*(*1*), 128–138. https://doi.org/10.1177/1359105311433910

Cohen, S., & Matthews, K. A. (1987). Social support, type A behavior, and coronary artery disease. *Psychosomatic Medicine, 49*, 325–330.

Coke, J. S., Batson, C. D., & McDavis, K. (1978). Empathic mediation of helping: A two-stage model. *Journal of Personality and Social Psychology, 36*, 752–766.

Cole, D. A., Martin, N. C., & Steiger, J. H. (2005). Empirical and conceptual problems with longitudinal trait-state models: Introducing a trait-state-occasion model. *Psychological Methods, 10*(1), 3–20. https://doi.org/10.1037/1082-989X.10.1.3

Coleridge, S. T. (1802). Letter to William Sotheby, July 13th. In E. L. Griggs (Ed.), *Collected letters of Samuel Taylor Coleridge* (Vol. 2). Oxford University Press. (Reprinted in 1956).

Coles, B. A. (2015). *Compassion fatigue and empathy in nurses caring for clients with HIV/AIDS.* (Publication No. 3730826). [Doctoral dissertation, University of Phoenix]. ProQuest Dissertations & Theses Global. DAI-B 77/03(E).

Coles, R. (1989). *Call of stories: Teaching and moral imagination*. Houghton-Mifflin.

Collier, V. U., MaCue, J. D., Markus, A., & Smith, L. (2002). Stress in medical residency: Status quo after a decade or reform? *Annals of Internal Medicine, 136*, 384–390.

Colligan, M. J., & Murphy, L. R. (1982). A review of mass psychogenic illness in work settings. In M. J. Colligan, J. W. Pennebaker, & L. R. Murphy (Eds.), *Mass psychogenic illness: A social psychological analysis* (pp. 33–52). Erlbaum.

Collins, F. S. (1999). Shattuck lecture—Medical and societal consequences of the human genome project. *New England Journal of Medicine, 341*, 28–37.

Colliver, J. A., Conlee, M. J., Verhulst, S. J., & Dorsey, J. K. (2010a). Rebuttals to critics of studies of the decline on empathy. *Academic Medicine, 85(12)*, 1813–1814. https://doi.org/10.1097/ACM.0b013e3181fa3576

Colliver, J. A., Conlee, M. J., Verhulst, S. J., & Dorsey, J. K. (2010b). Reports of the decline of empathy during medical education are greatly exaggerated: A reexamination of the research. *Academic Medicine, 85*(4), 588–593. https://doi.org/10.1097/ACM.0b013e3181d281dc

Colliver, J. A., Willis, M. S., Robbs, R. S., Cohen, D. S., & Swartz, M. H. (1998). Assessment of empathy in a standardized-patient examination. *Teaching and Learning in Medicine, 10*, 8–10.

Colman, A. M. (2001). *A dictionary of psychology*. Oxford University Press.

Comas-Diaz, L., & Jacobsen, F. M. (1991). Ethnocultural transference and countertransference in the therapeutic dyad. *American Journal of Orthopsychiatry, 61*, 392–402.

Comstock, L. M., Hooper, E. M., Goodwin, J. M., & Goodwin, J. S. (1982). Physician behaviors that correlate with patient satisfaction. *Journal of Medical Education, 57*, 105–112.

Connellan, J., Baron-Cohen, S., Wheelwright, S., Batki, A., & Ahluwalia, J. (2000). Sex differences in human neonatal social perception. *Infant Behavior & Development, 23*, 113–118.

Consorti, F., Notarangelo, M. A., Potasso, L. A., & Toscano, E. (2012). Developing professionalism in Italian medical students: An educational framework. *Advances in Medical Education and Practice, 3*, 55–60. https://doi.org/10.2147/AMEP.S31228

Cooper-Patrick, L., Gallo, J. J., & Gonzales, J. J. (1999). Race, gender and partnership in the patient-physician relationship. *Journal of the American Medical Association, 282*, 583–589.

Coplan, A. (2014). Understanding empathy: Its features and effects. In A. Coplan & P. Goldie (Eds.), *Empathy: Philosophical and psychological perspectives* (pp. 3–18). Oxford University Press.

Copland, A., & Goldie, P. (Eds.). (2014). *Understanding empathy: Its features and effects*. Oxford University Press.

Costa, P., Alves, R., Neto, I., Marvão, P., Portela, M., & Costa, M. J. (2014). Associations between medical student empathy and personality: A multi-institutional study. *PloS one, 9*(3), e89254. https://doi.org/10.1371/journal.pone.0089254

Costa, P., De Carvalho-Filho, M. A., Schweller, M., Thiemann, P., Salgueira, A., Benson, J., Costa, M. J., & Quince, T. (2017). Measuring medical students' empathy: Exploring the underlying constructs of and associations between two widely used self-report instruments in five countries. *Academic Medicine, 92(6)*, 860–867. https://doi.org/10.1097/ACM.0000000000001449

Costa, P., Magalhães, E., & Costa, M. J. (2013). A latent growth model suggests that empathy of medical students does not decline over time. *Advances in Health Sciences Education, 18*(3), 509–522. https://doi.org/10.1007/s10459-012-9390-z

Costa, P. T., Jr., & McCrea, R. B. (1992). *Revised NEO Personality Inventory (NEO PI-R) and NEO Five Factor Inventory (NEO-FFI): Professional manual*. Psychological Assessment Resources.

Coulehan, J. L., & Williams, P. (2001). Vanquishing virtue: The impact of medical education. *Academic Medicine, 76*, 598–605.

Coulmas, M. C. (2006). *A study of the effect of clinical experience on nursing empathy.* (Publication No. 3226809). [Doctoral dissertation, Capella University]. ProQuest Dissertations & Theses Global. DAI-B 67/07.

Courtenay, T. M. (2016). *Improving inpatient experience utilizing an empathy enhancement program.* (Publication No. 10295869). [Doctoral dissertation, University of Hawai'i at Manoa]. ProQuest Dissertations & Theses Global. DAI-A 81/1(E).

Cousins, N. (1985). How patients appraise physicians. *New England Journal of Medicine, 313*, 1422–1424.

Coutts, L. C., & Rogers, J. C. (2000). Humanism: Is its evaluation captured in commonly used performance measures? *Teaching and Learning in Medicine, 12*, 28–32.

Coutts-van Dijk, L. C., Bray, J. H., Moore, S., & Rogers, J. (1997). Prospective study of how students' humanism and psychosocial beliefs relate to specialty matching. *Academic Medicine, 72*, 1106–1108.

Crabb, W. T., Moracco, J. C., & Bender, R. C. (1983). A comparative study of empathy training with programmed instruction for lay helpers. *Journal of Counseling Psychology, 30*, 221–226.

Craig, K. D., & Weiss, S. M. (1971). Vicarious influences on pain-threshold determinations. *Journal of Personality and Social Psychology, 19*, 53–59.

Crandall, S. J., & Marion, G. S. (2009). Commentary: Identifying attitudes towards empathy: An essential feature of professionalism. *Academic Medicine, 84*(9), 1174–1176. https://doi.org/10.1097/ACM.0b013e3181b17b11

Cristy, B. L. (2001). Wounded healer: The impact of a therapist's illness on the therapeutic situation. *Journal of the American Academy of Psychoanalysis, 29*, 33–42.

Croft, R. L., Byrd, C. T., & Kelly, E. M. (2022). The influence of active listening on parents' perceptions of clinical empathy in a stuttering assessment: A preliminary study. *Journal of Communication Disorders, 100*, 106274. https://doi.org/10.1016/j.jcomdis.2022.106274

Cronbach, L. J. (1951). Coefficient alpha and the internal structure of tests. *Psychometrika, 16*, 297–334.

Cross, D. G., & Sharpley, C. F. (1982). Measurement of empathy with the Hogan Empathy Scale. *Psychological Reports, 50*, 62.

Crouse, B. B., & Mehrabian, A. (1977). Affiliation of opposite-sex strangers. *Journal of Research in Personality, 11*, 38–47.

Crump, W. J., Ziegler, C. H., & Fricker, R. S. (2018). A Residency Professional Identity Curriculum and a Longitudinal Measure of Empathy. *Journal of Regional Medical Campuses, 1*(4). https://doi.org/10.24926/jrmc.v1i4.1353

Crump, W. J., Ziegler, C. H., & Fricker, R. (2022). Do medical residents with rural upbringing show less decline in empathy during training? A report from a rural family medicine residency. *Marshall Journal of Medicine, 8*(1). https://doi.org/10.33470/2379-9536.1350

Cummings, S. A., Savitz, L. A., & Konrad, T. R. (2001). Reported response rates to mailed physician questionnaires. *Health Sciences Research, 35*, 1347–1355.

Cyphert, F. R., & Gant, W. L. (1970). The Delphi technique: A tool for collecting opinions in teacher education. *The Journal of Teacher Education, 21*, 417–425.

Cyrus, A., Salehi, B., Naziri, M., Sedeh, B. S., & Vosoulie, R. (2017). Empathic communication and essential instruction for medical students. *Journal of Biology and Today's World, 6*(6), 97–101. https://doi.org/10.15412/J.JBTW.01060601

D'Orazio, D. M. (2004). Letter to the editor. *Sexual Abuse: A Journal of Research and Treatment, 16*(2), 173–174. https://doi.org/10.1177/107906320401600207

Dalton, R., Sunblad, L., & Hylbert, S. (1976). Using principles of social learning in training for communication in empathy. *Journal of Counseling Psychology, 23*, 454–457.

Daly, M., & Wilson, M. (1988). *Homicide*. Aldine de Gruyter.

Damasio, A. (2003). *Looking for Spinoza: Joy, sorrow and the feeling brain*. Harcourt Brace.

Damasio, H., Grabowski, T., Frank, R., Galaburda, A. M., & Damasio, A. R. (1994). The return of Phineas Gage: Clues about the brain from the skull of a famous patient. *Science, 264*, 1102–1105.

Darwin, C. (1965). *The expression of emotion in man and animals*. St. Martin's Press. (Originally published in 1872).

Darwin, C. (1981). *The descent of man, and selection in relation to sex*. Princeton University Press. (Originally published in 1871).

DasGupta, S., & Charon, R. (2004). Personal illness narratives: Using reflective writing to teach empathy. *Academic Medicine, 79*, 351–356.

Davies, M. F. (2003). Confirmatory bias in the evaluation of personality descriptions: Positive test strategies and output inference. *Journal of Personality and Social Psychology, 85*(4), 736–744. https://doi.org/10.1037/0022-3514.85.4.736

Davis, M. H. (1983). Measuring individual differences in empathy: Evidence for a multidimensional approach. *Journal of Personality and Social Psychology, 44*, 113–126.

Davis, M. H. (1994). *Empathy: A social psychological approach*. Westview.

Davis, M. H., & Franzoi, S. L. (1991). Stability and change in adolescent self-consciousness and empathy. *Journal of Research in Personality, 25*, 70–87.

Davis, M. H., Luce, C., & Kraus, S. J. (1994). The heritability of characteristics associated with dispositional empathy. *Journal of Personality, 62*, 369–391.

Davis, M. R. (1985). Perception of affective reverberation component. In A. P. Goldstein & G. Y. Michaels (Eds.), *Empathy: Development, training, and consequences* (pp. 62–108). Erlbaum.

Davis, M. S. (1968). Physiological, psychological and demographic factors in patient compliance with doctor's orders. *Medical Care, 6*, 115–122.

Davison, A. N., & Peters, A. (1970). *Myelination*. Charles C Thomas.

Dawes, R. M. (1999). A message from psychologists to economists: Mere predictability doesn't matter like it should (without a good story appended to it). *Journal of Economic Behavior & Organization, 39*, 20–40.

Dawkins, R. (1999). *The selfish gene*. Oxford University Press.

Dawson, G. (1994). Development of emotional expression and emotion regulation in infancy: Contribution of the frontal lobe. In G. Dawson & K. W. Fischer (Eds.), *Human behavior and the developing brain* (pp. 346–379). Guilford.

Day, S. C., Norcini, J. J., Shea, J. A., & Benson, J. A., Jr. (1989). Gender differences in clinical competence of residents in internal medicine. *Journal of General Internal Medicine, 4*, 309–312.

de Oliveira, R., Montagna, E., Zaia, V., Torres, B. B., & Barbosa, C. P. (2019). The Development of Cognitive and Affective Skills Through a Sexual and Reproductive Health Medical Education Unit. *Sexual Medicine, 7*(3), 326–336. https://doi.org/10.1016/j.esxm.2019.06.008

de Quervain, D. J. F., Fischbacher, U., Treyer, V., Schellhammer, M., Schnyder, U., Buck, A., & Fehr, E. (2004). The neutral basis of altruistic punishment. *Science, 305(5688)*, 1254–1258. https://doi.org/10.1126/science.1100735

Dean, S., Foureur, M., Zaslawski, C., Newton-John, T., Yu, N., & Pappas, E. (2017). The effects of a structured mindfulness program on the development of empathy in healthcare students. *NursingPlus Open, 3*, 1–5. https://doi.org/10.1016/j.npls.2017.02.001

Deardroff, P. A., Finch, A. J., Jr., Kendall, P. C., Liran, F., & Indrisano, V. (1975). Empathy and socialization in repeat offenders, first offenders, and normals. *Journal of Counseling Psychology, 22*, 453–455.

Deardroff, P. A., Kendall, P. C., Finch, A. J., Jr., & Sitartz, A. M. (1977). Empathy, locus and control and anxiety in college students. *Psychological Reports, 40*, 1236–1238.

DeCasper, A. J., & Fifer, W. P. (1980). Of human bonding: Newborns prefer their mothers' voices. *Science, 208*, 1174–1176.

DeCasper, A. J., & Prescott, P. A. (1984). Human newborn's perception of male voices preference, discrimination, and reinforcing value. *Developmental Psychology, 17*, 481–491.

Decety, J. (2015). The neural pathways, development and functions of empathy. *Current Opinions in Behavioral Sciences, 3*, 1–3. https://doi.org/10.1016/j.cobeha.2014.12.001

Decety, J., & Chaminade, T. (2003). Neural correlates of feeling sympathy. *Neuropsychologia, 41*, 127–138.

Decety, J., & Cowell, J. M. (2015). Empathy, justice, and moral behavior. *AJOB Neuroscience, 6*(3), 3–14. https://doi.org/10.1080/21507740.2015.1047055

Decety, J., & Jackson, P. L. (2004). The functional architecture of human empathy. *Behavior and Cognitive Neuroscience Review, 3*(2), 71–100. https://doi.org/10.1177/1534582304267187

Decety, J., & Jackson, P. L. (2006). A social-neuroscience perspective on empathy. *Current Directions in Psychological Science, 15*, 54–58. https://doi.org/10.1111/j.0963-7214.2006.00406.x

Decety, J., & Lamm, C. (2006). Human empathy through the lens of social neuroscience. *The Scientific World Journal, 6*, 1146–1163. https://doi.org/10.1100/tsw.2006.221F

Dehning, S., Reiß, E., Krause, D., Gasperi, S., Meyer, S., Dargel, S., Müller, N., & Siebeck, M. (2014). Empathy in high-tech and high-touch medicine. *Patient Education and Counseling., 95*, 259–264. https://doi.org/10.1016/j.pec.2014.01.013

DeKruif. (1926). *Microb hunters*. Harcourt, Brace.

Del Canale, S., Louis, D. Z., Maio, V., Wang, X., Rossi, G., Hojat, M., & Gonnella, J. S. (2012). The relationship between physician empathy and disease complications: An empirical study of primary care physicians and their diabetic patients in Parma, Italy. *Academic Medicine, 87*(9), 1243–1249. https://doi.org/10.1097/ACM.0b013e3182628fbf

Delano Holden, J. (2017). *A toolkit to support nurse-patient communication through nurse-expressed empathy*. Publication No. 10271796). [Doctoral dissertation, Widener University]. ProQuest Dissertations & Theses Global. DAI-B 78/09(E).

Delgado-Bolton, R., San-Martin, M., Alcorta-Garza, A., & Vivanco, L. (2016). Medical empathy of physicians-in-training who are enrolled in professional training program: A comparative intercultural study in Spain. *Atención Primaria, 48*(*9*), 565–571. https://doi.org/10.1016/j.aprim.2015.10.005

Demos, E. (1988). Affect and the development of self: A new frontier. In A. Goldberg (Ed.), *Frontiers in self psychology: Progress in self psychology* (Vol. 3, pp. 27–33). Analytic Press.

Derbyshire, S. W. G. (2000). Exploring the pain "neuromatrix". *Current Review of Pain, 4*, 467–477.

Derntl, B., Finkelmeyer, A., Eickhoff, S., Kellermann, T., Falkenberg, D., Schneider, F., & Habel, U. (2010). Multidimensional assessment of empathic abilities: Neural correlates and gender differences. *Psychoneuroendocrinology, 35*(1), 67–82. https://doi.org/10.1016/j.psyneuen.2009.10.006

DeValck, C., Bensing, J., Bruynooghe, R., & Batenburg, V. (2001). Cure-oriented versus care-oriented attitudes in medicine. *Patient Education and Counseling, 45*, 119–126.

Di Blasi, Z., Harkness, E., Ernst, E., Georgiou, A., & Kleijnen, J. (2001). Influence of context effect on health outcomes: A systematic review. *Lancet, 357*, 757–762.

Di Lorenzo, R., Venturelli, G., Spiga, G., & Ferri, P. (2019). Emotional intelligence, empathy and alexithymia: a cross-sectional survey on emotional competence in a group of nursing students. *Acta Bio-Medica: Atenei Parmensis, 90*(4-S), 32–43. https://doi.org/10.23750/abm.v90i4-S.8273

Di Pellegrino, G., Fadiga, L., Fogassi, L., Gallese, V., & Rizzolutti, G. (1992). Understanding motor events: A neurophysiological study. *Experimental Brain Research, 91*, 176–180.

Díaz-Narváez, V. P., Alonso Palacio, L. M., Caro, S. E., Silva, M. G., Castillo, J. A., Bilbao, J. L., & Acosta, J. I. (2014). Empathic orientation among medical students from three universities in Barranquilla, Colombia and one university in the Dominican Republic. *Archivos Argentinos de Pediatria, 112*(*1*), 41–49. https://doi.org/10.5546/aap.2014.eng.41

Díaz-Narváez, V. P., Amezaga-Avitia, A. C., Sarabia-Alvarez, P. A., Lagos-Elgueta, M., Saavedra-Madrid, M., Silva-Reyes, P., Padilla, M., & Rodríguez-Hopp, M. P. (2018). Chilean Dentistry students, levels of empathy and empathic erosion: Necessary evaluation before a planned intervention: Levels of empathy, evaluation and intervention. *The Saudi Dental Journal, 30*(2), 117–124. https://doi.org/10.1016/j.sdentj.2017.11.004

Díaz-Narváez, V. P., Calzadilla-Nunez, A., Carrasco, D., Bustos, A., Zamorano, A., Silva, H., Lopez Tagle, E., & Hubermann, J. (2016). Levels of empathy among dental students in five Chilean universities. *Health, 8*, 32–41. https://doi.org/10.4236/health.2016.81005

Díaz-Narváez, V. P., Calzadilla-Núñez, A., Reyes-Reyes, A., Lastre Amell, G., Castellón-Montenegro, H., Andrade Valles, I., Fernández-Aragón, S., Fajardo-Ramos, E., Santander Díaz, K., Torres-Martínez, P., Muñoz Gámbaro, G., Borja González, J., & Arispe-Alburqueque, C. (2023). Empathy, psychometrics, cut-off points in nursing students from Latin America. *International Nursing Review, 70*(2), 185–193. https://doi.org/10.1111/inr.12783

Díaz-Narváez, V. P., Castillo, V. P., Reyes-Reyes, A., Padilla, M., Gonzalez-Martinez, F., Huberman, J., Calzadilla Núñez, A., Silva Vetri, M. G., Villalba, S. B., Ulloque, M. J., Erazo Coronado, A. M., López Tagle, E., Sánchez Jiménez, L., Bullen Cabrera, M., Salcedo Rioja, R., Gutiérrez, F., Bilbao Ramírez, J., Carrasco Mardones, D., Torres Martínez, P., & Sarabia-Alvarez, P. A. (2021). The Jefferson Sale of Empathy: Measurement properties, Underlying components, norms, and cutoff points in Dentistry students in Latin America, a multicentric study. *Intercencia, 46*(4), 169–176. https://repositorio.unphu.edu.do/handle/123456789/3660

Díaz-Narváez, V. P., Coronado, A. M. E., Bilbao, J. L., Gonzalez, F., Padilla, M., Howard, M., Silva, G., Alboleda, J., Bullen, M., Utsman, R., Fajardo, E., Alonso, L. M., & Cervantes, M. (2015a). Empathy levels of dental students of Central America and the Caribbean. *Health, 7*, 1678–1686. https://doi.org/10.4236/health.2015.712182

Díaz-Narváez, V. P., Gutierrez-Ventura, F. G., de Villalba, T. V., Salcedo-Rioja, M., Galzadilla-Nunez, A., & Hamdan-Rodriguiz, M. (2015b). Empathy levels of dentistry students in Peru and Argentina. *Health, 7*, 1268–1274. https://doi.org/10.4236/health.2015.710141

Diaz-Perez, A., Aragón, S. P. F., Narváez, V. P. D., Beleño, A. F., Navarro-Quiroz, E., & Cataño, C. L. M. (2018). Empathy in the curriculum for patient care. *Global Journal of Health Science, 10*(4), 93–99. https://doi.org/10.5539/gjhs.v10n4p93

Díaz Valentín, M. J., Garrido Abejar, M., Fuentes Chacón, R. M., Serrano Parra, M. D., Larrañaga Rubio, M. E., & Yubero Jiménez, S. (2019). Validation to the Spanish of the Jefferson empathy scale health professions students version and its psychometric properties in nursing students. *Nurse Education in Practice, 40*, 102629. https://doi.org/10.1016/j.nepr.2019.102629

Díez, N., García Del Barrio, L., Cristina Rodríguez-Díez, M., Martín-Lanas, R., Gea, A., & João Costa, M. (2022). Validation of the Jefferson Scale of Patient Perception of Physician Empathy Spanish (Spain) Version in Primary Care. *Family Medicine, 54*(8), 621–628. https://doi.org/10.22454/FamMed.2022.169675

DiLillo, M., Cicchetti, A., Lo Scalzo, A., Taroni, F., & Hojat, M. (2009). The Jefferson Scale of Physician Empathy: Preliminary psychometrics and group comparisons in Italian physicians. *Academic Medicine, 84*(9), 1198–1202. https://doi.org/10.1097/ACM.0b013e3181b17b3f

Dillard, J. P., & Hunter, J. E. (1989). On the use and interpretation of the Emotional Empathy Scale, the Self-Consciousness Scale, and the Self-Monitoring Scale. *Communication Research, 16*, 104–129.

DiLollo, V., & Berger, S. M. (1965). Effect of apparent pain in others on observers' reaction time. *Journal of Personality and Social Psychology, 2*, 573–575.

DiMascio, A., Boyd, R. W., & Greenblatt, M. (1957). Physiological correlates of tension and antagonism during psychotherapy: A study of "interpersonal physiology". *Psychosomatic Medicine, 19*, 99–104.

DiMatteo, M. R. (1979). A social-psychological analysis of physician-patient rapport toward a science of the art of medicine. *Journal of Social Issues, 35*, 12–33.

DiMatteo, M. R., Hays, R. D., & Prince, L. M. (1986). Relationship of physicians' nonverbal communication skills to patient satisfaction, appointment noncompliance, and physician workload. *Health Psychology, 5*, 581–594.

DiMatteo, M. R., Prince, I. M., & Taranta, A. (1979). Patients' perceptions of physicians' behavior: Determinants of patient commitment to the therapeutic relationship. *Journal of Community Health, 4*, 280–290.

DiMatteo, M. R., Sherbourne, C. D., Hays, R. D., Ordway, L., Kravitz, R. L., McGlynn, E. A., & Rogers, W. H. (1993). Physicians' characteristics influence patients' adherence to medical treatment: Results from the Medical Outcomes Study. *Health Psychology, 12*, 93–102.

DiMatteo, M. R., Taranta, A., Friedman, H. S., & Prince, L. M. (1980). Predicting patient satisfaction from physicians' nonverbal communication skills. *Medical Care, 17*, 376–387.

Dimberg, U., Thunberg, M., & Elmehed, K. (2000). Unconscious facial reactions to emotional facial expressions. *Psychological Science, 11*, 86–89.

Diseker, R. A., & Michielutte, R. (1981). An analysis of empathy in medical students before and following clinical experience. *Journal of Medical Education, 56*, 1004–1010.

Divinagarcia, R. M., Harkin, T. J., Bonk, S., & Schluger, N. W. (1998). Screening by specialists to reduce unnecessary test ordering in patients evaluated for tuberculosis. *Chest, 114*, 664–666.

Doherty, R. W. (1997). The emotional contagion scale: A measure of individual differences. *Journal of Nonverbal Behavior, 21*, 131–154.

Dohrenwend, A. M. (2018). Defining empathy to better teach, measure, and understand its impact. *Academic Medicine, 93*(12), 1754–1756. https://doi.org/10.1097/ACM.0000000000002427

Doidge, N. (2007). *The brain that changes itself: Stories of personal triumph from frontiers of brain science*. Penguin Books.

Domes, G., Heinrichs, M., Michel, A., Berger, C., & Herpertz, S. C. (2007). Oxytocin improves "mind-reading" in humans. *Biological Psychiatry, 61*(6), 731–733. https://doi.org/10.1016/j.biopsych.2006.07.015

Dorough, R. J. M. (2022). *The medicalization of communication: an analysis of the policies and educational practices surrounding patient and physician interaction.* (Publication No. 29331342). [Doctoral dissertation, The University of Texas at Arlington]. ProQuest Dissertations & Theses Global. DAI-A 83/12(E).

Dovidio, J. F. (1991). The empathy-altruistic hypothesis: Paradigm and promise. *Psychological Inquiry, 2*, 126–128.

Downie, R. S. (1991). Literature and medicine. *Journal of Medical Ethics, 17*, 93–96.

D'souza, P. C., Rasquinha, S. L., D'souza, T. L., Jain, A., Kulkarni, V., & Pai, K. (2020). Effect of a Single-Session Communication Skills Training on Empathy in Medical Students. *Academic Psychiatry: The Journal of the American Association of Directors of Psychiatric Residency Training and the Association for Academic Psychiatry, 44*(3), 289–294. https://doi.org/10.1007/s40596-019-01158-z

du Vaure, C. B., Lemogne, C., Bunge, L., Catu-Pinault, A., Hoertel, N., Ghasarossian, C., Vincens, M. E., Galam, E., & Jaury, P. (2017). Promoting empathy among medical students: A two-site randomized controlled study. *Journal of Psychosomatic Research, 103*, 102–107. https://doi.org/10.1016/j.jpsychores.2017.10.008

Dubnicki, C. (1977). Relationship among therapist empathy and authoritarianism. *Journal of Counseling and Clinical Psychology, 45*, 958–959.

Duff, P. (2002). Professionalism in medicine: An A–Z primer. *Obstetrics and Gynecology, 99*, 1127–1128.

Duke, P., Grosseman, S., Novack, D. H., & Rosenzweig, S. (2015). Preserving third-year medical students' empathy and enhancing self-reflection using small group "virtual hangout" technology. *Medical teacher, 37*(6), 566–571. https://doi.org/10.3109/0142159X.2014.956057

Dunstone, D. C., & Reames, H. R. J. (2001). Physician satisfaction revisited. *Social Science & Medicine, 52*, 825–837.

Durkheim, E. (1951). *Suicide: A study in sociology* (J.A. Spaulding & G. Simpson, Trans.). Glencoe, IL: Free Press.

Dymond, R. F. (1949). A scale for the measurement of empathic ability. *Journal of Consulting Psychology, 13*, 127–133.

Dymond, R. F. (1950). Personality and empathy. *Journal of Counseling Psychology, 14*, 343–350.

Dyrbye, L. N., Eacker, A. M., Harper, W., Power, D. V., Massie, F. S., Jr., Satele, D., Thomas, M. R., Sloan, J. A., & Shanafelt, T. D. (2012). Distress and empathy do not drive changes in

specialty preference among US medical students. *Medical Teacher, 34*(2), e116–e122. https://doi.org/10.3109/0142159X.2012.644830
Dziobek, I., Rogers, K., Fleck, S., Bahnemann, M., Heekeren, H. R., Wolf, O. T., & Convit, A. (2008). Dissociation of cognitive and emotional empathy in adults with Asperger Syndrome using multifaceted empathy test (MET). *Journal of Autism and Developmental Disorders, 38*(3), 464–473. https://doi.org/10.1007/s10803-007-0486-x
Eagly, A. H. (1987). *Sex differences in social behavior: A social role interpretation.* Erlbaum.
Eagly, A. H. (1995). The science and politics of comparing women and men. *American Psychologist, 50*, 145–158.
Eagly, A. H., & Crowley, M. (1986). Gender and helping behavior: A meta-analytic review of the social psychological literature. *Psychological Bulletin, 100*, 283–308.
Eagly, A. H., & Steffen, V. J. (1986). Gender and aggressive behavior: A meta-analytic review of the social psychological literature. *Psychological Bulletin, 100*, 309–330.
Eagly, A. H., & Wood, W. (1999). The origin of sex differences in human behavior: Evolved dispositions versus social roles. *American Psychologist, 54*, 408–423.
Eagly, A. H., & Wood, W. (2013). The nature-nurture debate: 25 years of challenges in the psychology of gender. *Perspectives on Psychological Science, 8*(3), 340–357. https://doi.org/10.1177/1745691613484767
Eaton, D. (2018). *The effect of participation in a dementia simulation on participants empathy.* (Publication No. 13421992). [Doctoral dissertation, Clarion University of Pennsylvania and Edinboro University]. ProQuest Dissertations & Theses Global. DAI-B 80/06(E).
Eddins-Folensbee, F. F., Harris, T. B., Miller-Wasik, M., & Thompson, B. (2012). Students versus faculty members as admission interviewers: Comparisons of ratings data and admission decisions. *Academic Medicine: Journal of the Association of American Medical Colleges, 87(4)*, 458–462. https://doi.org/10.1097/ACM.0b013e318249687d
Edmonds, D. (2015). *Would you kill the fat man? The trolley problem and what your answer tells us about right and wrong?* Princeton University Press.
Edwards, A. L. (1957). *The social desirability variable in personality assessment and research.* Dryden.
Edwards, M. T., & Zimet, C. N. (1976). Problems and concerns among medical students. *Journal of Medical Education, 51*, 619–625.
Edwards-Lee, T. A., & Saul, R. E. (1999). Neuropsychiatry of the right prefrontal lobe. In B. L. Miller & J. L. Cummings (Eds.), *The human prefrontal lobes: Functional and disorders.* Guilford Press.
Egan, G. (1975). *The skilled helper.* Brooks/Cole.
Egolf, B., Lasker, J., Wolf, S., & Potvin, L. (1992). Featuring health risks and mortality: The Roseto effect, a 50-year comparison of mortality rates. *American Journal of Public Health, 82*, 1089–1092.
Ehrlich, C. H., & Jaffe, C. (2002). Social support for dying. In J. D. Morgan (Ed.), *Social support: A reflection of humanity* (pp. 17–31). Baywood Publishing.
Eibel-Eibesfeldt, I. (1979). *The biology of peace and war.* Viking.
Eisenberg, A., Rosenthal, S., & Schlussel, Y. R. (2015). Medicine as a performing art: What we can learn about empathic communication from theater arts. *Academic Medicine, 90*(3), 272–276. https://doi.org/10.1097/ACM.0000000000000626
Eisenberg, N. (1983). The relation between empathy and altruism: Conceptual and methodological issues. *Academic Psychology Bulletin, 5*, 195–208.
Eisenberg, N. (1989). *Empathy and related emotional responses* (Vol. 44). Jossey-Bass.
Eisenberg, N., & Lennon, R. (1983). Sex differences in empathy and related capacities. *Psychological Bulletin, 94*(1), 100–131. https://doi.org/10.1037/0033-2909.94.1.100
Eisenberg, N., & Miller, P. A. (1987). The relation of empathy to prosocial and related behaviors. *Psychological Bulletin, 101*, 91–119.
Eisenberg, N., & Strayer, J. (1987a). Critical issues in the study of empathy. In N. Eisenberg & J. Strayer (Eds.), *Empathy and its development* (pp. 3–13). Cambridge University Press.

Eisenberg, N., & Strayer, J. (1987b). *Empathy and its development*. Cambridge University Press.

Eisenberg, N., Fabes, R. A., Murphy, B., Karbon, M., Maszk, P., Smith, M., O'Boyle, C., & Suh, K. (1994). The relations of emotionality and regulation to dispositional and situational empathy-related responding. *Journal of Personality and Social Psychology, 66*(4), 776–797. 10.1037//0022-3514.66.4.776.

Eisenberg-Berg, N., & Lennon, R. (1980). Altruism and the assessment of empathy in the preschool years. *Child Development, 51*, 552–557.

Eisenberg-Berg, N., & Mussen, P. (1978). Empathy and moral development in adolescence. *Developmental Psychology, 14*, 185–186.

Eisenberger, N., Leiberman, M., & Williams, K. (2003). Does rejection hurt? An fMRI study of social exclusion. *Science, 302*, 290–292.

Eisenthal, S. E., Emery, R., Lazare, A., & Udin, H. (1979). Adherence and negotiated approach in patienthood. *Archives of General Psychiatry, 36*, 393–398.

Ekman, P. (1992). An argument for basic emotions. *Cognition and Emotion, 6*, 169–200.

Ekman, P., & Friesen, W. V. (1974). Detecting deception from the body or face. *Journal of Personality and Social Psychology, 29*, 288–298.

Elam, C. L., & Johnson, M. M. S. (1992). An analysis of admission committee voting patterns. *Academic Medicine, 67*(10 Suppl), S72–S75.

Elizur, A., & Rosenheim, E. (1982). Empathy and attitudes among medical students: The effects of group experience. *Journal of Medical Education, 57*, 675–683.

Engel, G. L. (1977). The need for a new medical model: A challenge for biomedicine. *Science, 196*, 129–136.

Engel, G. L. (1990). The essence of the biopsychosocial model: From 17th to 20th century science. In H. Balner (Ed.), *A challenge for biomedicine?* (pp. 13–18). Swets & Zeitlinger, Inc.

Engler, C. M., Saltzman, G. A., Walker, M. L., & Wolf, F. M. (1981). Medical student acquisition and retention of communication and interviewing skills. *Journal of Medical Education, 56*, 572–579.

Englis, B. G., Vaughan, K. B., & Lanzetta, J. T. (1982). Conditioning of counter-empathetic emotional response. *Journal of Experimental and Social Psychology, 18*, 375–391.

Entman, S. S., Glass, C. A., Hickson, G. B., Githens, P. B., Whetten-Goldstein, K., & Sloan, F. A. (1994). The relationship between malpractice claims history and subsequent obstetric care. *Journal of the American Medical Association, 272*, 1588–1591.

Eom, S., & Kim, S. S. (2018). Factors associated with nurses' moral sensitivity. *Journal of Korean Academy of Psychiatric Mental Health Nursing, 27*(3), 199–207. https://doi.org/10.12934/jkpmhn.2018.27.3.199

Erera, P. I. (1997). Empathy training for helping professionals: Model and evaluation. *Journal of Social Work Education, 33*, 245–260.

Eres, R., Decety, J., Louis, W. R., & Molenberghs, P. (2015). Individual differences in local gray matter density are associated with differences in affective and cognitive empathy. *Neuroimage, 117*, 305–310. https://doi.org/10.1016/j.neuroimage.2015.05.038

Eron, L. D. (1958). The effect of medical education on attitudes: A follow-up study. *Journal of Medical Education, 33*, 25–33.

Eslinger, P. J. (1998). Neurological and neuropsychological bases of empathy. *European Neurology, 93*, 193–199.

Eslinger, P. J., Satish, U., & Grattan, L. M. (1996). Alterations in cognitive- and affective-based empathy after cerebral damage. *Journal of International Neuropsychological Society, 2*, 15–16.

Evans, B. J., Stanley, R. O., & Burrows, G. D. (1993). Measuring medical students' empathy skills. *British Journal of Medical Psychology, 66*, 121–133.

Eysenck, H. J., & Eysenck, S. B. G. (1975). *Manual of the Eysenck Personality Questionnaire (junior and adult)*. Hodder & Stoughton.

Fabrega, H., Ulrich, R., & Keshavan, M. (1994). Gender differences in how medical students learn to rate psychopathology. *Journal of Nervous and Mental Disease, 182*, 471–475.

Fahrbach, S. E., Morrell, I. I., & Pfaff, D. W. (1985). Role of oxytocin in the onset of estrogen-facilitated maternal behavior. In J. A. Amico & A. G. Robinson (Eds.), *Oxytocin: Clinical and laboratory studies* (pp. 372–388). Elsevier.

Falvo, D., & Tippy, P. (1988). Communicating information to patients. Patient satisfaction and adherence as associated with resident skill. *Journal of Family Medicine, 26*, 643–647.

Fan, Y., Duncan, N. W., de Greck, M., & Northoff, G. (2011). Is there a core neural network in empathy? An fMRI based quantitative meta-analysis. *Neuroscience & Biobehavioral Reviews, 35*(3), 903–911. https://doi.org/10.1016/j.neubiorev.2010.10.009

Farber, N. J., Novack, D. H., & O'Brien, M. K. (1997). Love, boundaries, and the patient-physician relationship. *Archives of Internal Medicine, 157*, 2291–2294.

Fashami, F. M., Nili, M., Mottaghi, M., & Farahani, A. V. (2023). Measuring Empathy in Iranian Pharmacy Students Using the Jefferson Scale of Empathy-Health Profession Student Version. *American journal of pharmaceutical education, 87*(2), ajpe8687. https://doi.org/10.5688/ajpe8687

Feighny, K. M., Arnold, L., Monaco, M., Munro, S., & Earl, B. (1998). In pursuit of empathy and its relation to physician communication skills: Multidimensional empathy training for medical students. *Annals of Behavioral Science and Medical Education, 5*, 13–21.

Feingold, A. (1990). Gender differences in effect of physical attractiveness on romantic attraction: A comparison across five research paradigms. *Journal of Personality and Social Psychology, 59*(5), 981–993. https://doi.org/10.1037/0022-3514.59.5.981

Feingold, A. (1992). Gender differences in mate selection preferences: A test of the parental investment model. *Psychological Bulletin, 112*(1), 125–139. https://doi.org/10.1037/0033-2909.112.1.125

Feingold, A. (1994). Gender differences in personality: A meta-analysis. *Psychological Bulletin, 116*, 429–456.

Feldman, C., & Kornfield, J. (1991). *Stories of the spirit, stories of the heart*. Harper Collins.

Feldman, R., Weller, A., Zagoor-Sharon, O., & Levine, A. (2007). Evidence for a neuroendocrinological foundation of human affiliation: Plasma oxytocin levels across pregnancy and the postpartum period predict mother-child bonding. *Psychological Science, 18*, 965–970.

Fenichel, O. (1945). *The psychoanalytic theory of neurosis*. W.W. Norton.

Ferguson, E., James, D., & Madeley, I. (2002). Factors associated with success in medical school: Systematic review of the literature. *British Medical Journal, 324*, 952–957.

Fernandez-Olano, C., Montoya-Fernandez, J., & Salinas-Sanchez, A. S. (2008). Impact of clinical interview training on the empathy level of medical students and medical and residents. *Medical Teacher, 30*(3), 322–324. https://doi.org/10.1080/01421590701802299

Ferrante, J. M., Chen, P. H., & Kim, S. (2007). The effect of patient navigation on time to diagnosis, anxiety, and satisfaction in urban minority women with abnormal mammograms: A randomized controlled trial. *Journal of Urban Health: Bulletin of the New York Academy of Medicine, 85*(1), 114–124. https://doi.org/10.1007/s11524-007-9228-9

Feshbach, N. D. (1982). Sex differences in empathy and social behavior in children. In N. Eisenberg (Ed.), *The development of prosocial behavior* (pp. 315–338). Academic Press.

Feshbach, N. D. (1989). Empathy training and prosocial behavior. In J. Groebel & R. A. Hinde (Eds.), *Aggression and war: Their biological and social bases* (pp. 101–111). Cambridge University Press.

Feshbach, N. D., & Roe, K. (1968). Empathy in six and seven year olds. *Child Development, 39*, 133–145.

Festinger, L. (1964). *Conflict, decision, and dissonance*. Stanford University Press.

Feudtner, C., Christakis, D. A., & Christakis, N. A. (1994). Do clinical clerks suffer ethical erosion? Students' perception of their ethical environment and personal development. *Academic Medicine, 69*, 670–679.

Ficklin, F. L., Browne, V. L., Powell, R. C., & Carter, J. E. (1988). Faculty and house staff members as role models. *Journal of Medical Education, 63*, 392–396.

Field, T. M., Woodson, R., Greenberg, R., & Cohen, D. (1982). Discrimination and imitation of facial expressions by neonates. *Science, 218*, 179–181.

Fields, S. K., Hojat, M., Gonnella, J. S., Mangione, S., Kane, G., & Magee, M. (2004). Comparisons of nurses and physicians on an operational measure of empathy. *Evaluation & the Health Professions, 27*(1), 80–94. https://doi.org/10.1177/0163278703261206

Fields, S. K., Mahan, P., Hojat, M., Tillman, P., & Maxwell, K. (2011). Measuring empathy in healthcare profession students using the Jefferson Scale of Physician Empathy: Health Provider-Student Version. *Journal of Interprofessional Care, 25*(4), 287–293. https://doi.org/10.3109/13561820.2011.566648

Fifer, W. P., & Moon, C. M. (1994). The role of mother's voice in the organization of brain function in the newborn. *Acta Pædiatrica Scandinavica, 397*, 86–93.

Figley, C. R. (1995). *Compassion fatigue: Coping with secondary traumatic stress disorder in those who treat the traumatized*. Brunner/Mazel.

Fine, V. K., & Therrien, M. E. (1977). Empathy in the doctor-patient relationship: Skill training for medical students. *Journal of Medical Education, 52*, 752–757.

Fishbein, M., & Ajzen, I. (1975). *Belief, attitude, intention, and behavior: An introduction to theory and research*. Addison-Wesley.

Fishbein, R. H. (1999). Scholarship, humanism, and the young physician. *Academic Medicine, 74*, 646–651.

Fjortoft, N., Van Winkle, L. J., & Hojat, M. (2011). Measuring empathy in pharmacy students. *American Journal of Pharmaceutical Education, 75(6)*, 109. https://doi.org/10.5688/ajpe756109

Flagler, E. (1997). Narrative ethics: A means to enrich medical education. *Annals of the Royal College of Physicians & Surgeons of Canada, 30*, 217–220.

Fleming, A. S., Corter, C., Stallings, J., & Steiner, M. (2002). Testosterone and prolactin are associated with emotional responses to infant cries in new fathers. *Hormones and Behavior, 42*, 399–413.

Fleming, A. S., Ruble, D., Krieger, H., & Wong, P. Y. (1997). Hormonal and experiential correlates of maternal responsiveness during pregnancy and the puerperium in human mothers. *Hormones and Behavior, 31*, 145–158.

Flores, G. (2002). Mad scientists, compassionate healers, and greedy egotists: The portrayal of physicians in the movies. *Journal of the American Medical Association, 94*, 635–658.

Flores, G., Gee, D., & Kastner, B. (2000). The teaching of cultural issues in US and Canadian medical schools. *Academic Medicine, 75*, 451–455.

Fonagy, P. (2001). *Attachment theory and psychoanalysis*. Other Press.

Fonagy, P., & Target, M. (1996). Playing with reality: I. Theory of mind and the normal development of psychic reality. *International Journal of Psychoanalysis, 77*, 217–233.

Foreback, J., Kusz, H., Lepisto, B. L., & Pawlaczyk, B. (2018). Empathy in internal medicine residents at community-based hospitals: A cross-sectional study. *Journal of Medical Education and Curricular Development, 5*. https://doi.org/10.1177/2382120518771352

Fornetti, M., & Barbosa, M. (2024). The association between empathy and artistic practice: A cross-sectional study with medical students. *MBC Medical Education., 24*, 1156. https://doi.org/10.1186/s12909-024-06146-y

Forouzan, I., & Hojat, M. (1993). Stability and change of interest in obstetrics and gynecology among medical students: Eighteen years of longitudinal data. *Academic Medicine, 68*, 919–922.

Forstater, A. T., Chauhan, N., Allen, A., Hojat, M., & Lopez, B. L. (2011). An emergency department shadowing experiences for emergency medicine residents: Can it prevent erosion of empathy? (Abstract). *Academic Emergency Medicine, 18*(s2, #3). https://doi.org/10.1111/j.1553-2712.2011.01188.x

Forsythe, M., Calnan, M., & Wall, B. (1999). Doctors as patients: Postal survey examining consultants and general practitioners adherence to guidelines. *British Medical Journal, 319*, 605–608.

Fox, C. M., Harper, A. P., Hyner, G. C., & Lyle, R. M. (1994). Loneliness, emotional expression, marital quality and major life events in women who developed breast cancer. *Journal of Community Health, 19*, 467–482.

Frances, A., First, M. B., & Pincus, H. A. (1995). *DSM-IV guidebook.* American Psychiatric Association.

Francis, V., & Morris, M. (1969). Gaps in doctor-patient communication: Patients' response to medical advice. *The New England Journal of Medicine, 280*, 535–540.

Frank, E., & Harvey, L. K. (1996). Preventive advice rates of women and men physicians. *Archives of Family Medicine, 5*, 215–219.

Fratiglioni, L., Wang, H. X., Ericsson, K., Maytan, M., & Winblad, B. (2000). Influence of social network on occurrence of dementia: A community-based longitudinal study. *Lancet, 355*, 1315–1319.

Free, N. K., Green, B. L., Grace, M. C., Chernus, L. A., & Whitman, R. M. (1985). Empathy and outcome in brief focal dynamic therapy. *American Journal of Psychiatry, 142*, 917–921.

Freeman, H. P., Muth, B., & Kerner, J. F. (1995). Expanding access to cancer screening and clinical follow-up among the medically underserved. *Cancer Practice, 3*, 19–30.

Freemon, B., Negrete, V. F., Davis, M., & Korsch, B. M. (1971). Gaps in doctor-patient communication: Doctor-patient interaction analysis. *Pediatric Research, 5*, 298–311.

Frenk, J. (1998). Medical care and health improvement: The critical link. *Annals of Internal Medicine, 129*, 419–420.

Fretz, B. R. (1966). Postural movement in a counseling dyad. *Journal of Counseling Psychology, 13*, 343.

Freud, S. (1955). Group psychology and the analysis of the ego. In J. Strachey (Ed.), *The standard edition of the complete psychological works of Sigmund Freud* (Vol. 18). Hogarth Press and the Institute of Psychoanalysis. (original work published in 1921).

Freud, S. (1958a). Recommendation to physicians practicing psychoanalysis. In J. Strachey (Ed.), *The standard edition of the complete psychological works of Sigmund Freud* (Vol. 12, pp. 109–120). Hogarth Press and the Institute of Psychoanalysis. (original work published in 1912).

Freud, S. (1958b). On beginning the treatment. In J. Starchey (Ed.), *The standard edition of the complete psychological works of Sigmund Freud* (Vol. 12, pp. 121–144). Hogarth Press and the Institute of Psychoanalysis. (original work published in 1913).

Freud, S. (1960). Jokes and their relation to the unconscious. In J. Strachey (Ed.), *The standard edition of the complete psychological works of Sigmund Freud(entire Vol. 8)*. Hogarth Press and the Institute of Psychoanalysis. (original work published in 1905).

Freud, S. (1964). An outline of psychoanalysis. In J. Strachey (Ed.), *The standard edition of the complete psychological works of Sigmund Freud* (Vol. 23, pp. 139–301). Hogarth Press and the Institute of Psychoanalysis. (original work published in 1938).

Friedman, E. (1990). The perlis of detachment. *Health Care Forum Journal, 33*, 9–10.

Friedman, H. S., Prince, L. M., Riggio, R. E., & DiMatteo, M. R. (1980). Understanding and assessing nonverbal expressiveness: The affective communication test. *Journal of Personality and Social Psychology, 39*, 333–351.

Friedrich, B., Evans-Lacko, S., London, J., Rhydderch, D., & Henderson, C. (2013). Anti-stigma training for medical students: The education not discrimination project. *British Journal of Psychiatry, Supplement, 55, s89–s94*. https://doi.org/10.1192/bjp.bp.112.114017

Frodi, A., & Macauley, J. (1977). Are women always less aggressive than men? A review of the experimental literature. *Psychological Bulletin, 84*, 634–660.

Fruen, M., Rothman, A., & Steiner, J. (1974). Comparisons of characteristics of male and female medical school applicants. *Journal of Medical Education, 49*, 137–145.

Fuertes, J. N., Boylan, L. S., & Fontanella, J. A. (2008). Behavioral indices in medical care outcomes: The working alliance, adherence, and related factors. *Journal of General Internal Medicine, 24*(1), 80–85. https://doi.org/10.1007/s11606-008-0841-4

Fukuyas, Y., Kataoka, H. U., Honda, M., Iwase, T., Ogawa, H., Sato, M., Watanabe, M., Fuji, C., Wada, J., DeSantis, J., Hojat, M., & Gonnella, J. A. (2021). The effect of Humanitude care methodology on improving empathy: A six-year longitudinal study of medical students in Japan. *BMC Medical Education, 21*, 316. https://doi.org/10.1186/s12909-021-02773-x

Fussel, F. W., & Bonney, W. C. (1990). A comparative study of childhood experience of psychotherapists and physicists: Implications for clinical practice. *Psychotherapy, 27*, 505–512.

Gabard, D. L., Lowe, D. L., Deusinger, S. S., Stelzner, D. M., & Crandall, S. J. (2013). Analysis of empathy in doctor of physical therapy students: A multi-site study. *Journal of Allied Health, 42*, 10–16.

Gabbard, G. O. (1994). On love and lust in erotic transference. *Journal of the American Psychoanalytic Association, 42*, 385–403.

Gabbard, G. O., & Nadelson, C. (1995). Professional boundaries in the physician-patient relationship. *Journal of the American Medical Association, 273*, 1445–1449.

Galam, E., Vauloup Soupault, C., Bunge, L., Buffel du Vaure, C., Boujut, E., & Jaury, P. (2017). 'Intern life': a longitudinal study of burnout, empathy, and coping strategies used by French GPs in training. *BJGP Open, 1*(2). https://doi.org/10.3399/bjgpopen17X100773

Galanter, M., Talbott, D., Gallegos, K., & Rubenstone, E. (1990). Combined alcoholics anonymous and professional care for addicted physicians. *American Journal of Psychiatry, 147*, 64–68.

Gallagher, H. L., & Frith, C. D. (2003). Functional imaging of 'theory of mind'. *Trends in Cognitive Sciences, 7*, 77–83.

Gallese, V. (2001). The 'shared manifold' hypothesis: From mirror neurons to empathy. *Journal of Conscious Studies, 8*, 33–50.

Gallese, V. (2003). The roots of empathy: The shared manifold hypothesis and the neural basis of intersubjectivity. *Psychopathology, 36*, 171–180.

Gallese, V., Fadiga, L., Fogassi, L., & Rizzolatti, G. (1996). Action cognition in the premotor cortex. *Brain, 119*, 593–609.

Gallese, V., Keysers, C., & Rizzolatti, G. (2004). A unifying view of the basis of social cognition. *Trends in Cognitive Sciences, 8*(9), 396–403. https://doi.org/10.1016/j.tics.2004.07.002

Gartrell, N., Herman, J., Olarte, S., Feldstein, M., & Localio, R. (1986). Psychiatrist-patient sexual contact: Results of a national survey: I. *Prevalence. American Journal of Psychiatry, 143*, 1126–1131.

Garza, J. M. (2015). *Physician assistant students' perceptions of mental illness: a correlational study of empathy, attitudes, and stigma levels.* (Publication No. 3728874). [Doctoral dissertation, The University of Texas - Pan American]. ProQuest Dissertations & Theses Global. DAI-B 77/03(E).

Gaufberg, E. H., Joseph, R. C., Pels, R. J., Wyshak, G., Wieman, D., & Nadelson, C. C. (2001). Psychosocial training in U.S. internal medicine and family practice residency programs. *Academic Medicine, 76*, 738–742.

Gazzola, V., Rizzolatti, G., Wicker, B., & Keysers, C. (2007). The anthropomorphic brain: The mirror neuron system responds to human and robotic actions. *Neuroimage, 35*(4), 1674–1684. https://doi.org/10.1016/j.neuroimage.2007.02.003

Geary, D. D. (1995). Sexual selection and sex differences is spatial cognition. *Learning and Individual Differences, 7*(4), 289–301. https://doi.org/10.1016/1041-6080(95)90003-9

Geisinger, K. F. (1994). Cross-cultural normative assessment: Translation and adaptation issues influencing the normative interpretation of assessment instruments. *Psychological Assessment, 6*, 304–312.

Geller, G., Tambor, E. S., Chase, G. A., & Holtzman, N. A. (1993). Measuring physicians' tolerance for ambiguity and its relationship to their reported practices regarding genetic testing. *Medical Care, 31*, 989–1001.

Gelmann, E. P., & Stewart, J. P. (1975). Faculty and students as admissions interviewers: Results of a questionnaire given to applicants. *Journal of Medical Education, 50*, 626–628.

Gendreau, P., Burke, D. M., & Grant, B. A. (1980). A second evaluation of the Rideau inmate volunteer program. *Canadian Journal of Criminology, 22*, 66–77.

Gerber, M., Colledge, F., Mucke, M., Schilling, R., Brand, S., & Ludyga, S. (2018). Psychometric properties of Shirom-Melamed Burnout Measure (SMBM) among adolescents: Results from three cross-sectional studies. *BMC Psychiatry, 18*, 226. https://doi.org/10.1186/s12888-018-1841-5

Ghardallou, M., Zedini, C., Sahli, J., Ajmi, T., Khairi, H., & Mtiraoui, A. (2022). Psychometric properties of a French version of the Jefferson Scale of Empathy. *International Journal of Medical Education, 13*, 205–214. https://doi.org/10.5116/ijme.62d2.8497

Ghetti, C., Chang, J., & Gosman, G. (2009). Burnout, psychological skills, and empathy: Balint training in obstetrics and gynecology residents. *Journal of Graduate Medical Education, 1*(2), 231–235. https://doi.org/10.4300/JGME-D-09-00049.1

Gholamzadeh, S., Khastavaneh, M., Khademian, Z., & Ghadakpour, S. (2018). The effects of empathy skills training on nursing students' empathy and attitudes toward elderly people. *BMC Medical Education, 18*(1), 198. https://doi.org/10.1186/s12909-018-1297-9

Gianakos, D. (1996). Empathy revisited. *Archives of Internal Medicine, 156*, 135–136.

Gibson, E. J., & Walk, R. D. (1960). The visual cliff. *Scientific American, 202*, 64–71.

Gillberg, C. (1992). The Emanuel Miller memorial lecture 1991: Autism and autistic-like conditions: Subclasses among disorders of empathy. *Journal of Child Psychology and Psychiatry, 33*, 813–842.

Gillberg, C. (1996). The long-term outcome of childhood empathy disorders. *European Child, and Adolescent Psychiatry, 5*(Suppl), 52–56.

Gilligan, C. (1982). *In a different voice: Psychological theory and women's development*. Harvard University Press.

Gilligan, C., & Attanucci, J. (1988). Two moral orientations: Gender differences and similarities. *Merrill-Palmer Quarterly, 34*, 223–237.

Giménez-Espert, M. D. C., & Prado-Gascó, V. J. (2020). Empathy in nurses: Spanish adaptation of the Jefferson scale of empathy (JSE) on nurses. *Contemporary Nurse, 56*(3), 255–265. https://doi.org/10.1080/10376178.2020.1813046

Giménez-Espert, M. D. C., Valero-Moreno, S., & Prado-Gascó, V. J. (2019). Evaluation of emotional skills in nursing using regression and QCA models: A transversal study. *Nurse Education Today, 74*, 31–37. https://doi.org/10.1016/j.nedt.2018.11.019

Girgis, A., & Sanson-Fisher, R. W. (1995). Breaking bad news: Consensus guidelines for medical practitioners. *Journal of Clinical Oncology, 13*, 2449–2456.

Gladding, S. T. (1978). Empathy, gender, and training as factors in the identification of normal infant cry-signals. *Perceptual & Motor Skills, 47*, 267–270.

Gladstein, G., & Feldstein, J. (1983). Using film to increase counselor empathic experiences. *Counselor Education and Supervision, 23*, 125–131.

Gladstein, G. A. (1977). Empathy and counseling outcome: An empirical and conceptual review. *The Counseling Psychologist, 6*, 70–79.

Gladstein, G. A., & associates. (1987). *Empathy and counseling: Explorations in theory and research*. Springer-Verlag.

Glaser, K., Hojat, M., Veloski, J. J., Blacklow, R. S., & Goepp, C. E. (1992). Science, verbal, or quantitative skills: Which is the most important predictor of physician competence? *Educational and Psychological Measurement, 52*(2), 395–406. https://doi.org/10.1177/0013164492052002015

Glaser, K. M., Markham, F. W., Adler, H. M., McManus, R. P., & Hojat, M. (2007). Relationships between scores on the Jefferson scale of physician empathy, patient perceptions of physician empathy, and humanistic approaches to patient care: A validity study. *Medical Science Monitor: International Medical Journal of Experimental And Clinical Research, 13*(7), CR291–CR294.

Gleichgerrcht, E., & Decety, J. (2013). Empathy in clinical practice: How individual dispositions, gender, and experience moderate empathic concern, burnout, and emotional distress in physicians. *PLoS One, 8*(4), e61526. https://doi.org/10.1371/journal.pone.0061526

Glynn, L. M., Christenfeld, N., & Gerin, W. (1999). Gender, social support, and cardiovascular response to stress. *Psychosomatic Medicine, 61*, 234–242.

Goldberg, P. E. (2000). The physician-patient relationship: Three psychodynamic concepts that can be applied to primary care. *Archives of Family Medicine, 9*, 1164–1168.

Golden, L. (1992). *Aristotle on tragic and comic mimesis*. Scholars Press.

Golden, T. (2002). Acknowledging the masculine and feminine in offering support. In J. D. Morgan (Ed.), *Social support: A reflection of humanity* (pp. 73–84). Baywood Publishing.

Goldstein, A. P., & Michaels, G. Y. (1985). *Empathy: Development, training, and consequences.* Erlbaum.

Goleman, D. (1995). *Emotional intelligence: Why it can matter more than I.Q.* Bantam Books.

Gonçalves-Pereira, M., Trancas, B., Loureiro, J., Papoila, A., & Caldas-De-Almeida, J. M. (2013). Empathy as related to motivations for medicine in a sample of first-year medical students. *Psychological Reports, 112*(1), 73–88. https://doi.org/10.2466/17.13.PR0.112.1.73-88

Gonnella, J. S., Callahan, C. A., Veloski, J. J., DeSantis, J., & Hojat, M. (2022). *Fifty years of findings from the Jefferson Longitudinal Study of Medical Education.* Springer. https://doi.org/10.1007/978-3-030-85379-2

Gonnella, J. S., & Hojat, M. (2001). Biotechnology and ethics in medical education of the new millennium: Physician roles and responsibilities. *Medical Teacher, 23*(4), 371–377. https://doi.org/10.1080/01421590120042982

Gonnella, J. S., Hojat, M., Erdmann, J. B., & Veloski, J. J. (1993a). What have we learned, and where do we go from here? *Academic Medicine, 68*(Suppl), S79–S87.

Gonnella, J. S., Hojat, M., Erdmann, J. B., & Veloski, J. J. (1993b). What have we learned, and where do we go from here? In J. S. Gonnella, M. Hojat, J. B. Erdmann, & J. J. Veloski (Eds.), *Assessment measures in medical school, residency, and practice: The connections* (pp. 155–173). Springer.

Gonnella, J. S., Hojat, M., & Veloski, J. J. (2011). AM last page: The Jefferson longitudinal study of medical education. *Academic Medicine, 86(3)*, 404. https://doi.org/10.1097/ACM.0b013e31820bb3e7

Gonnella, J. S., Mangione, S., Nasca, T. J., & Hojat, M. (2005). Empathy scores in medical school and ratings of empathic behavior in residency training 3 years later. *The Journal of Social Psychology, 145*(6), 663–672. https://doi.org/10.3200/SOCP.145.6.663-672

Gonullu, P., & Oztuna, D. (2012). A Turkish adaptation of the student version of the Jefferson Scale of Physician Empathy. *Marmara Medical Journal, 25*, 87–92.

Gonzalez, A., Kortlever, J., Rijk, L., Ring, D., Brown, L., & Reichel, L. (2020). Is there a correlation between the patient-doctor relationship questionnaire and other patient-reported experience measures? *Patient Experience Journal, 7*(1), 44–50. https://doi.org/10.35680/2372-0247.1399

Good, R. S. (1972). After office hours: The third ear. *Obstetrics & Gynecology, 40*, 760–762.

Goodchild, C. E., Skinner, T. C., & Parkin, T. (2005). The value of empathy in dietetic consultation: A pilot study to investigate its effect on satisfaction, autonomy and agreement. *Journal of Human Nutrition and Diet, 18*(3), 181–185. https://doi.org/10.1111/j.1365-277X.2005.00606.x

Goodwin, J. S., Hunt, W. C., Key, C. R., & Samet, J. M. (1987). The effect of marital status on stage, treatment, and survival of cancer patients. *Journal of the American Medical Association, 258*, 3125–3130.

Gorsuch, R. L. (1974). *Factor analysis*. W.B. Saunders.

Gosselin, E., Paul-Savoie, E., Lavoie, S., & Bourgault, P. (2017). Evaluation of Nurse Empathy Perceived by the Standardized Patient in Simulation: A French Validation of the Jefferson Scale of Patient Perceptions of Physician Empathy. *Journal of Nursing Measurement, 25*(2), 152–161. https://doi.org/10.1891/1061-3749.25.2.152

Goubert, L., Craig, K. D., Vervoort, T., Morley, S., Sullivan, M. J. L., Williams, C. A. C., Cano, A., & Crombez, G. (2005). Facing others in pain: The effects of empathy. *Pain, 118*(3), 285–288. https://doi.org/10.1016/j.pain.2005.10.025

Gough, H. G. (1987). *California Psychological Inventory administrator's guide.* Consulting Psychologist Press, Inc.

Gough, H. G., & Hall, W. B. (1977). A comparison of physicians who did or did not respond to a postal questionnaire. *Journal of Applied Psychology, 62*, 777–780.

Gould, S. J. (1981). *The mismeasurement of man*. W.W. Norton.

Gouveia, L., Lelorain, S., Brédart, A., Dolbeault, S., Bonnaud-Antignac, A., Cousson-Gélie, F., & Sultan, S. (2015). Oncologists' perception of depressive symptoms in patients with advanced cancer: accuracy and relational correlates. *BMC Psychology, 3(1)*, 6. https://doi.org/10.1186/s40359-015-0063-6

Gradiski, I. P., Borovecki, A., Ćurković, M., San-Martín, M., Delgado Bolton, R. C., & Vivanco, L. (2022). Burnout in International Medical Students: Characterization of Professionalism and Loneliness as Predictive Factors of Burnout. *International Journal of Environmental Research and Public Health, 19*(3), 1385. https://doi.org/10.3390/ijerph19031385

Grant, J. P. (1991). *The state of the world's children*. Oxford University Press.

Grattan, L. M., & Eslinger, P. J. (1989). Higher cognitive and social behavior: Changes in cognitive flexibility and empathy after lesions. *Neuropsychology, 3*, 185.

Gray, J. (1992). *Men are from Mars, women are from Venus: A practical guide for improving communication and getting what you want in a relationship*. Harper & Collins.

Green, A., Peters, T. J., & Webster, D. J. T. (1991). An assessment of academic performance and personality. *Medical Education, 25*, 343–348.

Green, J. A., & Gustafson, G. E. (1983). Individual recognition of human infants on the basis of cries alone. *Developmental Psychobiology, 16*, 485–493.

Greenberg, L. S., Watson, J. C., Elliot, R., & Bohart, A. C. (2001). Empathy. *Psychotherapy, 38*, 380–384.

Greenson, R. (1967). *The techniques and practice of psychoanalysis*. International University Press.

Greenson, R. R. (1960). Empathy and its vicissitudes. *International Journal of Psychoanalysis, 41*, 418–424.

Greif, E. B., & Hogan, R. (1973). The theory and measurement of empathy. *Journal of Counseling Psychology, 20*, 280–284.

Gross, E. B. (1992). Gender difference in physician stress. *Journal of the American Medical Women's Association, 29*, 57–68.

Grosseman, S., Hojat, M., Duke, P. M., Mennin, S., Rosenzweig, S., & Novack, D. (2014). Empathy, self-reflection, and curriculum choice. *The Interdisciplinary Journal of Problem-Based Learning, 8*(2), 35–41. https://doi.org/10.7771/1541-5015.1429

Grosseman, S., Novack, D. H., Duke, P., Mennin, S., Rosenzweig, S., Davis, T., & Hojat, M. (2014). Residents' and standardized patients' perspectives on empathy: Issues of agreement. *Patient Education and Counseling, 96*(*1*), 22–28. https://doi.org/10.1016/j.pec.2014.04.007

Grossman, M., & Wood, W. (1993). Sex differences in intensity of emotional experience: A social role interpretation. *Journal of Personality and Social Psychology, 65*, 1010–1022.

Gruen, R. J., & Mendelsohn, G. (1986). Emotional responses to affective displays in others: The distinction between empathy and sympathy. *Journal of Personality and Social Psychology, 51*, 609–614.

Gruin, P., Peng, T., Lopez, G., & Nagda, B. A. (1999). Context, identity, and intergroup relations. In D. A. Prentice & D. T. Miller (Eds.), *Cultural divides: Understanding and overcoming group conflict* (pp. 133–172). Russell Sage Foundation.

Guilera, T., Batalla, I., Forné, C., & Soler-González, J. (2019). Empathy and big five personality model in medical students and its relationship to gender and specialty preference: a cross-sectional study. *BMC Medical Education, 19*(1), 57. https://doi.org/10.1186/s12909-019-1485-2

Guillemin, F., Bombardier, C., & Beaton, D. (1993). Cross-cultural adaptation of health-related quality of life measures: Literature review and proposed guidelines. *Journal of Clinical Epidemiology, 46*, 1417–1432.

Gulanick, N., & Schmeck, R. (1977). Modeling praise and criticism in teaching empathic responding. *Counselor Education and Supervision, 16*, 284–290.

Gurfein, E. G. (2017). *Enhancing empathy and emotion regulation to decrease burnout: a pilot study of compassion cultivation for physicians in training.* (Publication No. 10193576). [Doctoral dissertation, Palo Alto University]. ProQuest Dissertations & Theses Global. DAI-A 81/1(E).

Gustafson, J. P. (1986). *The complex secret of brief psychotherapy*. W.W. Norton.

Guttman, H., & Laporte, L. (2002). Alexithymia, empathy, and psychological symptoms in family context. *Comprehensive Psychiatry, 43*, 448–455.

Guzzetta, R. A. (1976). Acquisition and transfer of empathy by the parents of early adolescents through structured learning training. *Journal of Community Psychology, 23*, 449–453.

Hafferty, F. W. (1998). Beyond curriculum reform: Confronting medicine's hidden curriculum. *Academic Medicine, 73*, 403–407.

Hajibabaee, F., Farahani, A. M., Ameri, Z., Salehi, T., & Hosseini, F. (2018). The relationship between empathy and emotional intelligence among Iranian nursing students. *International Journal of Medical Education, 9*, 239–243. https://doi.org/10.5116/ijme.5b83.e2a5

Håkansson Eklund, J., Holmström, I. K., Ollén Lindqvist, A., Sundler, A. J., Hochwälder, J., & Marmstål Hammar, L. (2019). Empathy levels among nursing students: A comparative cross-sectional study. *Nursing Open, 6*(3), 983–989. https://doi.org/10.1002/nop2.280

Hall, E. T. (1966). *The hidden dimension*. Doubleday.

Hall, J. A. (1978). Gender effects in decoding nonverbal cues. *Psychological Bulletin, 85*, 845–857.

Hall, J. A. (1984). *Nonverbal sex differences: Communication accuracy and expressive style*. Johns Hopkins University Press.

Hall, J. A. (1990). *Nonverbal sex differences: Accuracy of communication and expressive style*. John Hopkins University Press.

Hall, J. A. (1998). How big are nonverbal sex differences? The case of smiling and sensitivity to nonverbal cues. In D. J. Canary & K. Dindia (Eds.), *Sex differences and similarities in communication: Critical essays and empirical investigations of sex and gender in interaction* (pp. 155–177). Erlbaum.

Hall, J. A. (2005). The gender similarities hypothesis. *American Psychologist, 60(6)*, 581–592. https://doi.org/10.1037/0003-066X.60.6.581

Hall, J. A., Carter, J. D., & Horgan, T. G. (2000). Gender differences in the nonverbal communication of emotion. In A. H. Fischer (Ed.), *Gender and emotion: Social psychological perspectives* (pp. 97–117). Cambridge University Press.

Hall, J. A., & Dornan, M. C. (1988). Meta-analysis of satisfaction with medical care: Description of research domain and analysis of overall satisfaction level. *Social Science & Medicine, 27*, 637–644.

Hall, J. A., & Gunnery, S. D. (2013). Gender differences in nonverbal communication. In J. A. Hall & M. L. Knapp (Eds.), *Nonverbal communication (2, Handbook of communication science)* (pp. 639–669). deGruyter Mouton.

Hall, J. A., Irish, J. T., Roter, D. L., Ehrlic, C. M., & Miller, L. H. (1994). Gender in medical encounters: An analysis of physician and patient communication in a primary care setting. *Health Psychology, 13*, 384–392.

Hall, J. A., Roter, D. L., & Katz, N. R. (1988). Meta-analysis of correlates of provider behavior in medical encounters. *Medical Care, 26*, 657–675.

Hall, M., Hanna, L. A., Hanna, A., & McDevitt, C. (2015). Empathy in UK pharmacy students: Assessing differences by gender, level in the degree programme, part-time employment and medical status. *Pharmacy Education, 15*, 241–247. https://pharmacyeducation.fip.org/pharmacyeducation/article/view/393

Halpern, J. (2001). *From detached concern to empathy: Humanizing medical practice*. Oxford University Press.

Halsband, U., Schmitt, J., Weyers, M., Binkofski, F., Grutzner, G., & Freund, H. J. (2001). Recognition and imitation of pantomimed motor acts after unilateral parietal and premotor lesions: A perspective on apraxia. *Neuropsychology, 39*, 200–216.

Hamilton, N. G. (1984). Empathic understanding. In J. Lichtenberg, M. Bornstein, & D. Silver (Eds.), *Empathy II* (pp. 217–222). The Analytic Press.

Hamilton, W. D. (1964). The genetic evolution of social behavior. *Journal of Theoretical Biology, 7*, 1–52.

Han, S., Fan, Y., & Mao, L. (2008). Gender difference in empathy for pain: An electrophysiological investigation. *Brain Research, 1196*, 85–93. https://doi.org/10.1016/j.brainres.2007.12.062

Haney, C., Banks, C., & Zimbardo, P. (1973). Interpersonal dynamics in a simulated prison. *International Journal of Criminology and Penology, 1*, 69–97.

Haque, O. S., & Waytz, A. (2012). Dehumanization in medicine: Causes, solutions, and functions. *Perspectives on Psychological Sciences, 7(2)*, 176–186. https://doi.org/10.1177/1745691611429706

Hari, R., Forss, N., Avikainen, S., Kirveskari, E., Salenius, S., & Rizzolatti, G. (1998). Activation of human primary motor cortex during action observation: A neuromagnetic study. *Proceedings of the National Academy of Sciences of the United States of America, 95*, 15061–15065.

Harrigan, J. A., & Rosenthal, R. (1983). Physicians' head and body position as determinants of perceived rapport. *Journal of Applied Social Psychology, 13*, 496–509.

Harsch, H. H. (1989). The role of empathy in medical students' choice of specialty. *Academic Psychiatry, 13*, 96–98.

Hartup, W. W., & Stevens, N. (1999). Friendships and adaptation across the life span. *American Psychological Society, 8*, 76–79.

Harz, D., Begin, A. S., Alansari, R., Esparza, R., Zimmermann, C., Evans, B. D., Eisenberg, S., & Katz, J. T. (2023). The art of empathy: Teaching empathy through art. *The Clinical Teacher, 20*(5), e13643. https://doi.org/10.1111/tct.13643

Hasan, N., Al-Sharqawi, F., Dashti, M., AbdulAziz, A., Abdullah, M., Shukkur, M., & Bouhaimed, L. Thalib; Level of Empathy among Medical Students in Kuwait University, Kuwait. *Medical Principles and Practice, 22(4)*, 385–389. https://doi.org/10.1159/000348300

Hasan, S. H., Babar, M. G., Chen, K. K., Ahmed, S. I., & Mitha, S. (2013). An assessment of pharmacy students' empathy levels in Malaysia. *Journal of Advanced Pharmacy Education & Research, 3(4)*, 531–540.

Hass, J. S., Cook, E. F., Puopolo, A. L., Burnstin, H. R., Clearly, P. D., & Brennan, T. A. (2000). Is professional satisfaction of general internists associated with patient satisfaction? *Journal of General Internal Medicine, 15*, 122–128.

Hasse, R. F., & Tepper, D. T., Jr. (1972). Nonverbal components of empathic communication. *Journal of Counseling Psychology, 19*, 417–424.

Hatcher, S. L., Nadeau, M. S., Walsh, L. K., Reynolds, M., Gala, J., & Marz, K. (1994). The teaching of empathy for high school and college students: Testing Rogerian methods with the Interpersonal Reactivity Index. *Adolescence, 29*, 961–974.

Hebb, D. (1946). *The organization of behaviour*. John Wiley & Sons.

Hegazi, I., Hennessy, A., & Wilson, I. (2017). Empathy levels in medical students: do they really change over time? In M. Kondo (Ed.), *Empathy-An Evidence-based Interdisciplinary Perspective*. https://doi.org/10.5772/intechopen.69625

Heilman, K. M., Scholes, R., & Watson, R. T. (1975). Auditory affective agnosia: Disturbed comprehension of affective speech. *Journal of Neurology, Neurosurgery and Psychiatry, 38*, 69–72.

Hein, G., Engelmann, J. B., Vollberg, M. C., & Tobler, P. N. (2016). How learning shapes the empathic Pain. *Proceedings of the National Academy of Sciences, 113*(*1*), 80–85. https://doi.org/10.1073/pnas.1514539112

Hein, G., & Singer, T. (2008). I feel how you feel but not always: The empathic brain and its modulation. *Current Opinion in Neurobiology, 18*(2), 153–158. https://doi.org/10.1016/j.conb.2008.07.012

Heinrichs, M., & Domes, G. (2008). Neuropeptides and social behavior: Effects of oxytocin and vasopressin in humans. *Progress in Brain Research, 170*, 337–350. https://doi.org/10.1016/S0079-6123(08)00428-7

Heinrichs, M., Meinlschmidt, G., Wippich, W., Ehlert, U., & Hemmhammer, D. H. (2004). Selective Amnesic effects of oxytocin on human memory. *Physiology and Behavior, 83*(*1*), 31–38. https://doi.org/10.1016/j.physbeh.2004.07.020

Hekmat, H., Khajavi, F., & Mehryar, A. H. (1974). Psychoticism, neuroticism, and extraversion: The personality determinants of empathy. *Journal of Clinical Psychology, 30*, 559–561.

Hekmat, H., Khajavi, F., & Mehryar, A. H. (1975). Some personality correlates of empathy. *Journal of Counseling and Clinical Psychology, 43*, 89.

Hemmerdinger, H. M., Stoddart, A. D. R., & Lilford, R. J. (2007). A systematic review of tests of empathy in medicine. *BMC Medical Education, 7*, 24. https://doi.org/10.1186/1472-6920-7-24

Henderson, J. T., & Weisman, C. S. (2001). Physician gender effects on preventive screening and counseling: An analysis of male and female patients' health care experiences. *Medical Care, 39*, 1281–1292.

Henderson, S. (1974). Care-eliciting behavior in man. *The Journal of Nervous and Mental Disease, 159*, 172–181.

Hennen, B. K. (1975). Continuity of care in family practice. *The Journal of Family Practice, 2*, 371–372.

Henry-Tillman, R., Deloney, L. A., Savidge, M., Graham, C. J., & Klimberg, S. (2002). The medical student as patient navigator as an approach to teaching empathy. *The American Journal of Surgery, 183*, 659–662.

Herman, J. (2000). Reading for empathy. *Medical Hypotheses, 54*, 167–168.

Hess, U., Blairy, S., & Phillippot, P. (1999). Facial mimicry. In P. Phillippot, R. Feldman, & E. Coats (Eds.), *The social context of nonverbal behavior* (pp. 213–241). Cambridge University Press.

Hickson, G. B., Clayton, E. W., Entman, S. S., Miller, C. S., Githens, P. B., Whetten-Goldstein, K., & Sloan, F. A. (1994). Obstetricians' prior malpractice experience and patients' satisfaction with care. *Journal of the American Medical Association, 272*, 1583–1587.

Hickson, G. B., Clayton, E. W., Githens, P. B., & Sloan, F. A. (1992). Factors that prompted families to file medical malpractice claims following perinatal injuries. *Journal of the American Medical Association, 267*, 1359–1363.

Hill, E., Berthoz, S., & Frith, U. (2004). Brief report: Cognitive processing of own emotions in individuals with autistic spectrum disorder and in their relatives. *Journal of Autism and Developmental Disorders, 34*(2), 229–235. https://doi.org/10.1023/b:jadd.0000022613.41399.14

Hinshelwood, R. (1989). *A dictionary of Kleinian thought*. Free Association Press.

Hirshberg, C., & Barasch, M. I. (1995). *Remarkable recovery*. Riverside Books.

Hislop, T. G., Waxler, N. E., Coldman, A. J., Elwood, J. M., & Kan, L. (1987). The prognostic significance of psychosocial factors in women with breast cancer. *Journal of Chronic Diseases, 40*, 729–735.

Hittelman, J. H., & Dickes, R. (1979). Sex differences in neonatal eye contact time. *Merrill-Pamler Quarterly, 25*, 171–184.

Hobfolls, S. E., & Benor, D. (1981). Prediction of student clinical performance. *Medical Education, 15*, 231–236.

Hodges, S. D., & Wegner, D. M. (1997). Automatic and controlled empathy. In W. Ickes (Ed.), *Empathic accuracy* (pp. 311–339). Guilford.

Hoffman, M. L. (1977). Sex differences in empathy and related behaviors. *Psychological Bulletin, 84*, 712–722.

Hoffman, M. L. (1978). Psychological and biological perspectives on altruism. *International Journal of Behavioral Development, 1*, 323–339.

Hoffman, M. L. (1981). The development of empathy. In J. Rushton & R. Sorrentino (Eds.), *Altruism and helping behavior: Social personality and developmental perspectives* (pp. 41–63). Erlbaum.

Hoffman, M. L. (1982). The measurement of empathy. In C. E. Izard (Ed.), *Measuring emotions in infants and children* (pp. 279–296). Cambridge University Press.

Hoffman, S. B., Brand, F. R., Beatty, P. G., & Hamill, L. A. (1985). Geriatrix: A role-playing game. *Gerontologist, 25*, 568–572.

Hoffman, T. L., & Reif, S. D. (1978). *'Intro aging': Simulation game*. Charles B. Slack Inc.

Hogan, R. (1969). Development of an empathy scale. *Journal of Consulting and Clinical Psychology, 33*, 307–316.

Hogan, R. (1976). Moral conduct and moral character: A psychological perspective. *Psychological Bulletin, 79*, 217–232.

Hogan, R., & Dickstein, E. (1972). A measure of moral value. *Journal of Consulting and Clinical Psychology, 39*, 210–214.

Hogan, R., & Mankin, D. (1970). Determinants of interpersonal attraction: A clarification. *Psychological Reports, 26*, 235–238.

Hogan, R., Rossiter, C., & Catling, C. (2018). Cultural empathy in midwifery students: Assessment of an education program. *Nurse Education Today, 70*, 103–108. https://doi.org/10.1016/j.nedt.2018.08.023
Hogan, R., & Weiss, D. S. (1974). Personality correlates of superior academic achievement. *Journal of Consulting Psychology, 21*, 144–151.
Hojat, M. (1982a). Loneliness as a function of selected personality variables. *Journal of Clinical Psychology, 38*, 137–141.
Hojat, M. (1982b). Psychometric characteristics of the UCLA Loneliness Scale. *Educational and Psychological Measurement, 42*, 917–925.
Hojat, M. (1983). Comparison of transitory and chronic loners on selected personality variables. *British Journal of Psychology, 74*, 199–202.
Hojat, M. (1992). Social and economic factors in patients with coronary disease. *Journal of the American Medical Association, 268*, 195–196.
Hojat, M. (1993). The world's declaration of the rights of the child: Anticipated challenges. *Psychological Reports, 72*, 1011–1022.
Hojat, M. (1995). Developmental pathways to violence: A psychodynamic paradigm. *Peace Psychology Review, 1*, 177–196.
Hojat, M. (1996). Perception of maternal availability in childhood and selected psychosocial characteristics in adulthood. *Genetic, Social, And General Psychology Monographs, 122*, 425–450.
Hojat, M. (1997). The U.N. Convention: Lost in the clash of adverse opinions. *American Psychologist, 52*, 1384–1385.
Hojat, M. (1998). Satisfaction with early relationships with parents and psychosocial attributes in adulthood: Which parent contributes more? *Journal of General Psychology, 159*, 203–220.
Hojat, M. (2009). Ten approaches for enhancing empathy in health and human services cultures. *Journal Of Health And Human Services Association, 31*(4), 412–450.
Hojat, M. (2014). Assessments of empathy in medical school admissions: What additional evidence is needed? *International Journal Of Medical Education, 5*, 7–10. https://doi.org/10.5116/ijme.52b7.5294
Hojat, M. (2016). *Empathy in health professions education and patient care*. New York: Springer International Publishing. https://doi.org/10.1007/978-3-319-27625-0.
Hojat, M., Axelrod, D., Spandorfer, J., & Mangione, S. (2013a). Enhancing and sustaining empathy in medical students. *Medical Teacher, 35*(12), 996–1001. https://doi.org/10.3109/0142159X.2013.802300
Hojat, M., Bianco, J. A., Mann, D., Massello, D., & Calabrese, L. H. (2015a). Overlap between empathy, teamwork and integrative approach to patient care. *Medical Teacher, 37*(8), 755–758. https://doi.org/10.3109/0142159X.2014.971722
Hojat, M., Borenstein, B. D., & Shapurian, R. (1990). Perception of childhood dissatisfaction with parents and selected personality traits in adulthood. *The Journal of Genetic Psychology, 117*, 241–253.
Hojat, M., & Crandall, R. (Eds.). (1989). *Loneliness: Theory, research, and applications*. Sage.
Hojat, M., DeSantis, J., Cain, R., Speicher, M., Bragan, L., Shannon, S., & Calabrese, L. (2021). Attitudes toward osteopathic medicine scale: Development, psychometrics. *International Journal of Medical Education, 12*, 222–232. https://doi.org/10.5116/ijme.615c.2cfa
Hojat, M., DeSantis, J., & Gonnella, J. S. (2017). Patient perceptions of clinician's empathy: Measurement and psychometrics. *Journal of Patient Experience, 4*(2), 78–83. https://doi.org/10.1177/2374373517699273
Hojat, M., DeSantis, J., Ney, D., & DeCleene-Do, H. (2021). Empathy of medical students and compassionate care for dying patients: An assessment of "No One Dies Alone" program. *Journal of Patient Experience, 7*(6), 1164–1168. https://doi.org/10.1177/2374373520962605
Hojat, M., DeSantis, J., Shannon, S., Mortensen, L. H., Speicher, M., Bragan, L., LaNoue, M., & Calabrese, L. H. (2018). The Jefferson Scale of Empathy: A nationwide study of measurement properties, underlying components, latent variable structure, and national norm in medi-

cal students. *Advances in Health Profession Education, 23*, 899–920. https://doi.org/10.1007/s10459-018-9839-9

Hojat, M., DeSantis, J., Shannon, S. C., Speicher, M. R., Bragan, L., & Calabrese, L. H. (2020). Empathy as related to gender, age, race/ethnicity, academic background, and career interest: Results of a nationwide study of medical students. *Medical Education, 54*(6), 571–581. https://doi.org/10.1111/medu.14138

Hojat, M., Erdmann, J. B., & Gonnella, J. S. (2014). Personality assessments and outcomes in medical education and the practice of medicine. AMEE Guide No. 79. *Medical Teacher, 35*(7), e1267–e1301. https://doi.org/10.3109/0142159X.2013.785654

Hojat, M., Erdmann, J. B., Veloski, J. J., Nasca, T. J., Callahan, C., Julian, E., & Peck, J. (2000a). A validity study of the writing sample section of the Medical College Admission Test. *Academic Medicine, 75*, S25–S27.

Hojat, M., Fields, S. K., & Gonnella, J. S. (2003a). Empathy: An NP/MD comparison. *The Nurse Practioner, 28*, 45–47.

Hojat, M., Fields, S. K., Rattner, S. L., Griffiths, M., Cohen, M. J. M., & Plumb, J. (1997). Attitudes toward the physician-nurse alliance: Comparisons of medical and nursing students. *Academic Medicine, 72*, 1–3.

Hojat, M., Glaser, K., Xu, G., Veloski, J. J., & Christian, E. B. (1999a). Gender comparisons of medical students' psychosocial profile. *Medical Education, 33*, 342–349.

Hojat, M., Glaser, K. M., & Veloski, J. J. (1996). Associations between selected psychosocial attributes and ratings of physician competence. *Academic Medicine, 71*, S103–S105.

Hojat, M., & Gonnella, J. S. (2015). Eleven years of data on the Jefferson Scale of Empathy-Medical Student Version (JSE-S): Proxy norm data and tentative cutoff scores. *Medical Principles and Practice: International Journal of the Kuwait University, Health Science Centre, 24*(4), 344–350. https://doi.org/10.1159/000381954

Hojat, M., & Gonnella, J. S. (2017). What matters more about the Interpersonal Reactivity Index and the Jefferson Scale of Empathy? Their underlying constructs or their relationships with pertinent measures of clinical competence and patient outcomes? (invited commentary). *Academic Medicine, 92*(6), 743–745. https://doi.org/10.1097/ACM.0000000000001424

Hojat, M., Gonnella, J. S., Erdmann, J. B., Rattner, S. L., Veloski, J. J., Glaser, K., & Xu, G. (2000b). Gender comparisons of income expectations in the USA at the beginning of medical school during the past twenty-eight years. *Social Science & Medicine, 50*, 1665–1672.

Hojat, M., Gonnella, J. S., Erdmann, J. B., Veloski, J. J., Louis, D. Z., Nasca, T. J., & Rattner, S. L. (2000c). Physicians' perceptions of the changing health care system: Comparisons by gender and specialties. *Journal of Community Health, 25*, 455–471.

Hojat, M., Gonnella, J. S., Erdmann, J. B., & Vogel, W. H. (2003b). Medical students' cognitive appraisal of stressful life events as related to personality, physical well-being, and academic performance: A longitudinal study. *Personality and Individual Differences, 35*, 219–235.

Hojat, M., Gonnella, J. S., Mangione, S., Nasca, T. J., & Magee, M. (2003c). Physician empathy in medical education and practice: Experience with the Jefferson Scale of Physician Empathy. *Seminars in Integrative Medicine, 1*, 25–41.

Hojat, M., Gonnella, J. S., Mangione, S., Nasca, T. J., Veloski, J. J., Erdmann, J. B., Callahan, C. A., & Magee, M. (2002). Empathy in medical students as related to academic performance, clinical competence and gender. *Medical Education, 36*(6), 522–527. https://doi.org/10.1046/j.1365-2923.2002.01234.x

Hojat, M., Gonnella, J. S., Nasca, T. J., Fields, S. K., Alcorta-Gonzalez, A., Ibarra, D., & Torres-Ruiz, A. (2003d). Comparisons of American, Israeli, Italian and Mexican physicians and nurses on four dimensions of the Jefferson Scale of Attitudes toward Physician Nurse Collaboration. *International Journal of Nursing Studies, 40*, 426–435.

Hojat, M., Gonnella, J. S., Nasca, T. J., Mangione, S., Veloski, J. J., & Magee, M. (2002a). The Jefferson Scale of Physician Empathy: Further psychometric data and differences by gender and specialty at item level. *Academic Medicine [Supplement], 77*, S58–S60.

Hojat, M., Gonnella, J. S., Nasca, T. J., Mangione, S., Vergare, M., & Magee, M. (2002b). Physician empathy: Definition, components, measurement, and relationship to gender and specialty. *American Journal of Psychiatry, 159*, 1563–1569.

Hojat, M., Gonnella, J. S., & Veloski, J. (2010a). Rebuttals to critics of studies of decline on empathy. *Academic Medicine, 85*(12), 1812–1814. https://doi.org/10.1097/ACM.0b013e3181fa3576

Hojat, M., & Herman, M. W. (1985). Developing an instrument to measure attitudes toward nurses: Preliminary psychometric findings. *Psychological Reports, 56*, 571–579.

Hojat, M., & LaNoue, M. (2014). Exploration and confirmation of the latent variable structure of the Jefferson Scale of Empathy. *International Journal of Medical Education, 5*, 73–81. https://doi.org/10.1097/ACM.0b013e3181fa3576

Hojat, M., Louis, D. Z., Maio, V., & Gonnella, J. S. (2013b). Empathy and health care quality [Editorial]. *American Journal of Medical Quality, 28*(1), 6–7. https://doi.org/10.1177/1062860612464731

Hojat, M., Louis, D. Z., Markham, F. W., Wender, R., Rabinowitz, C., & Gonnella, J. S. (2011a). Physicians' empathy and clinical outcomes in diabetic patients. *Academic Medicine, 86*(3), 359–364. https://doi.org/10.1097/ACM.0b013e3182086fe1

Hojat, M., Louis, D. Z., Maxwell, K., & Gonnella, J. S. (2011b). The Jefferson Scale of Empathy (JSE): An update. *Health Policy Newsletter, 24*, 5–6.

Hojat, M., Louis, D. Z., Maxwell, K., Markham, F., Wender, R., & Gonnella, J. S. (2010b). Patient perceptions of physician empathy, satisfaction with physician, interpersonal trust, and compliance. *International Journal of Medical Education, 1*, 83–87. https://doi.org/10.5116/ijme.4d00.b701

Hojat, M., Maio, V., Markham, F. W., Louis, D., & Gonnella, J. S. (2019). Physician empathy and diabetes outcomes. *Journal of General Internal Medicine, 34*(*10*). https://doi.org/10.1007/s11606-019-05187-0

Hojat, M., Maio, V., Pohl, C. A., & Gonnella, J. S. (2023). Clinical empathy: Definition, measurement, correlates, group differences, erosion, enhancement, and healthcare outcomes. *Discover Health Systems., 2*, 8. https://doi.org/10.1007/s44250-023-00020-2

Hojat, M., Mangione, S., Gonnella, J. S., Nasca, T., Veloski, J. J., & Kane, G. (2001a). Empathy in medical education and patient care. *Academic Medicine, 76*(7), 669.

Hojat, M., Mangione, S., Kane, G., & Gonnella, J. S. (2005a). Relationships between scores of the Jefferson Scale of Physician Empathy (JSPE) and the Interpersonal Reactivity Index (IRI). *Medical Teacher, 27*(7), 625–628. https://doi.org/10.1080/01421590500069744

Hojat, M., Mangione, S., Nasca, T. J., Cohen, M. J. M., Gonnella, J. S., Erdmann, J. B., Veloski, J., & Magee, M. (2001b). The Jefferson Scale of Physician Empathy: Development and preliminary psychometric data. *Educational and Psychological Measurement, 61*(2), 349–365.

Hojat, M., Mangione, S., Nasca, T. J., Rattner, S. L., Erdmann, J. B., Gonnella, J. S., & Magee, M. (2004). An empirical study of decline of empathy in medical school. *Medical Education, 38*(*9*), 934–941. https://doi.org/10.1111/j.1365-2929.2004.01911.x

Hojat, M., Michalec, B., Veloski, J., & Tykocinski, M. L. (2015b). Can empathy, other personality attributes, and level of positive social influence in medical school identify potential leaders in medicine? *Academic Medicine, 90*(4), 505–510. https://doi.org/10.1097/ACM.0000000000000652

Hojat, M., Nasca, T. J., Cohen, M. J., Fields, S. K., Rattner, S. L., Griffiths, M., Ibarra, D., de Gonzalez, A. A., Torres-Ruiz, A., Ibarra, G., & Garcia, A. (2001c). Attitudes toward physician-nurse collaboration: A cross-cultural study of male and female physicians and nurses in the United States and Mexico. *Nursing Research, 50*, 123–128.

Hojat, M., Nasca, T. J., Gonnella, J. S., Frisby, A. J., Erdmann, J. B., & Veloski, J. J. (2003e). An operational measure of physician lifelong learning: Its development, components and preliminary psychometric data. *Medical Teacher, 25*, 433–437.

Hojat, M., Nasca, T. J., Magee, M., Feeney, K., Pascual, R., Urbano, F., & Gonnella, J. S. (1999b). A comparison of the personality profiles of internal medicine residents, physician role models, and the general population. *Academic Medicine, 74*, 54–60.

Hojat, M., Paskin, D. L., Callahan, C. A., Nasca, T. J., Louis, D. Z., Veloski, J., Erdmann, J. B., & Gonnella, J. S. (2007). Components of postgraduate competence: Analyses of 30 years of longitudinal data. *Medical Education, 41*(10), 982–989. https://doi.org/10.1111/j.1365-2923.2007.02841.x

Hojat, M., Robeson, M., Damjanov, I., Veloski, J. J., Glaser, K., & Gonnella, J. S. (1993). Students' psychosocial characteristics as predictors of academic performance in medical school. *Academic Medicine, 68*, 635–637.

Hojat, M., Robeson, M., Veloski, J. J., Blacklow, R. S., Xu, G., & Gonnella, J. S. (1994). Gender comparisons prior to, during, and after medical school using two decades of longitudinal data at Jefferson Medical College. *Evaluation and the Health Professions, 17*, 290–306.

Hojat, M., Samuel, S., & Thompson, T. L. (1995). Searching for the lost key under the light of biomedicine: A triangular biopsychosocial paradigm may cast additional light on medical education, research and patient care. In S. K. Majumdar, L. M. Rosenfeld, D. B. Nash, & A. M. Audet (Eds.), *Medicine & health care into the 21st century* (pp. 310–325). Pennsylvania Academy of Science.

Hojat, M., Shannon, S. C., DeSantis, J., Speicher, M., Braga, L., & Calabrese, L. (2020). Does empathy decline in the Clinical phase of medical education? A nationwide, multi-institutional, cross-sectional study of students at DO granting medical schools. *Academic Medicine, 95*(6), 911–918. https://doi.org/10.1097/ACM.0000000000003175

Hojat, M., Shannon, S., DeSantis, J., Speicher, M., Bragan, L., & Calabrese, L. (2019). National norms for the Jefferson Scale of Empathy: A nationwide project in osteopathic medical education and empathy (POMEE). *Journal of American Osteopathic Association, 119*(8), 520–532. https://doi.org/10.7556/jaoa.2019.091

Hojat, M., & Shapurian, R. (1986). Anxiety and its measurement: A study of psychometric characteristics of a short form of the Taylor Manifest Anxiety Scale in Iranian students. *Journal of Social Behavior and Personality, 1*, 621–630.

Hojat, M., Shapurian, R., Foroughi, D., Nayerahmadi, H., Farzaneh, M., Shafieyan, M., & Parsi, M. (2000d). Gender differences in traditional attitudes toward marriage and the family: An empirical study of Iranian immigrants in the United States. *Journal of Family Issues, 21*, 419–434.

Hojat, M., Shapurian, R., & Mehryar, A. H. (1986). Dimensionality of the short form of the Beck Depression Inventory. *Psychological Reports, 59*, 1069–1070.

Hojat, M., Shapurian, R., Nayerahmadi, H., Farzaneh, M., Foroughi, D., Parsi, M., & Azizi, M. (1999c). Premarital sexual, childrearing, and family attitudes of Iranian men and women in the United States and in Iran. *Journal of Psychology, 133*, 19–31.

Hojat, M., Spandorfer, J., Louis, D. Z., & Gonnella, J. S. (2011c). Empathic and sympathetic orientations toward patient care: Conceptualization, measurement, and psychometrics. *Academic Medicine, 86*(8), 989–995. https://doi.org/10.1097/ACM.0b013e31822203d8

Hojat, M., Spandorfer, J., Isenberg, G., Vergare, M., & Fassihi, R. (2012a). Psychometrics of the scale of attitudes toward physician-pharmacist collaboration: A study with medical students. *Medical Teacher, 34*, e833–e837.

Hojat, M., Veloski, J. J., & Gonnella, J. S. (2009a). Measurement and correlates of physicians' lifelong learning. *Academic Medicine, 84*(8), 1066–1074. https://doi.org/10.1097/ACM.0b013e3181acf25f

Hojat, M., Veloski, J. J., & Gonnella, J. S. (2010c). Physician lifelong learning: Conceptualization, measurement, and correlates in full-time clinicians and academic clinicians. In M. P. Caltone (Ed.), *Handbook of lifelong learning development* (pp. 37–78). Nova Science Publishers, Inc.

Hojat, M., Veloski, J. J., & Gonnella, J. S. (2012b). Physician lifelong learning: Conceptualization, measurement, and correlates in full-time clinicians, academic clinicians, and medical students. In G. J. Neimeyer & J. Taylor (Eds.), *Continuing professional development and lifelong learning: Issues, impacts and outcomes* (pp. 29–69). Nova Science Publishers, Inc.

Hojat, M., Veloski, J. J., Louis, D. Z., Xu, G., Ibarra, D., Gottlieb, J. E., & Erdmann, J. B. (1999d). Perceptions of medical seniors of the current changes in the United States health care system. *Evaluation and the Health Professions, 22*, 169–183.

Hojat, M., Veloski, J. J., & Zeleznik, C. (1985). Predictive validity of the MCAT for students with two sets of scores. *Journal of Medical Education, 60*, 911–918.

Hojat, M., Vergare, M., Isenberg, G., Cohen, M., & Spandorfer, J. (2015c). Underlying construct of empathy, optimism, and burnout in medical students. *International Journal of Medical Education, 6*, 12–16. https://doi.org/10.5116/ijme.54c3.60cd

Hojat, M., Vergare, M. J., Maxwell, K., Brainard, G., Herrine, S. K., Isenberg, G. A., Veloski, J., & Gonnella, J. S. (2009b). The devil is in the third year: A longitudinal study of erosion of empathy in medical school. *Academic Medicine, 84*(9), 1182–1191. https://doi.org/10.1097/ACM.0b013e3181b17e55

Hojat, M., & Vogel, W. H. (1989). Socioemotional bonding and neurobiochemistry. *Journal of Social Behavior and Personality, 2*, 135–144.

Hojat, M., Vogel, W. H., Zeleznik, C., & Borenstein, B. D. (1988). Effects of academic and psychosocial predictors of performance in medical school on coefficients of determination. *Psychological Reports, 63*, 383–394.

Hojat, M., Ward, J., Spandorfer, J., Arenson, C., Van Winkle, L. J., & Williams, B. (2015d). The Jefferson Scale of Attitudes Toward Interprofessional Collaboration (Jeff SATIC): Development and multi-institution psychometric data. *Journal of Intereprofessional Care, 29(3)*, 238–244. https://doi.org/10.3109/13561820.2014.962129

Hojat, M., & Xu, G. (2004). A visitor's guide to effect sizes: Statistical versus practical (clinical) importance of research findings. *Advances in Health Sciences Education, 9(3)*, 241–249. https://doi.org/10.1023/B:AHSE.0000038173.00909.f6

Hojat, M., Zuckerman, M., Gonnella, J. S., Mangione, S., Nasca, T., Vergare, M., & Magee, M. (2005b). Empathy in medical students as related to specialty interest, personality, and perception of mother and father. *Personality and Individual Differences, 39*(7), 1205–1215. https://doi.org/10.1016/j.paid.2005.04.007

Holden, C. (2004). Image studies show how brain thinks about pain. *Science, 303*, 1121.

Holland, J. C. (2001). Improving the human side of cancer care: Psycho-oncology's contribution. *Cancer Journal, 7*, 458–471.

Holland, J. C., Geary, N., Marchini, A., & Tross, S. (1987). An international survey of physician attitudes and practice in regard to revealing the diagnosis of cancer. *Cancer Investigation, 5*, 151–154.

Holleman, W. L. (2000). The play's the thing: Using literature and drama to teach about death and dying. *Family Medicine, 32*, 523–524.

Hollowell, E. E., & De Ville, K. A. (2003). *Physicians: Avoid treating family members*.

Holmes, C. A. (1992). The wounded healer. *International Journal of Communicative Psychoanalysis & Psychotherapy, 6*, 33–36.

Holtzman, J. M., Beck, J. D., & Coggin, P. G. (1978). Geriatric program for medical students: II. Impact of two educational experiences on students attitudes. *Journal of American Geriatric Society, 26*, 355–359.

Holtzman, J. M., Beck, J. D., & Ettinger, R. L. (1981). Cognitive knowledge and attitudes toward the aged dental and medical students. *Educational Gerontology, 6*, 195–207.

Holub, P. G. (2011). *The influence of narrative in fostering affective development of medical professionalism in an online class*. (Publication No 3439139). [Doctoral dissertation, Nova Southeastern University]. ProQuest Dissertations & Theses Global. DAI-A 72/03.

Hong, H., & Han, A. (2020). A systematic review on empathy measurement tools for care professionals. *Educational Gerontology, 46*(2), 72–83. https://doi.org/10.1080/03601277.2020.1712058

Hong, M., Bahn, G. H., Lee, W. H., & Moon, S. J. (2011). Empathy in Korean psychiatric residents. *Asia-Pacific Psychiatry, 3*(2), 83–90. https://doi.org/10.1111/j.1758-5872.2011.00123.x

Hong, M., Lee, W. H., Park, J. H., Yoon, T. Y., Moon, D. S., & Lee, S. M. (2012). Changes of empathy in medical college and medical school students: 1-year follow up study. *BMC Medical Education, 12*, 122. https://doi.org/10.1186/1472-6920-12-122

Hooper, E. M., Comstock, L. M., Goodwin, J. M., & Goodwin, J. S. (1982). Patient characteristics that influence physician behavior. *Medical Care, 20*, 630–638.

Hoover, R. N. (2000). Cancer: Nature, nurture, or both. *The New England Journal of Medicine, 343*, 135–136.

Hornblow, A. R., Kidson, M. A., & Jones, K. V. (1977). Measuring medical students' empathy: A validation study. *Medical Education, 11*, 7–12.

Hornblow, A. R., Kidson, M. A., & Ironside, W. (1988). Empathic processes: Perception by medical students of patients' anxiety and depression. *Medical Education, 22*, 15–18.

Hornstein, H. A. (1978). Promotive tension and prosocial behavior: A Lewinian analysis. In L. Wispe (Ed.), *Altruism, sympathy, and helping: Psychological and sociological principles* (pp. 177–207). Academic Press.

Horton, P. C. (1995). The comforting substrate and the right brain. *Bulletin of the Menninger Clinic, 59*, 480–486.

House, J. S., Landis, K. R., & Umberson, D. (1988). Social relationships and health. *Science, 241*, 540–544.

House, J. S., Robbins, C., & Metzner, H. L. (1982). The association of social relationships and activities with mortality: Prospective evidence from the Tecumseh Community Health Study. *American Journal of Epidemiology, 116*, 123–140.

Houston, W. R. (1938). The doctor himself as a therapeutic agent. *Annals of Internal Medicine, 11*, 1416–1425.

Howell, E. A., Gardiner, B., & Concato, J. (2002). Do women prefer female obstetricians? *Obstetrics and Gynecology, 100*, 827–828.

Howick, J., Moscrop, A., Mebius, A., Fanshawe, T. R., Lewith, G., Bishop, F. L., Mistiaen, P., Roberts, N. W., Dieninytė, E., Hu, X. Y., Aveyard, P., & Onakpoya, I. J. (2018). Effects of empathic and positive communication in healthcare consultations: a systematic review and meta-analysis. *Journal of the Royal Society of Medicine, 111*(7), 240–252. https://doi.org/10.1177/0141076818769477

Howick, J., Steinkopf, L., Ulyte, A., Roberts, N., & Meissner, K. (2017). How empathic is your healthcare practitioner? A systematic review and meta-analysis of patient surveys. *BMC Medical Education, 17*, 136. https://doi.org/10.1186/s12909-017-0967-3.

Hróbjartsson, A., & Gøtzsche, P. C. (2001). Is the placebo powerless? An analysis of clinical trials comparing placebo with no treatment. *The New England Journal of Medicine, 344*, 1594–1632.

Hsiao, C. Y., Tsai, Y. F., & Kao, Y. C. (2012). Psychometric properties of a Chinese version of the Jefferson Scale of Empathy—Health Profession Students. *Journal of Psychiatric and Mental Health Nursing, 12*, 866–873. https://doi.org/10.1111/jpm.12024

Hsieh, N. K., Herzig, K., Gansky, S. A., & Danley, D. (2006). Changing dentists' knowledge, attitudes and behavior regarding domestic violence through an interactive multimedia tutorial. *Journal of American Dental Association, 137(5)*, 596–603. https://doi.org/10.14219/jada.archive.2006.0254

Hu, L., & Bentler, P. M. (1998). Fit indices in covariance structure modeling: Sensitivity to underparameterized model misspecification. *Psychological Methods, 3*, 424–453.

Hu, S., & Lai, B. W. P. (2022). Increasing empathy for children in dental students using virtual reality. *International Journal of Paediatric Dentistry, 32*(6), 793–800. https://doi.org/10.1111/ipd.12957

Huang, L., Thai, J., Zhong, Y., Peng, H., Koran, J., & Zhao, X. D. (2019). The Positive Association Between Empathy and Self-Esteem in Chinese Medical Students: A Multi-Institutional Study. *Frontiers in Psychology, 10*, 1921. https://doi.org/10.3389/fpsyg.2019.01921

Hubel, D. H. (1967). Effect of distortion of sensory input on the visual system of kittens. *The Physiologist, 10*, 17–54.

Hubel, D. H., & Wiesel, T. N. (1963). Receptive fields of cell in striate cortex of young, visually inexperienced kittens. *Journal of Neurophysiology, 26*, 994–1002.
Hubel, D. H., & Wiesel, T. N. (1970). The period of susceptibility to the physiological effects of unilateral eye closure in kittens. *Journal of Physiology, 206*, 419–436.
Hudson, G. R. (1993). Empathy and technology in the coronary care unit. *Intensive and Critical Care Nursing, 9*, 55–61.
Humphrey, N. (1983). *Consciousness regained.* Oxford University Press.
Hunsdahl, J. B. (1967). Concerning Einfiühlung (empathy): A concept analysis of its origin and early development. *Journal of History of the Behavioral Sciences, 3*, 180–191.
Hunt, E., & Agnoli, F. (1991). The Whorfian hypothesis: A cognitive psychology perspective. *Psychological Review, 98*, 337–389.
Hurlemann, R., Patin, A., Onur, O. A., Cohen, M. X., Baumgartner, T., Metzler, S., Gallinat, J., Wagner, M., Maier, W., & Kendrick, K. M. (2010). Oxytocin enhances amygdala-dependent, socially reinforced learning ad emotional empathy in humans. *Journal of Neuroscience, 30*(14), 4999–5007. https://doi.org/10.1523/JNEUROSCI.5538-09.2010
Hurwitz, B. (2000). Narrative and the practice of medicine. *Lancet, 365*, 2086–2089.
Hyde, J. S. (1984). How large are gender differences in aggression? *Developmental Psychology, 20*, 722–736.
Hyde, J. S. (2005). The gender similarities hypothesis. *American Psychologist, 60*(*6*), 581–592. https://doi.org/10.1037/0003-066X.60.6.581
Hyyppa, M. T., Kronholm, E., & Mattlar, C. (1991). Mental well-being of good sleepers in a random sample population. *British Journal of Medical Psychology, 64*, 25–34.
Iacoboni, M. (2009a). Imitation, empathy, and mirror neurons. *Annual Review of Psychology, 60*, 653–670. https://doi.org/10.1146/annurev.psych.60.110707.163604
Iacoboni, M. (2009b). *Mirroring people: The science of empathy and how we connect with others*. Farrar, Straus & Giroux.
Iacoboni, M., Molnar-Szakacs, I., Gallese, V., Buccino, G., Mazziotta, J. C., & Rizzolatti, G. (2005). Grasping the intentions of others with one's own mirror neuron system. *PLoS Biology, 3*(3), e79. https://doi.org/10.1371/journal.pbio.0030079
Iacoboni, M., Woods, R. P., Brass, M., Bekkering, H., Mazziotta, J. C., & Rizzolatti, G. (1999). Cortical mechanisms of human imitation. *Science, 286*, 2526–2528.
Ickes, W. (1997). *Empathic accuracy*. Guilford Press.
Ickes, W., Gesn, P. R., & Graham, T. (2000). Gender differences in empathic accuracy: Differential ability of differential motivation? *Personal Relationships, 7*, 95–109. https://doi.org/10.1111/j.1475-6811.2000.tb00006.x
Igde, F. A., & Sahin, M. K. (2017). Changes in Empathy during Medical Education: An Example from Turkey. *Pakistan Journal of Medical Sciences, 33*(5), 1177–1181. https://doi.org/10.12669/pjms.335.13074
Ingelfinger, F. J. (1980). Arrogance. *The New England Journal of Medicine, 303*, 1507–1511.
Insel, T. R. (2000). Toward a neurology of attachment. *Review of General Psychology, 4*, 176–185.
Iqbal, M. Z., AlBuraikan, A. R., AlQarni, A. A., AlQahtani, H. A., AlOhail, A. M., & AlMusaileem, M. M. (2022). Measuring empathy in medical students: A cross-sectional study. *The Journal of the Pakistan Medical Association, 72*(6), 1101–1105. https://doi.org/10.47391/JPMA.3226
Isabella, R. A., & Belsky, J. (1991). Interaction synchrony and the origin of infant-mother attachment: A replication study. *Child Development, 62*, 373–384.
Ishikawa, H., Takayama, T., Yamazaki, Y., Skei, Y., & Katsumata, N. (2002). Physician-patient communication and patient satisfaction in Japanese cancer consultation. *Social Science & Medicine, 55*, 301–311.
Ivey, A. (1971). *Microcounseling: Innovations in interviewing training*. Charles C Thomas.
Ivey, A. E. (1974). Microcounseling and media therapy: State of the art. *Counselor Education and Supervision, 4*, 173–183.
Jack, D. C. (1993). *Silencing the self: Women and depression*. Harvard University Press.

Jackson, P. L., Brunet, E., Meltzoff, A. N., & Decety, J. (2006a). Empathy examined through the neural mechanisms involved in imagining how I feel versus how you feel pain. *Neuropsychologia, 44*, 754–761.

Jackson, P. L., & Decety, J. (2004). Motor cognition: A new paradigm to study self-other interactions. *Current Opinion in Neurobiology, 14*(2), 259–263. https://doi.org/10.1016/j.conb.2004.01.020

Jackson, P. L., Meltzoff, A. N., & Decety, J. (2005). How do we perceive the pain of others? A window into the neural process involved in empathy. *Neuroimage, 24*(3), 771–779. https://doi.org/10.1016/j.neuroimage.2004.09.006

Jackson, P. L., Rainville, P., & Decety, J. (2006b). To what extent do we share the pain of others? Insight from the neural bases of pain empathy. *Pain, 125*(*1-2*), 5–9. https://doi.org/10.1016/j.pain.2006.09.013

Jackson, S. W. (1992). The listening healer in the history of psychological healing. *American Journal of Psychiatry, 149*, 1623–1632.

Jackson, S. W. (2001). The wounded healer. *Bulletin of the History of Medicine, 75*, 1–36.

Jacoby, J. L., Smith, A. B., Barraco, R. D., Greenberg, M. R., Donoghue, E. A., Kane, B. G., Macfarlan, J. E., Crowley, L. M., Weaver, K. R., & Quinn, J. F. (2022). Do incoming residents vary in measures of emotional status even prior to residency training? *International Journal of Medical Education, 13*, 198–204. https://doi.org/10.5116/ijme.62cb.f308

Jaffe, D. S. (1986). Empathy, counteridentification, countertransference: A review with some personal perspectives on the "analytic instrument". *Psychoanalytic Quarterly, 15*, 215–243.

Jaffee, S., & Hyde, J. S. (2000). Gender differences in moral orientation: A meta-analysis. *Psychological Bulletin, 126*, 703–726.

James, W. (1890). *Principles of psychology*. Holt.

Jamison, R., & Johnson, J. E. (1975). Empathy and therapeutic orientation in paid and volunteer crisis phone workers, professional therapists, and undergraduate college students. *Journal of Community Psychology, 3*, 269–274.

Janssens, J. M. A. M., & Gerris, J. R. M. (1992). Child rearing, empathy and prosocial development. In J. M. A. M. Janssens & J. R. M. Gerris (Eds.), *Child rearing: Influence on prosocial development* (pp. 57–75). Swets & Zeitlinger.

Jarski, R. W., Gjerde, C. L., Bratton, B. D., Brown, D. D., & Matthes, S. S. (1985). A comparison of four empathy instruments in simulated patient-medical student interactions. *Journal of Medical Education, 60*, 545–551.

Jeffrey, D. (2016). Empathy, sympathy ans compassion in healthcare: Is there a problem? Is there a difference, Does it matter? *The Royal Society of Medicine, 109*(*12*), 446–452. https://doi.org/10.1177/0141076816680120

Jensen, N. (1994). The empathic physician. *Archives of Internal Medicine, 154*, 108.

Jessimer, M., & Markham, R. (1997). Alexithymia: A right hemisphere dysfunctional specific to recognition of certain facial expressions? *Brain and Cognition, 34*, 246–258.

Johnson, J. A., Cheek, J. M., & Smither, R. (1983). The structure of empathy. *Journal of Personality and Social Psychology, 45*, 1299–1312.

Johnston, M. A. C. (1992). A model program to address insensitive behaviors toward medical students. *Academic Medicine, 67*, 236–237.

Jones, A. H. (1987). Reflections, projections, and the future of literature-and-medicine. In D. Wear, M. Kohn, & S. Stocker (Eds.), *Literature and medicine: A claim for a discipline* (pp. 29–40). Society for Health and Human Values.

Jones, A. H. (1997). Literature and medicine: Narrative ethics. *Lancet, 349*, 1243–1246.

Joreskog, K. G. (1993). *Testing structural equation models*. In K. A. Bollen & J. S. Long (Eds.), *Testing structural equation models*. Sage.

Jose, P. E. (1989). The role of gender and gender role similarity in readers' identification with story characters. *Sex Roles, 21*, 697–713.

Juan, S. (2023). *The application of virtual simulation to promoting empathy in undergraduate nursing students.* (Publication No. 30420283). [Doctoral dissertation, Teachers College, Columbia University]. ProQuest Dissertations & Theses Global. DAI-A 84/11(E).

Jumroonrojana, K., & Zartrungpak, S. (2012). Development of the Jefferson Scale of Physician Empathy-student version (Thai version). *Journal of the Psychiatric Association of Thailand, 57*(2), 213–224. https://he01.tci-thaijo.org/index.php/JPAT/article/view/5229

Jung, C. G. (1964). *Man and his symbols*. Doubleday.

Kaiser, H. (1960). The application of electronic computer factor analysis. *Educational and Psychological Measurement, 20*, 141–151.

Kalisch, B. J. (1971). An experiment in the development of empathy in nursing students. *Nursing Research, 20*, 202–211.

Kalisch, B. J. (1973). What is empathy? *American Journal of Nursing, 73*, 1548–1552.

Kalliopuska, M. (1992a). Attitudes towards health, health behavior, and personality factors among school students very high on empathy. *Psychological Reports, 70*, 1119–1122.

Kalliopuska, M. (1992b). Self-esteem and narcissism among the most and least empathetic Finnish baseball players. *Perceptual & Motor Skills, 75*, 945–946.

Kalliopuska, M. (1994). Empathy related to living in towns versus the countryside. *Psychological Reports, 74*, 896–898.

Kandel, E. R. (1998). A new intellectual framework for psychiatry. *American Journal of Psychiatry, 155*, 457–469.

Kane, S. E. (2018). *The effects of a longitudinal patient experience on the enhancement of empathy in first and second year medical students.* (Publication No. 10809816). [Doctoral dissertation, City University of New York]. ProQuest Dissertations & Theses Global. DAI-A 79/10(E).

Kane, G. C., Gotto, J. L., Mangione, S., West, S., & Hojat, M. (2007). Jefferson Scale of Patient's Perceptions of Physician Empathy: Preliminary psychometric data. *Croatian Medicine Journal, 48*, 81–86.

Kanter, S. L. (2012). What are the most revealing interview questions? *Academic Medicine, 87*(4), 387–388. https://doi.org/10.1097/ACM.0b013e31824f619f

Kaplan, G. A., Salonem, J. T., & Cohen, R. D. (1988). Social connections and mortality from all causes and from cardiovascular disease: Prospective evidence from eastern Finland. *American Journal of Epidemiology, 128*, 370–380.

Kaplan, N. B., & Bloom, S. W. (1960). The use of sociological and social psychological concepts in physiological research. *Journal of Nervous and Mental Disease, 131*, 128–134.

Kaplan, R. M., Satterfield, J. M., & Kington, R. S. (2012). Building a better physician: The case for the new MCAT. *The New England Journal of Medicine, 366*(14), 1265–1268. https://doi.org/10.1056/NEJMp1113274

Kaplan, R. M., & Simon, H. J. (1990). Compliance in medical care: Reconsideration of self-predictions. *Annals of Behavioral Medicine, 12*, 66–71.

Karen, R. (1994). *Becoming attached.* Warner Books.

Karimi, F. Z., & Abdollahi, M. (2019). Factors Affecting Empathy with Patient among Healthcare Provider Students: A Structural Equation Modeling Study. *Indian Journal of Critical Care Medicine: Peer-Reviewed, Official Publication of Indian Society of Critical Care Medicine, 23*(9), 396–399. https://doi.org/10.5005/jp-journals-10071-23232

Karniol, R., Gabay, R., Ochion, Y., & Harari, Y. (1998). Is gender or gender-role orientation a better predictor of empathy in adolescence? *Sex Roles, 39*, 45–59.

Kassebaum, D. G., & Szenas, P. L. (1994). Factors influencing the specialty choice of 1993 medical school graduates. *Academic Medicine, 69*, 164–170.

Kassirer, J. P. (1998). Doctor discontent. *New England Journal of Medicine, 339*, 1543–1545.

Kataoka, H., Koide, N., Ochi, K., Hojat, M., & Gonnella, J. S. (2009). Measurement of empathy among Japanese medical students: Psychometrics and score differences by gender and level of medical education. *Academic Medicine, 84*(9), 1192–1197. https://doi.org/10.1097/ACM.0b013e3181b180d4

Kataoka, H. U., Koide, N., Hojat, M., & Gonnella, J. S. (2012). Measurement and correlates of empathy among female Japanese physicians. *BMC Medical Education, 12*, 48. https://doi.org/10.1186/1472-6920-12-48

Kataoka, H. U., Tokinobu, A., Fujii, C., Watanabe, M., & Obika, M. (2023). Eleven years of data on the Jefferson Scale of Empathy-Medical Student Version: Japanese norm data and tentative cutoff scores. *BMC Medical Education, 23*, 81. https://doi.org/10.1186/s12909-022-03977-5

Katz, J. (1984). *The silent world of doctor and patient*. Free Press.

Katz, R. L. (1963). *Empathy: Its nature and uses*. Free Press.

Kause, D. R., Robbins, A., Heidrich, R., Abrassi, I. B., & Anderson, L. A. (1980). The long-term effectiveness of interpersonal skills training in medical school. *Journal of Medical Education, 55*, 595–601.

Kay, J. (1990). Traumatic deidealization and the future of medicine. *Journal of the American Medical Association, 263*, 572–573.

Kazanowski, M., Perrin, K., Potter, M., & Sheehan, C. (2007). The silence of suffering: Breaking the sound barriers. *Journal of Holistic Nursing, 25(3)*, 195–203. https://doi.org/10.1177/0898010107305501

Kazmierczak, M., Rybicka, M., & Syty, P. (2024). Genetic variations as predictors of dispositional and dyadic empathy-a couple study. *Scientific Reports, 14*, 27411. https://doi.org/10.1038/s41598-024-78857-7

Keller, S., Shiflett, S. C., Schleifer, S. J., & Bartlett, J. A. (1994). *Human stress and immunity*. Academic Press.

Kelly, C. (2022). Improving empathy of occupational therapy students through reading literary narratives. *Journal of Occupational Therapy Education, 6*(4). https://doi.org/10.26681/jote.2022.060404

Kelly, C. P. (2021). *Empathic instruction through literary narratives: a quasi-experimental study of an occupational therapy course.* (Publication No. 28681265). [Doctoral dissertation, The University of Maine]. ProQuest Dissertations & Theses Global. DAI-A 83/3(E).

Kelman, H. C. (1958). Compliance, identification, and internalization: Three processes of attitude change. *Conflict Resolution, 2*, 51–60.

Kendall, P. C., & Wilcox, C. E. (1980). Cognitive behavioral treatment for impulsivity: Concrete versus conceptual training in non-self-controlled problem children. *Journal of Counseling and Clinical Psychology, 48*, 80–91.

Kennedy, S., Kiecolt-Glaser, J. K., & Glaser, R. (1988). Immunological consequences of acute and chronic stressors: Mediating role of interpersonal relationships. *British Journal of Medical Psychology, 61*, 77–85.

Kenny, D. T. (1995). Determinants of patient satisfaction with the medical consultation. *Psychology and Health, 10*, 427–437.

Kerr, N., & Tegge, A. M. (2017). Levels of empathy in undergraduate health-care-professions students. *International Journal of Human Caring, 21*(1), 41–45. https://doi.org/10.20467/1091-5710.21.1.41

Kerr, R. F., & Speroff, B. J. (1954). Validation and evaluation of the Empathy Test. *Journal of General Psychology, 50*, 269–276.

Kerr, W. A. (1947). *The empathy test: Form A*. Psychometric Affiliates.

Kestenbaum, R., Farber, E. A., & Sroufe, L. A. (1989). Individual differences in empathy among preschoolers: Relation to attachment history. In N. Eisenberg (Ed.), *Empathy and related emotional responses* (pp. 51–64). Jossey-Bass.

Ketterer, M. W., & Buckholtz, C. D. (1989). Somatization disorder. *Journal of the American Osteopathic Association, 89*, 489–490.

Keulen, M. H. F., Teunis, T., Kortlever, J. T. P., Vagner, G. A., Ring, D., & Reichel, L. M. (2020). Measurement of perceived physician empathy in orthopedic patients. *Journal of Patient Experience, 7*, 600–606. https://doi.org/10.1177/2374373519875842

Keverne, E. B., Nevison, C. M., & Martel, F. L. (1997). Early learning and social bond. *Annals of the New York Academy of Sciences, 807*, 329–339.

Keysers, C. (2011). *The empathic brain: How discovery of mirror neuron changes our understanding of human nature*. First published as a Kindle e-book, subsequently published by Social Brain Press in the U.S.

Keysers, C., Kohler, E., Umilta, M. A., Nanetti, L., Fogassi, L., & Gallese, V. (2003). Audiovisual mirror neurons and action recognition. *Experimental Brain Research, 153*, 628–636.

Keysers, C., & Perrett, D. I. (2004). Demystifying social cognition: A Hebbian perspective. *Trends in Cognitive Sciences, 8(11)*, 501–507. https://doi.org/10.1016/j.tics.2004.09.005

Keysers, C., Wicker, B., Gazzola, V., Anton, J. L., Fogassi, L., & Gallese, V. (2004). A touching sight: SII/VP activation during the observation and experience of touch. *Neuron, 42*, 335–346.

Khademalhosseini, M., Khademalhosseini, Z., & Mahmoodian, F. (2014). Comparison of empathy score among medical students in both basic and clinical levels. *Journal of Advances in Medical Education & Professionalism, 13*(2), 88–91.

Kiecolt-Glaser, J. K., Garner, W., Speicher, C. E., Penn, G. M., Holiday, J. E., & Glaser, R. (1984). Psychosocial modifiers of immunocompetence in medical students. *Psychosomatic Medicine, 46*, 7–14.

Kiersma, M. E., Chen, A. M. H., Yehle, K. S., & Plake, K. S. (2013). Validation of an empathy scale in pharmacy and nursing students. *American Journal of Pharmaceutical Education, 77*(5), 94. https://doi.org/10.5688/ajpe77594

Kim, S. S., Kaplowitz, S., & Johnston, M. V. (2004). The effects of physician empathy on patient satisfaction and compliance. *Evaluation and the Health Professions, 27*(3), 237–251. https://doi.org/10.1177/0163278704267037

Kimmelman, M., Giacobbe, J., Faden, J., Kumar, G., Pinckney, C. C., & Steer, R. (2012). Empathy in osteopathic medical students: A cross-sectional analysis. *Journal of the American Osteopathic Association, 112(6)*, 347–355. https://doi.org/10.7556/jaoa.2012.112.6.347

Kimura, D. (1999). Sex differences in the brain. *Scientific American,* May 13 issue.

King, S., & Holosko, M. J. (2012). The development and initial validation of the empathy scale for social workers. *Research on Social Work Practice, 22(2)*, 174–185. https://doi.org/10.1177/1049731511417136

Kinney, S. (2022). *The effects of abbreviated mindfulness-based interventions on empathy growth of prelicensure BSN students.* (Publication No. 28970879). [Doctoral dissertation, Capella University]. ProQuest Dissertations & Theses Global. DAI-A 83/9(E).

Kipper, D. A., & Ben-Ely, Z. (1979). The effectiveness of the psychodramatic double method, the reflection method, and lecturing in the training of empathy. *Journal of Clinical Psychology, 35*, 370–375.

Klaus, M., & Kennell, J. H. (1970). Mothers separated from their newborn infants. *Pediatric Clinics of North America, 17*, 1015–1037.

Klaus, M. H., Jerauld, R., Kreger, N. S., McAlpine, W., Steffa, M., & Kennell, J. H. (1972). Maternal attachment: Importance of the first post-partum days. *New England Journal of Medicine, 286*, 460–463.

Kleinman, A. (1988). *The illness narratives: Suffering, healing, and the human condition*. Basic Books.

Kleinman, A. (1995). *Writing at the margin: Discourse between anthropology and medicine*. University of California Press.

Kleinman, A., Eisenberg, L., & Good, B. (1978). Culture, illness, and care: Clinical lessons from anthropologic and cross-cultural research. *Annals of Internal Medicine, 88*, 251–258.

Klim, G. (2019). *Social empathy and associated factors among nurses: a mixed method study.* (Publication No. 13901527). [Doctoral dissertation, Loma Linda University]. ProQuest Dissertations & Theses Global. DAI-B 81/11(E).

Kline, R. B. (1998). *Principles and practice of structural equation modeling*. Guilford Press.

Kliszcz, J., Hebanowski, M., & Rembowski, J. (1998). Emotional and cognitive empathy in medical schools. *Academic Medicine, 73*, 541.

Kliszcz, J., Nowicka-Sauer, K., Trzeciak, B., Nowak, P., & Sadowska, A. (2006). Empathy in health care providers–validation study of the Polish version of the Jefferson Scale of Empathy.

Advances in Medical Sciences, 51, 219–225. http://www.advms.pl/ms_2006/Kliszcz_J_et%20al_Empathy%20in%20health%20care%20providers.pdf
Knafo, A., Zahn-Waxler, C., Van Hule, C., Robinson, J. L., & Rhee, S. H. (2008). The developmental origins of disposition toward empathy: Genetic and environmental contributions. *Emotion (Washington, D.C.), 8*(6), 737–752. https://doi.org/10.1037/a0014179
Knapp, B. L. (1984). *A Jungian approach to literature*. Southern Illinois University.
Knight, J. A. (1981). *Doctor-to-be: Coping with trials and triumphs of medical school*. Appleton-Century.
Koenig, H. G. (2002). *Spirituality in patient care*. Templeton Foundation Press.
Kohler, E., Keysers, C., Umilta, M. A., Fogassi, L., Gallese, V., & Rizzolatti, G. (2002). Hearing sounds, understanding actions: Action representation in mirror neurons. *Science, 297*, 846–848.
Kohn, L. T., Corrigan, J. M., & Donaldson, M. S. (2000). *To err is human: Building a safe health system*. National Academy Press.
Kohut, H. (1959). Introspection, empathy and psychoanalysis. *Journal of American Psychoanalysis, 7*, 459–483.
Kohut, H. (1971). *Analysis of the self: A systematic approach to the psychoanalytic treatment of narcissistic personality disorders*. International Universities Press.
Kohut, H. (1984). Introspection, empathy, and the semicircle of mental health. In J. Lichtenberg, M. Bornstein, & D. Silver (Eds.), *Empathy* (Vol. 1, pp. 81–100). Erlbaum.
Kolb, B., & Taylor, L. (1981). Affective behavior in patients with localized cortical excisions: Role of lesion site and side. *Science, 214*, 81–89.
Kolenikov, S., & Bollen, K. A. (2012). Testing negative error variances: Is a Heywood case a symptom of misspecification? *Sociological Methods & Research, 1*(1), 124–167. https://doi.org/10.1177/0049124112442138
Komor, T. L. (2024). *Does baseline empathy level of undergraduate nursing students affect empathic responses and change in empathy following participation in a simulation? A mixed method study.* (Publication No. 31243640). [Doctoral dissertation, State University of New York at Binghamton]. ProQuest Dissertations & Theses Global. DAI-A85/12(E).
Konner, M. (2004). The ties that bind [Comment]. *Nature, 429*, 705. https://doi.org/10.1038/429705a
Konrath, S. H., O'Brien, E. H., & Hsing, C. (2011). Changes in dispositional empathy in American college students over time: A meta-analysis. *Personality and Social Psychology Review: An Official Journal of the Society for Personality and Social Psychology, Inc, 15*(2), 180–198. https://doi.org/10.1177/1088868310377395
Korsch, B. M., Gozzi, E. K., & Francis, V. (1968). Gaps in doctor-patient interaction and patient satisfaction. *Pediatrics, 42*, 855–871. https://doi.org/10.1542/peds.42.5.855
Kosfeld, M., Heinrichs, M., Zak, P., Fischbacher, U., & Fehr, E. (2005). Oxytocin increases trust in humans. *Nature, 435*, 673–676. https://doi.org/10.1038/nature03701
Kožený, J., Tišanská, L., & Hoschl, C. (2013). Assessing empathy among Czech medical students: A cross-sectional study. *Československá Psychologie, 57*, 246–254.
Kramer, C. (1974). *Folk linguistics. Psychology Today, 8*, 82–85.
Kramer, D., Ber, R., & Moore, M. (1987). Impact of workshop on students' and physicians' rejecting behaviors in patient interviews. *Journal of Medical Education, 62*, 904–910.
Kramer, D., Ber, R., & Moore, M. (1989). Increasing empathy among medical students. *Medical Education, 23*, 168–173.
Krasner, M. S., Epstein, R. M., Beckman, H., Suchman, A. L., Chapman, B., Mooney, C. J., & Quill, T. E. (2009). Association of an educational program in mindful communication with burnout, empathy, and attitudes among primary care physicians. *Journal of the American Medical Association, 302*(12), 1284–1293. https://doi.org/10.1001/jama.2009.1384
Krebs, D. (1975). Empathy and altruism. *Journal of Personality and Social Psychology, 32*, 1134–1146.
Kremer, J. F., & Dietzen, L. L. (1991). Two approaches to teaching accurate empathy to undergraduates: Teacher-intensive and self-directed. *Journal of College Student Development, 32*, 69–75.

Krevans, J., & Gibbs, J. C. (1996). Parents' use of inductive discipline: Relations to children's empathy and prosocial behavior. *Child Development, 67*, 3263–3277.

Kring, A. M., & Gordon, A. L. (1998). Sex differences in emotion. *Journal of Personality and Social Psychology, 74*, 686–703.

Krishna Bahadur, G. C., Arjyal, A., Douglas, A. H., Subedi, M., & Gongal, R. (2022). A quantitative evaluation of empathy using JSE-S Tool, before and after a Medical Humanities Module, amongst first-year medical students in Nepal. *BMC Medical Education, 22*(1), 159. https://doi.org/10.1186/s12909-022-03188-y

Kristensen, T., Ejersted, C., Ahnfeldt-Mollerup, P., Søndergaard, J., & Charles, J. A. (2022). Profiles of GPs with high and low self-reported physician empathy-personal, professional, and antibiotic prescribing characteristics. *BMC Primary Care, 23*(1), 243. https://doi.org/10.1186/s12875-022-01847-z

Kugiumutzakis, G. (1998). Neonatal imitation in the intersubjective companion space. In S. Braten (Ed.), *Intersubjective communication and emotion in early ontogeny* (pp. 63–88). Cambridge University Press.

Kumagai, A. K. (2008). A conceptual framework for the use of illness narratives in medical education. *Academic Medicine, 83*(7), 653–658. https://doi.org/10.1097/ACM.0b013e3181782e17

Kunyk, D., & Olson, J. K. (2001). Clarification of conceptualizations of empathy. *Journal of Advanced Nursing, 35*, 317–325.

Kupfer, D. J., Drew, F. L., Curtis, E. K., & Rubinstein, D. N. (1978). Personality style and empathy in medical students. *Journal of Medical Education, 53*, 507–509.

Kurtines, W., & Hogan, R. (1972). Sources of conformity in unspecialized college students. *Journal of Abnormal Psychology, 80*, 49–51.

Kurtz, R. R., & Grummon, D. L. (1972). Different approaches to the measurement of therapist empathy and their relationship to therapy outcomes. *Journal of Consulting and Clinical Psychology, 39*, 106–115.

La France, M. (1979). Nonverbal synchrony and rapport: Analysis by the cross-lag panel technique. *Social Psychology Quarterly, 42*, 66–70.

La France, M. (1982). Posturre mirroring and rapport. In M. Davis (Ed.), *Interaction rhythms: Periodicity in communication behavior* (pp. 279–298). Human Sciences Press.

LaFrance, M., Hecht, M. A., & Paluck, E. L. (2003). The contingent smile: A meta-analysis of sex differences in smiling. *Psychological Bulletin, 129*, 305–334.

Lakin, J. L., Jefferis, V. E., Cheng, C. M., & Chartland, T. L. (2003). The chameleon effect as social glue: Evidence for the evolutionary significance of nonconscious mimicry. *Journal of Nonverbal Behavior, 27*, 145–162.

Lal, A., Tharyan, A., & Tharyan, P. (2020). The prevalence, determinants and the role of empathy and religious or spiritual beliefs on job stress, job satisfaction, coping, burnout, and mental health in medical and surgical faculty of a teaching hospital: A cross-sectional survey. *La Revue de Medecine Interne, 41*(4), 232–240. https://doi.org/10.1016/j.revmed.2019.12.005

Lamm, C., Batson, D., & Decety, J. (2007). The neural substrate of human empathy: Effects of perspective-taking and cognitive appraisal. *Journal of Cognitive Neuroscience, 19*(1), 42–58. https://doi.org/10.1162/jocn.2007.19.1.42

LaMonica, E. L. (1981). Construct validity of an empathy instrument. *Research in Nursing & Health, 4*, 389–400.

LaMonica, E. L., Carew, D. K., Winder, A. E., Haase, A. M., & Blanchard, K. H. (1976). Empathy training as the major thrust of a staff development program. *Nursing Research, 25*, 447–451.

Lamont, L. M., & Lundstrom, W. J. (1977). Identifying successful industrial salesmen by personality and personal characteristics. *Journal of Marketing Research, 14*, 517–529.

Lamothe, M., Boujut, E., Zenasni, F., & Sultan, S. (2014). To be or not to be empathic: The combined role of empathic concern and perspective taking in understanding burnout in general practice. *BMC Family Practice, 15*, 15. https://doi.org/10.1186/1471-2296-15-15

Lancaster, T., Hart, R., & Gardner, S. (2002). Literature and medicine: Evaluating a special study module using the nominal group technique. *Medical Education, 36*, 1071–1076.

Lane, F. E. (1986). Utilizing physician empathy with violent patients. *American Journal of Psychotherapy, 40*, 448–456.

Lanzetta, J. T., & Englis, B. G. (1989). Expectation of cooperation and competition and their effects on observers' vicarious emotional response. *Journal of Personality and Social Psychology, 56*, 543–554.

Lanzetta, J. T., & Kleck, R. E. (1970). Encoding and decoding nonverbal affect in humans. *Journal of Personality and Social Psychology, 16*, 12–19.

LaRocco, J. M., House, J. S., & French, J. R. P. (1980). Social support, occupational stress, and health. *Journal of Health and Social Behavior, 21*, 202–218.

Larson, D. (1993). *The helper's journey: Working with people facing grief, loss, and life-threatening illness*. Research Press.

Larson, E. B., & Yao, X. (2005). Clinical empathy as emotional labor in the patient-physician relationship. *Journal of the American Medical Association, 293*(9), 1100–1106. https://doi.org/10.1001/jama.293.9.1100

Laskowski, C., & Pellicore, K. (2002). The wounded healer archetype: Applications to palliative care practice. *American Journal of Hospice & Palliative Care, 19*, 403–407.

Lawrence, E. J., Shaw, P., Baker, D., Baron-Cohen, S., & David, A. S. (2004). Measuring empathy: Reliability and validity of the Empathy Quotient. *Psychological Medicine, 34*(5), 911–919. https://doi.org/10.1017/s0033291703001624

Layton, J. M. (1979). The use of modeling to teach empathy to nursing students. *Research in Nursing & Health, 2*, 163–176.

Layton, J. M., & Wykle, M. H. (1990). A validity study of four empathy instruments. *Research in Nursing & Health, 13*, 319–325.

Lazarus, R. S. (1982). Thoughts on the relations between emotion and cognition. *American Psychologist, 37*, 1019–1024.

Lee, B. K., Bahn, G. H., Lee, W. H., Park, J. H., Yoon, T. Y., & Baek, S. B. (2009). The relationship between empathy and medical education system, grades, and personality in medical college students and medical school students. *Korean Journal of Medical Education, 21*(2), 117–124. https://doi.org/10.3946/kjme.2009.21.2.117

Leiper, R., & Casares, P. (2000). An investigation of the attachment organization of clinical psychologists and its relationship to clinical practice. *British Journal of Medical Psychology, 73*, 449–464.

Lelorain, S., Brédart, A., Dolbeault, S., Cano, A., Bonnaud-Antignac, A., Cousson-Gélie, F., & Sultan, S. (2014). How can we explain physician accuracy in assessing patient distress? A multilevel analysis in patients with advanced cancer. *Patient Education and Counseling, 94*(3), 322–327. https://doi.org/10.1016/j.pec.2013.10.029

Lelorain, S., Brédart, A., Dolbeault, S., Cano, A., Bonnaud-Antignac, A., Cousson-Gélie, F., & Sultan, S. (2015). How does a physician's accurate understanding of a cancer patient's unmet needs contribute to patient perception of physician empathy? *Patient Education and Counseling, 98*(6), 734–741. https://doi.org/10.1016/j.pec.2015.03.002

Lelorain, S., Bredart, A., Dolbeault, S., & Sultan, S. (2012). A systematic review of the associations between empathy measures and patient outcomes in cancer care. *Psycho-Oncology, 21*, 1255–1264. https://doi.org/10.1002/pon.2115

Lelorain, S., Sultan, S., Zenasni, F., Catu-Pinault, A., Juar, P., Boujut, E., & Rigal, L. (2013). Empathic concern and professional characteristics associated with clinical empathy in French general practitioners. *European Journal of General Practice, 19*(1), 23–28. https://doi.org/10.3109/13814788.2012.709842

Lemogne, C., Buffel du Vaure, C., Hoertel, N., Catu-Pinault, A., Limosin, F., Ghasarossian, C., Le Jeunne, C., & Jaury, P. (2020). Balint groups and narrative medicine compared to a control condition in promoting students' empathy. *BMC Medical Education, 20*(1), 412. https://doi.org/10.1186/s12909-020-02316-w

Leombruni, P., Di Lillo, M., Miniotti, M., Picardi, A., Alessandri, G., Sica, C., Zizzi, F., Castelli, L., & Torta, R. (2014). Measurement properties and confirmatory factor analysis of the

Jefferson Scale of Empathy in Italian medical students. *Perspectives on Medical Education.*, *3*(6), 419–430. https://doi.org/10.1007/s40037-014-0137-9
Lerner, A. (1978). *Poetry in the therapeutic experience*. Pergamon Press.
Lerner, A. (2001). Poetry therapy. In R. J. Corsini (Ed.), *Handbook of innovative therapies* (pp. 472–479). John Wiley & Sons.
Lerner, M. J., & Meindl, J. R. (1981). Justice and altruism. In J. P. Rushton & J. R. Sorrentino (Eds.), *Altruism and helping behavior: Social, personality, and developmental perspectives* (pp. 213–232). Erlbaum.
Letourneau, C. (1981). Empathy and stress: How they affect parental aggression. *Social Work, 26*, 383–389.
Levasseur, J., & Vance, A. R. (1993). Doctors, nurses, and empathy. In H. M. Spiro, M. G. Mccrea Curnen, E. Peschel, & D. S. James (Eds.), *Empathy and practice of medicine* (pp. 76–84). Yale University Press.
Levenson, R. W., & Ruef, A. M. (1992). Empathy, a physiological substrate. *Journal of Personality and Social Psychology, 63*, 234–246.
Levine, L. E., & Hoffman, M. L. (1975). Empathy and cooperation in 4-year olds. *Developmental Psychology, 4*, 533–534.
Levinson, W. (1994). Physician-patient communication: A key to malpractice prevention. *Journal of the American Medical Association, 272*, 1619–1620.
Levinson, W., Gorawara-Bhat, R., & Lamb, J. (2000). A study of patient clues and physician responses in primary care and surgical settings. *Journal of the American Medical Association, 284*, 1021–1027.
Levinson, W., Roter, D., Mullooly, J. P., Dull, V. T., & Frankel, R. (1997). Physician-patient communication: The relationship with malpractice claims among primary care physicians and surgeons. *Journal of the American Medical Association, 277*, 553–559.
Levy, D. (Ed.). (1999). *Medical milestones from the National Heart, Lung, and Blood Institute's Framingham Heart Study*. Center for Bio-Medical Communication.
Levy, J. (1997). A note on empathy. *New Ideas in Psychology, 15*, 179–184.
Lewin, K. (1936). *A dynamic theory of personality*. McGraw-Hill.
Lewinsohn, R. (1998). Medical theories, science, and the practice of medicine. *Social Science & Medicine, 46*, 1261–1270.
Lewis, J. M. (1998). For better or worse: Interpersonal relationships and individual outcome. *American Journal of Psychiatry, 155*, 582–589.
Lewis, T., Amini, F., & Lannon, R. (2000). *A general theory of love*. Vintage Books.
Li, C. Q., Ma, Q., Liu, Y. Y., & Jing, K. J. (2018a). Are parental rearing patterns and learning burnout correlated with empathy amongst undergraduate nursing students? *International Journal of Nursing Sciences, 5*(4), 409–413. https://doi.org/10.1016/j.ijnss.2018.07.005
Li, D., Xu, H., Kang, M., & Ma, S. (2018b). Empathy in Chinese eight-year medical program students: differences by school year, educational stage, and future career preference. *BMC Medical Education, 18*(1), 241. https://doi.org/10.1186/s12909-018-1348-2
Li, L., Wang, J., Hu, X., & Xu, C. (2015). Empathy in Chinese pharmacy undergraduates: Implication for integrating humanities into professional pharmacy education. *Indian Journal of Pharmaceutical Education and Research, 49(1)*, 31–39. https://doi.org/10.5530/ijper.49.1.5. https://archives.ijper.org/article/208
Liang, A., Gao, C., Xu, W., Shen, Y., Liu, C., Lu, Z., & Yang, Y. (2022). Individual factors in dignified care: A cross-sectional study of critical care nurses. *Journal of Nursing Management, 30*(7), 3286–3294. https://doi.org/10.1111/jonm.13765
Libert, Y., Canivet, D., Ménard, C., Van Achte, L., Farvacques, C., Merckaert, I., Liénard, A., Klastersky, J., Reynaert, C., Slachmuylder, J. L., Durieux, J. F., Delvaux, N., & Razavi, D. (2017). Predictors of physicians' communication performance in a decision-making encounter with a simulated advanced-stage cancer patient: A longitudinal study. *Patient Education and Counseling, 100*(9), 1672–1679. https://doi.org/10.1016/j.pec.2017.02.025

Licciardone, J. C., Tran, Y., Ngo, K., Toledo, D., Peddireddy, N., & Aryal, S. (2024). Physician empathy and chronic pain outcomes. *JAMA Network, 7*(4), e246026. https://doi.org/10.1001/jamanetworkopen.2024.6026

Lichtenstein, P., Holm, N. V., Verkasalo, P. K., Iliadou, A., Kaprio, J., Koskenvuo, M., Pukkala, E., Skytthe, A., & Hemminki, K. (2000). Environmental and heritable factors in the causation of cancer: Analyses of cohort twins from Sweden, Denmark, and Finland. *New England Journal of Medicine, 343*, 78–85.

Lieberman, M. D. (2007). Social cognitive neuroscience: A review of core processes. *Annual Review of Psychology, 58*, 259–289. https://doi.org/10.1146/annurev.psych.58.110405.085654

Lief, H. I., & Fox, R. C. (1963). Training for "detached concerns" in medical students. In H. I. Lief, V. F. Lief, & N. R. Lief (Eds.), *The psychological basis of medical practice* (pp. 12–35). Harper & Row.

Lief, H. I., Lief, V. F., & Lief, N. R. (Eds.). (1963). *The psychological basis of medical practice*. Harper & Row.

Lieu, T. A., Schroeder, S. A., & Altman, D. F. (1989). Specialty choice at one medical school: Recent trends and analysis of predictive factors. *Academic Medicine, 64*, 622–629.

Likert, R. (1932). A technique for the measurement of attitudes. *Archives of Psychology, 140*, 5–35.

Lilienfeld, R. (1978). *The rise of systems theory: An ideological analysis*. John Wiley & Sons.

Lim, B. T., Moriarty, H., & Huthwaite, M. (2011). "Being-in-role": A teaching innovation to enhance empathy communication skills in medical students. *Medical Teacher, 33*(12), e663–e669. https://doi.org/10.3109/0142159X.2011.611193

Lim, B. T., Moriarty, H., Huthwaite, M., Gray, L., Pullon, S., & Gallagher, P. (2013). How well do medical students rate and communicate clinical empathy? *Medical Teacher, 35*(2), e946–e951. https://doi.org/10.3109/0142159X.2012.715783

Lima, F. F., & Osorio, F. D. L. (2021). Empathy: Assessment instruments and psychometric quality- a systematic literature review with a meta-analysis of the past ten years. *Frontiers in Psychology, 12*, 781346. https://doi.org/10.3389/psyg.2021.781346

Lin, C., Li, L., Wan, D., Wu, Z., & Yan, Z. (2012). Empathy and avoidance in treating patients living with HIV/AIDS (PLWHA) among service providers in China. *AIDS Care, 24*(11), 1341–1348. https://doi.org/10.1080/09540121.2011.648602

Lin, I. H., Wang, C. Y., Lin, Y. N., Chen, H. C., & Lin, L. F. (2022). Simulation-based holistic education in physiotherapy interns to increase empathy toward older adults and individuals with disabilities. *BMC Geriatrics, 22*(1), 795. https://doi.org/10.1186/s12877-022-03500-x

Linley, P. A., & Joseph, S. (2007). Therapy work and therapists' positive and negative well-being. *Journal of Social and Clinical Psychology, 26*(3), 385–403. https://doi.org/10.1521/jscp.2007.26.3.385

Linn, L. S. (1974). Care vs. cure: How the nurse practitioner views the patient. *Nursing Outlook, 22*, 641–644.

Linn, L. S. (1975). A survey of the "care-cure" attitudes of physicians, nurses, and their students. *Nursing Forum, 14*, 145–161.

Linn, L. S., Cope, D. W., & Leake, B. (1984). The effect of gender and training of residents on satisfaction ratings by patients. *Journal of Medical Education, 59*, 964–966.

Linn, L. S., DiMatteo, M. R., Cope, D. W., & Robbins, A. (1987). Measuring physicians' humanistic attitudes, values, and behaviors. *Medical Care, 25*, 504–515.

Linn, L. S., Yager, J., Cope, D., & Leake, B. (1985). Health status, job satisfaction, job stress, and life satisfaction among academic and clinical faculty. *Journal of the American Medical Association, 254*, 2775–2782.

Lipner, R. S., Blank, L. L., Leas, B. F., & Fortna, G. S. (2002). The value of patient and peer ratings in recertification. *Academic Medicine, 77*, S64–S66.

Litvack-Miller, W., McDougall, D., & Romney, D. M. (1997). The structure of empathy during middle childhood and its relationship to prosocial behavior. *Genetic, Social, and General Psychology Monographs, 123*, 303–324.

Liu, Q., Tao, J., Gao, L., He, X., Wang, Y., Xia, W., & Huang, L. (2021). Attitudes of Front-Line Nurses Toward Hospice Care During the COVID-19 Pandemic. *The American Journal of Hospice & Palliative Care, 38*(2), 204–210. https://doi.org/10.1177/1049909120968533

Lockett, J. M. (2021). *The effect of empathy training on associate degree nursing students' empathy.* (Publication No. 28316507). [Doctoral dissertation, Capella University]. ProQuest Dissertations & Theses Global. DAI-A 82/8(E).

Logan, A., Yule, E., Hughes, J., Peters, D., Hadley, M., Betts, B., Jones, L., & Froude, E. (2022). The impact of face-to-face mental health consumer-led teaching on occupational therapy student empathy levels: Two group comparison design. *Australian Occupational Therapy Journal, 69*(6), 703–713. https://doi.org/10.1111/1440-1630.12833

Loggia, M. L., Mogil, J. S., & Bushnell, C. M. (2008). Empathy hurts: Compassion for another increases both sensory and affective components of pain perception. *Pain, 136*, 68–176.

Lombardi, M. J. (2016). *Fostering humanism in medicine: a mixed methods study on the influence of humanism in medicine workshops on medical student empathy.* (Publication No. 10132967). [Doctoral dissertation, Rowan University]. ProQuest Dissertations & Theses Global. DAI-A 81/1(E).

Lone, M. M., Adnan, S., Habib, M. E., Lone, M. H., Sajjad, I., Ishtiaq, M., & Abidi, S. Y. A. (2024). Empathy unmasked: The compassion quotient of dental students. *BMC Medical Education, 24*, 1106. https://doi.org/10.1186/s12909-024-06093-8

Lopez, G. E., Gurin, P., & Nagda, B. A. (1998). Education and understanding structural causes for group inequalities. *Political Psychology, 19*, 305–329.

Lott, D. A. (1998). Brain development, attachment and impact on psychic vulnerability. *Psychiatric Times, 15*(*5*) https://www.psychiatrictimes.com/view/brain-development-attachment-and-impact-psychic-vulnerability

Lounsburg, M. L., & Bates, J. E. (1982). The cries of infants of differing levels of perceived temperamental difficultness: Acoustic properties and effects on listeners. *Child Development, 53*, 677–686.

Lu, M. C. (1995). Why it was hard for me to learn compassion as a third-year medical student. *Cambridge Quarterly of Healthcare Ethics, 4*, 454–458.

Luborsky, L., Chandler, M., Auerbach, A. H., Cohen, J., & Bacharach, H. M. (1971). Factors influencing the outcome of psychotherapy: A review of quantitative research. *Psychological Bulletin, 75*, 145–185.

Ludmerer, K. M. (1999). *Time to heal. American medical education from the turn of the century to the era of managed care*. Oxford University Press.

Luscher, T. F., & Vetter, W. (1990). Adherence to medication. *Journal of Human Hypertension, 4*(Suppl. 1), 43–46.

Lutchmaya, S., Baron-Cohen, S., & Raggatt, P. (2002). Foetal testosterone and vocabulary size in 18 and 24-month old infants. *Infant Behavior & Development, 24*, 418–424.

Lwow, M., Canetti, L., & Muszkat, M. (2020). Gender differences in the effect of medical humanities program on medical students' empathy: a prospective longitudinal study. *BMC Medical Education, 20*(1), 413. https://doi.org/10.1186/s12909-020-02333-9

Lynch, J. J. (1977). *The broken heart: The consequences of loneliness*. Basic books.

Maccoby, E. E., & Jacklin, C. N. (1974). *The psychology of sex differences*. Stanford University Press.

MacKay, R., Hughes, J. R., & Carver, E. J. (Eds.). (1990). *Empathy in the helping relationship*. Springer.

MacLean, H., Braschi, E., Archibald, D., Sanchez-Campos, M., Jebanesan, D., Koszycki, D., & Gonsalves, C. (2020). A pilot study of a longitudinal mindfulness curriculum in undergraduate medical education. *Canadian Medical Education Journal, 11*(4), e5–e18. https://doi.org/10.36834/cmej.56726

MacLean, P. D. (1967). The brain in relation to empathy and medical education. *Journal of Nervous and Mental Disease, 144*, 374–382.

MacLean, P. D. (1990). *The triune brain evolution*. Plenum Press.

Macmillan, M. B. (2000). Restoring Phineas Gage: A 150th retrospective. *Journal of History of Neurosciences, 9*, 42–62.

MacPherson, H., Mercer, S. W., Scullion, T., & Thomas, K. J. (2003). Empathy, enablement, and outcome: An exploratory study on acupuncture patient's perceptions. *Journal of Alternative & Complementary Medicine, 9*, 869–876.

Magalhäes, E., Costa, P., & Costa, M. (2012). Empathy of medical students and personality: Evidence from the Five-Factor Model. *Medical Teacher, 34*, 807–812.

Magalhäes, E., Salgueira, A. P., Costa, P., & Costa, M. J. (2011). Empathy in senior year and first year medical students: A cross-sectional study. *BMC Medical Education, 11*, 52. https://doi.org/10.1186/1472-6920-11-52

Magee, M., & Hojat, M. (1998). Personality profiles of male and female positive role models in medicine. *Psychological Reports, 82*, 547–559.

Magee, M., & Hojat, M. (2001). Impact of health care system on physicians' discontent. *Journal of Community Health, 26*, 357–365.

Magee, M., & Hojat, M. (2010). Rocking chair and empathy: A pilot study. *Family Medicine, 42*(7), 467.

Maheux, B., & Beland, F. (1989). Students' perceptions of values emphasized in three medical schools. *Journal of Medical Education, 61*, 308–316.

Maheux, B., Beaudoin, C., Berkson, L. C. L., Des Marchais, J., & Jean, P. (2000). Medical faculty as humanistic physicians and teachers: The perceptions of students at innovative and traditional medical schools. *Medical Education, 34*, 630–634.

Maheux, B., Duford, F., Beland, F., Jacques, A., & Levesque, A. (1990). Female medical practitioners: More preventive and patient oriented? *Medical Care, 28*, 87–92.

Main, M., & Solomon, J. (1990). Procedures for identifying infants as disorganized/disoriented during the Ainsworth strange situation. In M. Greenberg, D. Cicchetti, & E. M. Cummings (Eds.), *Attachment in the preschool years: Theory, research and intervention* (pp. 121–160). University of Chicago Press.

Makoul, G. (1998). Perpetuating passivity: Reliance and reciprocal determinism in physician-patient interaction. *Journal of Health Communication, 3*, 233–259.

Makoul, G. (2001). Essential elements of communication in medical encounters: The Kalamazoo consensus statement. *Academic Medicine, 76*, 390–393.

Makoul, G., & Strauss, A. (2003). Building therapeutic relationships during patient visits. *Journal of General Internal Medicine, 18*(Suppl. 1), 275.

Malno, R. B., Boag, T. J., & Smith, A. A. (1957). Physiological study of personal interaction. *Psychosomatic Medicine, 19*, 105–119.

Mandel, E. D., & Schweinle, W. E. (2012). A study of empathy decline in physician assistant students at completion of first didactic year. *The Journal of Physician Assistant Education, 23*(4), 16–24. https://doi.org/10.1097/01367895-201223040-00005

Mandell, H., & Spiro, H. (1987). *When doctors get sick*. Plenum.

Mangione, S., Chakraborti, C., Staltari, G., Harrison, R., Tunkel, A. R., Liou, K. T., Cerceo, E., Voeller, M., Bedwell, W. L., Fletcher, K., & Kahn, M. J. (2018). Medical Students' Exposure to the Humanities Correlates with Positive Personal Qualities and Reduced Burnout: A Multi-Institutional U.S. Survey. *Journal of general internal medicine, 33*(5), 628–634. https://doi.org/10.1007/s11606-017-4275-8

Mangione, S., Kane, G. C., Caruso, J. W., Gonnella, J. S., Nasca, T. J., & Hojat, M. (2002). Assessment of empathy in different years of internal medicine training. *Medical Teacher, 24*, 370–373.

Mann, L., Wise, T. N., Trinidad, A., & Kohanski, R. (1994). Alexithymia, affect recognition, and the five-factor model of personality in normal subjects. *Psychological Reports, 74*, 563–567.

Manning, R., Levine, M., & Collins, A. (2007). The Kitty Genovese murder and social psychology of helping: The parable of the 38 witnesses. *American Psychologist, 62*, 555–562.

Mansen, T. J. (1993). Role-taking abilities of nursing education administrators and their perceived leadership effectiveness. *Journal of Professional Nursing, 9*, 347–357.

Marcus, E. R. (1999). Empathy, humanism, and the professionalization process of medical education. *Academic Medicine, 74*, 1211–1215.

Markham, B. (1979). Can a behavioral science course change medical students' attitudes? *Journal of Psychiatric Education, 3*, 44–54.

Markham, F., & Kass, B. S. (2023). The importance of physician empathy in clinical outcomes needs more study. *International Journal of Community Medicine & Public Health., 3*(2), 106.

Markus, H. R., & Kitayama, S. (1991). Culture and the self: Implications for cognition, emotion, and motivation. *Psychological Review, 98*, 224–253.

Marmot, M. G., & Syme, S. L. (1976). Acculturation and coronary heart disease in Japanese-Americans. *American Journal of Epidemiology, 104*, 225–247.

Marsh, A. A. (2012). Empathy and compassion: A cognitive neuroscience. In J. Decety (Ed.), *From bench to bedside* (pp. 191–205). MIT Press.

Marshall, W. L., & Maric, A. (1996). Cognitive and emotional components of generalized empathy deficits in child molesters. *Journal of Child Sexual Abuse, 5*, 101–111.

Marshall, P. A., & O'Keefe, J. P. (1994). Medical students' first person narrative of a patient's story of AIDS. *Social Science & Medicine, 40*, 67–76.

Marte, A. L. (1988). How does it feel to be old? Simulation game provides "into aging" experience. *Journal of Continuing Education in Nursing, 19*, 166–168. https://doi.org/10.3928/0022-0124-19880701-06

Martin, R. (2007). *The psychology of humor: An integrative approach*. Elsevier Academic Press.

Martin, G. B., & Clark, R. D. (1982). Distress crying in neonates: Species and peer specificity. *Developmental Psychology, 18*, 3–9.

Martin, R. A., & Lefcourt, H. M. (1983). Sense of humor as a moderator of the relation between stress and mood. *Journal of Personality and Social Psychology, 45*, 1313–1324.

Marx, B. P., Heidt, J. M., & Gold, S. D. (2005). Perceived uncontrollability and unpredictability, self-regulation, and sexual revictimization. *Review of General Psychology, 9(1)*, 67–90. https://doi.org/10.1037/1089-2680.9.1.67

Maslach, C. (1993). Burnout: A multidimensional perspective. In W. B. Schaufeli, C. Maslach, & F. T. Marek (Eds.), *Professional burnout: Recent developments in theory and research*. Taylor & Francis.

Mathad, M. D., Pradhan, B., & Sasidharan, R. K. (2017). Effect of Yoga on Psychological Functioning of Nursing Students: A Randomized Wait List Control Trial. *Journal of Clinical and Diagnostic Research, 11*(5), KC01–KC05. https://doi.org/10.7860/JCDR/2017/26517.9833

Matravers, D. (2014). Empathy as a route to knowledge. In A. Coplan & P. Goldie (Eds.), *Empathy: Philosophical and psychological perspectives* (pp. 19–30). Oxford University Press.

Matthews, D. A., & Feinstein, A. R. (1989). A new instrument for patients' rating of physician performance in the hospital setting. *Journal of General Internal Medicine, 4*, 14–22.

Matthews, D. A., Suchman, A. L., & Branch, W. T. (1993). Making "connexions": Enhancing the therapeutic potential of patient-clinician relationships. *Annals of Internal Medicine, 118*, 973–977.

Matthews, K. A., Batson, C. D., Horn, J., & Rosenman, R. H. (1981). Principles in his nature which interest him in the fortune of others: The heritability of empathic concern for others. *Journal of Personality, 49*, 237–247.

Maurer, R. E., & Tindall, J. H. (1983). Effect of postural congruence on client's perception of counselor empathy. *Journal of Counseling Psychology, 30*, 158–163.

Mayerson, E. W. (1976). *Putting the ill at ease*. Harper & Row.

Mays, L. C., Carter, A. S., Eggar, H. L., & Pajer, K. A. (1991). Reflection on stillness: Mother's reaction to the still-face situation. *Journal of Academy of Child and Adolescent Psychiatry, 30*, 22–28.

McClintock, M. K. (1971). Menstrual synchrony and suppression. *Nature, 229*, 244–245.

McEwen, B. S. (1998). Protective and damaging effects of stress mediators. *New England Journal of Medicine, 338*, 171–179.

McKellar, P. (1957). *Imagining and thinking: A psychological analysis*. Basic Books.

McKenna, L., Boyle, M., Brown, T., Williams, B., Molloy, A., Lewis, B., & Molloy, L. (2011). Levels of empathy in undergraduate midwifery students: An Australian cross-sectional study. *Women and Birth: Journal of the Australian College of Midwives, 24*(2), 80–84. https://doi.org/10.1016/j.wombi.2011.02.003

McKenna, L., Boyle, M., Brown, T., Williams, B., Molloy, A., Lewis, B., & Molloy, L. (2012). Levels of empathy in undergraduate nursing students. *International Journal of Nursing Practice, 18*, 246–251. https://doi.org/10.1111/j.1440-172X.2012.02035.x

McKinlay, J. B., & McKinlay, S. M. (1981). Medical measures and the decline of mortality. In P. Conrad & R. Kern (Eds.), *The sociology of health and illness: Critical perspectives* (pp. 12–30). St. Martin's Press.

McKnight-Chelius, R. (2017). *The relationships among emergency nurses' perceptions of nurse empathy, compassion fatigue, compassion satisfaction, and emergency patients' perception of nurse empathy.* Publication No. 10282345). [Doctoral dissertation, Widener University]. ProQuest Dissertations & Theses Global. DAI-B 78/10(E).

Mclean, M. (2004). The choice of role models by students at a culturally diverse South African medical school. *Medical Teacher, 26*, 133–141.

McLellan, J. D., Jansen-McWilliams, L., Comer, D. M., Gardner, W. P., & Kelleher, K. J. (1999). The Physician Belief Scale and psychosocial problems in children: A report from the pediatric research in office settings and the ambulatory sentinel practice network. *Journal of Developmental & Behavioral Pediatrics, 20*, 24–30.

McLellan, M. F., & Husdon Jones, A. (1996). Why literature and medicine? *Lancet, 348*, 109–111.

McManus, I. C. (1995). Humanity and the medical humanities. *Lancet, 346*, 1143–1145.

McManus, S., Killeen, D., Hartnett, Y., Fitzgerald, G., & Murphy, K. C. (2020). Establishing and evaluating a Balint group for fourth-year medical students at an Irish University. *Irish Journal of Psychological Medicine, 37*(2), 99–105. https://doi.org/10.1017/ipm.2019.28

McMillan, J. R., Clifton, A. K., McGrath, D., & Gale, W. S. (1977). Women's language: Uncertainty or interpersonal sensitivity and emotionality. *Sex Roles, 3*, 545–559.

McMillan, L. R., & Shannon, D. M. (2011). Psychometric analysis of the JSPE nursing student version R: Comparison of senior BSN students and medical students' attitudes toward empathy in patient care. *International Scholarly Research Network Nursing*, 726063. https://doi.org/10.5402/2011/726063

McTighe, A. J. (2014). *Effect of Medical Education on Empathy in Osteopathic Medical Students*. [Unpublished doctoral dissertation]. Philadelphia College of Osteopathic Medicine.

McVey, L. J., Davis, D. E., & Cohen, H. J. (1989). The aging game: An approach to education in geriatrics. *Journal of the American Medical Association, 262*, 1507–1509.

Mead, G. H. (1934). *Mind, self and society*. University of Chicago Press.

Means, J. J. (2002). Mighty prophet/wounded healer. *Journal of Pastoral Care, 56*, 41–49.

Meeuwesen, L., Schaap, C., & Van der Staak, C. (1991). Verbal analysis of doctor-patient communication. *Social Science & Medicine, 32*, 1143–1150.

Mehrabian, A. (1969). Significance of posture and position in the communication of attitude and status relationships. *Psychological Bulletin, 71*, 359–372.

Mehrabian, A. (1972). *Nonverbal communication*. Aldine-Atherton.

Mehrabian, A. (1996). *The Balanced Emotional Empathy Scale (BEES)*. Unpublished document. Information www.kaaj.com/psych/scales/emp.html

Mehrabian, A. (1997). Relations among personality scales of aggression, violence, and empathy: Validational evidence bearing on the Risk of Eruptive Violence Scale. *Aggressive Behavior, 23*, 433–445.

Mehrabian, A., & Epstein, N. A. (1972). A measure of emotional empathy. *Journal of Personality, 40*, 525–543.

Mehrabian, A., & O'Reilly, E. (1980). Analysis of personality measures in terms of basic dimensions of temperament. *Journal of Personality and Social Psychology, 38*, 492–503.

Mehrabian, A., Young, A. L., & Sato, S. (1988). Emotional empathy and associated individual differences. *Current Psychology: Research & Reviews, 7*, 221–240.

Melamed, S., Shirom, A., Toker, S., Berliner, S., & Sharira, I. (2006). Burnout and risk of cardiovascular disease: Evidence, possible causal paths, and promising research directions. *Psychological Bulletin, 132*(3), 327–353. https://doi.org/10.1037/0033-2909.132.3.327

Mello, M. M., Studdert, D. M., DesRoches, C. M., Peugh, J., Zapert, K., Brennan, T. A., & Sage, W. M. (2004). Caring for patients in a malpractice crisis: Physician satisfaction and quality of care. *Health Affairs, 23*(4), 42–53. https://doi.org/10.1377/hlthaff.23.4.42

Meltzoff, J., & Kornreich, M. (1970). *Research in psychotherapy*. Atherton.

Meltzoff, A. N., & Moore, M. K. (1977). Imitation of facial and manual gestures by human neonates. *Science, 198*, 75–78.

Meltzoff, A. N., & Moore, M. K. (1983). Newborn infants imitate adult facial gestures. *Child Development, 54*, 702–709.

Meltzoff, A. N., & Prinz, W. (2002). *The imitative mind: Development, evolution, and brain bases*. Cambridge University Press.

Melzack, R. (1990). Phantom limb and the concept of neuromatrix. *Trends in Neurosciences, 13*, 88–92.

Mengel, M. B. (1987). Physician ineffectiveness due to family-of-origin issues. *Family Systems Medicine, 5*, 176–190.

Menks, F. (1983). The use of a board game to simulate the experience of old age. *Gerontologist, 23*, 565–568.

Mercer, S. W. (2004). The consultation and relational empathy (CARE) measure: development and preliminary validation and reliability of an empathy-based consultation process measure. *Family Practice, 21*, 699–705.

Mercer, S. W., Maxwell, M., Heaney, D., & Watt, G. C. M. (2004). The consultation and rational empathy (CARE) measure: Development and preliminary validation and reliability of an empathy-based consultation process measure. *Family Practice, 21*(6), 699–705. https://doi.org/10.1093/fampra/cmh621

Mercer, S. W., McConnachie, A., Maxwell, M., Heaney, D., & Watt, G. C. (2005). Relevance and practical use of the Consultation and Relational Empathy (CARE) measure in general practice. *Family Practice, 22*(3), 328–334. https://doi.org/10.1093/fampra/cmh730

Mercer, S. W., & Reynolds, W. J. (2002). Empathy and quality of care. *British Journal of General Practice, 52*, S9–S12.

Mercer, S. W., Watt, G. C. M., & Reilly, D. (2001). Empathy is important for enablement. *British Medical Journal, 322*, 865.

Merlyn, S. (1998). Improving doctor-patient communication: Not an option, but a necessity. *British Medical Journal, 316*, 1922.

Mestre, M. V., Samper, P., Frias, M. D., & Tur, A. M. (2009). Are women more empathic than men? A longitudinal study in adolescence. *The Spanish Journal of Psychology, 12*(1), 76–83. https://doi.org/10.1017/S1138741600001499

Metcalfe, J., & Mischel, W. (1999). A hot/cool system analysis of delay of gratification: Dynamics of willpower. *Psychological Review, 106*, 3–19.

Meyers, A. R. (1987). Lumping it: The hidden denomination of the medical malpractice crisis. *American Journal of Public Health, 77*, 1544–1548.

Michalec, B. (2010). As assessment of medical student school stressors on preclinical students' level of clinical empathy. *Current Psychology, 29*, 210–221. https://doi.org/10.1007/s12144-010-9081-y

Michalec, B., Veloski, J. J., Hojat, M., & Tykocinski, M. L. (2015). Identifying potential engaging leaders within medical education: The role of positive influence on peers. *Medical Teacher, 37*(7), 677–683. https://doi.org/10.3109/0142159X.2014.947933

Michalska, M. J., Kinzler, K. D., & Decety, J. (2013). Age-related sex differences in explicit measures of empathy do not predict brain responses across childhood and adolescence. *Developmental Cognitive Neuroscience, 3*, 22–32. https://doi.org/10.1016/j.dcn.2012.08.001

Milgram, S. (1963). Behavioral study of obedience. *Journal of Abnormal and Social Psychology, 67*, 371–378.

Milgram, S. (1968). Some conditions of obedience and disobedience to authority. *Human Relations, 6*, 259–276.

Miller, K. (2002). *Communication theories: Perspective, processes, and context*. McGraw-Hill.

Miller, M. T. (2016). *Comparison of empathy scores in RN-BSN students before and after compassionate care course*. (Publication No. 10016589). [Doctoral dissertation, Carlow University]. ProQuest Dissertations & Theses Global. DAI-B 77/07(E).

Miller, M. N., & McGowen, K. R. (2000). The Painful truth: Physicians are not invincible. *Southern Medical Journal, 91*, 966–972.

Miller, P. A., & Eisenberg, N. (1988). The relation of empathy to aggressive and externalizing/antisocial behavior. *Psychological Bulletin, 103*, 324–344.

Milner, K., Squire, L. R., & Kanel, E. R. (1998). Cognitive neuroscience and the study of memory. *Neuron, 20*, 445–468.

Miniotti, M. (2022). Empathy for patient care in medical students: new evidence on the importance of self-transcendence. *Psychology, Health & Medicine, 27*(5), 1035–1041. https://doi.org/10.1080/13548506.2020.1842897

Misra-Hebert, A. D., Isaacson, J. H., Kohn, M., Hull, A. L., Hojat, M., Papp, K. K., & Calabrese, L. (2012). Improving empathy of physicians through guided reflective writing. *International Journal of Medical Education, 3*, 71–77. https://doi.org/10.5116/ijme.4f7e.e332

Mizobe, M., Kataoka, H., Yamagami, H., Ito, C., Koyama, Y., Yawata, E., & Shiga, T. (2019). A night on call or an overnight shift does not reduce residents' empathy: a randomized crossover multicenter survey. *BMC Medical Education, 19*(1), 391. https://doi.org/10.1186/s12909-019-1822-5

Mocny-Pachońska, K., Łanowy, P., Trzcionka, A., Skaba, D., & Tanasiewicz, M. (2020). Gender related changes of empathy level among Polish dental students over the course of training. *Medicine, 99*(1), e18470. https://doi.org/10.1097/MD.0000000000018470

Modi, A., Fascelli, M., Daitch, Z., & Hojat, M. (2017). Evaluating the Relationship between participation in student-run free clinics and changes in empathy in medical students. *Journal of Primary Care and Community Health, 8*(3), 122–126. https://doi.org/10.1177/2150131916685199

Montanari, P. (2012). *Psychometric Analysis of the Jefferson Scale of Empathy (JSE) Health Professional Students (HPS) Version: An Italian Validation Study with Undergraduate Nursing Students*. [Unpublished doctoral dissertation]. University of L'Aquila, Italy.

Montgomery Hunter, K., Charon, R., & Coulehan, J. L. (1995). The study of literature in medical education. *Academic Medicine, 70*, 787–794.

Moore, B. E., & Fine, B. D. (1968). *A glossary of psychoanalytic terms and concepts*. American Psychoanalytic Association.

Moore, D. B. (1996). Illegal action-official reaction: Affect theory, criminology, and the criminal justice system. In D. L. Nathanson (Ed.), *Knowing feeling: Affect, script, and psychotherapy* (pp. 346–378). W.W. Norton.

Moore, P. J., Adler, N. E., & Robertson, P. A. (2000). Medical malpractice: The effect of doctor-patient relations on medical patient perceptions and malpractice intentions. *Western Journal of Medicine, 173*, 244–250.

Morelli, S. A., Rameson, L. T., & Lieberman, M. D. (2014). The neural components of empathy: Predicting daily prosocial behavior. *Social Cognitive and Affective Neuroscience, 9*(1), 39–47. https://doi.org/10.1093/scan/nss088

Moreno, J. L. (1934). *Who shall survive?* Nervous and Mental Disease Publishing Co.

Moreto, G. (2015). *Evaluating Empathy In Undergraduate Medical Students At São Paulo University Using Two Instruments*. [Unpublished doctoral dissertation]. São Paulo University, Brazil.

Moreto, G., Santos, I. S., Blasco, P. G., Pessini, L., & Lotufo, P. A. (2018). Assessing Empathy among Medical Students: A Comparative Analysis Using Two Different Scales in a Brazilian Medical School. *Educación Médica, 19*, 162–170.

Morgan, J. D. (Ed.). (2002). *Social support: A reflection of humanity*. Baywood Publishing Company.

Mori, M. S., Vigh, A., Miayata, T., & Yoshihara, S. (1990). Oxytocin is the major prolactin releasing factor in the posterior pituitary. *Endocrinology, 125*, 1009–1013.

Morrison, I., Lloyd, D., di Pellegrino, G., & Roberts, N. (2004). Vicarious responses to pain in anterior cingulated cortex: Is empathy a multisensory issue? *Cognitive & Affective Behavioral Neuroscience, 4*(2), 270–278. https://doi.org/10.3758/cabn.4.2.270

Morse, D. S., Edwardsen, E. A., & Gordon, H. S. (2008). Missed opportunities for interval empathy in long cancer communication. *Archives of Internal Medicine, 168(17)*, 1853–1858. https://doi.org/10.1001/archinte.168.17.1853

Morse, J. M., Anderson, G., Bottorff, J. L., Yonge, O., O'Brien, B., Solberg, S. M., & McIlveen, K. H. (1992). Exploring empathy: A conceptual fit for nursing practice? *Image: Journal of Nursing Scholarship, 24*, 273–280.

Morse, J. M., & Mitcham, C. (1997). Coempathy: The contagion of physical distress. *Journal of Advanced Nursing, 26*, 649–657.

Moser, R. S. (1984). Perceived role-taking behavior and course grades in junior year college nursing students. *Journal of Nursing Education, 23*, 294–297.

Moss, H. A. (1967). Sex, age, and state as determinants of mother-infant interaction. *Merrill-Palmer Quarterly, 13*, 19–36.

Mostafa, A., Hoque, R., Mosrafa, M., Rana, M., & Mostafa, F. (2014). Empathy in undergraduate medical students of Bangladesh: Psychometric analysis and differences by gender, academic year, and specialty preference. *International Scholarly Research Notices Psychiatry*, 375439. https://doi.org/10.1155/2014/375439

Moyers, T. B., & Miller, W. (2013). Is low therapist empathy toxic? *Psychology of Addictive Behaviors, 27*, 878–884.

Mullins-Nelson, J. L., Salekin, R. T., & Leistico, A. R. (2006). Psychopathy, empathy, and perspective-taking ability in a community sample: Implications for the successful psychotherapy concept. *International Journal of Forensic Mental Health, 5*, 133–149.

Mumford, L. (1967). *The myth of the machine*. Harcourt, Brace & World.

Murray, H. A. (1938). *Explorations in personality*. Prentice-Hall.

Mussen, P., & Eisenberg-Berg, N. (1977). *Roots of caring, sharing, and helping: The development of prosocial behavior in children*. W.H. Freeman.

Musson, D. M. (2009). Personality and medical education. *Medical Education, 43*(5), 395–397. https://doi.org/10.1111/j.1365-2923.2009.03358.x

Naftulin, D. H., Ware, J. E., Jr., & Donnelly, F. A. (1973). The Doctor Fox lecture: A paradigm of educational seduction. *Journal of Medical Education, 48*, 630–635.

Naguib, G. H., Sindi, A. M., Attar, M. H., Alshouibi, E. N., & Hamed, M. T. (2020). A Cross-Sectional Study of Empathy Among Dental Students at King Abdulaziz University. *Journal of Dental Education, 84*(1), 22–26. https://doi.org/10.21815/JDE.019.160

Nasr Esfahani, M., Behzadipour, M., Jalili Nadoushan, A., & Shariat, S. V. (2014). A pilot randomized controlled trial on the effectiveness of inclusion of a distant learning component into empathy training. *Medical Journal of the Islamic Republic of Iran, 28*(65), 1–6.

Nathanson, D. L. (Ed.). (1996). *Knowing feeling: Affect, script, and psychotherapy*. W.W. Norton.

Nauta, W. J. H., & Feirtag, M. (1986). *Fundamental neuroanatomy*. W.H. Freeman.

Nazam, B., & Ozcakir, A. (2017). Turkish version of the Jefferson scale of Empathy psychometric properties. *European Scientific Journal, 13*(20), 101–111. https://doi.org/10.19044/esj.2017.v13n20p101

NBOME. (2011). *Fundamental Osteopathic Medical Competency Domains: Guidelines for Osteopathic Medical Licensure and the Practice of Osteopathic Medicine*. National Board of Osteopathic Medical Examiners. https://www.nbome.org/docs/NBOME%20Fundamental%20Osteopathic%20Medical%20Competencies.pdf

Nelson, D. W., & Baumgarte, R. (2004). Cross-cultural misunderstandings reduce empathic responding. *Journal of Applied Social Psychology, 34*, 391–401. https://doi.org/10.1111/j.1559-1816.2004.tb02553.x

Nembhard, I. M., David, G., Ezzeddine, I., Betta, D., & Radin, J. (2023). A systemic review of Research on empathy in health care. *Health Services Research, 58*, 250–263. https://doi.org/10.1111/1475-6773.14016

Neubauer, R. B., & Neubauer, A. (1990). *Nature's thumbprint: The new genetics of personality*. Addison-Wesley.

Neumann, M., Edelhäuser, F., Tauschel, D., Fischer, M. R., Wirtz, M., Woopen, C., Haramati, A., & Scheffer, C. (2011). Empathy decline and its reasons: A systematic review of studies with medical students and residents. *Academic Medicine, 86*(8), 996–1009. https://doi.org/10.1097/ACM.0b013e318221e615

Neumann, M., Scheffer, C., Tauschel, D., Lutz, G., Wirtz, M., & Edelhäuser, F. (2012). Physician empathy: Definition, outcome-relevance and its measurement in patient care and medical education. *GMS Zeitschrift Für Medizinische Ausbildung, 29*(1), Doc11. https://doi.org/10.3205/zma000781

Neuwirth, Z. E. (1997). Physician empathy—Should we care? *Lancet, 350*, 606.

Newberg, A., & Waldman, R. (2010). Yawn, it's one of the best things you can do for your brain. In *How god changes your*. Ballantine books/Random House.

Newman, T. B. (2003). The power of stories over statistics. *British Medical Journal, 327*, 1224–1427.

Newton, B. W. (2010). Rebuttals to critics of studies of decline on empathy [Letter to the editor]. *Academic Medicine, 85*(12), *1812–1814*. https://doi.org/10.1097/ACM.0b013e3181fa36e7

Newton, B. W. (2023). Perspective chapter: Having heart-the different facets of empathy. In S. Ventura (Ed.), *Empathy: Advanced research and applications* (pp. 29–49). IntechOpen.

Newton, B. W., Savidge, M. A., Barber, L., Cleveland, E., Clardy, J., Beeman, G., & Hart, T. (2000). Differences in medical students' empathy. *Academic Medicine, 75*, 1215.

Newton, N., & Newton, M. (1967). Psychologic aspects of lactation. *New England Journal of Medicine, 277*, 1179–1188.

Newton, N., Feeler, D., & Rawlins, C. (1968). Effect of lactation on maternal behavior in mice with comparative data on humans. *Lying-in: Journal of Reproductive Medicine, 1*, 257–262.

Nguyen, V. P., & Newton, B. W. (2019). Anecdote or Reality: Are People from the South and/or rural areas of the USA more empathetic? *Medical Science Educator, 29*(1), 277–284. https://doi.org/10.1007/s40670-019-00693-6

Nicholas, D. (2002). Social support of the bereaved: Some practical suggestions. In J. D. Morgan (Ed.), *Social support: A reflection of humanity* (pp. 33–43). Baywood Publishing.

Nightingale, S. D., Yarnold, P. R., & Greenberg, M. S. (1991). Sympathy, empathy, and physician resource utilization. *Journal of General Internal Medicine, 6*, 420–423.

Nolte, J. (1993). *The human brain: An introduction to its functional anatomy* (3rd ed.). Mosby.

Noll, D.R., Ginsberg T., Elahi, A., Cavalieri,T. A. (2016). Effective patient-physician communication based on osteopathic philosophy in caring for elderly patients. *Journal of American Osteopathic Association, 116*(1), 42–47.

Nonnenkamp, D. J. (2013). *A quantitative study of the impact of an empirically validated empathy training program on pre-med students.* (Publication No. 3605751). [Doctoral dissertation, Saint Louis University]. ProQuest Dissertations & Theses Global. DAI-A 75/04(E).

Norsica, I., Demuru, E., & Palagi, E. (2016). She more than he: Gender bias supports the empathic nature of yawn contagion in Homo Sapiens. *Royal Society Open Science, 3*(2), 150459. https://doi.org/10.1098/rsos.150459

Novack, D. H. (1987). Therapeutic aspects of the clinical encounter. *Journal of General Internal Medicine, 2*, 346–355.

Novack, D. H., Epstein, R. M., & Paulsen, R. H. (1999). Toward creating physician-healers: Fostering medical students' self-awareness, personal growth, and well-being. *Academic Medicine, 74*, 516–520.

Nummenmaa, L., Hirvonen, J., Parkkola, R., & Hietanen, J. (2008). Is emotional contagion special? An fMRI study on neural system for affective and cognitive empathy. *Neuroimage, 43*(3), 571–580. https://doi.org/10.1016/j.neuroimage.2008.08.014

Nunes, P., Williams, S., Sa, B., & Stevenson, K. (2011). A study of empathy decline in students from five health disciplines during their first year of training. *International Journal of Medical Education, 2*, 12–17. https://doi.org/10.5116/ijme.4d47.ddb0

O'Conner, J. P., Nash, D. B., Buehler, M. L., & Bard, M. (2002). Satisfaction higher for physician executives who treat patients, survey finds. *Physician Executive, 28*, 16–21.

O'Sullivan, J., & Whelan, T. A. (2011). Adversarial growth in telephone counsellors: Psychological and environmental influences. *British Journal of Guidance & Counselling, 39*(4), 307–323. https://doi.org/10.1080/03069885.2011.567326

Oatley, K. (2004). Scripts, transformation, and suggestiveness of emotions in Shakespeare and Chekhov. *Review of General Psychology, 8*(4), 323–340. https://doi.org/10.1037/1089-2680.8.4.323

Ochsner, K. N., Zaki, J., Hanelin, J., Ludlow, D. H., Knierim, K., Ramachandran, T., Glover, G. H., & Mackey, S. C. (2008). Your pain or mine? Common and distinct neural systems supporting the perception of pain in self and others. *Social Cognitive and Affective Neuroscience, 3*(2), 144–160. https://doi.org/10.1093/scan/nsn006

Ogle, J., Bushnell, J., & Caputi, P. (2013). Empathy is related to clinical competence in medical care. *Medical Education, 47*(8), 824–831. https://doi.org/10.1111/medu.12232

Olinick, S. L. (1984). A critique of empathy and sympathy. In J. Lichtenbergh, M. Borenstein, & D. Silver (Eds.), *Empathy I* (pp. 137–166). Analytic Press.

Oliver, J. (1939). An ancient poem on the duties of a physician, Part 1. *Bulletin of the History of Medicine, 7*, 315.

Olson, J., & Hanchett, E. (1997). Nurse-expressed empathy, patient outcomes, and development of a middle-range theory. *Image—The Journal of Nursing Scholarship, 29*, 71–76.

Ong, L. M., DeHaes, J. M., Hoos, A. M., & Lammies, F. B. (1995). Doctor-patient communication: A review of the literature. *Social Science & Medicine, 40*, 903–918.

Oppenheim, A. (1992). *Questionnaire design: Interviewing and attitude measurement*. Printer Publishing.

Orlando, I. (1961). *The dynamic nurse-patient relationship*. Putman.

Orlando, I. (1972). *The discipline and teaching of nursing process*. Putman.

Ornish, D. (1998). *Love and survival: The scientific basis for the healing power of intimacy*. Harper Collins.

Orr, F. (2017). *I know how it feels: a voice-hearing simulation to enhance nursing students' empathy and self-efficacy*. (Publication No. 31100612). [Doctoral dissertation, University of Technology Sydney, Australia]. ProQuest Dissertations & Theses Global. DAI-A 85/10(E).

Orth-Gomer, K., & Johnson, J. V. (1987). Social network integration and mortality: A six-year follow-up study of random sample of the Swedish population. *Journal of Chronic Diseases, 40*, 949–957.

Ortmeyer, C. F. (1974). Variations in mortality, morbidity, and health care by marital status. In L. L. Erhardt & J. E. Beln (Eds.), *Mortality and morbidity in the United States* (pp. 159–184). Harvard University Press.

Osim, J. H., Essien, E. A., Aniekan Okegbe, J., & Udofia, O. (2019). The Jefferson Scale of Physician Empathy: A Preliminary Study of Validity and Reliability among Physicians in Nigerian Tertiary Hospital. *Acta Medica International, 6*(1), 22–27. https://doi.org/10.4103/ami.ami_70_18

Osler, W. (1932). *Aequanimitas with other addresses to medical schools, nurses, and practitioners of medicine*. Blakiston.

Osofsky, J. D., & O'Connell, E. J. (1977). Patterning of newborn behavior in an urban population. *Child Development, 48*, 532–536.

Ouzouni, C., & Nakakis, K. (2012). An exploratory study of student nurses' empathy. *Health Science Journal, 6*, 534–552.

Ozturk, M., & Demirci, H. (2020). Turkish validation of the Jefferson scale of empathy for nurses seeking kidney donations in intensive care units. *The Aging Male: The Official Journal of the*

International Society for the Study of the Aging Male, 23(5), 564–570. https://doi.org/10.1080/13685538.2018.1544238

Pacala, J. T., Boult, C., Bland, C., & O'Brien, J. (1995). Aging game improves medical students' attitudes toward caring for elderly. *Gerontology and Geriatrics Education, 15*, 45–57.

Pacala, J. T., Boult, C., & Hepburn, K. (2006). Ten years' experience conducting the Aging game workshop: was it worth it? *Journal of American Geriatric Society, 54*(1), 144–149. https://doi.org/10.1111/j.1532-5415.2005.00531.x

Page, K. M., & Novak, M. A. (2002). Empathy leads to fairness. *Bulletin of Mathematical Biology, 64*, 1101–1116.

Panizzi Woodley, K. T. C. (2012). *A repeated measures quantitative prospective inquiry into the change in medical student self-reported empathy in clinical rotations.* (Publication No. 3550376). [Doctoral dissertation, The University of Alabama at Birmingham]. ProQuest Dissertations & Theses Global. DAI-A 74/05(E).

Papadakis, M. A., Teherani, A., Banach, M. A., Knettler, T. R., Rattner, S. L., Stern, D. T., Veloski, J. J., & Hodgson, C. S. (2005). Disciplinary action by ethical boards and prior behavior in medical school. *New England Journal of Medicine, 353*(25), 2673–2682. https://doi.org/10.1056/NEJMsa052596

Papousek, M., Papousek, H., & Symmes, D. (1991). The meanings of melodies in motherese in tone and stress languages. *Infant Behavior & Development, 14*, 415–440.

Park, K. H., Roh, H., Suh, D. H., & Hojat, M. (2015). Empathy in Korean medical students: Findings from a nationwide survey. *Medical Teacher, 37*(10), 943–948. https://doi.org/10.3109/0142159X.2014.956058

Parlow, J., & Rothman, A. (1974). Attitudes toward social issues in medicine of five health science facilities. *Social Science & Medicine, 8*, 351–358.

Paro, H., Daud-Gallotti, R. M., Tiberio, I. C., Pinto, R. M. C., & Martins, M. A. (2012). Brazilian version of the Jefferson Scale of Empathy: Psychometric properties and factor analysis. *BMC Medical Education, 12*, 73. https://doi.org/10.1186/1472-6920-12-73

Pascalis, O., DeSchonen, S., Morton, J., Deruella, C., & Fabre-Grenet, M. (1995). Mother's face recognition by neonates: A replication and extension. *Infant Behavior & Development, 18*, 79–85.

Patterson, C. H. (1984). Empathy, warmth, and genuineness in psychotherapy: A review of reviews. *Psychotherapy, 21*, 431–438.

Paulhus, D. L. (1991). Measurement and control of response bias. In J. P. Robinson, P. R. Shaver, & L. S. Wrightsman (Eds.), *Measures of personality and social psychological attitudes* (pp. 17–59). Academic Press.

Peabody, F. W. (1984). The care of the patient. *Journal of the American Medical Association, 252*, 813–818.

Pearl, R. (2024). *ChatGPT MD*. Robert Pearl, MD & ChatGPT.

Pecukonis, E. V. (1990). A cognitive/affective empathy training program as a function of ego development in aggressive adolescent females. *Adolescence, 25*, 59–76.

Pedersen, R. (2009). Empirical research on empathy in medicine: A critical review. *Patient Education and Counseling, 76*(3), 307–322. https://doi.org/10.1016/j.pec.2009.06.012

Pedersen, C. A., Ascher, J. A., Monroe, Y. L., & Prange, A. J. J. (1982). Oxytocin induces maternal behavior in virgin female rats. *Science, 216*, 648–649.

Pedersen, C. A., & Prange, A. J. J. (1979). Induction of maternal behavior in virgin rats after intracerebroventicular administration of oxytocin. *Proceedings of the National Academy of Sciences of the United States of America, 76*, 6661–6665.

Pellegrino, E. (1979). *Humanism and the physician*. University of Tennessee Press.

Pennebaker, J. W. (1990). *Opening up: The healing power of confining in others*. William Morrow.

Pennebaker, J. W., Kiecolt-Glaser, J. K., & Glaser, K. (1988). Disclosure of traumas and immune function: Health implications for psychotherapy. *Journal of Consulting and Clinical Psychology, 56*, 239–245.

Pennington, R. E., & Pierce, W. L. (1985). Observations of empathy of nursing-home staff: A predictive study. *International Journal of Aging and Human Development, 21*, 281–291.

Penninx, B. W., van Tilburg, T., & Kriegsman, D. M. (1997). Effects of social support and personal coping resources on mortality in older age: The Longitudinal Aging Study, Amsterdam. *American Journal of Epidemiology, 146*, 510–519.

Perls, F. S. (1969/1992). *Gestalt therapy verbatim*. The Gestalt Journal Press, Inc..

Perry, R. J., Rosen, H. R., Kramer, J. H., Beer, J. S., Levenson, R. L., & Miller, B. L. (2001). Hemispheric dominance for emotions, empathy and social behaviour: Evidence from right and left handers with frontotemporal dementia. *Neurocase, 7*, 145–160.

Peschel, E. R. (1980). *Medicine and literature*. Neale Watson.

Peter, E., & Gallop, R. (1994). The ethic of care: A comparison of nursing and medical students. *Image—The Journal of Nursing Scholarship, 26*, 47–50.

Piaget, J. (1967). *Six psychological studies*. Random House.

Pietro, K. (2023). *Examining empathy during an initial nutrition counseling session through video-cued narrative reflection*. (Publication No. 30426358). [Doctoral dissertation, University of New Hampshire]. ProQuest Dissertations & Theses Global. DAI-A 84/12(E).

Pigman, G. W. (1995). Freud and the history of empathy. *International Journal of Psychoanalysis, 76*, 237–256.

Pinkston, M. M. (2008). *Increasing empathy in medical school students towards individuals living with HIV/AIDS and medication adherence*. (Publication No. 3328710). [Doctoral dissertation, University of Missouri-Kansas City]. ProQuest Dissertations & Theses Global. DAI-A 81/1(E).

Piumatti, G., Abbiati, M., Baroffio, A., & Gerbase, M. W. (2020). Empathy trajectories throughout medical school: Relationships with personality and motives for studying medicine. *Advances in Health Sciences Education: Theory and Practice, 25*(5), 1227–1242. https://doi.org/10.1007/s10459-020-09965-y

Piumatti, G., Costa, M. J., Ardenghi, S., Baroffio, A., Elorduy, M., Gerbase, M. W., Gustin, M. P., Palés, J., Quince, T., Rampoldi, G., Strepparava, M. G., Thiemann, P., Virumbrales, M., & Costa, P. S. Cross-national Psychometric Evaluation of the Jefferson Scale of Empathy-Medical Student Version. *Evaluation & the Health Professions*. https://doi.org/10.1177/01632787241296540

Platek, S. M., Critton, S. R., Myers, T. E., & Gallup, G. G. (2003). Contagious yawning: The role of self awareness and mental state attribution. *Cognitive Brain Research, 17*, 223–227.

Platek, S. M., Keenan, J. P., Gallup, G. G., & Mohamed, F. B. (2004). Where am I? The neurological correlates of self and other. *Cognitive Brain Research, 19*(2), 114–122. https://doi.org/10.1016/j.cogbrainres.2003.11.014

Platek, S. M., Mohamed, F. B., & Gallup, G. G. (2005). Contagious yawning and the brain. *Cognitive Brain Research, 23*(2-3), 448–452. https://doi.org/10.1016/j.cogbrainres.2004.11.011

Platt, F. W., & Keller, V. F. (1994). Empathic communication: A teachable and learnable skill. *Journal of General Internal Medicine, 9*, 222–226.

Plutchik, R. (1987). Evolutionary bases of empathy. In N. Eisenberg & J. Strayer (Eds.), *Empathy and its development* (pp. 38–46). Cambridge University Press.

Podhorecka, M., Pyszora, A., Woźniewicz, A., Husejko, J., & Kędziora-Kornatowska, K. (2022). Empathy as a Factor Conditioning Attitudes towards the Elderly among Physiotherapists-Results from Poland. *International Journal of Environmental Research and Public Health, 19*(7), 3994. https://doi.org/10.3390/ijerph19073994

Pohl, C. A., Hojat, M., & Arnold, L. (2011). Peer nominations as related to academic attainment, empathy, and specialty interest. *Academic Medicine, 86*(6), 747–751. https://doi.org/10.1097/ACM.0b013e318217e464

Polgar, C., & Thomas, S. (1988). *Introduction to research in health sciences*. Churchill Livingston.

Pollak, O. (1976). *Human behavior and the helping professions*. Spectrum Publications.

Pollak, K. I., Arnold, R. M., Jeffreys, A. S., Alexander, S. C., Olsen, M. K., Abernethy, A. P., Sugg Skinner, C., Rodriguez, K. L., & Tulsky, J. A. (2007). Oncologist communication about emotions during visits with patients with advanced cancer. *Journal of Clinical Oncology, 25*(36), 5748–5752. https://doi.org/10.1200/JCO.2007.12.4180

Poole, A. D., & Sanson-Fisher, R. W. (1980). Long-term effects of empathy training on the interview skills of medical students. *Patient Counseling and Health Education, 2*, 125–127.

Potash, J. S., Chen, J. Y., Lam, C. L., & Chau, V. T. (2014). Art-making in a family medicine clerkship: How does it affect medical student empathy? *BMC Medical Education, 14*, 247. https://doi.org/10.1186/s12909-014-0247-4

Powell, A. S., Boakes, J. P., & Slater, P. (1988). Hostility and the medical student: How a trait measure influences perception of medical specialties. *Medical Education, 22*, 222–230.

Pratiwi, H., Kristina, S. A., Widayanti, A. W., & Prabandari, Y. S. (2022). Educational Interventions to Improve Pharmacy Students' Empathy Towards Geriatrics: A Systematic Review. *Indonesian Journal of Pharmacy, 33*(2), 174–185. https://doi.org/10.22146/ijp.3837

Preston, S. D., & deWaal, F. B. M. (2002). Empathy: It's ultimate and proximate bases. *Behavioral and Brain Sciences, 25*, 1–20.

Preusche, I., & Wagner-Menghin, M. (2013). Rising to the challenge: Cross-cultural adaptation and psychometric evaluation of the adapted German version of the Jefferson Scale of Physician Empathy for students (JSPE-S). *Advances in Health Science Education: Theory and Practice, 18*(4), 573–587. https://doi.org/10.1007/s10459-012-9393-9

Price, B. H., Daffner, K. R., Stowe, R. M., & Mesulam, M. (1990). The compartmental learning disabilities of early frontal lobe damage. *Brain, 113*, 1383–1393.

Prinz, W. (1997). Perception and action planning. *European Journal of Cognitive Psychology, 9*, 129–154.

Pumilia, C. V. (2002). Psychological impact of the physician-patient relationship on compliance: A case study and clinical strategies. *Progress in Transplantation, 12*, 10–16.

Puryear, J. B., & Lewis, L. A. (1981). Description of the interview process in selecting students for admission to U.S. medical school. *Journal of Medical Education, 56*, 881–885.

Quail, M., Brundage, S. B., Spitalnick, J., Allen, P. J., & Beilby, J. (2016). Student self-reported communication skills, knowledge and confidence across standardised patient, virtual and traditional clinical learning environments. *BMC Medical Education, 16*, 73. https://doi.org/10.1186/s12909-016-0577-5

Quill, T. E. (1987). Medical resident education: A cross-sectional study of the influence of the ambulatory preceptor as a role model. *Archives of Internal Medicine, 147*, 971–973.

Radley, C. (1992). Imagining ethics: Literature and practice of ethics. *Journal of Clinical Ethics, 3*, 38–45.

Rafaqat, W., Sami, A., Ibrahim, M. T., Ibad, H., Awais, S., Memon, A., Shahbaz, F. F., Ahmed, D., Zindani, S., Leghari, A. L., & Saleem, S. (2022). Impact of Perfectionism and Resilience on Empathy in Medical Students: A Cross-Sectional Study. *Journal of Patient Experience, 9*, 23743735221106603. https://doi.org/10.1177/23743735221106603

Rahimi-Madiseh, M., Tavakol, M., Dennick, R., & Nasiri, J. (2010). Empathy in Iranian medical students: A preliminary psychometric analysis and differences by gender and year of medical school. *Medical Teacher, 32*(11), e471–e478. https://doi.org/10.3109/0142159X.2010.509419

Rahm, E. T. (2006). Tracking the subprocesses of decision-based action in the human frontal lobes. *Neuroimage, 30*(2), 656–667. https://doi.org/10.1016/j.neuroimage.2005.09.045

Raja, B. A. J., Khandhadiya, K., Guru, S. C., & Mahajan, U. (2024). Physician empathy during crisis: A survey of doctors in COVID-19 pandemic (COPE study). *Medical Journal Armed Forces India, 80*(3), 335–345. https://doi.org/10.1016/j.mjafi.2022.08.012

Rakel, D. P., Hoeft, T. J., Barrett, B. P., Chewning, B. A., Craig, B. M., & Niu, M. (2009). Practitioner empathy and the duration of the common cold. *Family Medicine, 41*(7), 494–501.

Rankin, K. P., Gorno-Tempini, M. L., Allison, S. C., Stanley, C. M., Glenn, S., Weiner, M. W., & Miller, B. L. (2006). Structural anatomy of empathy in neurodegenerative disease. *Brain : a journal of neurology, 129*(Pt 11), 2945–2956. https://doi.org/10.1093/brain/awl254

Rankin, K. P., Kramer, J. H., & Miller, B. L. (2005). Patterns of cognitive and emotional empathy in frontotemporal lobar degeneration. *Cognitive Behavioral Neurology, 18*(1), 28–36. https://doi.org/10.1097/01.wnn.0000152225.05377.ab

Raudonis, B. M. (1993). The meaning and impact of empathic relationships in hospice nursing. *Cancer Nursing, 16*, 304–309.

Ray, O. (2004). How the mind hurts and heals the body. *American Psychologist, 59*(1), 29–40. https://doi.org/10.1037/0003-066X.59.1.29

Raynolds, P., Boyd, P. T., & Blacklow, R. S. (1994). The relationships between social ties and survival among black and white breast cancer patients: National Cancer Institute, Cancer Survival Study Group. *Cancer Epidemiology, Biomarkers & Prevention, 3*, 253–259.

Reed, V. A., Jernstedt, C., & Reber, E. S. (2001). Understanding and improving medical student specialty choice: Synthesis of the literature using decision theory as a referent. *Teaching and Learning in Medicine, 13*, 117–129.

Reik, T. (1948). *Listening with the third ear: The inner experience of a psychoanalyst*. Farrar, Straus.

Reiser, M. F., Reeves, R. B., & Armington, J. (1955). Effects of variation in laboratory procedure and experimenter upon the ballistoeargram, blood pressure, and heart rate in healthy young men. *Psychosomatic Medicine, 17*, 185–199.

Reisetter, B. C. (2002). *Relationship between psychosocial physician characteristics and physician price awareness*. (Publication No. 3069120). [Doctoral dissertation, The University of Mississippi]. ProQuest Dissertations & Theses Global. DAI-B 63/10.

Reisetter, B. C., Bently, J. P., & Wilkin, N. E. (2005). Relationship between psychosocial physician characteristics and physician price awareness. *Journal of Pharmaceutical Marketing & Management, 17*(1), 51–76. https://doi.org/10.3109/J058v17n01_05

Reiter-Palmon, R., & Connelly, M. S. (2000). Item selection counts: A comparison of empirical key and rational scale validities in theory-based and non-theory-based item pools. *Journal of Applied Psychology, 85*, 143–151.

Rempel, J. K., Holmes, J. G., & Zanna, M. P. (1985). Trust in close relationships. *Journal of Personality and Social Psychology, 49*, 95–112.

Reniers, R. L. E. P., Corcoran, R., Drake, R., Shryane, N. M., & Völlm, B. A. (2011). The QCAE: a questionnaire of cognitive and affective empathy. *Journal of Personality Assessment, 93*(1), 84–95. https://doi.org/10.1080/00223891.2010.528484

Reverby, S. (1987). A caring dilemma: Womanhood and nursing in historical perspective. *Nursing Research, 36*, 1–5.

Reynolds, W. J. (2000). *The measurement and development of empathy in nursing*. Ashgate.

Rezayat, A. A., Shahini, N., Asl, H. T., Jarahi, L., Behdani, F., Shojaei, S. R. H., & Abadi, J. S. A. (2018). Empathy score among medical students in Mashhad, Iran: Study of the Jefferson Scale of Physician Empathy. *Electronic Physician, 10*(7), 7101–7106. https://doi.org/10.19082/7101

Richard, F. D., Bond, C. F., Jr., & Stokes-Zoota, J. J. (2003). One hundred years of social psychology quantitatively described. *Review of General Psychology, 7*, 331–363.

Richard, G. V., Nakamoto, D. M., & Lockwood, J. H. (2001). Medical career choices: Traditional and new possibilities. *Journal of the American Medical Association, 285*, 2249–2250.

Richards, H. L., Fortune, D. G., Weildmann, A., Sweeney, S. K. T., & Griffiths, C. E. M. (2004). Detection of psychological distress in patients with psoriasis: Low consensus between dermatologist and patient. *British Journal of Dermatology, 151(6)*, 1227–1233. https://doi.org/10.1111/j.1365-2133.2004.06221.x

Richter, C. P. (1957). On the phenomenon of sudden death in animals and man. *Psychosomatic Medicine, 19*, 191–198.

Ridley, M., & Dawkins, R. (1981). The natural selection of altruism. In J. P. Rushton & R. M. Sorrentino (Eds.), *Altruism and helping behavior: Social, personality, and developmental perspectives* (pp. 19–39). Erlbaum.

Riess, D. L. (2018). *Effects of simulated clinical experiences on empathy, self-confidence, and satisfaction in nursing students*. (Publication No. 10829752). [Doctoral dissertation, Walden University]. ProQuest Dissertations & Theses Global. DAI-A 81/1(E).

Riess, H., Kelley, J. M., Bailey, R., Konowitz, P. M., & Gray, S. T. (2011). Improving empathy and relational skills in otolaryngology residents: A pilot study. *Otolaryngology-Head and Neck Surgery, 144(1)*, 120–122. https://doi.org/10.1177/0194599810390897

Riess, H., Kelley, J., Bailey, R., Dunn, E., & Phillips, M. (2012). Empathy training for resident physicians: A randomized controlled trial of a neuroscience-informed curriculum. *Journal of General Internal Medicine, 27(10)*, 1280–1286. https://doi.org/10.1007/s11606-012-2063-z

Riggio, R. E., Tucker, J., & Coffaro, D. (1989). Social skills and empathy. *Personality and Individual Differences, 10*, 93–99.

Rizzolatti, G., & Arbibi, M. A. (1998). Language within our grasp. *Trends in Neuroscience, 21*, 188–194.

Rizzolatti, G., & Craighero, L. (2004). The mirror-neuron system. *Annual Review of Neuroscience, 27*, 169–192.

Rizzolatti, G., Fadiga, L., Gallese, V., & Fogassi, L. (1996). Premotor cortex and the recognition of motor action. *Cognitive Brain Research, 3*, 131–141.

Roberts, B. W., & DelVecchio, W. F. (2000). The rank-order consistency of personality traits from childhood to old age: A quantitative review of longitudinal studies. *Psychological Bulletin, 126*, 3–25.

Robertson, A. D., Moore, M., McFadden, L., Steere, E. L., Barnes, J., & Shrader, S. (2022). Implementation and evaluation of simulations in a required course to improve empathy of pharmacy students. *Currents in Pharmacy Teaching & Learning, 14*(11), 1404–1410. https://doi.org/10.1016/j.cptl.2022.09.021

Robinson, J. L., Zahn-Waxler, C., & Emde, R. N. (1994). Patterns of development in early empathic behavior: Environmental and child constitutional influences. *Social Development, 3*, 125–145.

Robinson, J. P. (1978). General attitudes toward people. In J. P. Robinson & P. R. Shaver (Eds.), *Measures of social psychological attitudes* (pp. 587–627). Institute for Social Research.

Rodewald, E. E. (2012). *Attachment style and empathy in health care counseling: is there an association?* (Publication No. 3491500). [Doctoral dissertation, Capella University]. ProQuest Dissertations & Theses Global. DAI-B 73/05.

Rodriguez, M. S., & Cohen, S. (1998). Social support. In H. S. Friedman (Ed.), *Encyclopedia of mental health* (pp. 535–544). Academic Press.

Roe, A. (1957). Early determinants of vocational choice. *Journal of Consulting Psychology, 4*, 212–217.

Roe, K. V. (1977). A study of empathy in young Greek and U.S. children. *Journal of Cross-Cultural Psychology, 8*, 493–502.

Rogers, C. R. (1959). A theory of therapy: Personality and interpersonal relationships as developed in the client-centered framework. In S. Koch (Ed.), *Psychology, a study of science: Foundations of the person and the social context* (pp. 184–256). McGraw-Hill.

Rogers, C. R. (1975). Empathic: An unappreciated way of being. *Counseling Psychologist, 5*, 2–11.

Rogers, C. R., Gendlin, E., Kiesler, D., & Truax, C. B. (1967). *The therapeutic relationship and its impact*. University of Wisconsin Press.

Roghmann, K. J., Hengst, A., & Zastowny, T. R. (1979). Satisfaction with medical care: Its measurement and relation to utilization. *Medical Care, 17*, 461–479.

Roh, M. S., Hahm, B. J., Lee, D. H., & Suh, D. H. (2010). Evaluation of empathy among Korean medical students: A cross-sectional study using Korean version of the Jefferson Scale of Physician Empathy. *Teaching and Learning in Medicine: An International Journal, 22(3)*, 167–171. https://doi.org/10.1080/10401334.2010.488191

Rohrer, J. (2021). *Teaching compassion skills to students of behavior analysis via telehealth.* (Publication No. 28493962). [Doctoral dissertation, Endicott College]. ProQuest Dissertations & Theses Global. DAI-A 82/11(E).

Rokeach, M. (1973). *The nature of human values*. Free Press.

Romano, J. M., Jensen, M. P., Turner, J. A., Good, A. B., & Hops, H. (2000). Chronic pain patient-partner interactions: Further support for a behavioral model of chronic pain. *Behavior Therapy, 31*, 415–440.

Román-Sánchez, D., Paramio-Cuevas, J. C., Paloma-Castro, O., Palazón-Fernández, J. L., Lepiani-Díaz, I., de la Fuente Rodríguez, J. M., & López-Millán, M. R. (2022). Empathy, Burnout, and Attitudes towards Mental Illness among Spanish Mental Health Nurses. *International Journal of Environmental Research and Public Health, 19*(2), 692. https://doi.org/10.3390/ijerph19020692

Rosenberg, D. A., & Silver, H. K. (1984). Medical student abuse—An unnecessary and preventable cause of stress. *Journal of the American Medical Association, 251*, 739–742.

Rosenberg, M. (1957). *Occupation and values*. Free Press.

Rosenberg, M. (1965). *Society and adolescent self-image*. Princeton University Press.

Rosenberg, M. J., & Hovland, C. I. (1960). Cognitive, affective, and behavioral components of attitudes. In M. J. Hovland & M. J. Rosenberg (Eds.), *Attitude organization and change* (pp. 1–14). Yale University Press.

Rosenfeld, H. M. (1965). Effect of an approval-seeking induction on interpersonal proximity. *Psychological Reports, 17*, 120–122.

Rosenhan, D. L. (1973). On being sane in insane places. *Science, 179*, 250–258.

Rosenow, E. C. (1999). The challenge of becoming a distinguished clinician. *Mayo Clinic Proceedings, 74*, 635–637.

Rosenthal, R., Hall, J. A., DiMatteo, M. R., Rogers, P. L., & Archer, D. (1979). *Sensitivity to nonverbal communication: The PONS test*. Johns Hopkins University Press.

Rosenthal, S., Howard, B., Schlussel, Y. R., Herrigel, D., Smolarz, B. G., Gable, B., Vasquez, J., Grigo, H., & Kaufman, M. (2011). Humanism at heart: Preserving empathy in third-year medical students. *Academic Medicine, 86(3)*, 350–358. https://doi.org/10.1097/ACM.0b013e318209897f

Rosenzweig, J., Blaizot, A., Cougot, N., Pegon-Machat, E., Hamel, O., Apelian, N., Bedos, C., Munoz-Sastre, M. T., & Vergnes, J. N. (2016). Effect of a Person-Centered Course on the Empathic Ability of Dental Students. *Journal of Dental Education, 80*(11), 1337–1348. https://doi.org/10.1002/j.0022-0337.2016.80.11.tb06219.x

Ross, R. (2017). *"This will only hurt a bit" evaluating the usage of patient focused empathy amongst general surgery residents.* (Publication No. 10757883). [Doctoral dissertation, Rutgers The State University of New Jersey, Graduate School of Applied and Professional Psychology]. ProQuest Dissertations & Theses Global. DAI-A 79/04(E).

Ross, E. D., & Mesulam, M. M. (1979). Dominant language functions of the right hemisphere? Prosody and emotional gesturing. *Archives of Neurology, 36*, 144–148.

Ross, J. B., & McLaughlin, M. M. (1949). *The portable medieval reader*. Penguin Books USA Inc.

Roter, D., Lipkin, M., & Korsgaard, A. (1991). Sex differences in patients' and physicians' communication during primary care medical visits. *Medical Care, 29*, 1088–1093.

Roter, D. L., & Hall, J. A. (1997). Gender differences in patient-physician communication. In S. J. Gallant, G. P. Keita, & R. Royak-Schater (Eds.), *Health care for women: Psychological, social, and behavioral influences* (pp. 57–71). American Psychological Association.

Roter, D. L., Hall, J. A., & Aoki, Y. (2002). Physician gender effects in medical communication. *Journal of the American Medical Association, 288*, 756–764.

Roter, D. L., Hall, J. A., Kern, D. E., Baker, L. R., Cole, K. A., & Roca, R. P. (1995). Improving physicians' interviewing skills and reduction in patients' emotional distress: A randomized clinical trial. *Archives of Internal Medicine, 155*, 1877–1884.

Roter, D. L., Hall, J. A., Merisca, R., Nordstrom, B., Cretin, D., & Svarstad, B. (1998). Effectiveness of interventions to improve patient compliance: A meta-analysis. *Medical Care, 36*, 1138–1161.

Rovezzi-Carroll, S., & Fitz, P. A. (1984). Predicting allied health major fields of study with selected personality characteristics. *College Student Journal, 18*, 43–51.

Ruby, P., & Decety, J. (2004). How would you feel versus how would you think she would feel? A neuroimaging study of perspective taking with social emotions. *Journal of Cognitive Neuroscience, 16*(6), 988–999. https://doi.org/10.1162/0898929041502661

Rueckert, L., & Naybar, N. (2008). Gender differences in empathy: The role of the right hemisphere. *Brain and Cognition, 67*(2), 162–167. https://doi.org/10.1016/j.bandc.2008.01.002

Ruiz-Hernández, J. A., López-García, C., Llor-Esteban, B., Galián-Muñoz, I., & Benavente-Reche, A. P. (2016). Evaluation of the users violence in primary health care: Adaptation of an instrument. *International Journal of Clinical and Health Psychology, 16*(3), 295–305. https://doi.org/10.1016/j.ijchp.2016.06.001

Runyan, C., Savageau, J. A., Potts, S., & Weinreb, L. (2016). Impact of a family medicine resident wellness curriculum: a feasibility study. *Medical Education Online, 21*, 30648. https://doi.org/10.3402/meo.v21.30648

Rushton, J. P. (1981). The altruistic personality. In P. J. Rushton & R. M. Sorrentino (Eds.), *Altruism and helping behavior: Social, personality, and developmental perspectives* (pp. 251–266). Erlbaum.

Rushton, J. P. (2004). Genetic and environmental contributions to pro-social attitudes: A twin study of social responsibility. *Proceedings of the Royal Society of Biological Sciences, 271*(1557), 2583–2585. https://doi.org/10.1098/rspb.2004.2941

Rushton, J. P., Chrisjohn, R. D., & Fekker, G. C. (1981). The altruistic personality and the self-report Altruism Scale. *Personality and Individual Differences, 2*, 293–302.

Rushton, J. P., Fulker, D. W., Neale, M. C., Nias, D. K. B., & Eysenck, H. J. (1986). Altruism and aggression: The heritability of individual differences. *Journal of Personality and Social Psychology, 50*, 1192–1198.

Russek, L. G., & Schwartz, G. E. (1997). Perceptions of parental caring predict health status in midlife: A 35-year follow up of the Harvard Mastery of Stress study. *Psychosomatic Medicine, 59*, 144–149.

Russell, D., Peplau, L. A., & Cutrona, C. B. (1980). The revised UCLA Loneliness Scale: Concurrent and discriminant validity evidence. *Journal of Personality and Social Psychology, 39*, 472–480.

Rutter, M., Caspi, A., Fergusson, D., Horwood, L. J., Goodman, R., Maughan, B., Moffitt, T. E., Meltzer, H., & Carroll, J. (2005). Sex differences in developmental reading ability: New findings from 4 epidemiological studies. *Journal of the American Medical Association, 291*(16), 2007–2012. https://doi.org/10.1001/jama.291.16.2007

Sackett, D. H., & Haynes, R. B. (1976). *Compliance with therapeutic regimens*. Johns Hopkins University Press.

Safdar, B., Heins, A., Homel, P., Miner, J., Neighbor, M., De Sandre, P., & Todd, K. (2009). Impact of physician and patient gender on pain management in the emergency department-A multicenter study. *Pain Medicine, 10*(2), 364–372. https://doi.org/10.1111/j.1526-4637.2008.00524.x

Sage, W. M. (2002). Putting the patient in patient safety: Linking patient complaints and malpractice risk. *Journal of the American Medical Association, 287*, 3003–3005.

Sagi, A., & Hoffman, M. L. (1976). Empathic distress in newborns. *Developmental Psychology, 12*, 175–176.

Salk, L. (1960). The effects of normal heartbeat sound on the behavior of the newborn infant: Implications for mental health. *World Mental Health, 12*, 168–175.

Salovey, P., & Mayer, J. D. (1990). Emotional intelligence. *Imagination, Cognition, and Personality, 9*, 185–211.

Sandler, G. (1980). The importance of the history in the medical clinic and the cost of unnecessary tests. *American Heart Journal, 100*, 928–931.

Sandoval, A. M., Hancock, D., Poythress, N., Edens, J. F., & Lilienfeld, S. (2000). Construct validity of the Psychopathic Personality Inventory in a correctional sample. *Journal of Personality Assessment, 74*, 262–281.

San-Martín, M., Delgado-Bolton, R., & Vivanco, L. (2017a). Role of a Semiotics-Based Curriculum in Empathy Enhancement: A Longitudinal Study in Three Dominican Medical Schools. *Frontiers in Psychology, 8*, 2018. https://doi.org/10.3389/fpsyg.2017.02018

San-Martín, M., Delgado-Bolton, R., & Vivanco, L. (2017b). Professionalism and occupational well-being: Similarities and differences among Latin American health professionals. *Frontiers in Psychology, 8*, 63. https://doi.org/10.3389/fpsyg.2017.00063

Sanson-Fisher, R., & Maguire, P. (1980). Should skills in communication with patients be taught in medical schools? *Lancet, 2*, 523–526.

Sanson-Fisher, R. W., & Poole, A. D. (1978). Training medical students to empathize: An experimental study. *Medical Journal of Australia, 1*, 473–476.

Sapolsky, R. M. (2004). *Why zebras don't get ulcers* (3rd ed.). Times Books.

Schachter, S. (1959). *The psychology of affiliation*. Stanford University Press.

Schafer, R. (1959). Generative empathy in the treatment situation. *Psychoanalytic Quarterly, 28*, 342–373.

Schaflen, A. E. (1964). The significance of posture in communication systems. *Psychiatry, 27*, 316–331.

Schlesinger, M. (2002). A loss of faith: The sources of reduced political legitimacy for the American medical profession. *Milbank Quarterly, 80*, 185–235.

Schmidmaier, M., Rupp, J., Cvetanova, D., & Mayer, S. (2024). *Perceived Empathy of Technology Scale (PETS): Measuring Empathy of Systems Toward the User*. In *Proceedings of the 2024 CHI Conference on Human Factors in Computing Systems (CHI '24)* (pp. 1–18). Association for Computing MachineryArticle 456. https://doi.org/10.1145/3613904.3642035

Schmidt, C. W., & Baker, L. R. (1986). Psychotherapy in ambulatory practice. In L. R. Barker, J. R. Burton, & P. D. Zieve (Eds.), *Principles of ambulatory medicine* (pp. 133–139). Williams & Wilkins.

Schmitt, D. P. (2012). When the difference is in the detail: A critique of Zentner and Mitura (2012) "Stepping out of the caveman's shadow: Nations' gender gap predicts degree of sex differentiation in mate preferences". *Evolutionary Psychology, 10(4)*, 720–726. https://doi.org/10.1177/147470491201000406

Schneiderman, L. J. (2002). Empathy and the literary imagination. *Annals of Internal Medicine, 137*, 627–629.

Schoenbach, V., Kaplan, B. H., Fredman, L., & Kleinbaum, D. G. (1986). Social ties and mortality in Evans County, Georgia. *American Journal of Epidemiology, 123*, 577–591.

Schore, A. N. (1996). *Affect regulation and the origin of the self: The neurobiology of emotional development*. Erlbaum.

Schroeder, T. (1925). The psycho-analytic method of observation. *International Journal of Psychoanalysis, 6*, 155–170.

Schulte-Ruther, M., Markowitsch, H., Fink, G., & Piefke, M. (2007). Mirror neuron and theory of mind mechanisms involved in face-to-face interactions: A functional magnetic resonance imaging approach to empathy. *Journal of Cognitive Neuroscience, 19*(*8*), 1354–1372. https://doi.org/10.1162/jocn.2007.19.8.1354

Schutle-Ruther, M., Markowitsch, H. J., Shah, N. J., Fink, G. R., & Piefke, M. (2008). Gender differences in brain networks supporting empathy. *Neuroimage, 42(1)*, 393–403. https://doi.org/10.1016/j.neuroimage.2008.04.180

Schutte, N. S., Malouff, J. M., Bobik, C., Coston, T. D., Greeson, C., Jedlicka, C., Rhodes, E., & Wendorf, G. (2001). Emotional intelligence and interpersonal relations. *Journal of Social Psychology, 141*, 523–536.

Schwaber, E. (1981). Empathy: A mode of analytic listening. *Psychoanalytic Inquiry, 1*, 357–392.

Schwartz, B., & Bohay, R. (2012). Can patient help teach professionalism and empathy to dental students? Adding patient video to lecture course. *Journal of Dental Education, 76*(*2*), 174–184.

Schwartz, B. D., Horst, A., Fisher, J. A., Michels, N., & Van Winkle, L. J. (2020). Fostering Empathy, Implicit Bias Mitigation, and Compassionate Behavior in a Medical Humanities Course. *International Journal of Environmental Research and Public Health, 17*(7), 2169. https://doi.org/10.3390/ijerph17072169

Schweller, M., Costa, F. O., Antônio, M. Â., Amaral, E. M., & de Carvalho-Filho, M. A. (2014). The impact of simulated medical consultations on the empathy levels of students at one medical school. *Academic Medicine, 89(4)*, 632–637. https://doi.org/10.1097/ACM.0000000000000175

Scourfield, J., Martin, N., Lewis, G., & McGuffin, P. (1999). Heritability of social cognitive skills in children and adolescents. *British Journal of Psychiatry, 175*, 564.

Seaberg, D. C., Godwin, S. A., & Perry, S. J. (1999). Teaching empathy in an emergency medicine residency. *Academic Emergency Medicine, 6*, 485.

Seaberg, D. C., Godwin, S. A., & Perry, S. J. (2000). Teaching patient empathy: The ED visit program. *Academic Emergency Medicine, 7*, 1433–1436.

Seeman, T. E., Berkman, L. F., & Kohout, F. (1993). Intercommunity variation in the association between social ties and mortality in elderly: A comparative analysis of three communities. *Annals of Epidemiology, 3*, 325–335.

Seeman, T. E., & Syme, L. (1987). Social network and coronary artery disease: A comparison of the structure and function of social relations and predictors of disease. *Psychosomatic Medicine, 49*, 341–354.

Seifritz, E., Esposito, F., Neuhoff, J. G., Lüthi, A., Mustovic, H., Dammann, G., von Bardeleben, U., Radue, E. W., Cirillo, S., Tedeschi, G., & Di Salle, F. (2003). Differential sex-independent amygdala response to infant crying and laughing in parents versus nonparents. *Biological Psychiatry, 54*, 1367–1375.

Self, D. J., Schrader, D. E., Baldwin, D. C., Jr., & Wolinsky, F. D. (1993). The moral development of medical students: A pilot study of the possible influence of medical education. *Medical Education, 27*, 26–34.

Seo, H. Y., Lee, D. W., Nam, S., Cho, S. J., Yoon, J. Y., Hong, Y. C., & Lee, N. (2020). Burnout as a Mediator in the Relationship between Work-Life Balance and Empathy in Healthcare Professionals. *Psychiatry Investigation, 17*(9), 951–959. https://doi.org/10.30773/pi.2020.0147

Seo, J. W., Kyung, H. P., Ha, Y. P., Kyung, H. S., Song, Y. P., Tae, H. K., HyeRin, R., & Junho, C. (2016). Empathy and quality of life in Korean emergency physicians. *Journal of The Korean Society of Emergency Medicine, 27*(2), 150–156. http://www.jksem.org/journal/view.php?number=2020

Shallice, T. (2001). "Theory of Mind" and the prefrontal cortex. *Brain, 124*, 247–248.

Shamasundar, M. R. C. (1999). Reflections: Understanding empathy and related phenomena. *American Journal of Psychotherapy, 53*, 232–245.

Shamay-Tsoory, S. G., Tomer, R., Berger, B. D., & Aharon-Peretz, J. (2003). Characterization of empathy deficit following prefrontal brain damage: The role of the right ventromedial prefrontal cortex. *Cognitive Neuroscience, 15*, 324–337.

Shamay-Tsoory, S. G., Tomer, R., Goldsher, D., Berger, B. D., & Aharon-Peretz, J. (2004). Impairment in cognitive and affective empathy in patients with brain lesions: Anatomical and cognitive correlates. *Journal of Clinical and Experimental Neuropsychology, 26(8)*, 1113–1127. https://doi.org/10.1080/13803390490515531

Shapiro, A. K., & Shapiro, E. (1984). Patient-provider relationships and the placebo effect. In J. D. Matarazzo, S. M. Weiss, J. A. Herd, N. E. Miller, & S. M. Weiss (Eds.), *Behavioral health: A handbook of health enhancement and disease prevention* (pp. 371–383). Wiley-Interscience.

Shapiro, D. E., Boggs, S. R., Melamed, B. G., & Graham-Pole, J. (1992). The effect of varied physician affect on recall, anxiety, and perceptions in women at risk of breast cancer: An analogue study. *Health Psychology, 11*, 61–66.

Shapiro, J. (2002). How do physicians teach empathy in the primary care setting? *Academic Medicine, 77*, 323–328.

Shapiro, J., & Hunt, L. (2003). All the world's a stage: The use of theatrical performance in medical education. *Medical Education, 37*, 922–927.

Shapiro, J., Morrison, E., & Boker, J. (2004). Teaching empathy to first year medical students: Evaluation of an elective literature and medical course. *Education for Health, 17*, 73–84.

Shapiro, R. S., Simpson, D. E., & Lawrence, S. L. (1989). Survey of sued and non-sued physicians and suing patients. *Annals of Internal Medicine, 149*, 2190–2196.

Shapiro, T. (1974). The development and distortions of empathy. *Psychoanalytic Quarterly, 43*, 4–25.

Shapurian, R., & Hojat, M. (1985). Psychometric characteristics of a Persian version of the Eysenck Personality Questionnaire. *Psychological Reports, 57*, 631–639.

Shariat, S. V., & Habibi, M. (2013). Empathy in Iranian medical students: Measurement model of the Jefferson Scale of Empathy. *Medical Teacher, 35*(*1*), e913–e918. https://doi.org/10.3109/0142159X.2012.714881

Shariat, S. V., Eshtad, E., & Ansari, S. (2010). Empathy and its correlates in Iranian physicians: A preliminary psychometric study of the Jefferson Scale of Physician Empathy. *Medical Teacher, 32*(*10*), e417–e421. https://doi.org/10.3109/0142159X.2010.498488

Shariat, S. V., & Kaykhavoni, A. (2010). Empathy in medical residents at Iran University of Medical Sciences. *Iranian Journal of Psychiatry and Clinical Psychology, 16*, 248–256. http://ijpcp.iums.ac.ir/article-1-1090-en.html

Sharma, R., Sapkota, A., Acharya, A., Luintel, P., Paudel, L., Sharma, S., & Pradhan, S. N. (2022). A cross-sectional study on empathy and its association with stress in medical students. *International Journal of Occupational Safety and Health, 12*(3), 224–229. https://doi.org/10.3126/ijosh.v12i3.44432

Shaver, P., & Hazan, C. (1989). Being lonely, falling in love: Perspectives from attachment theory. In M. Hojat & R. Crandall (Eds.), *Loneliness: Theory, research, and applications* (pp. 105–124). Sage.

Sheehan, C. A., Perrin, K. O., Potter, M. L., Kazanowski, M. K., & Bennett, L. A. (2013). Engendering empathy in baccalaureate nursing students. *International Journal of Caring Sciences, 6*(*3*), 456–464. https://internationaljournalofcaringsciences.org/docs/19.%20Sheedan.pdf

Sheehan, K. H., Sheehan, D. V., White, K., Leibowitz, A., & Baldwin, D. C., Jr. (1990). A pilot study of medical student 'abuse': Student perceptions of mistreatment and misconduct in medical school. *Journal of the American Medical Association, 263*, 533–537.

Shelton, W. (1999). Can virtue be taught? *Academic Medicine, 74*, 671–674.

Sherif, C. W., Sherif, M., & Nebergall, R. E. (1965). *Attitudes and attitude change: The social judgment-involvement approach*. W.B. Saunders.

Sherman, J. J., & Cramer, A. (2005). Measurement of changes in empathy during dental school. *Journal of Dental Education, 69*(*3*), 338–345.

Sherman, J. J., & Cramer, A. P. (2010). Rebuttals to critics of studies of decline on empathy. *Academic Medicine, 85*(*12*), 1813–1814. https://doi.org/10.1097/ACM.0b013e3181fa3877

Sherrard, S. (2007). *Empathy in psychology interns and medical residents: An investigation of the cognitive and emotional components of empathy.* (Publication No. 3253152). [Doctoral dissertation, George Fox University]. ProQuest Dissertations & Theses Global. DAI-B 68/02.

Shirom, A., & Melamed, S. (2006). A comparison of the construct validity of two burnout measures in two groups of professionals. *International Journal of Stress Management, 13*(2), 176–200. https://doi.org/10.1037/1072-5245.13.2.176

Shorey, H. S., & Snyder, C. R. (2006). The role of adult attachment styles in psychopathology and psychotherapy outcomes. *Review of General Psychology, 10*(*1*), 1–20. https://doi.org/10.1037/1089-2680.10.1.1

Shorter, E. (1986). *Bedside manners: The troubled history of doctors and patients*. Viking.

Siegel, D. J. (1999). *The developing mind: How relationships and the brain interact to shape who we are*. Guilford.

Sieratzki, J. S., & Woll, B. (1996). Why do mothers cradle babies on their left? *Lancet, 347*, 1746–1748.

Sierles, F. S., Vergare, M., Hojat, M., & Gonnella, J. S. (2004). Academic performance of psychiatrists compared other specialists before, during, and after medical school. *American Journal of Psychiatry, 161*(*8*), 1477–1482. https://doi.org/10.1176/appi.ajp.161.8.1477

Silver, H. K. (1982). Medical students and medical school. *Journal of the American Medical Association, 247*, 309–310.

Silver, H. K., & Glicken, A. D. (1990). Medical student abuse: Incidence, severity, and significance. *Journal of the American Medical Association, 263*, 527–532.

Simmons, J. M. P., Robie, P. W., Kendrick, S. B., Schumacher, S., & Roberge, L. P. (1992). Residents' use of humanistic skills and content of resident discussions in a support group. *American Journal of the Medical Sciences, 303*, 227–232.

Simner, M. L. (1971). Newborn response to the cry of another infant. *Developmental Psychology, 5*, 136–140.

Simpson, M., Buckman, R., Stewart, M., Maguire, P., Kipkin, M., Novack, D., & Till, J. (1991). Doctor-patient communication: The Toronto consensus statement. *British Medical Journal, 303*, 1385–1387.

Sims, A. (1988). *Symptoms in the mind: An introduction to descriptive psychotherapy*. Baillier, Tindall, W.B. Saunders.

Singer, T., & Frith, C. (2005). The painful side of empathy. *Nature Neuroscience, 8(7)*, 845–846. https://doi.org/10.1038/nn0705-845

Singer, T., Seymour, B., O'Doherty, J., Kaube, H., Dolan, R. J., & Frith, C. D. (2004). Empathy for pain involves the affective but not sensory components of pain. *Science, 303(5661)*, 1157–1162. https://doi.org/10.1126/science.1093535

Singer, T., Seymour, B., O'Doherty, J., Stephan, K. E., Dolan, R. J., & Frith, C. (2006). Empathic neural responses are modulated by the perceived fairness of others. *Nature, 439(7075)*, 466–469. https://doi.org/10.1038/nature04271

Skeff, K. M., & Mutha, S. (1998). Role models: Guiding the future of medicine. *New England Journal of Medicine, 339*, 2015–2017.

Skelton, J. R., Macleod, J. A. A., & Thomas, C. P. (2000). Teaching literature and medicine to medical students: Part II. Why literature and medicine? *Lancet, 356*, 2001–2003.

Skogevall, S. (2023). *Telephone nurses' work with persons calling healthcare services frequently.* (Publication No. 30663515). [Doctoral dissertation, Malardalen University, Sweden]. ProQuest Dissertations & Theses Global. DAI-A 85/1(E).

Slipp, S. (2000). Subliminal stimulation research and its implications for psychoanalytic theory and treatment. *Journal of the American Academy of Psychoanalysis, 28*, 305–320.

Sloan, F. A., Mergenhagen, P. M., Burfield, W. B., Bovjerg, R. R., & Hassan, M. (1989). Medical malpractice experience of physicians: Predictable or haphazard? *Journal of the American Medical Association, 262*, 3291–3297.

Smith, B. H. (1981). Narrative versions, narrative theories. In W. J. T. Mitchell (Ed.), *On narrative* (pp. 209–232). University of Chicago Press.

Smith, G. R. (1991). *Somatization disorder in the medical setting*. American Psychiatric Press.

Smith, K. E., Norman, G. J., & Decety, J. (2017). The complexity of empathy during medical school training: evidence for positive changes. *Medical Education, 51*(11), 1146–1159. https://doi.org/10.1111/medu.13398

Smith, R. C. (1984). Teaching interviewing skills to medical students: The issue of countertransference. *Journal of Medical Education, 59*, 582–588.

Smolarz, B. G. (2005). *Determining the relationship between medical student empathy and undergraduate college major* (Publication No. 1459590). [Master's thesis, Albany Medical College] ProQuest Dissertations & Theses Global. MAI 47/02M.

Smotherman, W. P., & Robinson, S. R. (1994). Milk as the proximal mechanism for behavioral change in the newborn. *Acta Pædiatrica Scandinavica, 397*, 64–70.

Smyth, J., Stone, A., Hurewitz, A., & Kaell, A. (1999). Effects of writing about stressful experiences on symptom reduction in patients with asthma or rheumatoid arthritis: A randomized trial. *Journal of the American Medical Association, 281*, 1304–1309.

Sng, G., Tung, J., Ping, Y. S., Lee, S. S., Win, M. T., Hooi, S. C., & Samarasekera, D. D. (2016). Complex and novel determinants of empathy change in medical students. *Korean Journal of Medical Education, 28*(1), 67–78. https://doi.org/10.3946/kjme.2016.11

Sochting, I., Skoe, E. E., & Marcia, J. E. (1994). Care-oriented moral reasoning and prosocial behavior: A question of gender role orientation. *Sex Roles, 31*, 131–147.

Soenens, B., Duriez, B., Vansteenkiste, M., & Goossens, L. (2007). The intergeneration transmission of empathy-related responding in adolescence: The role of maternal support. *Personality and Social Psychology Bulletin, 33(3)*, 299–311. https://doi.org/10.1177/0146167206296300
Soler-Gonzalez, J., San-Martín, M., Delgado-Bolton, R., & Vivanco, L. (2017). Human connections and their roles in the occupational well-being of healthcare professionals: A study on loneliness and empathy. *Frontiers in Psychology, 8*, 1475. https://doi.org/10.3389/fpsyg.2017.01475
Solomon, R. C. (1976). *The passion*. Anchor/Doubleday.
Sommer, R. (1969). *Personal space*. Prentice-Hall.
Soncini, F., Silvestrini, G., Poscia, A., Clorba, V., Conti, A., Murru, C., & Ziglio, A. (2013). Public health physicians and empathy: Are we really empathic? The Jefferson Scale applied to Italian resident doctors in public health. *European Journal of Public Health, 23*(Suppl. 1), 264–265. https://doi.org/10.1093/eurpub/ckt124.068
Sorce, J. F., Emde, R. N., Campos, J., & Klinnert, M. D. (1985). Maternal emotional signaling: Its effect on the visual cliff behavior of 1-year-olds. *Developmental Psychology, 21*, 195–200.
Sotile, W. M., & Sotile, M. O. (1996). *The medical marriage: A couple's survival manual*. Carol Publication.
Souror, Y. R., Aljehani, D. K., & Alshaikh, M. H. (2020). Empathy of dental students towards children after behaviour guidance lectures and clinical experience. *European Journal of Dental Education: Official Journal of the Association for Dental Education in Europe, 24*(3), 458–464. https://doi.org/10.1111/eje.12523
Southard, E. E. (1918). The empathic index in the diagnosis of mental diseases. *Journal of Abnormal Psychology, 13*, 199–214.
Sox, H. C. (2002). Medical professionalism in the new millennium: A physician charter. *Annals of Internal Medicine, 136*, 243–246.
Speedling, E. J., & Rose, D. N. (1985). Building an effective doctor-patient relationship: From patient satisfaction to patient participation. *Social Science & Medicine, 21*, 115–120.
Spelke, E. S. (2005). Sex differences in intrinsic aptitude for mathematics and science? A critical review. *American Psychologist, 60*(9), 950–958. https://doi.org/10.1037/0003-066X.60.9.950
Spiegel, D. (1990). Can psychotherapy prolong cancer survival? *Psychosomatics, 31*, 361–366.
Spiegel, D. (1993). *Living beyond limits: New hope and help for facing life-threatening illness*. Times Books.
Spiegel, D. (1994). Health caring: Psychological support for patients with cancer. *Cancer, 74*, 1453–1457.
Spiegel, D. (2004). Mind matters—Group therapy and survival in breast cancer. *The New England Journal of Medicine, 345(24)*, 1767–1768. https://doi.org/10.1056/NEJM200112133452409
Spiegel, D., & Bloom, J. R. (1983). Group therapy and hypnosis reduce metastatic breast carcinoma pain. *Psychosomatic Medicine, 45*, 333–339.
Spiegel, D., Bloom, J. R., Kraemer, H. C., & Gottheil, E. (1989). Effect of psychosocial treatment on survival of patients with metastatic breast cancer. *Lancet, 2*, 888–891.
Spiegel, D., Bloom, J. R., & Yalom, I. D. (1981). Group support for patients with metastatic breast cancer. *Archives of General Psychiatry, 38*, 527–533.
Spinella, M. (2002). A relationship between smell identification and empathy. *International Journal of Neuroscience, 112*, 605–612.
Spiro, H. (1992). What is empathy and can it be taught? *Annals of Internal Medicine, 116*, 843–846.
Spiro, H. (1998). *The power of hope: A doctor's perspective*. Yale University Press.
Spiro, H. (2009). Commentary: The practice of empathy. *Academic Medicine, 84(9)*, 1177–1179. https://doi.org/10.1097/ACM.0b013e3181b18934
Spiro, H. M. (1986). *Doctors, patients and placebos*. Yale University Press.
Spiro, H. M., McCrea Curnen, M. G. M., Peschel, E., & St. James, D. (1993). *Empathy and the practice of medicine: Beyond pills and the scalpel*. Yale University Press.
Spreng, R. N., McKinnon, M. C., Mar, R. A., & Levine, B. (2009). The Toronto Empathy Questionnaire: Scale development and initial validation of a factor analytic solution to

multiple empathy measures. *Journal of Personality Assessment, 91*(1), 62–71. https://doi.org/10.1080/00223890802484381

Squier, R. W. (1990). A model of empathic understanding and adherence to treatment regimens in practitioner-patient relationships. *Social Science & Medicine, 30*, 325–339.

Srivastava, A. K., Tiwari, K., Vyas, S., Semwal, J., & Kandpal, S. D. (2017). Teaching clinical empathy to undergraduate medical students of Dehradun: A quasi-experimental study. *Indian Journal of Community Health, 29*(3), 258–263. https://doi.org/10.47203/IJCH.2017.v29i03.008

Stamps, P. L., & Boley Cruz, N. T. (1994). *Issues in physician satisfaction: New perspectives*. Health Administration Press.

Stansfield, R. B., Schwartz, A., O'Brien, C. L., Dekhtyar, M., Dunham, L., & Quirk, M. (2016). Development of a metacognitive effort construct of empathy during clinical training: A longitudinal study of the factor structure of the Jefferson Scale of Empathy. *Advances in Health Sciences Education : Theory and Practice, 21*, 5–17. https://doi.org/10.1007/s10459-015-9605-1

Starcevic, V., & Piontek, C. M. (1997). Empathic understanding revisited: Conceptualization, controversies, and limitations. *American Journal of Psychotherapy, 51*, 317–328.

Starfield, B., Wray, C., Hess, K., Gross, R., Birk, P., & D'Lugoff, B. (1981). The influence of patient-practitioner agreement on outcome of care. *American Journal of Public Health, 71*, 127–131.

Starr, J. A., Holmes, M. B., Riley, E., McDonnell, B., Driscoll, L., Camarinos, J., Grabowska, W., & Harbaugh, A. G. (2020). A Quantitative Measurement of Physical Therapists' Empathy and Exploration of the Relationship With Practice Setting and Work Engagement. *Evaluation & the Health Professions, 43*(4), 255–263. https://doi.org/10.1177/0163278719864687

Starr, P. (1982). *Social transformation of American medicine*. Basic Books.

Staub, E. (1978). *Positive social behavior and morality: Social and personal influences* (Vol. 1). Academic Press.

Staudenmayer, H., & Lefkowitz, M. S. (1981). Physician-patient psychological characteristics influencing medical decision-making. *Social Science & Medicine, 15*, 77–81.

Stebbins, C. A. (2005). *Enhancing empathy in medical students using FLEX Care™ communication training*. (Publication No. 3172245). [Doctoral dissertation, Iowa State University]. ProQuest Dissertations & Theses Global. DAI-A 81/1(E).

Stein, M. D., Fleisman, J., Mor, V., & Dresser, M. (1993). Factors associated with patient satisfaction among HIV-infected persons. *Medical Care, 31*, 182–188.

Steinbrook, R. (2002). Nursing in the crossfire. *New England Journal of Medicine, 346*, 1757–1766.

Steiner, J. F. (2005). The use of stories in clinical research and health policy. *Journal of the American Medical Association, 294*(22), 2901–2904. https://doi.org/10.1001/jama.294.22.2901

Stephan, W. G., & Finlay, K. (1999). The role of empathy in improving inter-group relations. *Journal of Social Issues, 55*, 729–743.

Stepien, K. A., & Baernstien, A. (2006). Educating for empathy: A review. *Journal of General Internal Medicine, 21*(5), 524–530. https://doi.org/10.1111/j.1525-1497.2006.00443.x

Ster, M. P., Ster, B., Petek, D., & Gorup, E. C. (2014). Validation of Slovenian version of Jefferson Scale of Empathy for students. *Slovenian Journal of Public Health, 53*(1), 89–100. https://doi.org/10.2478/sjph-2014-0010

Stern, D. (1985). *The interpersonal world of the infant: A view from psychoanalysis and developmental psychology*. Basic Books.

Stern, D. T., Frohna, A. Z., & Gruppen, L. D. (2005). The prediction of professional behaviour. *Medical Education, 39*(1), 75–82. https://doi.org/10.1111/j.1365-2929.2004.02035.x

Stern, J. A., & Cassidy, J. (2018). Empathy from infancy to adolescence: An attachment perspective on the development of individual differences. *Developmental Review, 47*, 1–22. https://doi.org/10.1016/j.dr.2017.09.002

Stern, J.A., Baily, N. A., Castello, M. A., Hellwin, A. F., Mitchell, J., & Allen, J. P. (2024). Empathy across three generations: From maternal and peer support in adolescence to adult parenting and child outcomes. *Child Development, 95*(5), 1628–1640. https://doi.org/10.1111/cdev.14109

Stern, J. A., Castello, M. A., Kansky, J., Fowler, C., Loeb, E. L., & Allen, J. P. (2021). Here for you: Attachment and growth of empathic support for friends in adolescence. *Child Development, 92(6)*, e1326–e1341. https://doi.org/10.1111/cdev.13630

Sternberg, R. J. (2004). Culture and intelligence. *American Psychologist, 59*, 325–338.

Stewart, M. A. (1996). Effective physician-patient communication and health outcomes: A review. *Canadian Medical Association Journal, 152*, 1423–1433.

Stewart-Williams, S., & Thomas, A. G. (2013). The ape that thought it was a peacock: Does evolutionary psychology exaggerate human sex differences? *Psychological Inquiry, 24(3)*, 137–168. https://doi.org/10.1080/1047840X.2013.804899

Stiles, W., Putman, S., Wolfe, M., & James, S. (1979). Interaction exchange structure and patient satisfaction with medical interview. *Medical Care, 17*, 667–679.

Stokes, J. (1980). Grief and the performing arts: A brief experiment in humanistic medical education. *Journal of Medical Education, 55*, 215.

Stotland, E. (1969). Exploratory investigation of empathy. In L. Berkowitz (Ed.), *Advances in experimental social psychology* (pp. 271–314). Academic Press.

Stotland, E. (1978). Fantasy-empathy research: An integration. In E. Stotland, K. E. Matthews Jr., S. E. Sherman, R. O. Hansson, & B. Z. Richardson (Eds.), *Empathy, fantasy, and helping* (pp. 103–122). Sage.

Stotland, E., Mathews, K. E., Jr., Sherman, S. E., Hansson, R. O., & Richardson, B. Z. (1978). *Empathy, fantasy and helping* (Vol. 65). Sage.

Strauss, M. B. (1968). *Familiar medical quotations*. Little, Brown.

Street, R. L., Makoul, G., Arora, N. K., & Epstein, R. M. (2009). How does communication heal? Pathways linking clinician-patient communication to health outcomes. *Patient Education and Counseling, 74*(3), 295–301. https://doi.org/10.1016/j.pec.2008.11.015

Streit, U. (1980). Attitudes toward psycho-social factors in medicine: An appraisal of the ATSIM scale. *Medical Education, 14*, 259–266.

Streit-Forest, U. (1982). Differences in empathy: A preliminary analysis. *Journal of Medical Education, 57*, 65–67.

Stuss, D. T. (2001). The right frontal lobes are necessary for theory of mind. *Brain, 124*, 279–286.

Su, R., Rounds, J., & Armstrong, P. I. (2009). Men and things, women and people: A meta-analysis of sex differences in interests. *Psychological Bulletin, 135*(6), 859–884. https://doi.org/10.1037/a0017364

Suchman, A. L., Markakis, K., Beckman, H. B., & Frankel, R. (1997). A model of empathic communication in the medical interview. *Journal of the American Medical Association, 277*, 678–682.

Suh, D. H., Hong, J. S., Lee, D. H., Gonnella, J. S., & Hojat, M. (2012). The Jefferson Scale of Physician Empathy: A preliminary psychometric study and group comparisons in Korean physicians. *Medical Teacher, 34*(6), e464–e468. https://doi.org/10.3109/0142159X.2012.668632

Sullivan, P. (1990). Pay more attention to your own health, physicians warned. *Canadian Medical Association Journal, 142*, 1309–1310.

Sultan, S., Attali, C., Gilberg, S., Zenasni, F., & Hartemann, A. (2011). Physicians' understanding of patients' personal representations of their diabetes: Accuracy and association with self-care. *Psychology and Health, 26(Suppl 1), 101–117.* https://doi.org/10.1080/08870441003703226

Sulzer, S. H., Feinstein, N. W., & Wendland, C. L. (2016). Assessing empathy development in medical education: a systematic review. *Medical Education, 50*(3), 300–310. https://doi.org/10.1111/medu.12806

Sundling, V., Dulmen, S., & Eide, H. (2016). Communication self-efficacy in optometry: the mediating role of mindfulness. *Scandinavian Journal of Optometry and Visual Science, 9*(2), 8–12. https://doi.org/10.5384/sjovs.vol9i2p8-12

Suppiah Cavert, M. (2020). *Continuing medical education (CME): an exploration of method in teaching empathy to first year residents in a Singapore hospital.* (Publication No. 28018299). [Doctoral dissertation, The University of Liverpool, United Kingdom]. ProQuest Dissertations & Theses Global. DAI-A 81/12(E).

Surbone, A. (1992). Truth telling to the patient. *Journal of American Medical Association, 268*, 1661–1662.

Surrey, J. L., & Bergman, S. J. (1994). Gender differences in rational development: Implications for empathy in the doctor-patient relationship. In L. S. More & M. A. Milligan (Eds.), *The empathic practitioner: Empathy, gender, and medicine* (pp. 113–131). Rutgers University Press.

Sutherland, J. A. (1993). The nature and evolution of phenomenological empathy in nursing: An historical treatment. *Archives of Psychiatric Nursing, 7*, 369–376.

Swain, J. E., Lorberlaum, J. P., Kose, S., & Strathearn, L. (2007). Brain basis of early parent-infant interactions: Psychology, physiology, and in vivo functional neuroimaging studies. *Journal of Child Psychology and Psychiatry, 48*(3-4), 262–287. https://doi.org/10.1111/j.1469-7610.2007.01731.x

Szalita, A. B. (1976). Some thoughts on empathy. The eighteenth annual Frieda Fromm-Reichmann memorial lecture. *Psychiatry, 39*, 142–152.

Tai, Y. F., Scherfler, C., Brooks, D. J., Sawamoto, N., & Castiello, U. (2004). The human premotor cortex is 'mirror' only for biological actions. *Current Biology, 14*(2), 117–120. https://doi.org/10.1016/j.cub.2004.01.005

Takooshian, H. (2014). Fifty years later: What have we learnt from the 1964 Kitty Genovese tragedy? *The General Psychologist, 49*(1–2), p1-2, p34. https://assets.ctfassets.net/z36oungqq8ay/5Q2rY8eMe3TzPxI2vKPJY5/5a182163379e4ddc4bf623ac395ed6c9/Vol49_Issue1_2015.pdf

Tamayo, C. A., Rizkalla, M. N., & Henderson, K. K. (2016). Cognitive, behavioral and emotional empathy in pharmacy students: targeting programs for curriculum modification. *Frontiers in Pharmacology, 7*, 96. https://doi.org/10.3389/fphar.2016.00096

Tamsukhin, S. M. (2022). *Measuring empathy of undergraduate dietetics students at two southwestern Ohio universities.* (Publication No. 29704808). [Doctoral dissertation, University of Cincinnati]. ProQuest Dissertations & Theses Global. DAI-B 84/3(E).

Tannen. (1990). *You just don't understand: Women and men in conversation.* Ballantine.

Taragin, M. I., Sonnenberg, F. A., Karns, M. E., Trout, R., Shapiro, S., & Carson, J. L. (1994). Does physician performance explain interspecialty differences in malpractice claim rates? *Medical Care, 32*, 661–667.

Tausch, R. (1988). The relationship between emotions and cognitions: Implications for therapist empathy. *Person-Centered Review, 3*, 277–291.

Tavakol, S., Dennick, R., & Tavakol, M. (2011a). Empathy in UK medical students: Differences by gender, medical year and specialty interest. *Education for Primary Care, 22*(5), 297–303. https://doi.org/10.1080/14739879.2011.11494022

Tavakol, S., Dennick, R., & Tavakol, M. (2011b). Psychometric properties and confirmatory factor analysis of the Jefferson Scale of Physician Empathy. *BMC Medical Education, 11*, 54. https://doi.org/10.1186/1472-6920-11-54

Taylor, S. E., Klein, L. C., Gruenewald, T. L., Gurung, R. A. R., & Fernandes-Taylor, S. (2003). Affiliation, social support and biobehavioral response to stress. In J. Suls & K. A. Wallston (Eds.), *Social psychological foundations of health and illness* (pp. 314–331). Blackwell.

Taylor, S. E., Klein, L. C., Lewis, B. P., Gruenewald, T. L., Gurung, R. A., Regan, A. R., & Updegraff, J. (2000). Biobehavioral responses to stress in females: Tend-and-befriend, not fight-or-flight. *Psychological Review, 107*(3), 411–429. https://doi.org/10.1037/0033-295x.107.3.411

Therrien, M. E. (1979). Evaluating empathy skills training for parents. *Social Work, 24*, 417–419.

Thom, D. H., Hall, M. A., & Pawlson, L. G. (2004). Measuring patients' trust in physicians when assessing quality of care. *Health affairs (Project Hope), 23*(4), 124–132. https://doi.org/10.1377/hlthaff.23.4.124

Thomas, L. (1985). *The youngest science*. Oxford University Press.

Thompson, B. M., Hearn, G. N., & Collins, M. J. (1992). Patient perceptions of health professional interpersonal skills. *Australian Psychologist, 27*, 91–95.

Thorndike, E. L. (1926). *The measurement of intelligence*. Teacher's College, Columbia University.

Tisdale, C. E., Black, A. C., Jain, S., Lowther, E., Madeline, L., Troup, C., Nathaniel, T., & Fowler, L. A. (2020). The Impact of Meeting Patients with Neurological Disorders on Medical

Student Empathy. *Medical Science Educator, 30*(4), 1561–1568. https://doi.org/10.1007/s40670-020-01102-z

Titchener, E. B. (1909). *Lectures on the experimental psychology of the thought-processes*. Macmillan.

Titchener, E. B. (1915). *A beginner's psychology*. Macmillan.

Tomkins, S. S. (1962). *Affect, imagery, consciousness: I. The positive effects*. Springer.

Tomkins, S. S. (1963). *Affect, imagery, consciousness: II. The negative effects*. Springer.

Tomkins, S. S. (1987). Script theory. In J. Aronoff, A. J. Rubin, & R. A. Zucker (Eds.), *The emergence of personality* (pp. 147–216). Springer.

Tooby, J., & Cosmides, L. (1990). On the universality of human nature and the uniqueness of the individual: The role of genetic and adaptation. *Journal of Personality, 58*, 17–67.

Tranel, D., Bechara, A., & Denburg, N. L. (2002). Asymmetric functional roles of right and left ventromedial prefrontal cortices in social conduct, decision-making, and emotional processing. *Cortex, 38*, 589–612.

Trautmann Banks, J. (2002). The story inside. In R. Charon & M. Montello (Eds.), *Stories matter: The role of narrative in medical ethics* (pp. 219–226). Routledge.

Triandis, H. C. (1995). *Individualism & collectivism*. Westview Press.

Trivers, R. L. (1972). Parental investment and sexual selection. In B. Campbell (Ed.), *Sexual selection and the descent of man* (pp. 136–179). Aldine.

Trommsdorff, G. (1991). Child-rearing and children's empathy. *Perceptual & Motor Skills, 72*, 387–390.

Trommsdorff, G. (1995). Person-context relations as developmental conditions for empathy and prosocial action: A cross-cultural analysis. In T. A. Kindermann & J. Valsiner (Eds.), *Development of person-context relations* (pp. 189–208). Erlbaum.

Tronick, E., Als, H., Adamson, L., Wise, S., & Brazelton, T. B. (1978). The infant's response to entrapment between contradictory messages in face-to-face interaction. *Journal of the American Academy of Child Psychiatry, 17*, 1–13.

Trout, D. L., & Rosenfeld, H. M. (1980). The effect of postural lean and body congruence on the judgment of psychotherapeutic rapport. *Journal of Nonverbal Behavior, 4*, 176–190.

Trout, J. D. (2010). *Why empathy matters: The science and psychology of better judgment*. Penguin.

Truax, C. B., Altmann, H., & Millis, W. A. (1974). Therapeutic relationships provided by various professionals. *Journal of Community Psychology, 2*, 33–36.

Truax, C. B., & Carkhuff, R. (1967). *Towards effective counseling and psychotherapy: Training and practice*. Aldine.

Tucker, D., Luu, P., & Derryberry, D. (2005). Love hurts: The evolution of empathic concern through the encephalization of nociceptive capacity. *Development and Psychopathology, 17*(3), 699–713. https://doi.org/10.1017/S0954579405050339

Turner, J. A., Deyo, R. A., Loeser, J. D., von Korff, M., & Fordyce, W. E. (1994). The importance of placebo effect on pain treatment and research. *Journal of the American Medical Association, 271*, 1609–1614.

Twenge, J. M. (1997). Changes in masculine and feminine traits over time: A meta-analysis. *Sex Roles, 36*, 305–325. https://doi.org/10.1007/BF02766650

Uchino, B. N., Cacioppo, J. T., & Kiecolt-Glaser, J. K. (1996). The relationship between social support system and physiological processes: A review with emphasis on underlying mechanisms and implications for health. *Psychological Bulletin, 119*, 488–531.

Umilta, M. A., Kohler, E., Gallese, V., Fogassi, L., Fadiga, L., Keysers, C., & Rizzolatti, G. (2001). I know what you are doing: A neurophysiological study. *Neuron, 31*, 155–165.

Underwood, B., & Moore, B. (1982). Perspective-taking and altruism. *Psychological Bulletin, 91*, 143–173.

Uvnas-Moberg, K. (1997). Physiological and endocrine effects of social contact. *Annals of the New York Academy of Sciences, 807*, 146–163.

Valeriani, M., Betti, V., Le Pera, D., De Armas, L., Miliucci, R., Restuccia, D., Avenanti, A., & Aglioti, S. M. (2008). Seeing the pain of others while being in pain: a laser-evoked potentials study. *NeuroImage, 40*(3), 1419–1428. https://doi.org/10.1016/j.neuroimage.2007.12.056

Vallabh, K. (2011). Psychometrics of the student version of the Jefferson Scale of Physician Empathy (JSPE-S) in final-year medical students in Johannesburg in 2008. *South African Journal of Bioethics and Law, 4*, 63–68. http://www.sajbl.org.za/index.php/sajbl/article/view/164/140

Valliant, G. E. (1977). *Adaptation to life*. Little, Brown.

Van Honk, J., Schutter, D., Bos, P., Kruijt, A., Lentjes, E., & Baron-Cohen, S. (2011). Testosterone administration impairs cognitive empathy in women depending on second-to-fourth digit ratio. *Proceedings of the National Academy of Sciences of the United States of America, 108*(8), 3448–3452. https://doi.org/10.1073/pnas.1011891108

Van Orum, W., Foley, J. M., Burns, P. R., DeWolfe, A. S., & Kennedy, E. C. (1981). Empathy, altruism, and self-interest in college students. *Adolescence, 16*, 799–808.

Van Winkle, L. J., Bjork, B. C., Chandar, N., Cornell, S., Fjortoft, N., Green, J. M., La Salle, S., Lynch, S. M., Viselli, S. M., & Burdick, P. (2012a). Interprofessional workshop to improve mutual understanding between pharmacy and medical students. *American Journal of Pharmaceutical Education, 76*(8), 150. https://doi.org/10.5688/ajpe768150

Van Winkle, L. J., Burdick, P., Bjork, B. C., Chandar, N., Green, J. M., Lynch, S. M., & Robson, C. (2014). Critical thinking and reflection on community service for a medical biochemistry course raise students' empathy, patient-centered orientation, and examination scores. *Medical Science Educator, 24*, 279–290. https://doi.org/10.1007/s40670-014-0049-7

Van Winkle, L. J., Fjortoft, N., & Hojat, M. (2011). Validation of an instrument to measure pharmacy and medical students' attitudes toward physician-pharmacist collaboration. *American Journal of Pharmaceutical Education, 75*(9), 178. https://doi.org/10.5688/ajpe759178

Van Winkle, L. J., Fjortoft, N., & Hojat, M. (2012b). Impact of a workshop about aging on the empathy scores of pharmacy and medical students. *American Journal of Pharmaceutical Education, 76*(1), 9. https://doi.org/10.5688/ajpe7619

Van Winkle, L. J., La Salle, S., Richardson, L., Bjork, B. C., Burdick, P., Chandar, N., Green, J. M., Lynch, S. M., Robson, C., & Viselli, S. M. (2013). Challenging medical students to confront their biases: A case study simulation approach. *Medical Science Educator, 23*, 217–224. https://doi.org/10.1007/BF03341624

Van Zanten, M., Boulet, J. R., Norcini, J., & McKinley, D. (2005). Using standardised patient assessment to measure professional attributes. *Medical Education, 39*, 20–29. https://doi.org/10.1111/j.1365-2929.2004.02029.x

Varkey, P., Chutka, D. S., & Lesnick, T. G. (2006). The aging game: Improving medical students' attitudes toward caring for the elderly. *Journal of the American Medical Directors Association, 7*(4), 224–229. https://doi.org/10.1016/j.jamda.2005.07.009

Vaughan, K. B., & Lanzetta, J. T. (1981). The effect of modification of expressive displays on vicarious emotional arousal. *Journal of Experimental Social Psychology, 17*, 16–30.

Velicer, W. F., & Fava, J. L. (1998). Effects of variables and subject sampling on factor pattern recovery. *Psychological Methods, 3*, 231–251.

Veloski, J. J., & Hojat, M. (2006). Measuring specific elements of professionalism: Empathy, teamwork, and lifelong learning. In D. T. Stern (Ed.), *Measuring Medical Professionalism* (pp. 117–145). Oxford University Press.

Verbrugge, L. M. (1979). Marital status and health. *Journal of Marriage and the Family, 41*, 267–285.

Verweij, H., Waumans, R. C., Smeijers, D., Lucassen, P. L., Donders, A. R., van der Horst, H. E., & Speckens, A. E. (2016). Mindfulness-based stress reduction for GPs: results of a controlled mixed methods pilot study in Dutch primary care. *The British Journal of General Practice: The Journal of the Royal College of General Practitioners, 66*(643), e99–e105. https://doi.org/10.3399/bjgp16X683497

Viviani, P. (2002). Motor competence in the perception of dynamic events: A tutorial. In W. Prinz & B. Hommel (Eds.), *Common mechanisms in perception and action* (pp. 406–442). Oxford University Press.

Voinescu, B. I., Szentagotai, A., & Coogan, A. (2009). Residents' clinical empathy: Gender and specialty comparisons—A Romanian study. *Acta Medica Academica, 38*(1), 11–15. https://www.ama.ba/index.php/ama/article/view/50

Vossen, H. G. M., Piotrowski, J. T., & Valkenburg, P. M. (2015). Development the adolescent measure of empathy and sympathy (AMES). *Personality and Individual Differences, 74*, 66–71. https://doi.org/10.1016/j.paid.2014.09.040

Voyer, D., Voyer, S., & Bryden, M. P. (1995). Magnitude of sex differences in spatial abilities: A meta-analysis and consideration of critical variables. *Psychological Bulletin, 117*(2), 250–270. https://doi.org/10.1037/0033-2909.117.2.250

Wagner, H. L., Buck, R., & Winterbotham, M. (1993). Communication of specific emotions: Gender differences in sending accuracy and communication measures. *Journal of Nonverbal Behavior, 17*, 29–53.

Wagoner, N. E., Suriano, J. R., & Stoner, J. A. (1986). Factors used by program directors to select residents. *Journal of Medical Education, 61*, 10–21.

Wahjudi, J. W., Findyartini, A., & Kaligis, F. (2019). The relationship between empathy and stress: a cross-sectional study among undergraduate medical students. *Korean Journal of Medical Education, 31*(3), 215–226. https://doi.org/10.3946/kjme.2019.132

Waisman, M. (1966). Listening with the third ear in eczematous eruptions. *Medical Times, 94*, 1108–1113.

Wallace, D. S., Paulson, R. M., Lord, C. G., & Bond, C. F., Jr. (2005). Which behaviors do attitudes predict? Meta-analyzing the effects of social pressure and perceived difficulty. *Review of General Psychology, 9(3)*, 214–227. https://doi.org/10.1037/1089-2680.9.3.214

Walton, H. J. (1987). Personality assessment of future doctors. *Journal of the Royal Society of Medicine, 80*, 27–30.

Wang, C., Wu, Q., Feng, M., Wan, Q., & Wu, X. (2017). International Nursing: Research on the correlation between empathy and China's Big Five Personality Theory: Implications for nursing leaders. *Nursing Administration Quarterly, 41*(2), E1–E10. https://doi.org/10.1097/NAQ.0000000000000219

Wang, C. X. Y., Pavlova, A., Boggiss, A. L., O'Callaghan, A., & Consedine, N. S. (2023). Predictors of Medical Students' Compassion and Related Constructs: A Systematic Review. *Teaching and Learning in Medicine, 35*(5), 502–513. https://doi.org/10.1080/10401334.2022.2103816

Ward, J., Cody, J., Schaal, M., & Hojat, M. (2012). The empathy enigma: An empirical study of decline in empathy among undergraduate nursing students. *Journal of Professional Nursing, 28(1)*, 34–40. https://doi.org/10.1016/j.profnurs.2011.10.007

Ward, J., Schaal, M., Sullivan, J., Bowen, M. E., Erdmann, J. B., & Hojat, M. (2008). The Jefferson Scale of Attitudes toward Physician-Nurse Collaboration: A study with undergraduate nursing students. *Journal of Interprofessional Care, 22(4)*, 375–386. https://doi.org/10.1080/13561820802190533

Ward, J., Schaal, M., Sullivan, J., Bowen, M. E., Erdmann, J. B., & Hojat, M. (2009). Reliability and validity of the Jefferson Scale of Empathy in undergraduate nursing students. *Journal of Nursing Measurement, 17*(1), 73–88. https://doi.org/10.1891/1061-3749.17.1.73

Wasserman, R. C., Inui, T. S., Barriatua, R. D., Carter, W. B., & Lippincott, P. (1984). Pediatric clinicians' support for patients makes a difference: An outcome-based analysis of clinician-parent interaction. *Pediatrics, 74*, 1047–1053.

Watson, J. B. (1924). *Behaviorism*. W.W. Norton.

Watson, J. C. (2002). Re-visioning empathy. In D. Cain & J. Seeman (Eds.), *Humanistic psychotherapies: Handbook of research and practice* (pp. 445–471). American Psychological Association.

Watson, P. J., Grisham, S. O., Trotter, M. V., & Biderman, M. D. (1984). Narcissism and empathy: Validity evidence for the Narcissistic Personality Inventory. *Journal of Personality Assessment, 48*, 301–305.

Watts, D. (2012). Cure for the common cold. *New England Journal of Medicine, 367*, 1184–1185.

Waxler-Morrison, N., Anderson, J. M., & Richardson, E. (1990). *Cross-cultural caring: A handbook for health professionals in Western Canada*. University of British Columbia Press.

Wear, D., & Aultman, J. M. (2005). The limits of narrative: Medical student resistance to confronting inequality and oppression in literature and beyond. *Medical Education, 39(10)*, 1056–1065. https://doi.org/10.1111/j.1365-2929.2005.02270.x

Wear, D., & Nixon, L. L. (2002). Literary inquiry and professional development in medicine: Against abstraction. *Perspectives in Biology and Medicine, 45*, 104–124.

Weaver, M. J., Ow, C. L., Walker, D. J., & Degenhardt, E. F. (1993). A questionnaire for patients' evaluations of their physicians' humanistic behaviors. *Journal of General Internal Medicine, 8*, 135–139.

Webb, C. (1996). Caring, curing, coping: Toward an integrated model. *Journal of Advanced Nursing, 23*, 960.

Weijters, B., Baumgartner, H., & Schillewaert, N. (2013). Reversed item bias: An integrated model. *Psychological Methods, 18*(3), 320–334. https://doi.org/10.1037/a0032121

Weinberg, M. K., & Tronik, E. Z. (1996). Infant affective reaction to the resumption of maternal interaction after the still-face. *Child Development, 67*, 905–914.

Weinberg, M. K., Tronick, E. Z., & Cohn, J. F. (1999). Gender differences in emotional expressivity and self-regulation during early infancy. *Developmental Psychology, 35*, 175–188.

Weisman, C. S., & Teitlebaum, M. A. (1985). Physician gender and the physician-patient relationship: Recent evidence and relevant questions. *Social Science & Medicine, 20*, 1119–1127.

Weiss, R. F., Boyer, J. L., Lombardo, J. P., & Stich, M. H. (1973). Altruistic drive and altruistic reinforcement. *Journal of Personality and Social Psychology, 25*, 390–400.

Weisse, C. S., Melekis, K., & Hutchins, B. (2019). Providing end-of-life care: Increased empathy and self-efficacy among student caregivers in residential homes for the dying. *The American Journal of Hospice & Palliative Care, 36*(6), 538–545. https://doi.org/10.1177/1049909118820844

Weissman, J. S., Betancourt, J., Campbell, E. G., Park, E. R., Kim, M., Clarridge, B., Blumenthal, D., Lee, K. C., & Maina, A. W. (2005). Resident physicians' preparedness to provide cross-cultural care. *Journal of the American Medical Association, 294*(9), 1058–1067. https://doi.org/10.1001/jama.294.9.1058

Weissman, S. H., Haynes, R. A., Killan, C. D., & Robinowitz, C. (1994). A model to determine the influence of medical school on students' career choices. *Academic Medicine, 69*, 58–59.

Wellman, B. (1998). Social network. In H. S. Friedman (Ed.), *Encyclopedia of mental health* (pp. 525–544). Academic Press.

Wellman, H. (1991). *The child's theory of mind*. Bradford Books/MIT Press.

Wen, D., Ma, X., Li, H., Liu, Z., Xian, B., & Liu, Y. (2013a). Empathy in Chinese medical students: Psychometric characteristics and differences by gender and year of medical education. *BMC Medical Education, 13*, 130. https://doi.org/10.1186/1472-6920-13-130

Wen, D., Ma, X., Li, H., & Xian, B. (2013b). Empathy in Chinese physicians: Preliminary psychometrics of the Jefferson Scale of Physician Empathy (JSE) [Letter to the editor]. *Medical Teacher, 35*, 609–610.

Weng, H. C., Steed, J. F., Yu, S. W., Liu, Y. T., Hsu, C. C., Yu, T. J., & Chen, W. (2011). The effect of surgeon empathy and emotional intelligence on patient satisfaction. *Advances in Health Sciences Education, 16*, 591–600. https://doi.org/10.1007/s10459-011-9278-3

Werner, A., & Schneider, J. M. (1974). Teaching medical students interactional skills: A research-based course in doctor-patient relationship. *New England Journal of Medicine, 290*, 1232–1237.

West, C. P., Dyrbye, L. N., Rabatin, J. T., Call, T. G., Davidson, J. H., Multari, A., Romanski, S. A., Hellyer, J. M., Sloan, J. A., & Shanafelt, T. D. (2014). Intervention to promote physician well-being, job satisfaction, and professionalism: A randomized clinical trial. *JAMA Internal Medicine, 174*(4), 527–533. https://doi.org/10.1001/jamainternmed.2013.14387

West, C. P., Huschka, M. M., Novotny, P. J., Sloan, J. A., Kolars, J. C., Habermann, T. M., & Shanafelt, T. D. (2006). Association of perceived medical errors with resident distress and empathy. *Journal of American Medical Association, 296*(9), 1071–1078. https://doi.org/10.1001/jama.296.9.1071

West, C. P., Tan, A. D., Habermann, T. M., Sloan, J. A., & Shanafelt, T. D. (2009). Association of resident fatigue and distress with perceived medical errors. *Journal of American Medical Association, 302*(12), 1294–1300. https://doi.org/10.1001/jama.2009.1389

Wester, W. C., & Smith, A. H. J. (1984). *Clinical hypnosis: A multidisciplinary approach.* Lippincott.

Westerman, M. A. (2005). What is interpersonal behavior? Post-cartesian approach to problematic interpersonal pattern and psychotherapy process. *Review of General Psychology, 9*(1), 16–34. https://doi.org/10.1037/1089-2680.9.1.16

Wetzel, A. P., Mazmanian, P. E., Hojat, M., Kreutzer, K. O., Carrico, R. J., Carr, C., Veloski, J., & Rafiq, A. (2010). Measuring medical students' orientation toward lifelong learning: a psychometric evaluation. *Academic medicine, 85*(*10 Suppl*), S41–S44. https://doi.org/10.1097/ACM.0b013e3181ed1ae9

White, K. L. (1991). *Healing the schism: Epidemiology, medicine, and the public's health.* Springer-Verlag.

Whittemore, P. B., Burstein, A. G., Loucks, S., & Schoenfeld, L. S. (1985). A longitudinal study of personality changes in medical students. *Journal of Medical Education, 60*, 404–405.

Whorf, B. L. (1956). *Language, thought, and reality: Selected writings of Benjamin Lee Whorf.* John Wiley & Sons.

Wicker, B., Keysers, C., Plailly, J., Royet, J. P., Gallese, V., & Rizzolatti, G. (2003). Both of us disgusted in my insula: The common neural basis of seeing and feeling disgust. *Neuron, 40*, 655–664.

Wickramasekera, I. E., & Szylk, J. P. (2003). Could empathy be a predictor of hypnotic ability? *International Journal of Clinical & Experimental Hypnosis, 51*, 390–399.

Wiehe, V. R. (2003). Empathy and narcissism in a sample of child abuse perpetrators and a comparison sample of foster parents. *Child Abuse & Neglect, 27*, 541–555.

Wiesenfeld, A. R., Whitman, P. B., & Malatesta, C. Z. (1984). Individual differences among adult women in sensitivity to infants: Evidence in support of an empathy concept. *Journal of Personality and Social Psychology, 46*, 118–124.

Wiklund, I., Oden, A., & Sanne, H. (1988). Prognostic importance of somatic and psychosocial variables after a first myocardial infarction. *American Journal of Epidemiology, 128*(4), 786–795.

Wilkes, M., Milgrom, E., & Hoffman, J. R. (2002). Toward more empathic medical students: A medical student hospitalization experience. *Medical Education, 36*, 528–533.

Williams, B., & Beovich, B. (2020). A systematic review of psychometric assessment of the Jefferson Scale of Empathy using the COSMIN Risk of Bias checklist. *Journal of Evaluation in Clinical Practice, 26*(4), 1302–1315. https://doi.org/10.1111/jep.13293

Williams, B., Boyle, M., Brightwell, R., Devenish, S., Hartley, P., McCall, M., McMullen, P., Munro, G., O'Meara, P., & Webb, V. (2012). Paramedic empathy levels: Results from seven Australian universities. *International Journal of Emergency Services, 1*(2), 111–121. https://doi.org/10.1108/20470891211275902

Williams, B., Boyle, M., Brightwell, R., Devenish, S., Hartley, P., McCall, M., McMullen, P., Munro, G., & O'Meara, P. (2015). Undergraduate paramedic students' empathy levels: A two-year longitudinal study. *Journal of Nursing Education and Practice, 5*, 58–64. https://doi.org/10.5430/jnep.v5n1p58

Williams, B., Boyle, M., & Earl, T. (2013a). Measurement of empathy levels in undergraduate parametric students. *Prehospital and Disaster Medicine, 28*(2), 145–149. https://doi.org/10.1017/S1049023X1300006X

Williams, B., Brown, T., Boyle, M., & Dousek, S. (2013b). Psychometric testing of the Jefferson Scale of Empathy Health Profession Students' version with Australian paramedic students. *Nursing and Health Sciences, 15*, 45–50. https://doi.org/10.1111/j.1442-2018.2012.00719.x

Williams, B., Brown, T., Boyle, M., McKenna, L., Palermo, C., & Etherington, J. (2014a). Levels of empathy in undergraduate emergency health, nursing, and midwifery students: A longitudinal study. *Advances in Medical Education and Practice, 5*, 299–306. https://doi.org/10.2147/AMEP.S66681

Williams, B., Brown, T., & McKenna, L. (2013c). DVD empathy simulations: An interventional study. *Medical Education, 47(11)*, 1142–1143. https://doi.org/10.1111/medu.12343

Williams, B., Brown, T., McKenna, L., Boyle, M., Palermo, C., Nestel, D., Brightwell, R., McCall, L., & Russo, V. (2014b). Empathy levels among health professional students: A cross-sectional study at two universities in Australia. *Advances in Medical Education and Practice, 5*, 107–113. https://doi.org/10.2147/AMEP.S57569

Williams, B., Sadasivan, S., Kadirvelu, A., & Olaussen, A. (2014c). Empathy level among first year Malaysian medical students: An observational study. *Advances in Medical Education and Practice, 5*, 149–156. https://doi.org/10.2147/AMEP.S58094

Williams, B., Sifris, A., & Lynch, M. (2016). A psychometric appraisal of the Jefferson Scale of Empathy using law students. *Psychology Research and Behavior Management, 9*, 171–178. https://doi.org/10.2147/PRBM.S108036

Williams, C. A. (1989). Empathy and burnout in male and female helping professionals. *Research in Nursing & Health, 12*, 169–178.

Williams, R. B., Barefoot, J. C., Califf, R. M., Haney, T. L., Saunders, W. B., & Pryor, D. B. (1992). Prognostic importance of social and economic resources among medically treated patients with angiographically documented coronary artery disease. *Journal of the American Medical Association, 267*, 524.

Willingham, W. W., & Cole, N. S. (1997). *Gender and fair assessment*. Erlbaum.

Wilmer, H. A. (1968). The doctor-patient relationship and issues of pity, sympathy and empathy. *British Journal of Medical Psychology, 41*, 243–248.

Wilson, S. E., Prescott, J., & Becket, G. (2012). Empathy levels in first- and third-year students in health and non-Health disciplines. *American Journal of Pharmaceutical Education, 76*(2), 24. https://doi.org/10.5688/ajpe76224

Windholz, M. J., Marmar, C. R., & Horowitz, M. J. (1985). A review of research in conjugal bereavement: Impact on health and efficacy of intervention. *Comprehensive Psychiatry, 26*, 433–447.

Winefield, H. R., & Chur-Hansen, A. (2000). Evaluating the outcome of communication skill teaching for entry-level medical students: Does knowledge of empathy increase? *Medical Education, 34*, 90–94.

Winnicott, D. W. (1987). *Babies and their mothers*. Addison-Wesley.

Wispe, L. (1978). *Altruism, sympathy, and helping: Psychological and sociological principles*. Academic Press.

Wispe, L. (1986). The distinction between sympathy and empathy: To call forth a concept, a word is needed. *Journal of Personality and Social Psychology, 50*, 314–321.

Wittstein, I. S., Thiemann, D. R., Lima, J. A. C., Baughman, K. L., Schulman, S. P., & Chapman, H. C. (2005). Neurohormunal features of myocardial stunning due to sudden emotional stress. *New England Journal of Medicine, 352(6)*, 539–548. https://doi.org/10.1056/NEJMoa043046

Wolf, E. S. (1980). The dutiful physician: The central role of empathy in psychoanalysis, psychotherapy, and medical practice. *Hillside Journal of Clinical Psychiatry, 2*, 41–56.

Wolf, S. (1992). Prediction of myocardial infarction over a span of 30 years in Roseto, Pennsylvania. *Integrative Physiological & Behavioral Science, 27*, 246–257.

Wolf, T. M., Balson, P. M., Faucett, J. M., & Randall, H. M. (1989). A retrospective study of attitude change during medical education. *Medical Education, 23*, 19–23.

Wolfgang, A. (1979). *Nonverbal behavior: Applications and cultural implications*. Academic Press.

Wood, W., & Eagly, A. H. (2002). A cross-cultural analysis of the behavior of women and men: Implications for the origin of sex differences. *Psychological Bulletin, 128*, 699–727.
Wood, W., & Eagly, A. H. (2010). Gender. In S. T. Fiske, D. T. Gilbert, & G. Lindzey (Eds.), *The handbook of social psychology* (Vol. 1, 5th ed., pp. 629–667). McGraw-Hill.
World Health Organization. (1948). *World Health Organization Constitution: Basic documents*. World Health Organization.
Worly, B. (2013). Professionalism education of OB/GYN resident physicians: What makes a difference? *Open Journal of Obstetrics and Gynecology, 3(1A)*, 137–141. https://doi.org/10.4236/ojog.2013.31A026
Wright, S. (1996). Examining what residents look for in their role models. *Academic Medicine, 71*, 290–292.
Wu, W., Ma, X., Liu, Y., Qi, Q., Guo, Z., Li, S., Yu, L., Long, Q., Chen, Y., Teng, Z., Li, X., & Zeng, Y. (2022). Empathy alleviates the learning burnout of medical college students through enhancing resilience. *BMC Medical Education, 22(1)*, 481. https://doi.org/10.1186/s12909-022-03554-w
Xia, L., Hongyu, S., & Xinwei, F. (2011). Study on correlation between empathy ability and personality characteristics of undergraduate nursing students. *Chinese Nursing Research, 32*, 2933–2935.
Yaden, M. E., Yaden, D. B., Buffone, A. E. K., Eichstaedt, J. C., Crutchley, P., Smith, L. K., Cass, J. L., Callahan, C. A., Rosenthal, S. R., Ungar, L. H., Schwartz, H. A., & Hojat, M. (2020). Linguistic analysis of empathy in medical school admission essays. *International journal of medical education, 11*, 186–190. https://doi.org/10.5116/ijme.5f2d.0359
Yaghmaei, M., Monajemi, A., & Soltani-Arabshahi, K. (2014). The effect of storytelling course on medical students' empathy toward patients. *International Journal of Body, Mind & Culture, 1*(2), 127–134. https://doi.org/10.22122/ijbmc.v1i2.12
Yamada, Y., Fujimori, M., Shirai, Y., Ninomiya, H., Oka, T., & Uchitomi, Y. (2018). Changes in physicians' intrapersonal empathy after a communication skills training in Japan. *Academic Medicine: Journal of the Association of American Medical Colleges, 93*(12), 1821–1826. https://doi.org/10.1097/ACM.0000000000002426
Yang, K. T., & Yang, J. H. (2013). A study of the effect of a visual arts-based program on the scores of Jefferson Scale of Physician Empathy. *BMC Medical Education, 13*, 142. https://doi.org/10.1186/1472-6920-13-142
Yang, N., Xiao, H., Wang, W., Li, S., Yan, H., & Wang, Y. (2018). Effects of doctors' empathy abilities on the cellular immunity of patients with advanced prostate cancer treated by orchiectomy: the mediating role of patients' stigma, self-efficacy, and anxiety. *Patient preference and adherence, 12*, 1305–1314. https://doi.org/10.2147/PPA.S166460
Yarnold, P. R., Bryant, F. B., Nightingale, S. D., & Martin, G. J. (1996). Assessing physician empathy using the Interpersonal Reactivity Index: A measurement model and cross-sectional analysis. *Psychology, Health & Medicine, 1*, 207–221.
Yarnold, P. R., Greenberg, M. S., & Nightingale, S. D. (1991). Comparing resource use of sympathetic and empathetic physicians. *Academic Medicine, 66*, 709–710.
Yarnold, P. R., Martin, G. J., & Soltysik, R. C. (1993). Androgyny predicts empathy for trainees in medicine. *Perceptual & Motor Skills, 77*, 576–578.
Yates, S. (2001). Finding your funny bone: Incorporating humour into medical practice. *Australian Family Physician, 30*, 22–24.
Ye, Q., Zhong, X., Zhou, Q., Hua, L., & Li, G. (2024). Empathy fatigue among physicians and its influencing factor: A cross-sectional survey from southwest China. *BMC Psychiatry, 24*, 780. https://doi.org/10.1186/s12888-024-06217-w
Yedidia, M. J., Gillespie, C. C., Kachur, E., Schwartz, M. D., Ockene, J., Chepaitis, A. E., Snyder, C. W., Lazare, A., & Lipkin, M., Jr. (2003). Effect of communications training on medical student performance. *Journal of the American Medical Association, 290*, 1157–1165.

Yeo, S. (2019). Differences and changes in the empathy of Korean medical students according to gender and vocational aptitude, before and after clerkship. *Korean Journal of Medical Education, 31*(4), 343–355. https://doi.org/10.3946/kjme.2019.144

Younger, J. B. (1990). Literary works as a mode of knowing. *Journal of Nursing Scholarship, 22*, 39–43.

Youssef, F. F., Nunes, P., Sa, B., & Williams, S. (2014). An exploration of changes in cognitive and emotional empathy among medical students in the Caribbean. *International Journal of Medical Education, 5*, 185–192. https://doi.org/10.5116/ijme.5412.e641

Yu, H., Jiang, A., & Shen, J. (2016). Prevalence and predictors of compassion fatigue, burnout and compassion satisfaction among oncology nurses: A cross-sectional survey. *International Journal of Nursing Studies, 57*, 28–38. https://doi.org/10.1016/j.ijnurstu.2016.01.012

Yu, J., & Kirk, M. (2009). Evaluation of empathy measurement tools in nursing: Systematic review. *Journal of Advanced Nursing, 65*(9), 1790–1806. https://doi.org/10.1111/j.1365-2648.2009.05071.x

Yu, J., Lee, S., Kim, M., Lim, K., Chang, K., & Lee, M. (2020). Relationships Between Perspective-Taking, Empathic Concern, and Self-rating of Empathy as a Physician Among Medical Students. *Academic Psychiatry: The Journal of The American Association of Directors of Psychiatric Residency Training and the Association for Academic Psychiatry, 44*(3), 316–319. https://doi.org/10.1007/s40596-019-01114-x

Yuguero, O., Forné, C., Esquerda, M., Pifarré, J., Abadías, M. J., & Viñas, J. (2017). Empathy and burnout of emergency professionals of a health region: A cross-sectional study. *Medicine, 96*(37), e8030. https://doi.org/10.1097/MD.0000000000008030

Yuguero, O., Melnick, E. R., Marsal, J. R., Esquerda, M., & Soler-Gonzalez, J. (2018). Cross-sectional study of the association between healthcare professionals' empathy and burnout and the number of annual primary care visits per patient under their care in Spain. *BMJ Open, 8*(7), e020949. https://doi.org/10.1136/bmjopen-2017-020949

Zachariae, R., Pedersen, C. G., Jensen, A. B., Ehrnrooth, E., Rossen, P. B., & von der Maase, H. (2003). Association of perceived physician communication style with patient satisfaction, distress, cancer-related self-efficacy, and perceived control over the disease. *British Journal of Cancer, 88*, 658–665.

Zahedi, F. (2011). The challenge of truth telling across cultures: A case study. *Journal of Medical Ethics and History of Medicine, 4*, 11–19.

Zahn-Waxler, C., & Radke-Yarrow, M. (1990). The origin of empathic concern. *Motivation and Emotion, 14*, 107–130.

Zahn-Waxler, C., Radke-Yarrow, M., & King, R. A. (1979). Child rearing and children's prosocial initiations toward victims of distress. *Child Development, 50*, 319–330.

Zahn-Waxler, C., Robinson, J. L., & Emde, R. N. (1992). The development of empathy in twins. *Developmental Psychology, 28*, 1038–1047.

Zeldow, P. B., & Daugherty, S. R. (1987). The stability and attitudinal correlates of warmth and caring in medical students. *Medical Education, 21*, 353–357.

Zeleznik, C., Hojat, M., Goepp, C. E., Amadio, P., Kowlessar, O. D., & Borenstein, B. D. (1988). Measurement of certainty in medical school examination: A pilot study on non-cognitive dimensions of test-taking behavior. *Journal of Medical Education, 63*, 881–891.

Zeleznik, C., Hojat, M., & Veloski, J. J. (1983). Levels of recommendation for students and academic performance in medical school. *Psychological Reports, 52*, 851–858.

Zell, E., Krizan, Z., & Teener, S. R. (2015). Evaluating similarities and differences using metasynthesis. *American Psychologist, 70(1)*, 10–20. https://doi.org/10.1037/a0038208

Zenasni, F., Boujut, E., de Vaure, C. B., Catu-Pinault, A., Tavani, J. L., Rigal, L., Jaury, P., Magnier, A. M., Falcoff, H., & Sultan, S. (2012). Development of a French-language version of the Jefferson Scale of Physician Empathy and association with practice characteristics and burnout in a sample of general practitioners. *The International Journal of Person Centered Medicine, 2(4)*, 759–766.

Zentner, M., & Mitura, K. (2012). Stepping out of the caveman's shadow: Nations' gender gap predicts degree of sex differentiation in mate preferences. *Psychological Science, 23*(*10*), 1176–1185. https://doi.org/10.1177/0956797612441

Zhang, X., Pang, H., & Duan, Z. (2023). Educational efficacy of medical humanities in empathy of medical students and health professionals: a systematic review and meta-analysis. *BMC Medical Education, 23*(*1*), 925. https://doi.org/10.1186/s12909-023-04932-8

Zhang, Y. (2021). *Empathy among nursing undergraduates at a Chinese private university.* (Publication No. 28714514). [Doctoral dissertation, Chapman University]. ProQuest Dissertations & Theses Global. DAI-A 83/2(E).

Zhou, Q., Eisenberg, N., Losoya, S. H., Fabes, R. A., Reiser, M., Guthrie, I. K., & Shepard, S. A. (2002). The relations of parental warmth and positive expressiveness to children's empathy-related responding and social functioning: A longitudinal study. *Child Development, 73*, 893–915.

Zhou, Q., Valiente, C., & Eisenberg, N. (2003). Empathy and its measurement. In S. J. Lopez & C. R. Snyder (Eds.), *Positive psychological assessment: A handbook of models and measures* (pp. 269–284). American Psychological Association.

Zimbardo, P. (2007). *Lucifer effect: Understanding how good people turn evil.* Random House.

Zinn, W. (1990). Transference phenomenon in medical practice: Being whom the patient needs. *Annals of Internal Medicine, 113*, 298.

Zuckerman, M. (2002). Zuckerman-Kuhlman Personality Questionnaire (ZKPQ): An alternative five-factor model. In B. DeRaad & M. Perugini (Eds.), *Big five assessment* (pp. 377–396). Hogrefe & Huber.

Zuckerman, M., DePauls, B. M., & Rosenthal, R. (1981). Verbal and nonverbal communication of deception. In L. Berkowitz (Ed.), *Advances in experimental social psychology* (Vol. 14). Academic Press.

Zuger, A. (2004). Dissatisfaction with medical practice. *New England Journal of Medicine, 350*(1), 69–75. https://doi.org/10.1056/NEJMsr031703

Name Index

M. Hojat, *Clinical Empathy*, https://doi.org/10.1007/978-3-031-87413-0

G

P

Subject Index

M. Hojat, *Clinical Empathy*, https://doi.org/10.1007/978-3-031-87413-0

D

N

O

Q

R

S

T

MIX
Papier aus verantwortungsvollen Quellen
Paper from responsible sources
FSC® C105338

If you have any concerns about our products,
you can contact us on
ProductSafety@springernature.com

In case Publisher is established outside the EU,
the EU authorized representative is:
Springer Nature Customer Service Center GmbH
Europaplatz 3, 69115 Heidelberg, Germany

Printed by Libri Plureos GmbH
in Hamburg, Germany